HEALTH CARE

for the

Older Woman

HEALTH CARE

for the

Older Woman

edited by

Morton A. Stenchever

Professor and Chairman of Obstetrics and Gynecology
University of Washington School of Medicine, Seattle

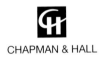

CHAPMAN & HALL

New York • Albany • Bonn • Boston • Cincinnati • Detroit • London • Madrid • Melbourne
Mexico City • Pacific Grove • Paris • San Francisco • Singapore • Tokyo • Toronto • Washington

Library of Congress Cataloging-in-Publication Data

Health care for the older woman / edited by Morton A. Stenchever.
            p.   cm.
    Includes bibliographical references and index.
    ISBN 0-412-05401-9 (alk. paper)
    1. Aged women—Health and hygiene. 2. Aged women—Diseases.
  3. Aged women—Medical care. I. Stenchever, Morton A.
    [DNLM: 1. Women's Health—United States. 2. Aging. 3. Genital
Diseases, Female—in old age.   WA 309 H434 1995]
RA564.85.H396 1996
618.97'0082—dc20
DNLM/DLC   96-21175
for Library of Congress   CIP

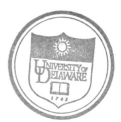

To my wife, Diane.

Contents

Preface

It is a fact that the population of the United States and most developed countries is aging. Women now spend about one third of their lives in the postreproductive years. It therefore has become a major responsibility of physicians offering care to these individuals to see that proper health maintenance and early disease intervention take place. The overall goals should be to ensure excellent physical and mental function and to achieve the highest quality of life for as long as possible.

The contributors to this book represent experts in a variety of disciplines in the hopes of giving physicians who care for older women a total picture of their health care needs and the means by which physicians can offer care. The topics vary from the biology and ethics of aging to the treatment programs that are available for managing the special problems of older individuals. This book should have applicability not only to obstetricians and gynecologists but to all health care providers who are responsible for the health needs of older women.

It is hoped that this book will not only help the practitioner care for older women but will also make it possible for the physician to continue enjoying the doctor–patient relationship with persons in their later years. As the number of these patients increases, so will the opportunities available to physicians. Older women deserve excellent and specialized care so that they may continue to enjoy life to the fullest measure of their physical and emotional capabilities.

Morton A. Stenchever, MD

Contributors

George N. Aagaard, MD
Dean Emeritus and Professor Emeritus, Department of Medicine and Pharmacology, University of Washington School of Medicine, Seattle, Washington

Joanna M. Cain, MD
Professor, Department of Obstetrics and Gynecology, Division of Gynecologic Oncology, University of Washington, Seattle, Washington

M. Elaine Cress, PhD
Research Assistant Professor, Medicine/Gerontology, University of Washington, Seattle, Washington

Felicity A. Green, OT
Occupational Therapist, University of Washington, Seattle, Washington

M. Wayne Heine, MD
Professor, Department of Obstetrics and Gynecology, University of Arizona Health Sciences Center, Tucson, Arizona

Albert R. Jonsen, PhD
Chairman and Professor, Department of Medical History and Ethics, University of Washington, Seattle, Washington

Gretchen Lentz, MD
Assistant Professor, Department of Obstetrics and Gynecology, University of Washington, Seattle Washington

Wylie Burke, MD, PhD
Associate Professor, Department of Medicine, University of Washington, Seattle, Washington

Gurkamal S. Chatta, MD
Instructor, Department of Medicine, University of Washington, Seattle, Washington

David C. Dale, MD
Professor, Department of Medicine, University of Washington, Seattle, Washington

Julia R. Heiman, PhD
Professor, Department of Psychiatry and Behavioral Sciences, University of Washington, Seattle, Washington

Nancy S. Jecker, PhD
Associate Professor, Department of Medical History and Ethics, University of Washington, Seattle, Washington

Joseph F. Lang, MD
Chief Resident, Department of Obstetrics and Gynecology, University of Aizona Health Sciences Center, Tucson, Arizona

George M. Martin, MD
Professor, Department of Pathology, University of Washington School of Medicine, Seattle, Washington

Donald E. Moore, MD
Associate Professor, Department of Obstetrics and Gynecology, University of Washington School of Medicine, Seattle, Washington

Lauren Nathan, MD
Assistant Professor, Department of Obstetrics and Gynecology, UCLA School of Medicine, Los Angeles, California

Linda Pinsky, MD
Acting Instructor, Department of Medicine, University of Washington School of Medicine, Seattle, Washington

Marvin C. Rulin, MD
Chief, Division of Gynecology, Professor Obstetrics, Gynecology, and Reproductive Services, University of Pittsburgh School of Medicine, Magee-Womens Hospital, Pittsburgh, Pennsylvania

Louis Vontver, MD
Professor and Vice Chairman, Department of Obstetrics and Gynecology, University of Washington, Seattle, Washington

Roger Moe, MD
Associate Professor, Department of Surgery, University of Washington, Seattle, Washington

Roy M. Pitkin, MD
Professor, Department of Obstetrics and Gynecology, UCLA School of Medicine, Los Angeles, California

Wendy H. Raskin, MD, PhD
Associate Professor, Department of Medicine, University of Washington, Seattle, Washington

Morton A. Stenchever, MD
Professor and Chairman, Department of Obstetrics and Gynecology, University of Washington School of Medicine, Seattle, Washington

Edward A. Walker, MD
Associate Professor, Departments of Psychiatry and Behavioral Sciences, and Obstetrics and Gynecology, University of Washington, Seattle, Washington

HEALTH CARE

for the

Older Woman

Chapter 1

The Aging of a Woman

Morton A. Stenchever, MD

Life expectancy has risen steadily during the past century. In fact, during the last 20 years the total life expectancy for the United States population has increased from 70.8 to 75.7 years, with women enjoying an improvement from 74.9 to 79.1 years. Biologists have estimated that the probable life expectancy for humans is about 85 years, even though longer life is certainty possible for and observable in many. The challenge for society in general and medicine in particular, then, is to find ways to postpone pathology and morbidity as long as possible, so that each individual can attain a length of life as close to the biological norm and in as healthy a state as possible. Achieving these goals will help to ensure each individual not only a long life, but one of quality.

In women over the age of 65, the leading causes of death are heart disease (1,735/100,000) and cancer (871.2/100,000). Other common causes are stroke (423/100,000), chronic obstructive pulmonary disease (167/100,000), pneumonia and influenza (211.1/100,000), diabetes (116.2/100,000) and accidents (70.7/100,000). Clearly, preventive and interventional means are available to address and reduce or at least postpone many of these.

Table 1.1 presents the most recent (1990) death rates by site and type of cancer for the different age categories of older women. Attention to these also offers direction for research, application of preventive measures, and patient education initiatives.

Currently, about 9.5% of women and 7.0% of men in the United States are over 60 years of age. By the year 2025, it is estimated that the percentages will increase to 12.5% and 11.5%, respectively. It will be of great value for society to keep these individuals healthy and productive as long as possible, or society will surely suffer major economic and social disasters.

Health Care Goals

In caring for the older woman, health care objectives should be designed to delay morbidity and to improve or maintain quality of life. With this in mind, the following goals seem appropriate: encouraging healthy practices, preventing disease, and addressing psychological and psychosocial issues.

Encouraging Healthy Practices (Table 1.2)

Dietary habits that promote good nutrition should be outlined and discussed at each annual visit. If a weight problem is noted, suggestions for correction should be offered. Where appropriate, a nutritionist may be consulted.

Table 1.1 Death Rates (Deaths per 100,000 Population) in Females Aged 65 and Over (1990)

Age group	Type of cancer	Death rate
65–74	Respiratory	181.7
	Digestive organs	153.0
	Breast	111.7
	Genital organs	71.0
	Lymphatic and heme (excluding leukemia)	39.5
	Urinary	19.8
	Leukemia	18.8
75–84	Respiratory	194.5
	Digestive organs	293.3
	Breast	146.3
	Genital organs	95.3
	Lymphatic and heme (excluding leukemia)	71.2
	Urinary	38.5
	Leukemia	38.8
85 and over	Respiratory	142.8
	Digestive organs	497.6
	Breast	196.8
	Genital organs	115.6
	Lymphatic and heme (excluding leukemia)	90.0
	Urinary	68.5
	Leukemia	65.0

The patient should be encouraged to get at least eight hours of sleep each night.

An exercise program that takes into consideration the patient's abilities and interests should be suggested and encouraged. Even very elderly and partially disabled patients may benefit from daily short walks, swimming, dancing, or other forms of light exercise. Exercise tones the body, improves the patient's sense of well-being, and relieves stress.

Hormone replacement therapy should be offered and encouraged for all women who have no contraindications. In addition to alleviating the psychomotor symptoms of hot flashes and night sweats, hormone replacement therapy reduces the risks of osteoporosis and arteriosclerotic heart disease, improves pelvic supports and bladder function, and improves subcutaneous connective

Table 1.2 Health Practices that Should Be Encouraged by the Physician

Good nutrition
Adequate sleep
Exercise
Hormone replacement therapy
Smoking cessation
Limiting alcohol use
Reviewing prescription and other medications and drugs
Using seat belts
Wearing safe footwear
Moving about with caution
Avoiding strenuous tasks and activities

tissue. While estrogen replacement is key, progesterone should be supplemented when the woman has an intact uterus.

If the patient smokes, she should be encouraged to stop. Programs to accomplish this should be discussed, benefits outlined (even if the patient has been a long-time, heavy smoker), and the proper action plan or referral made to accomplish this. Likewise, if the patient abuses alcohol, the problems associated with respect to health and relationships should be discussed and means of controlling the abuse reviewed. Several definitions exist for excessive use of alcohol; many of these are relative, depending on other aspects of the patient's life. A useful guideline for potential alcohol abuse is 45 drinks per month, with a drink being defined as an ounce of whiskey, a glass of beer, or a glass of wine. Other danger criteria are binge drinking, consisting of more than five drinks at a sitting, and repetitive drinking to inebriation.

Use of illegal drugs should be discouraged and a plan to stop discussed. Reasons for such drug use should be sought and, if identified, dealt with by appropriate treatment or counseling. Likewise, the overuse of prescription drugs should be noted and discouraged because this practice may be equally dangerous and destructive.

Various safety issues should also be discussed with the patient. She should be reminded to use her seat belt when riding in motor vehicles. She should be encouraged to wear sturdy, comfortable shoes in an effort to prevent stumbling and falling. She should be cautioned not to move too quickly on waxed and wet surfaces. Finally, she should be advised to avoid tasks or activities that are no longer safely within her capabilities, such as heavy lifting.

Preventing Disease (Table 1.3)

There are several aspects to disease prevention. In addition to promoting a healthy lifestyle, the physician should use appropriate screening tests, diagnose and treat diseases as early as possible, and offer appropriate immunizations. To date, a number of screening tests have been found to be useful and many are also cost-effective. The issue of the sensitivity and specificity of a given test must always be considered. On the one hand, setting the level of a test high enough to detect almost all cases of a given illness will likely identify many false positives. On the other hand, setting the level low enough to eliminate most false positives will probably fail to detect several actual illnesses. Screening tests useful for disease detection in older women are the following: the Papanicolaou (Pap) stain test for cervical cancer; mammography for breast cancer; the Hemoccult test and flexible sigmoidoscopy for colon and rectal cancer; a complete blood cell count (CBC) for anemia and some blood dyscrasias; blood glucose level testing for diabetes mellitus; measuring serum lipids for hypercholesterolemia and hyperlipemia; testing for thyroid-stimulating hormone (TSH) for hypothyroidism; the serologic test for syphyllis (STS); measuring blood urea nitrogen (BUN) testing for the human immunodeficiency virus (HIV); and creatinine for certain renal diseases; and chest radiography for smokers.

An important and, unfortunately, common problem in older women is that of urinary incontinence. It becomes more prevalent with aging and may affect as many as 30% of older women.

Table 1.3 Disease Prevention Measures

Use appropriate screening tests
Evaluate for incontinence
Diagnose disease early
Maintain an immunization record and offer appropriate immunizations

Patients should be questioned about the possibility of their having urinary incontinence. If it is found to be present, it should be evaluated and treated.

Diagnosing disease states early is made possible in many cases by seeing the patient at reasonable intervals, performing a careful interim history, completing a thorough physical examination, ordering appropriate screening tests, and offering patient education appropriate for the patient to make her aware of the danger signals of common diseases.

The physician should maintain an immunization record for each patient. Suggested immunizations for women in the older age group include influenza vaccine annually in autumn, Pneumovax vaccine given only once, diphtheria–tetanus booster every 10 years, and a polio booster, depending on when the individual was immunized. If the patient is planning a trip to a foreign country, she should be given protective vaccinations or prophylaxis for diseases that may be encountered. Information about what measures are necessary may be obtained by contacting the Centers for Disease Control (CDC) or referring the patient to a travel medicine clinic.

Considering Psychological and Psychosocial Issues (Table 1.4)

A number of psychosocial issues should be considered and discussed at the annual health maintenance visit. These include sexuality and sexual functions, loss and grief, prevention of abuse, and depression.

Sexuality involves many aspects including the woman's state of health and vigor, her selfimage, the availability of a partner and his health and vigor, and the importance that the couple places on sexual activities within the context of their relationship. Clearly, these circumstances will differ for each woman and each couple, but it is reasonable for the physician to make inquiries and offer advice so that the patient and her partner may achieve sexual fulfillment within the context of their abilities and wishes. As an example, the physician may learn within the context of the discussion with the patient that coitus is no longer possible because the spouse is suffering impotence. Further discussion might reveal that this began when he was placed on antihypertensive therapy with a beta blocker. Discussion with the husband's doctor might lead to a change in medication with a return of function.

Loss is a part of living and may include the loss of a close friend or loved one, a body part, a job, an ability or function, or a pet. Whatever the loss, if that which is lost is important to the individual it will probably be accompanied by a grief reaction. According to Lindemann, grief is usually accompanied by a definite syndrome that includes both somatic and psychological components. The individual suffering the loss often exhibits a tightening of the throat and chest, a choking sensation and dry cough, shortness of breath, frequent sighing, an empty feeling, muscle weakness, tension, and mental pain. The individual often experiences disorders of the sensorium and may tend to isolate herself from others. Previous emotional problems may recur and psychosomatic illnesses may flare up. Decisions and actions that may be potentially destructive in a physical, emotional, or economic sense may be made or taken. The type of loss suffered by the individual will determine the degree and type of reaction experienced. Loss of a loved one usually causes a

Table 1.4 Psychological and Psychosocial Issues

Sexuality and sexual function
Loss and grief
Death and dying
Abuse and intimidation
Depression

grief reaction that lasts 6 to 18 months but tends to be longer in certain instances such as the loss of a child or the loss of a spouse by a very old person. In general, the grief reaction tends to resolve when the patient can place the loss within the context of her total life experience and find other individuals and pursuits to relate to. Since older patients may have fewer life options, grief resolution may be more difficult and time-consuming. A sensitive physician can be very useful in helping an individual through such a period.

Loss of a body part has a special potential for provoking grief. This seems particularly true for the loss of organs or body parts that serve a necessary function such as an eye or a limb, or organs that are tied to the individuals personal identity such as a breast, uterus, or ovary. Drummond and Field, in discussing a woman's adjustment to the loss of a uterus, point out four stages of incorporation previously described by Roberts: impact, retreat, acknowledgment, and reconstruction. The impact stage occurs when the patient is told she must lose an organ. If she is symptomatic this stage may be short; if she is not, she must be given time to assimilate the information or depression may result. The retreat stage is the stage in which the patient accepts the fact that she must lose the organ. During this stage she may seek second opinions and investigate the possibility of alternative types of therapy. This is a healthy pursuit and should be encouraged by the doctor. In the acknowledgment stage, she will discuss the planned procedure, ask questions about alternative approaches, and talk about the postoperative period from the point of view of what she will experience and what will be done. The final or reconstruction stage involves her redefinition of herself without the organ, including what she will be like, how she will function, and how she will be perceived and treated by others, especially those close to her.

A particular type of grief and loss situation involves the possible loss of the patient's own life. Kubler-Ross changed our perception of the death process in 1969 when she described five stages that an individual goes through in accepting the inevitability of death. These are denial, anger, bargaining, depression, and acceptance. Denial is the state that occurs when the individual first learns that she has an illness from which she will probably not recover. She may deny ever having been given the information and may isolate herself from others particularly those who may possess the information. This period can vary widely in duration and depends on the individual's symptoms and how well she has been prepared by life experiences to deal with such information. The anger stage usually follows and is often directed at staff and family alike. Staff suffer because they are the messengers of the dreaded news and family because they will survive and go on living. Because of the anger vented, both staff and family members tend to avoid the patient, which is, of course, just the opposite of what she wants and needs. The bargaining stage follows and is useful because it allows her to correct old grievances and put her affairs in order. She is apparently doing good deeds in the hope of being given, presumably by God, more time. Depression may occur at any stage and should be expected by the physician. It may be dealt with by the most appropriate means, depending on the patient's condition and life expectancy when it occurs. The final stage, acceptance, will eventually occur when the patient has worked through the earlier stages if she lives long enough. Kubler-Ross did not believe that this stage represented surrender to symptoms, but rather an acceptance of the inevitable after all preparations have been made by the patient.

Abuse of the elderly is common and may be physical or emotional. It may also involve neglect. About 2.5 million elderly are abused in one way or another in the United States each year. The perpetrator is often a family member and the victim is often an elderly female living with the family. Care-givers are often involved in the abuse. The physician should ask open-ended questions such as the following. Has anyone hurt you recently or in the past? Has anyone been cruel to you or tried to intimidate or frighten you lately? Has anyone tried to extort money from you? If the patient implies that she is a victim of abuse or intimidation, her rights may be discussed and referral made, to a social service agency.

While mild transient depression is common in individuals suffering bereavement, loss, or disappointment, serious organic depression is also quite common, occurring in 10% to 20% of individuals at some time in their lives. A major depressive disorder can be diagnosed if the depression lasts for more than 2 weeks and any five of the following are present: depressed mood, loss of interest or pleasure in most activities, significant weight loss or gain (change in appetite), insomnia or hypersomnia, psychomotor retardation or agitation, fatigue or energy loss, feelings of worthlessness and guilt, diminished ability to think or concentrate, and recurrent thoughts of death.

The probable diagnosis of depression can be managed by psychiatric referral or by treatment with antidepressive drugs with or without concurrent counseling. The decision on which course of management to choose depends on the severity of the patient's symptoms and the physician's comfort in using the available drug therapy. The important issue, however, is to make the diagnosis and plan an appropriate course of management.

Summary

The physician who accepts the responsibility for the health care of the older woman has an important task to fulfill. With the objectives of delaying morbidity as long as possible and improving or maintaining quality of life, attention must be given to a large variety of physical and psychosocial conditions. The annual health maintenance visit is an ideal opportunity to address these issues. This book discusses in detail these various aspects of health care for the older woman so that these objectives can be fulfilled for all women.

References

1. American College of Obstetricians and Gynecologists. Committee Opinion, Committee on Gynecology Practice, #128 Routine cancer screening, October 1993, Washington, DC.
2. American College of Obstetricians and Gynecologists. *The Role of the Obstetrician and Gynecologist in Primary Preventive Care,* 1993, Washington, DC.
3. Brown GW, Harris T, Copeland JR: Depression and loss. *Br J Psychiatry* 1977;130:1–18.
4. Bryny RL: Establishing guidelines for preventive medicine. *Contemp Obstet Gynecol* 1988;31:43.
5. Cancer facts and figures—1994. American Cancer Society. New York, N.Y.
6. Centers for Disease Control, Promotion Health/Preventing Disease: *Objectives for the Nation, Health Resource Administration.* Publication No. F00009, Fall 1980. Atlanta, GA.
7. Current Population Reports. *Population projections of the United States, by age, sex, race, and Hispanic origin: 1992–2050.* United States Department of Commerce, November 1992. Washington, DC.
8. Drummond J, Field PA: Emotional and sexual sequelae following hysterectomy. *Health Care Women Int* 1984;5:261–271.
9. Ehrlich P, Anetzberger G: *Survey of state public health departments on procedures for reporting elder abuse.* Public Health Reports 1991;106:151–154.
10. Fiore MC, Novotny TE, Pierce JP, et al: Methods used to quit smoking in the United States. *JAMA* 1990;263:2760–2765.
11. Fries JF, Crapo LM: *Vitality and Aging.* San Francisco, WH Freeman, 1981.
12. Giordano NH, Giordanano JA: Elder abuse: A review of the literature. *Soc Work* 1984;29:232–236.
13. Gordon TJ, Gerjuoy H, Anderson M, eds.: *Life-Extending Technologies: A Technology Assessment.* New York, Pergamon Press, 1979.
14. Hammond DC. Screening for sexual dysfunction. *Clin Obstet Gynecol* 1984;27:732–737.
15. Henderson BE, Paganini-Hill A, Ross RK: Decreased mortality in users of estrogen replacement therapy. *Arch Intern Med* 1991;151:75–78.
16. Hermanson B, Omenn GS, Kronmal RA, Gersh BJ: Beneficial six-year outcome of smoking cessation in older men and women with coronary artery disease. Results from the CASS registry. *N Engl J Med* 1988;319:1365–1369.
17. Kubler-Ross E: *On Death and Dying.* New York, Macmillan, 1969.
18. Lewis M: Older women and health: An overview, in Golub S, Freedman RJ (eds.): *Health Needs of Women as they Age.* New York, The Haworth Press, 1985; pp. 1–16.

19. Lindemann E: Symptomatology and management of acute grief. *Am J Psychiatry* 1944;101:141–148.
20. Masters WH, Johnson VE: *Human Sexual Inadequacy.* Boston, Little, Brown, 1970.
21. Masters WH, Johnson VE: *Human Sexual Response.* Boston, Little, Brown, 1966.
22. Pillemer K, Suitor JJ: Violence and violent feelings: What causes them among family caregivers? *J Gerontol* 1992;47:S165–S172.
23. Quackenbush J: The death of a pet: How it can affect owners. *Vet Clin North Am Small Anim Pract* 1985;15:395–402.
24. Ripley HS: Depression and the life span-epidemiology, in Usdin G. (ed.): *Depression: Clinical, Biological and Psychological Perspectives.* New York, Brummer/Mazel, 1977.
25. Select Committee on Aging: Domestic Violence Against the Elderly. Hearings before the Subcommittee on Human Services. House of Representatives. April 21, 1980. Washington, DC, US Government Printing Office, 1980.
26. Semmens JP, Semmens EC: Sexual function in the menopause. *Clin Obstet Gynecol* 1984;27:717–723.
27. Stampfer MJ, Colditz GA: Estrogen replacement therapy and coronary heart disease: A quantitative assessment of the epidemiologic evidence. *Prev Med* 1991:20:47–63.
28. Statistical abstract of the United States—1993. United States Department of Commerce ed 113. 1993. Washington, DC.

Chapter 2

Ethical Issues in the Health Care of the Older Woman

Nancy S. Jecker, PhD, and *Albert R. Jonsen, PhD*

In the years ahead, physicians will serve an increasing number of elderly patients.[1] This will be true not only for physicians with special expertise, interest, or commitment to geriatric care, but for physicians of diverse specialties, skills, and interests. The fact that life expectancy for women is on average 7.5 years higher than for men[2] means that women will be disproportionately represented in the oldest and fastest growing age groups. To meet new demands, physicians will clearly need to hone medical skills and knowledge concerning care of the aged, and care of the aged female, in particular. Beyond this, physicians will be challenged to fine-tune medical ethical principles to suit a new patient population, reconceptualize dominant attitudes toward the elderly, and strengthen their commitment to care for older patients.

This chapter focuses on the ethical aspects of clinical geriatric care. Our strategy for charting these issues will be threefold. First, we sketch a series of cases that bring to the fore important medical ethical questions involving care of elderly patients. Second, we note alternative conceptions about the aged and clarify how these can affect the interpretation and application of medical ethical principles. Finally, we propose ways in which age is objectively and subjectively significant and suggest how physicians might differentiate between the real significance of age and ageist assumptions.

Cases Illustrative of Geriatric Ethical Issues

A currently favored approach for assessing ethical issues of the following kind is to frame them in terms of competing ethical principles. In the first pair of cases, an initial framing of ethical issues can be made in terms of traditional principles of autonomy and beneficence.[3] Autonomy refers to the capacity to act on the basis of principles that are one's own. This implies an absence of internal constraints, such as fear, duress, or impaired cognitive functioning, as well as an absence of external constraints, such as coercion or threats by others. By contrast, the principle of beneficence enjoins us to promote a person's best interests. This may require either actions that produce benefits, the omission of actions that produce harm, or the avoidance of harm that is not outweighed by benefits. The related concept of paternalism specifies that beneficence is appropriate even in situations where it conflicts with respecting a person's autonomous choice. Although professionals and nonprofessionals alike are under a duty to refrain from actions that harm others, physicians possess a special duty to do good for patients. For example, failure to benefit a stranger when one is in a position to do so is less morally serious than failure on the part of a physician to benefit his or her own patient.

Case One

Mrs. A, a 76-year-old with diabetes, has already had a below-the-knee amputation and refuses to consent to similar surgery on her other leg. Recently, she has had repeated hospital stays for sepsis of this leg and other complications. She now is brought to the emergency room in an obtunded state due to hyperosmolar coma. Following discussions with Mrs. A's son, surgery is performed on the leg. Mrs. A recovers and, with rehabilitation, adjusts well to a second prosthesis. Medicare billings total more than $62,000.[4]

Case Two

Mrs. B, age 85, was treated 5 years earlier for basal cell carcinoma of the vulva by local excision. She was depressed about her condition, seemed to respond negatively to the information given her, and wondered aloud repeatedly, "Why should this happen to an old woman who just wants to live out her last years in peace?" Now, metastatic lesions have been discovered. The physician considers chemotherapy, but decides against it and decides not to tell Mrs. B of the findings, believing that it would be more than she could bear. "At her age, she doesn't have much time left even if we arrested the disease," reasons the physician; "Why make her last months miserable with futile treatment or with the knowledge that she is dying?"[5]

The cases of Mrs. A and Mrs. B dramatize the potential conflict between autonomy and beneficence. In the first case, it appears that Mrs. A's best interests are promoted by amputating her leg in order to prevent spreading of sepsis. But this is done against her wishes in a situation where, due to coma, she is unable to protest. Here, the principle of beneficence prevails against the principle of autonomy. Hence, the conflict is resolved in accordance with the principle of paternalism.

In the second case, Mrs. B's preferences are also not determinative of treatment. Mrs. B's physician presumably judges that the deleterious effects of disclosing medical information would be overwhelming and may result in inappropriate and cruel prolonging of Mrs. B's suffering. Unlike in Mrs. A's case, in this case there may or may not be an actual conflict between the patient's wishes and serving the patient's best interests. By assigning priority to beneficence, the physician dissipates the tension between competing principles and precludes the possibility of practical conflict.

The second set of cases displays conflicting, but different ethical imperatives. Here, a central issue is quality of life and care of chronic diseases, rather than prolongation of life and treatment of potentially life-threatening conditions. Three competing conceptions of quality of life may be operative[6]: (1) quality of life understood as subjective satisfaction and as a patient's own subjective perception of life quality; (2) quality of life judged by an onlooker, such as a physician or family member, who assesses the patient's condition; and (3) quality of life interpreted as achievement of certain attributes a culture deems necessary for life quality, such as a certain level of physical or mental functioning.

Case Three

At age 90, Mrs. C is bedridden, blind, and has never fully recovered her mental faculties after striking her head in a fall. She is cared for in a comparatively inadequate nursing home. Except for an occasional respiratory infection and arthritic pain, she seems in no distress. She sometimes recognizes her husband, but his attempts to speak to her are usually unintelligible. Six years ago Mrs. C had given a talk at her church on the misery of prolonging the life of the dying elderly, particularly in nursing homes, and made an eloquent plea for "a dignified and simple way to choose death." Now her husband and physician face the problem of determining whether her present situation is a violation of the concept of "death with dignity" that she seemed to advocate.[7]

Case Four

Mrs. D is a 67-year-old retired store clerk who suffers from mild urinary stress incontinence. On this particular visit to her physician, she complains, in a whisper, of loss of sexual libido and discomfort during coitus, but says she prefers not to discuss it. She consistently finds discussing her sexual life or disclosing gynecological symptoms excruciatingly difficult. Two years earlier, she was treated surgically for vaginal phimosis, although she had never complained of the obvious discomfort caused from inspissated smegma collecting beneath the prepuce. Her doctor is now uncertain whether to insist upon discussing her sexual concerns or to accept her clearly expressed wish to terminate the discussion.

In Mrs. C's case, historical evidence suggests that life quality does not meet Mrs. C's own subjective standards, and both her physician and spouse are concerned to respect this subjective measure as far as possible. Mrs. D more clearly conveys a present dissatisfaction with her quality of life. Since Mrs. D is extremely reluctant to discuss sexual issues, the mere broaching of them raises the suspicion that her sexual discomfort and loss of libido matter deeply to her. In both Mrs. C's and Mrs. D's cases, patients, physicians, or family members may forfeit their own assessment of life quality by succumbing to cultural stereotypes and values. For example, Mrs. D or her physician may not expect a 67-year-old woman to enjoy a regular and active sexual life. The concerns Mrs. C's husband and physician voice about the quality of Mrs. C's life in a nursing home may be based, in part, on the fact that Mrs. C's life falls below acceptable cultural standards of what qualifies as a worthwhile life.

These ethical aspects obviously warrant further discussion. For example, what we have said so far clearly has implications for clinical ethical decisions concerning Do Not Resuscitate (DNR) orders and withdrawal of care. However, we now turn our attention to some unique issues in geriatric medical ethics. Our aim is to underscore the myriad ways in which ethical principles may be vitiated when negative attitudes toward aging impinge upon treatment decisions.

Negative Conceptions of the Elderly

Properly balancing medical ethical principles and standards is part of sound ethical decision-making, but not the whole of it. In geriatric care, in particular, the attitudes of both physicians and patients toward aging may have a pernicious influence on clinical decisions. Even if important ethical considerations are clarified, the interpretation and application of these considerations can be sullied at the start by negative stereotyping by the elderly themselves or by others. Such stereotyping can infect the entire assessment and place in jeopardy the very values ethical principles aim to protect.

Although controversy exists about the extent and manner in which negative attitudes toward the elderly operate in clinical decision-making,[4,8–12] there is mounting evidence that (1) age is a risk factor for inadequate treatment[13]; (2) variations in patterns of care are related to age[14–16]; and (3) scarce medical resources are less likely to be distributed to older or female patients who are equally medically needy.[17–20] Moreover, despite the difficulty of documenting the precise nature and scope of these problems, to the extent that negative stereotyping is legion in the larger society, both physicians and patients may take for granted certain assumptions about the elderly and incorporate these into their treatment choices. We would do well, then, to explore negative conceptions of the elderly and see how they might influence ethical assessment.

"Ageism," a term first coined by Robert Butler in the late 1960s,[21] refers to a subjective experience of "deep seated uneasiness on the part of the young and middle-aged—a personal revulsion to and distaste for growing old . . . and fear of powerlessness, uselessness, and death." Whereas racism and sexism involve systematic stereotyping of and discrimination against people because of skin color and gender, ageism accomplishes this with chronological age. For example, elderly people are characterized as senile, physically weak and fragile, rigid in thought and manner, and old-fashioned in morality and skills. Attributing negative characteristics to older individuals enables younger individuals to distance themselves and subtly cease identifying with elders as human beings.

So defined, ageist attitudes impart a negative tinge to perceptions of the elderly made by the nonelderly. However, it is important to extend Butler's analysis to incorporate negative stereotypes the elderly *themselves* may harbor. Only then can we fully comprehend the magnitude of ageism and its potential to wreak havoc on otherwise careful ethical argument. Age bias directed at oneself involves internalizing negative attitudes toward aging and, therefore, rejecting personal traits and life events that make age salient (eg, qualities such as wrinkles or graying hair, and hallmark events such as birthdays or becoming a grandparent). A negative stance toward personal aging produces alienation by literally distancing a person from certain aspects of the self that are experienced as revolting and distasteful.

The following illustrations of ageist attitudes are culled from recent literature.

1. *The Equation of an Individual's Value with Life Years Remaining.* Because older individuals have, on average, fewer years remaining, the lives of elderly persons are deemed less valuable.

2. *The View that Life Has Already Been Lived.* Old age is regarded as "borrowed time" or "icing on the cake" because the old have already lived a full life.[22-25]

3. *The Hasty Generalization.* Declining physiological functions that are statistically concomitant with aging are assumed to be present in each aging individual. For example, since many nursing home residents are cognitively impaired, every resident is assumed to be.[8,26]

4. *The Sexual Standard.* Senescence is viewed as synonymous with loss of sexual libido, and it is considered normal and desirable for regular sexual activity to cease in later years.[27]

5. *The Devaluation of Later Years.* Older years are thought to be of lower quality than younger years.[28]

6. *The View that Aging Is a Disease.* Age and disease are regarded as one process. Clinical changes associated with aging are negatively evaluated as "deterioration, disorganization, disintegration," even when there is nothing degenerative about these changes unless one assumes that young adulthood represents the paradigm of health.[29-33]

These ageist attitudes present difficulties when interposed between ethical principles and the concrete cases to which these principles apply. For example, an ageist stance can work against the application of an ethical principle or skew its proper interpretation. Ageist starting points can also parade as makeshift principles themselves, gaining legitimacy because of the widespread cultural norms they reflect. Finally, in an opposite fashion, the effort to avoid even the appearance of ageism can discourage frank probing of ways in which age is genuinely relevant.

Interpreting and Utilizing Ethical Principles

Autonomy and Beneficence

Having summarily stated examples of ageist attitudes, we are now in a position to assess how these attitudes can infiltrate otherwise acceptable ethical assessment. To this end, it will be useful to return to the four cases outlined earlier. With respect to each case, we should attempt to say exactly how attributions of ageist assumptions may impugn otherwise sound reasoning.

Let us consider, first, the case of Mrs. A, the 76-year-old with sepsis of the leg. One question that arises in connection with this case is the basis for the physician's decision to treat against the patient's prior wishes. Respecting Mrs. A's wishes would presumably call for not amputating the leg and allowing her to die (eg, from infection that may be present when she arrives at the emergency room in a coma). It may be fear of death or the view that the death of one's patient constitutes a personal failure that underlies the physician's decision to treat. One philosopher eloquently describes this as "the fear of one's own death as it peers out at one from the face of debilitated patients. . . . A physical, stomach-wrenching fear [that] can cause some to withdraw and 'do nothing' and others to continue aggressive therapy beyond the point of making sense."[34] If fear of death is operative, the antidote is mustering courage: the courage to confront ethical decisions. Courage can be aided by consulting with colleagues or an ethics committee or by education. But, in the end, it must emanate from within, from self-awareness and from letting go of fear.

An alternative explanation of the outcome in Mrs. A's case would occur if we attribute to her physician an ageist viewpoint, such as that because a greater proportion of elderly people are cognitively impaired, Mrs. A must be. If this assumption is entertained, the physician may reason in the following way. "The principle of autonomy requires that I respect my patient's capacity to make her own rational choice about treatment. But the scope of this principle is obviously limited to persons who actually possess the capacity for autonomous choice. Mrs. A is old and probably not in full possession of this capacity. Her persistent refusal to accept my recommendation for appropriate treatment is further evidence of an impaired state. Hence, my responsibility as her physician is to promote her interests to the best of my ability." The upshot of this reasoning may be a consultation with family members that excludes Mrs. A, followed by an agreement between the physician and family concerning the treatment course that best promotes Mrs. A's interests.

In this case, ageism stands in the way of sound ethical reasoning. The application of the principle of autonomy is obstructed, because the physician is inclined to judge that older people are not in possession of the capacity for autonomous choice. What makes this judgment unwarranted is that it may or may not apply to Mrs. A. Unless and until Mrs. A is evaluated for competency and diagnosed as incompetent, she should not be assumed to be so. Being old is associated with a greater frequency of cognitive impairment, but that does not imply that this particular individual is cognitively compromised. Second, even if informal assessment provides some evidence of incompetence, competence is task-specific. For example, incompetence in performing mathematical calculations or remembering the day of the week may not be germane to assessing competence to decide between treatment options. What is critical in the latter case is just that Mrs. A fully comprehend the nature of the options before her and the risks and benefits associated with each. Finally, although consulting with family members may be advisable, so long as Mrs. A is competent, the decision rests with her, not with her son or other family members.

In connection with the first case, it is also important to focus on the statement that the costs of care for Mrs. A totaled $62,000 in Medicare funds. To what extent should her physician take this into account? Suppose that, rather than treating against Mrs. A's wishes, the physician is considering not treating on the following grounds. "An investment of public monies in Mrs. A will probably yield a lower return than alternative investments of Medicare dollars. That money can be better spent elsewhere."

Even if the decision not to treat is ethically sound, this reasoning does not support it. Such reasoning can be faulted on several grounds. First, it displays the ageist view that an individual's worth is simply a function of years remaining. But surely this assumption does not reflect our considered judgments. For example, the murder of an older person is not considered less of a crime than the murder of a younger person, nor does it receive a lighter penalty.[35] This suggests that we regard all persons as possessing an underlying worth and dignity, regardless of the number of future years a person will live. Second, the physician's role is to advocate the patient's interests, not to decide how public resources should be distributed. Dispersing Medicare funds is a decision rightly made at the level of public policy by the larger society and not left to the discretion of individual practitioners. Although physicians do not owe more care than a patient is legally or ethically entitled to receive, care supported by public funding should not be withheld on the grounds that dispersing it is unjust. Physicians who oppose present policies should enter into public debates, but they should not usurp a decision that rightly rests with the public at large.[36–40]

Finally, let us consider how ageist assumptions may enter into Mrs. A's *own* decision to forgo care. Suppose we attribute to *her* a poor self-image and lack of self-esteem and the consequent belief that at her age she does not deserve publicly funded medical care aimed at prolonging life. How might this belief skew the outcome of Mrs. A's deliberations? Suppose Mrs. A does wish to continue living; however, she declines treatment because she judges that a woman of her age does not *deserve* to have her life extended.

Here, it is helpful to begin by focusing on the ageist assumption itself and exposing it as unfounded. To do this, we need to explain why it is wrong to suppose that after reaching the marker of a "full life span," individuals have no claim to life-extending care. To begin with, it is far from clear to what a "full life span" refers or whether it refers to the same thing for every individual. Second, even assuming that this considerable difficulty can be surmounted, a further difficulty remains—namely, that although having lived a full life span may make a person's death easier to accept in *hindsight,* it hardly makes any *manner* of death acceptable.[41,42] In the case of an individual like Mrs. A who desires to live and whose future holds out the hope of many good years, it would be wrong to deny routine antibiotic care simply because she is old. Although Mrs. A's claim to medical care is not unlimited, Mrs. A should reject the idea that old age per se makes her ethically ineligible for routine treatment.

Let us turn now to the case of Mrs. B, the 85-year-old with recurrent carcinoma. In this case, it is important to distinguish between the process of weighing competing ethical principles, on the one hand, and the process of guarding against ageist assumptions inimical to these principles, on the other hand. To illustrate this, let us suppose that Mrs. B entertains the ageist assumption that since she does not have much time left, it follows that her life is not worth much. If we suppose that Mrs. B is apprised of her situation, this assumption will be inimical both to autonomy and to beneficence. It is contrary to both because it undervalues the importance of all of Mrs. B's interests, including her capacity to make self-directed choices. For example, on these grounds, Mrs. B will be considerably less motivated to protect her own welfare and to struggle with making an autonomous choice between options. She will be less likely to protect any of her interests should they be threatened by others.

Next, suppose that we assign to Mrs. B's physician the view that 85-year-olds are cognitively impaired and so stand in need of special protection. On these grounds, the choice is made to withhold information about Mrs. B's condition from her. The outcome of this reasoning favors beneficence, but ageism itself does not *support* beneficence. Mrs. B's best interests are not protected by ageist assumptions, because her interests include being treated with respect, but ageism prompts others to regard her as childlike and incompetent. Mrs. B's interest in developing and sustaining self-esteem and self-confidence are also ill-served. Hence, even where ageism leads to favoring one ethical principle over another, it fails to *uphold* ethical principles.

Finally, suppose that ageist assumptions are not held by either Mrs. B or her physician. How should the principles of beneficence and autonomy be weighed against one another? To begin with, the physician should make a careful assessment as to whether his suspicion that knowledge of recurrent cancer would "be more than Mrs. B could bear" is genuinely warranted. If she is diagnosed as depressed, this factor should be taken into consideration. It may be decisive, but it is not necessarily decisive. This will depend on how depressed the patient is diagnosed as being. It may be possible, for example, to bring a mild depression under control to the point where, with counseling and assistance, Mrs. B is able to face her situation and make autonomous choices. Alternatively, if Mrs. B is not clinically depressed but is nonetheless anxious and fearful about facing death, she should be told of the situation and assisted.

What about the other argument, suggested by the physician's remark that it is best "not to make her last months miserable with futile treatment or the knowledge that she is dying"? First, it is important to probe the medical judgment that chemotherapy for this patient would be "futile." Although the efficacy of chemotherapy in older patients is controversial, there is evidence to suggest that its value has been understated.[13,43] It may well be that the choice is between gaining a small benefit (eg, a few months' more time purchased at the price of an unpleasant chemotherapy regimen versus not undergoing therapy) and perhaps dying sooner. If the choice can be framed appropriately in this way, then confronting the patient with options may be crucial to clarifying the patient's values and goals. For example, Mrs. B may wish to be alive a few more months to witness the birth of her first great-grandchild or to attend the wedding of her only granddaughter. Protecting her true interests may not be possible without exploring with her where her interests lie.

Even if we accept the suggestion that beneficence as well as autonomy support disclosing information to a competent patient, it is still important for the physician to make efforts to prevent the knowledge of terminal illness from making Mrs. B's last months miserable. For instance, it would be appropriate for the physician to tell Mrs. B about her situation while concomitantly attending to her emotional needs. One physician, who works with terminally ill geriatric cancer patients,[44] recommends that palliative care at this point include the following:

1. *Empathy:* Acknowledging the patient's emotional reaction.

2. *Legitimation:* Affirming that the patient's emotions are legitimate by underscoring the fact that these emotions are common and reasonable emotions to experience under the circumstances.

3. *Support:* Explicit affirmation by the physician that he or she will be with the patient and provide care throughout the entire course of the illness.

4. *Partnership:* Offering assistance in decision-making.

5. *Respect:* Expressing regard for the patient—for example, by an honest compliment praising the patient's openness, courage, or honesty.

Quality of Life

As caring for large numbers of elderly patients becomes a central mission of health care professionals, the present emphasis on acute care and crisis intervention is likely to shift to chronic care and to improving the patient's quality of life. The three remaining ageist assumptions are (4) the sexual standard, (5) the devaluation of later years, and (6) the view that age is a disease. These pose special problems for clinical decisions involving chronic conditions that threaten the quality of a patient's life without presenting a threat to life itself.

For example, Mrs. D, who finds coitus painful and experiences a loss of libido, may be prevented from seeking assistance because she falsely believes that old age is synonymous with loss of libido or that her discomfort during intercourse is nature's way of telling her that sex at her age is no longer possible. Simple medical treatment, such as estrogen therapy or vaginal cream, may ameliorate her discomfort and make sexual activity more enjoyable.[45] Yet even if Mrs. D combats her embarrassment and discusses her difficulties with her physician, ageist assumptions may keep her from following through and complying with her doctor's recommendations.[46]

It is important to begin by spelling out the reasons for rejecting the ageist stereotype Mrs. D holds. First, although deprivation of sexual stimulation can result in loss of erotic desire, senescence need not be accompanied with deprivation of sexual stimulation. Although physiological changes in genitalia in postmenopausal women can make coitus uncomfortable (eg, by shrinkage in the diameter of the introitus and diminished secretion of vaginal fluid), these conditions can be treated and sexual activity made possible. Finally, sexual activity in later years is desirable for the same reason it is desirable at any age: it improves the quality of a person's life, for example, by imparting a sense of well-being and vitality and by strengthening feelings of love for another human being. On these grounds, it is important to do what is possible to make sexual relations possible for elderly patients who wish them. One way of doing this is to unmask ageist assumptions. Otherwise, even if aging does not actually interfere with sexual functioning, a view of aging that rejects sexuality as inappropriate prevents sexual relations from occurring.[47] Another way of making sexual relations possible is to perform medical procedures, such as surgery, in a way that preserves capacity for intercourse wherever possible. Finally, practical issues should be addressed: if nursing home resident romances develop, opportunities for privacy and intimacy should be afforded; for elderly patients with special disabilities such as stroke, a footboard or trapeze can assist mobility.[48–51]

Physicians should also be aware that ageist standards can be an especially heavy burden for the older woman. In our society, women are encouraged to believe that loss of youth represents loss of beauty and that physical beauty is an important gauge of personal worth. Moreover, women are often considered sexually ineligible much earlier than men. Whereas men remain eligible sexual partners as long as they can perform coitus, women are at a disadvantage because their sexual candidacy often depends upon meeting much stricter standards related to looks and age.[52] To the extent that Mrs. D or her spouse internalize these cultural standards, the likelihood of rich and meaningful intimacy is reduced.

Whereas Mrs. D appears in relatively good health, the case of Mrs. C—the bedridden, blind, and cognitively impaired 90-year-old—challenges us to identify the extent to which an acceptable quality of life is possible with multiple serious impairments. Mrs. C is especially vulnerable to becoming the victim of ageist assumptions, because she is not in a position to defend herself against them. The devaluation of life, because it is the life of a 90-year-old, or the related pejorative assumption that aging itself is a pathology, may impede ethically responsible care.

One way for Mrs. C's physician to improve the quality of Mrs. C's daily life is by assisting with locating a more adequate nursing home or extended-care facility. Alternatively, home care may be a feasible option if a spouse or offspring is able to assist with care, perhaps in conjunction with community-based assistance. In considering how to improve Mrs. C's situation, it is important to recall the distinction made earlier between subjective satisfaction with life, the evaluation of life quality by third parties, and the evaluation of life quality implied by society's values. The pleasure of life in old age, even life with multiple impairments, is liable to be misjudged by those who are neither old nor impaired.[53] Finally, it is important to distinguish between the views espoused by Mrs. C 6 years earlier, and her present subjective satisfaction.

Despite the fact that no specific treatment decision faces Mrs. C's physician, it is important to consider what role quality of life judgments should have in future decisions. While quality of life is sometimes an acceptable basis for limiting treatment, the judgment of life quality would ideally come from patients themselves. However, even though this is not possible in Mrs. C's case, poor life quality may nonetheless be an acceptable ground for limiting future care.[54] This will be so if the quality of Mrs. C's life falls below a minimal threshold and the intervention would only preserve this condition.[55] The minimal threshold would include, for example, loss of qualities necessary for human interaction. In the process of making such an assessment, it is important to denude ageist stereotypes hidden beneath the surface of seemingly benign judgments. As far as possible, third-party assessments should reflect the subjective standard patients themselves would apply if they were able.

The Salience of Age

> That direct stare which passes between the young and the old is high up among the classic confrontations. It prefaces one of the great dialogues of opposites, and contains a frank admission of helplessness on either side, for nothing can be done to blot out the detail of what has been, or block in the detail of what is to come. On the one side is the clean sheet and on the other the crammed page. . . .[56]

Defusing ageist assumptions is not the only reason to attend specifically to medical ethical issues in geriatrics. It is also important to take stock of the multitude of ways in which having lived a long life distinguishes a person. It would be a mistake to suppose that age is never appropriately salient or that the old are no different from the young.

Caring for the elderly places special responsibilities on physicians, because diagnosis and communication with the elderly are more likely to pose a challenge. The elderly are more likely than other age groups to present with atypical or altered symptoms that make diagnosis difficult. They are more likely to present with qualities that make effective communication difficult, such as dementia (10%), impaired hearing (22%), and visual handicaps (15%).[29] In addition, as a group, elderly people have a high incidence of noncompliance. For example, one study revealed that 43% of elderly patients were noncompliant with their medication regimens and 90% of these patients underused their medication.[57] In another study, 59% of participating outpatients over 60 years of age had taken medications incorrectly, with 26% of the errors considered dangerous.[58] These and other medical factors set the elderly apart from other age groups and place upon physicians a duty to attend to special needs. For example, once a prescription is written for an elderly patient, the physician's responsibilities are not discharged. Physicians are additionally responsible to confirm compliance; enlist others to assist with medication where appropriate; maintain simple and short therapeutic regimens where possible; monitor compliance in nonobtrusive ways if indicated; facilitate compliance by compensating for problems, such as diminution of senses, confusion, and memory loss; and communicate effectively the importance of medication, especially in asymptomatic patients.[59]

In addition to these and other physiological differences that are sometimes present in old age, the subjective experience of aging distinguishes the elderly. Although the subjective experience of aging is not the subject of medicine, appreciating it is part of treating the patient as a full person. Medicine mistakenly objectifies patients when it regards them as bodies with symptoms, rather than attending to the inner experience of being in a particular body. Likewise, medicine mistakenly objectifies older patients when it stereotypes the elderly or imposes a predetermined meaning upon old age, rather than comprehending aging in the individual.

A patient's subjective experience of aging is evoked by augmenting objective medical methods with methods that aim to interpret the patients' subjective life. Employing such an approach in medical history taking, for example, involves interpreting the chronological fact of age not only by asking, "How old are you?" but also by asking, "What is life now like for you?"[60] Acknowledging subjective components of aging recognizes that a person's biography and personal history are part of what makes individuals what they are. By contrast, ignoring these dimensions falsifies a reality that is part of a person in his or her fullness.[22]

If medicine aims to enlarge its perspective and find a place for a subjective focus, the possibility of morally grounding the physician–patient relationship is made possible. Moral grounding hinges not only on articulating and interpreting moral principles, it is also a matter of human beings and human interactions realizing the values these principles protect. In medicine, the visible body and the objective data it produces easily loom large, occluding human subjective aspects that animate the body. A more humane approach to geriatric medicine requires laying bare personal and idiosyncratic human qualities that enlighten us about each other and enable us to discover one another as persons.

These possibilities are especially potent in the long-term care of elderly patients. The rewards of caring for geriatric patients are more likely to be found in the ongoing therapeutic relationship than in dramatic cues or heroic outcomes.[61] Geriatric medicine thus holds out the hope of an alternative model for the physician–patient relationship and a new and richer medical ethic.[62,63]

References

1. Campion EW: The oldest old. *JAMA* 1994;330:1819–20.
2. Jecker NS: Age-based rationing and women. *JAMA* 1991;266:3012–3015.
3. Beauchamp TL, Childress JF: *Principles of Biomedical Ethics,* ed. 4. New York, Oxford University Press, 1994.
4. Wetle TT: Ethical aspects of decision making for and with the elderly, in Kapp MB, Pies HE, Doudera AE (eds.): *Legal and Ethical Aspects of Health Care for the Elderly.* Ann Arbor, Health Administration Press, 1985, pp. 258–267.
5. Gadow S: Medicine, ethics, and the elderly. *Gerontologist* 1980;20:680–685.
6. Pearlman R, Jonsen A: The use of quality of life considerations in medical decision making. *J Am Geriatr Soc* 1985;33:344–352.
7. Veatch RM: *Case Studies in Medical Ethics.* Cambridge, Harvard University Press, 1977, pp 340–342.
8. Crockett W, Hummert ML: Perceptions of aging and the elderly. *Annu Rev Gerontol Geriatr* 1987;7:217–239.
9. Greene MG, Adelman R, Charon R, et al: Ageism in the medical encounter: An exploratory study of the doctor–elderly patient relationship. *Language and Communication* 1986;6:113–124.
10. Kosberg JI: The importance of attitudes on the interaction between health care providers and geriatric populations. *Interdiscipl Topics Gerontol* 1983;17:132–143.
11. Ward RA; The marginality and salience of being old: When is age relevant? *Gerontologist* 1984;24:227–232.
12. Damrasch SP, Fischman SH: Medical students' attitudes toward sexually active older people. *J Am Geriatr Soc* 1985;33:852–855.
13. Wetle T: Age as a risk factor for inadequate treatment. *JAMA* 1987;258:516.
14. Greenfield S, Blanco DM, Elashoff RM, et al: Patterns of care related to age of breast cancer patients. *JAMA* 1987;257:2766–2770.
15. Samet J, Hunt WC, Key C, et al: Choice of cancer therapy varies with age of patient. *JAMA* 1986;255:3385–3390.
16. Wagner A: Cardiopulmonary resuscitation in the aged. *N Engl J Med* 1984;310:1129–1130.
17. Eggers PW: Effect of transplantation on the medicare end-stage renal disease program. *N Engl J Med* 1988;318:223–229.
18. Held PJ, Pauly MV, Bovbjerg RB, et al: Access to kidney transplantation: Has the United States eliminated income and racial differences? *Arch Intern Med* 1988;148:2594–2600.
19. Kjellstrand CM: Age, sex, and race inequality in renal transplantation. *Arch Intern Med* 1988;148:1305–1309.
20. Kilner JF: Selecting patients when resources are limited: A study of U.S. medical directors of kidney dialysis and transplantation facilities. *Am J Public Health* 1988;78:144–147.
21. Butler RN: Age-ism: Another form of bigotry. *Gerontologist* 1969;9:243–246.
22. Callahan D: *Setting Limits: Medical Goals in an Aging Society.* New York, Simon & Schuster, 1987.
23. Callahan D: On defining a natural death. *Hastings Cent Rep* 1977;7:32–37.
24. Somerville MA: Should the grandparents die?: Allocation of medical resources with an aging population. *Law Med Health Care* 1986;14:158–163.

25. MacIntyre A: The right to die garrulously, in Purtill RL (ed.): *Moral Dilemmas.* Belmont, Wadsworth, 1985.

26. Leslie LA: Changing factors and changing needs in women's health care. *Nurs Clin North Am* 1986;21:111–123.

27. Starr BD: Sexuality and aging. *Annu Rev Gerontol* 1985;5:97–126.

28. Schelling TC: The life you save may be your own, in Chase S (ed.): *Problems in Public Expenditure Analysis.* Washington, D.C., Brookings Institution, 1968, pp. 127–176.

29. Rowe JW: Health care for the elderly. *N Eng J Med* 1985;312:828.

30. Jecker NS: Towards a theory of age group justice. *J Med Philosophy* 1989;14:655–676.

31. Caplan A: The 'unnaturalness' of aging—A sickness unto death?, in Caplan A, Engelhardt HT, McCartney JJ (eds.): *Concepts of Health and Disease Interdisciplinary Perspectives.* Reading, Massachusetts, Addison-Wesley, 1981.

32. Rosenfeld A: *Prolongevity.* New York, Knopf, 1976.

33. Gelein JL: Aged women and health. *Nurs Clin North Am* 1982;17:179–185.

34. Thomasma DC: Ethical judgments of quality of life in the care of the aged. *J Am Geriatr Soc* 1984;32:525–527.

35. Bell N: Ethical considerations in the allocation of scarce medical resources. Ph.D. dissertation, University of North Carolina, Chapel Hill, 1978.

36. Jecker NS: Fidelity to patients and resources constraints, in Campbell CS, Lustig BA (eds.): *Duties to Others.* Boston, Kluwer, 1994:293–308.

37. Angell M: Cost containment and the physician. *JAMA* 1985;254:1203–1207.

38. Morreim HE: Cost containment: Challenging fidelity and justice. *Hastings Cent Rep* 1988;18:20–25.

39. Jecker NS: Integrating medical ethics with normative theory. *Theor Med* 1990;11:125–139.

40. Daniels N: The ideal advocate and limited resources. *Theor Med* 1987;8:69–80.

41. Miles SH, Sachs GA: Intimate strangers: Roommates in nursing homes, in Kane RA, Caplan AL (eds.): *Everyday Ethics: Resolving Dilemmas in Nursing Home Life.* New York, Springer, 1990: pp. 90–97.

42. Cassel CK, Neugarten BL: The goals of medicine in an aging society, in Binstock RH, Post SG (eds.): *Too Old for Health Care?* Baltimore, The Johns Hopkins University Press, 1991, pp. 75–91.

43. Begg CB, Cohen FL, Ellerton J: Are the elderly predisposed to toxicity from cancer chemotherapy? *Cancer Clin Trials* 1980;3:369–374.

44. Kinzel T: Relief of emotional symptoms in elderly patients with terminal cancer. *Geriatrics* 1988;43:61–66.

45. Breen JL, Lebow M, Boffard D: Practice of gynecology in the elderly. *Clin Ther* 1985;7:400–405.

46. Pucino F, Beck CL, Seifert RL, et al: Pharmacogeriatrics. Pharmacotherapy 1985;5:314–326.

47. Nadelson CC: Geriatric sex problems: Discussion. *J Geriatr Psychiatry* 1984;17:139–147.

48. Meyers WA: Sexuality in the older individual. *J Am Acad Psychoanal* 1985;13:511–520.

49. Renshaw DC: Geriatric sex problems. *J Geriatr Psychiatry* 1984;17:123–138.

50. Renshaw DC: Sex, age, and values. *J Am Geriatr Soc* 1985;33:635–643.

51. Thienhaus OJ: Practical overview of sexual function and advancing age. *Geriatrics* 1988;43:63–67.

52. Sontag S: The double standard of aging. *Occas Pap Gerontol* 1975.

53. Avron J: Benefit and cost analysis in geriatric care: Turning age discrimination into health policy. *N Engl J Med* 1984;310:1294–1301.

54. Jonsen AR, Siegler M, Winslade WJ: *Clinical Ethics,* ed. 3. New York, McGraw-Hill, 1992.

55. Schneiderman LJ, Jecker NS, Jonsen AR: Medical futility: Its meaning and ethical implications. *Ann Intern Med* 1991;112:949–954.

56. Blythe R: *The View in Winter: Reflections on Old Age.* New York, Harcourt Brace Jovanovich, 1979.

57. Cooper JK, Love DW, Raffoul PR: Intentional prescription nonadherance (noncompliance) by the elderly. *J Am Geriatr Soc* 1982;30:329–333.

58. Shaw PG: Common pitfalls in geriatric drug prescribing. *Drugs* 1982;23:324–328.

59. Robertson W: The problem of patient compliance. *Am J Obstet Gynecol* 1985;152:948–952.

60. Gadow S: Introduction to Part II, in Gadow S, Cole T (eds.): *What Does It Mean To Grow Old?* Durham, Duke University Press, 1986.

61. Cassel CK: The meaning of health care in old age, in Gadow S, Cole T (eds.): *What Does It Mean To Grow Old?* Durham, Duke University Press, 1986.

62. Agich GJ: *Autonomy and Long-Term Care.* New York, Oxford University Press, 1993.

63. Moddy HR: *Ethics in an Aging Society.* Baltimore, The Johns Hopkins University Press, 1992.

Chapter 3

The Biology of Aging

George M. Martin, MD

The demographic data, reviewed in an earlier chapter of this book and considered in more detail elsewhere,[1] reveal major gains in life expectancies for human populations, particularly for the female. We are now witnessing exponential increases in the proportions of those segments of our population that are over the age of 65, particularly those over the age of 80. Moreover, the developing societies around the world are almost certain to witness similar dramatic changes in their demographics.[2] Thus, to an increasing degree, gynecologists and other health professionals should be aware of the state of our knowledge concerning the biology of aging. In this chapter I attempt to provide a concise review of this field as of 1994, including some discussion of topics particularly germane to the human female, such as the biology of reproductive aging and current views as to the reasons females generally outlive their spouses.

By way of introduction, I must caution the reader that a rigorous program of research on the basic mechanisms of aging is of relatively recent vintage. The National Institute on Aging is one of the newest branches of the National Institutes of Health (NIH), having been established in 1974. While we know a great deal about the phenomenology of aging, including age-related disease, we still have comparatively little understanding of the fundamental mechanisms.

Some Definitions

Some gerontologists (particularly plant biologists) use the term *aging* to refer to all of the structural and functional alterations observable during the course of life, from birth to death.[3] Mammalian gerontologists, however, differentiate between such changes associated with development and those that follow sexual maturation and the emergence of a young adult phenotype. They often use the term *aging* synonymously with *senescence* (or, more properly, *senescing*). In this chapter, we shall define aging as a constellation of changes in structure and function of an organism (usually deteriorative, but sometimes adaptive), generally beginning after sexual maturation, such that there is a slow, insidious, and progressive decline in the efficiency of homeostasis and a decreasing probability of a successful reaction to injury. In the language of thermodynamics, there appears to be an inexorable increase in entropy or, put another way, an increase in the degree of molecular disorder. In any case the net result for large populations of organisms is an exponential increase in the probability of death per unit time. This is shown schematically in Figure 3.1. A hypothetical population of organisms that do not exhibit aging is represented by *A* in Figure 3.1, in which there is no change in the death rate over time. Populations exhibiting biological aging would follow trajectories indicated by *B* and *C*, the former representing a comparatively long-lived species in

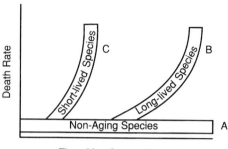

Figure 3.1. Schematic diagrams of death rates, over time, for a hypothetical population of nonaging organisms (*A*) and two populations exhibiting intrinsic biological aging (*B* and *C*), although with contrasting life spans.

which the exponential rise in death rate is delayed and the initial slope is less steep in comparison with species *C*. These oversimplified diagrams (see below) refer to organisms with iteroparous types of reproduction—that is to say, repeated episodes of reproduction. Virtually all mammals are of that type. Organisms with semelparous types of reproduction ("big bang" reproduction)[4] typically exhibit—immediately following their single, massive reproductive efforts—very rapid and roughly synchronized structural and physiological deteriorations resulting in patterns of approximately synchronized death of populations, often interpreted as "programmed" aging. Such patterns of aging are characteristic of certain species of migrating salmon, flowering plants, octopuses, and marsupial mice.

Recent research into iteroparous populations of invertebrates (fruit flies and medflies)[5,6] has shown that when exceedingly large populations of subjects are considered (millions of individual organisms), subpopulations of very old individuals depart from strict Gompertz kinetics in that, paradoxically, their mortality rates appear to decrease over time. The same pattern may obtain for man.[7] These observations could be related to behavioral changes in such organisms, by which environmental hazard functions are reduced. For example, very old flies cease to fly, becoming virtually immobilized. Perhaps some very old human subjects also experience behavioral and environmental changes such that the risks of exposure to trauma, infections, and other events that precipitate mortality are decreased. Perhaps of even greater significance for the case of human subjects is their substantial degrees of constitutional genetic heterogeneity. For example, it has recently been reported that centenarians are much more likely to bear the apolipoprotein E ε2 allele, an unusual polymorphic allele in Western Caucasian populations.[8] While such intrinsic genetic variation is unlikely to explain late life departures from the Gompertz function in populations of genetically inbred fruit flies, some component of the variance in such inbred organisms could be related to de novo meiotic mutations, recombination, and/or differential outcomes of such poorly understood epigenetic mechanisms as parental genomic imprinting.[9]

Evolutionary Biology and Aging

Why did aging evolve in biological systems? After all, given such incredible biological achievements as embryogenesis and the development of central nervous systems capable of higher cognition, by comparison the design of molecular machinery suitable for the indefinite maintenance of an adult structure seems facile. Most evolutionary biologists believe that aging evolved on the basis of one or both of the following nonadaptive mechanisms.[10,11] Probably the favored idea is that of antagonistic pleiotropy. According to that notion, various alleles at a number of genetic loci, selected because they confer enhanced reproductive fitness during the early phase of the life span, have negative effects late in the life span, when the force of natural selection is comparatively weak, since reproduction declines or ceases. One specific example cited in a classic paper by Williams[12] concerned genes with effects on the efficiency of incorporation of calcium into bones of young organisms; he argued that alleles selected for enhanced efficiency might contribute to the development of calcific depositions in the arterial walls later in life, thus contributing to senescence. The second idea simply suggests that mutations with late-life effects accumulate during biological evolution because natural selection against such accumulations is not sufficiently strong.[13] There is some experimental evidence in fruit flies to support these ideas.[14] Whatever the mechanisms, in the last few years two independent laboratories have shown that it is possible to indirectly select lines of long-lived flies by serially selecting for females exhibiting comparatively high fecundity *late* in the life span.[15,16] Both laboratories began with different isolates of genetically heterogeneous wild-type lines of *Drosophila melanogaster.* Many genes seem to be contributing to the increased life span.[17] A few of these genes are now being characterized. Could they prove to be of relevance to the life span of other species, including man? While it is indeed possible that there may be some common denominators, a priori, there are no compelling reasons why the specific kinds of antagonistically pleiotropic genes and accumulated mutations should be identical.[18,19] Furthermore, we must remember that all phenotypes are the result of the interactions of the genetic constitution and the environment. It is possible that the nature of a particular gene action vis-à-vis its effect upon aging could vary substantially in contrasting environmental settings.

How Many Genes?

The most obvious arguments that rates of aging are subject to genetic controls derive from observations on the variations of maximal life-span potentials of various species, including those within specific taxonomic groups. For example, there is more than a thirtyfold difference in maximal life spans among mammalian species.[20] Note that I have emphasized *maximal* life span. It is well-established that, for many populations, *mean* life span is subject to wide fluctuations as functions of even modest alterations in environment, while, with the single exception so far of caloric restriction regimes (discussed below), effects of nonlethal alterations in environment on the maximal life span of a cohort appear to be relatively small. The maximal life-span potential indeed appears to be a constitutional feature of speciation, although there is the potential for plasticity.

How many genes might be involved in the determination of varying rates of aging and varying longevities among species and within a species? There are no satisfactory answers to this question. In the fruit fly selection experiments noted above, while there were genetic elements contributing to long life span on all of the chromosomes of *Drosophila,* the total number of genes involved is unknown. Studies of the fossil remains of the hominid precursors of man, coupled with known correlations between brain size and longevity and estimates of rates of point mutation, have suggested that during the comparatively rapid period of evolution to *Homo sapiens* perhaps 200 to 300 genes were involved, supporting a polygenic basis for the modulation of life span.[21,22] There are reasons to believe, however, that the important changes in speciation involved chromosomal rearrangements rather than point mutations.[23] My own approach to this question involved a system-atic analysis of the known mutations in man that had overlapping phenotypic effects—to some extent—with the senescent phenotype of man, as we see it in the clinics and on the autopsy table.[24] The conclusion was that, as an upper limit, perhaps 7,000 loci could be involved, assuming a total of 100,000 genes in man. However, since there was evidence of certain single-gene syndromes with rather profound, multiple effects on the phenotype ("segmental progeroid syndromes"), such as the Werner syndrome,[25] it was speculated that only a small proportion of such loci (perhaps as few as 70 genes) might be of *major* importance in determining differential rates of aging in our species. That study is also subject to many uncertainties, however. It is nonetheless reasonable to conclude that the control of how we age is subject to rather complex genetic controls. Another conclusion, of special significance to the clinician, is that human beings, who are exceptionally heterogeneous in terms of both genetic and environmental influences, are likely to vary substantially in their patterns of aging. It is fair to say that no two individuals ever have or ever will age in precisely the same fashion. Thus, every time a clinician contemplates an intervention in a geriatric patient, the clinician should consider that he or she is embarking on a new experiment.

Molecular and Cell Biology of Aging

Rather than simply cataloging the numerous molecular and cellular alterations that occur in aging organisms, in this section I review a selective subset of these within the framework of a few of the many theories of aging. For a more complete treatment, see Warner and coworkers.[26] For the reader who wants to quickly learn the current status of "the bottom line," suffice it to say that there is no compelling evidence supporting a given theory of aging, although the general notion that oxidative alterations to macromolecules are of major importance (the "free radical theory of aging") has been gaining favor. Moreover, we are unlikely to discover a single mechanism or process of aging. Instead, one should think in terms of multiple processes of aging. At issue is exactly how many independent mechanisms are involved primarily. One interpretation of the caloric restriction experiments (see below) is that there may be comparatively few such processes. Such a conclusion is at odds with the evolutionary and genetic considerations discussed above. We will require a great deal more research to learn which interpretation is closer to the truth.

The Free Radical Theory of Aging

Chemical free radicals are atoms or groups of atoms (for example, the hydroxyl ion) characterized by the presence of at least one unpaired electron. They are highly reactive moieties, capable of interacting with a variety of biologically important macromolecules. According to the free radical theory of aging—perhaps currently the most popular of the molecular theories of aging—such radicals are responsible for a host of oxidative alterations that are the root causes of cell alteration and cell death in aging aerobic organisms.[27,28] In all aerobic organisms, the cytochrome oxidase system of respiration evolved in order to quadrivalently reduce molecular oxygen. There is, however, a slight but significant "leakage" in the system in which univalently reduced oxygen leads to the generation of active oxygen radicals.[29] While specific enzymatic protective mechanisms have presumably evolved to protect against such products (eg, the two major forms of superoxide dismutase, catalase, and glutathione peroxidase),[29] some degree of damage to cell organelles may nevertheless ensue, according to the theory. Moreover, there are numerous other biochemical reactions that produce active radicals as products of intermediary metabolism. Under some circumstances an attack by chemical free radicals can lead to a chain reaction (for example, lipid peroxidation), resulting in extensive damage to the membranes of cells and cell organelles. Such reactions have been postulated as the basis for the appearance, during aging, of lipofuscin pigments ("wear-and-tear" pigments, "aging pigments").[30] These pigments (Fig. 3.2) can be found in a number of cell types and in an amazing variety of aging organisms, ranging from fungi to man.[31] Their rates of accumulation appear to be related to intrinsic biological aging and not merely to chronological time.[32,33] Lipofuscin pigments are thus candidates for biological markers of aging and may be interpreted as evidence in support of the free radical theory of aging. One type of relatively direct test of the theory, involving the treatment of experimental animals with antioxidants,

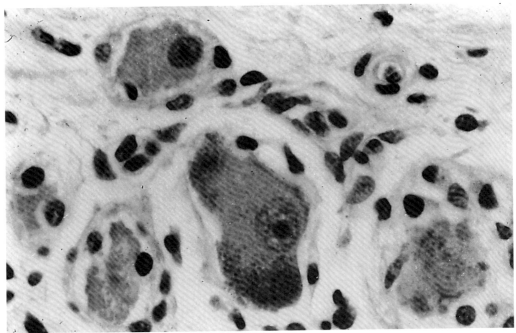

Figure 3.2. A light micrograph of a neuron of a spinal ganglion from an 88-year-old patient who died of Alzheimer's disease. There are masses of lipofuscin pigment within the cytoplasm that, with the hematoxylin and eosin (H&E) stain, appeared yellow-brown. These pigments also exhibit a characteristic fluorescence.

however, has not resulted in convincing life-span extensions.[34] An alternative approach involving the synthesis of transgenic organisms overexpressing a combination of free radical scavenging enzymes, however, has been successful—at least in fruit flies.[35] Lines of flies overexpressing cDNA constructs for either superoxide dismutase 1 or catalase did not exhibit evidence of enhanced life spans. Flies overexpressing *both* constructs did exhibit extensions of the maximal life span (up to 33%).[35] This result is not surprising in that overexpression of superoxide dismutase 1 (SOD-1) would be expected to generate excess hydrogen peroxide, a generator of the highly reactive hydroxyl radical; addition of excess catalase would obviate this problem. Readers who desire a more sophisticated analysis of the general issue of free radical generation, disease, and aging should consult the text of Halliwell and Gutteridge.[36]

Caloric restriction is a more established experimental approach for the enhancement of longevity, including maximal life spans.[37] This was initially interpreted by some as evidence in support of the free radical theory, as the assumption was that the metabolic rates of the calorically restricted animals were reduced. Direct measurements, however, have failed to show reductions in oxygen uptake per lean body mass.[38,39] Thus, the best established method for the enhancement of life span does not appear to alter the metabolic rate, and hence the flux of oxygen free radicals. It is possible, however, that caloric restrictions could decrease the "leakiness" of the cytochrome oxidase system.

There is as yet no compelling evidence that caloric restriction increases the life spans of human populations. With the exception of some small ongoing studies on nonhuman primates,[40] all studies have utilized animal species (mostly rodents) that undergo comparatively rapid rates of sexual maturation, have comparatively large numbers of progeny, and have relatively short life spans. This is in contrast to the life history strategies of higher primates such as man. One should therefore entertain some skepticism about the extent to which the rodent experiments can be extrapolated to man.[41]

Somatic Mutational Theories of Aging

Somatic mutations are structural alterations in genes (either alterations in the primary nucleotide sequences of DNA or alterations in gene dosage) that occur in the cells of the body (soma). Their frequencies may or may not be correlated with mutations in the germ line. There are many different types of somatic mutation and these may result from a number of different molecular mechanisms.[42] One potential mechanism is, in fact, damage to DNA by active oxygen species. We know relatively little about the molecular details of such injury and its genetic consequences, although recent results suggest that a certain class of mutations (doublet transitions from C-C to T-T) may serve as "signature" mutations of oxidative damage.[43,44]

Do somatic mutations of any kind accumulate during aging in mammals? For the case of the peripheral blood T lymphocytes of man, there is evidence that mutations at the X-linked locus, hypoxanthine-guanine phosphoribosyltransferase (HPRT) do indeed accumualte during aging.[45] No evidence for the accumulation of such HPRT mutations could be found in the somatic cells (renal tubular epithelium and interstitial fibroblasts of skeletal muscle) of very old mice, however.[46] Thus, the positive findings in man may simply be related to chronological time rather than to intrinsic biological aging, since the maximal life span of man is about 20 or 30 times that of the house mouse. Of course, it is difficult to make any generalizations at this time because so few genetic loci have been examined and in only a few cell types.

In the mutation research noted above, the lesions were presumably point mutations and intragenic deletions or rearrangements. Chromosomal mutations, involving larger scale mutations, do indeed accumulate in the tissues of aging mice at very high frequencies.[47] In addition, alterations in the numbers of chromosomes are seen. There are several possible etiologies for such aberrations, including free radical damage, viral-induced cell fusion, transposon-mediated rearrangements, premature centromere division (perhaps related to abnormalities in centromeric proteins), and gene amplification. With respect to the latter mechanism, it has been proposed that a variety of agents that interrupt DNA synthesis can result, via a sort of "stuttering" of reinitiation, in extra strands of DNA with resulting recombinational pathways leading to many different types of chromosomal lesions.[48] There have also been many studies showing increased frequencies of chromosomal aberrations in somatic cells from aging human subjects, mostly peripheral blood lymphocytes, including demonstrations of increased sensitivies of cells from older donors to agents that break chromosomes.[49]

A line of research that supports an important role of chromosomal pathology in aging comes from studies of a rare but striking progeroid syndrome, the Werner syndrome (sometimes referred to as "progeria of the adult"). The disorder is inherited as an autosomal recessive gene and is characterized by a failure to undergo the usual adolescent growth spurt and by the premature onset and rapid progression of graying of the hair, loss of hair, atrophic changes and ulceration of skin, ocular cataracts, osteoporosis, diabetes mellitus, several forms of arteriosclerosis, hypogonadism, and a susceptibility to neoplasia (particularly mesenchymal neoplasms).[25] Somatic cells from such subjects are prone to develop chromosomal deletions, inversions, and reciprocal translocations.[50] Intragenic mutations also appear to be predominately deletions.[51,52]

Arguments against a universal role for somatic mutations in aging come from experiments in insects.[53] For the case of recessive mutations, their effects on life span could be tested in a species of wasps (*Habrobracon*), males of which may be either haploid or diploid. The life spans of haploids and diploids are the same, but in control experiments ionizing radiation was much more effective in reducing the life span in the haploids.[54] Thus, it seems unlikely that the accumulation of recessive mutations are of importance in the natural senescence of the wasp. A caveat, however, is that a number of critically important loci may, in fact, be diploid in the predominately haploid organism. Moreover, the results do not rule out the possibility that aging in the wasp might be due to some combination of recessive and dominant mutations; the diploid organism, having double the number of target genes, would be more susceptible to dominant mutations, while the haploid organism would be more susceptible to recessive mutations.

Protein Synthesis Error Catastrophe Theory

Although essentially "pronounced dead" by at least one distinguished gerontologist,[55] this particularly elegant idea still has not been rigorously tested, in my opinion, in certain critical settings—for example, in a variety of obligate postreplicative mammalian cells in vivo.

In his original formulation, Orgel[56] argued that errors in the synthesis of proteins that were themselves involved in the synthesis of other proteins would lead to an exponential increase in subsequent error rates, leading to massive accumulations of abnormal proteins in the cells of very aged organisms. In a later publication, Orgel pointed out that such error catastrophes were by no means inevitable, a crucial variable being the efficiency with which proteolytic enzymes were able to recognize and degrade the abnormal protein synthetic machinery.[57] These ideas stimulated a great number of experiments, the bulk of which argue against the accumulation of biosynthetic errors during aging.[55] Abnormal proteins definitely accumulate; however, they result from posttranslational alterations.[58] One such type of alteration, the glycation of proteins, has recently been postulated to play an important role in aging and is discussed further below.

Glycation of Proteins and DNA

Glycation is currently the preferred biochemical nomenclature for "nonenzymatic glycosylation" reactions. Glycation of proteins involves reactions between reducing sugars and the primary amino groups of proteins. The first product of the reaction is a comparatively labile Schiff base derivative of the protein. This slowly undergoes an isomerization reaction to form the relatively stable ketoamine adduct via an Amadori rearrangement.[59] The most familiar example to physicians would be the glycation of hemoglobins at the N-termini of their beta chains by glucose and its phosphorylated derivatives, assays of which are used for the monitoring of the level of control of diabetic patients.[60]

Cerami and coworkers[61] have proposed that glucose-mediated glycation of proteins are major mediators of aging. His group has also emphasized the potential role of glycations of DNA in mutagenesis.[62]

Support for a role for glycation reactions in aging comes from the observations of reduced levels of glycated hemoglobins in long-lived, calorically restricted rodents.[63]

Clonal Senescence

Clonal senescence may be defined as the gradual attenuation of the growth of proliferating colonies of somatic cells (derived from single parental cells), culminating in populations of cells that are still viable, but "reproductively dead."[64] This is the basic phenomenology of the famous "Hayflick limit."[65] It is apparent that this phenomenon cannot be of relevance to the aging of most species of insects, since their somatic cells—with the exception of the lineages leading to the production of gametes—are obligately postreplicative. In mammals, however, the maintenance of the integrity of many tissues is dependent on an orderly replacement of effete cells. It is therefore possible that the clonal senescence of certain critical cell types may contribute to the development of components of senescence. Furthermore, the senescent phenotype of mammals is characterized by a marked decline in proliferative homeostasis, with the appearance of tissue atrophy side by side with multiple foci of inappropriate proliferation.[66] It is therefore possible that aberrations in cell–cell interaction, consequent to clonal senescence, contribute to the precursors of age-related neoplasia.

That the phenomenon of clonal senescence, as studied in cell culture, may in fact be of relevance to cell aging in vivo is supported by three lines of evidence. Most important, perhaps, is the observation that the life spans of cultured somatic cells from a series of mammalian species of contrasting maximal life-span potentials exhibit clear positive correlations with in vivo life spans.[67] Second, although there is considerable variance, cultured cells from older donors exhibit less growth potential than those from younger donors.[68,69] Finally, cultured somatic cells from patients with the striking progeroid disorder noted above (the Werner syndrome) exhibit marked deficiencies of growth potential.[68]

The mechanisms of the clonal senescence of normal diploid somatic cells are unknown. Two contrasting views are that it results from various forms of cell injury or that it represents a more physiological process, such as terminal differentiation resulting from regulated alterations in gene expression. Formally, the process appears to obey stochastic laws. The progeny of single cells show great variations in their growth potentials.[70,71] While the growth histories of mass cultures are quite predictable for given strains, the growth potential of an individual cell within a group of morphologically "young" cells (those that have not yet developed certain morphological alterations associated with senescent cells, notably greatly enlarged cytoplasmic masses) is not predictable.

The limited replicative life span of normal diploid somatic cells is dominant in crosses with cell lines of indefinite growth potentials.[72] Such experiments have defined four distinct complementation groups among such "immortal" cell lines, most of which are derived from cancer cells.[72] These exciting results, although not reproducible by some workers,[73] are likely to prove of great significance in unraveling an important aspect of oncogenesis—the escape from a limited life span of at least a proportion of cells within a population of neoplastic cells. There is some evidence that the dominance of the aging phenotype in culture may be related to specific alterations in gene expression and the appearance of specific proteins associated with the plasma cell membrane.[74,75,76] The block in the mitotic cell cycle of the senescent cells appears to be in late G_1,[77] but is potentially reversible, however.[78]

Recent research on the molecular structure of the ends of chromosomes (telomeric repeat sequences) have suggested a mechanism whereby normal somatic cells may eventually cease replicating, whereas cells may replicate indefinitely.[79,80] Because of the nature of semiconservative DNA replication, a special type of reverse transcriptase, "telomerase," is thought to have evolved in order to provide both an RNA template and a protein catalyst for the synthesis of the 3′ ends of DNA; without such an enzyme complex there would be a gradual loss of sequences at the ends of chromosomes, eventually resulting either in the loss of subtelomeric genes or the activation or repression of subtelomeric genes.[81] Telomerase has been found in both the germ line and in a number of cancer cell types, but has not been identified in normal somatic cells. While the absence of telomerase in normal cells is an attractive hypothesis for why normal cells undergo clonal senescence, the current evidence does not yet differentiate between a causal relationship and a simple correlation. Regardless of its role in replicative senescence, however, telomerase emerges as an exciting target for new modalities of cancer therapy, since inhibitors of telomerase would presumably have no effects on normal tissues, with the exception of germ cells of the testes and ovaries.

Neuroendocrine Mechanisms of Aging

The examples of rapid, synchronized, postreproductive death noted above for the case of some animal species with semelparous modes of reproduction suggest the possibility that some degree of neuroendocrine-regulated aging may be retained in iteroparous species. A number of gerontologists, in fact, believe that neuroendocrine alterations are of paramount and primary significance in the determination of the life spans of mammals. The conceptions have varied from positively acting "death hormones" (such substances have yet to be isolated)[82] to the notion of a gradual loss of sensitivity to feedback inhibition within the hypothalamus.[83] Finch[84] has pointed to the possibility of a neuroendocrine cascade of alterations leading to senescence.

Organ System Changes During Aging

Age-related alterations have been observed in all of the organ systems, as might be expected, given the above discussion of potentially pervasive cellular and molecular mechanisms of aging. The immune system has been covered in a separate chapter. Here, we briefly review a few other key systems, concentrating on what is known about major phenotypic changes in our own species. For more comprehensive coverage, textbooks such as that of Hazzard and coworkers[85] should be consulted.

The Female Reproductive System

In comparison with other primates, the human female is unusual in undergoing menopause at a comparatively early phase of the overall life span (see the review by Harman and Talbert).[86] Presumably, such early menopause evolved because it conferred an overall enhancement of reproductive fitness.

Although the complete cessation of menses is considered a landmark qualitative marker of aging, there are signs of aging of the reproductive system beginning after the age of 30, including anovulatory cycles, spontaneous abortions, infertility, and the appearance of aneuploid progeny.[87] At the cellular level, the most dramatic feature of ovarian aging is the depletion of primary ovarian follicles (Figure 3.3). The ovary is essentially devoid of oocytes by the beginning of menopause.

Epidemiologists have uncovered a statistically significant increased risk of relatively premature death, from all causes, among women with early natural menopause compared to a control group

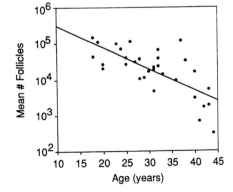

Figure 3.3 A replot of the data of Block[88] showing an exponential decline in the numbers of human ovarian primordial follicles as a function of age.

with natural menopause between the ages of 50 and 54.[89] Logistic repression analysis ruled out contributions of smoking, overweight, underweight, reproductive history, and use of replacement estrogens. While these results will have to be confirmed with other population groups and by longitudinal study designs, they are consistent with the proposition that rates of reproductive aging, in particular the rates of loss of primordial follicles, may be coupled, to some degree, with aging rates in other systems.

The Neuroendocrine System

In experimental rodents, there are many lines of evidence that document major alterations in the neuroendocrine milieu accompanying the transition to female infertility.[90] Measurements of circadian patterns of norepinephrine and serotonin turnover rates, alpha$_1$-adrenergic receptors, and the pulsatile release of luteinizing hormone suggest a critical role for the suprachiasmatic-preoptic region of the hypothalamus, thought to be a master "pacemaker" of biological rhythms.

The dynamic coupling of aging of the neuroendocrine and reproductive systems can be modulated by environmental manipulations. Of potentially great clinical significance are observations for a "feed-back" role of estrogens. Thus, physiological doses of estrogens can accelerate age-related alterations and, conversely, estrogen deprivation can delay the loss of reproductive function of aging rodents.[91,92]

Are there alterations of the suprachiasmatic nucleus of aging human subjects? The answer appears to be yes.[93] Such alterations could partially explain, for example, the sleep disturbances that are so commonly observed in older patients. The suprachiasmatic alterations, including cell loss, may be particularly striking in dementia of the Alzheimer's type. Although most clinicians have been taught to regard Alzheimer's disease as being distinct from normative aging, all of the classic histopathological stigmata of that disorder (neuritic plaques, neurofibrillary tangles, amyloid angiopathy) can be found, although to a lesser degree, in the hippocampus and neocortex of older individuals who, by crude clinical criteria, appear to be cognitively intact.[94]

There is a great deal of current research regarding the potential modulation of postmenopausal estrogen treatments on the risk of developing Alzheimer's disease. Initial reports of a protective effect[95,96] have not been confirmed.[97] Thus, in 1994, no definitive conclusions can be made. Clinicians should follow this story closely, however, as it will be of increasing concern to their patients.

Special Senses

Physicians are well aware of age-related alterations in the visual and auditory systems, but are less well informed about alterations in the vestibular, gustatory, olfactory, and somatosensory systems.[98] About 80% of older subjects exhibit abnormalities in the senses of smell and taste, presenting a major problem in the nutritional management of patients.

Cardiovascular System

This system, particularly the arterial components, can be considered the Achilles' heel of aging in our species. For those of us who manage to survive into our nineties, the vast majority will die as a result of major cardiovascular diseases.[31] We do not understand the cellular and molecular basis of this vulnerability, although progress has been made in elucidating such abnormalities as a diminished response to beta-adrenergic modulation.[99] As people age, there is a gradual increase in vascular stiffness, increases in systolic, diastolic, and mean arterial pressures, left ventricular hypertrophy, and decreases in early diastolic filling rates.[100] When subjected to maximal exercise, there is a diminution of the heart rate response. In the absence of clinically detectable coronary artery disease, a normal cardiac output may be maintained via an enhanced end-diastolic volume (Starling's mechanism); this is an excellent example of what may prove to be a large array of "second line" or "third line" compensatory mechanisms that aging organisms invoke in their constant attempts to maintain homeostasis.

The Respiratory System

Significant age-related structural changes in the pulmonary system include the following: (1) loss of the alveolar elastic recoil; (2) alterations in chest wall structure with decreased respiratory muscle strength; (3) loss of alveolar surface area; (4) an increase in the thickness of the media and intima of pulmonary arteries; and (5) a decrease in the number of cilia lining the airways.[101] The functional consequences of these alterations include a decrease in the dynamic lung volumes, less uniform alveolar ventilation, a decreased response to hypoxia and hypercapnia, decreased vital capacity, and decreased arterial partial pressure of oxygen (PO_2).[101] Chronic obstructive pulmonary disease is common by age 65, and the prevalence of pulmonary infections is increased in the elderly and the consequences of such infections are more serious.[102] Annual influenza vaccines are now recommended for patients over the age of 65.

The Urinary Tract

Pathologists are quite familiar with a number of anatomic alterations in the aged kidney. These include loss of tissue mass, progressive hyalinization (sclerosis) of glomerular units, diminished numbers of nephrons, thickened basement membranes of tubules and vasculature, interstitial fibrosis, arteriolosclerosis, and atherosclerosis. The functional consequences of these lesions include decreased renal blood flow, decreased glomerular filtration rate, impaired ability to concentrate or to dilute the urine, impaired reabsorption of glucose, and altered endocrine functions (renin–angiotensin; vitamin D metabolism; response to vasopressin).[103–105] A core problem in the interpretation of these alterations, vis-à-vis their relationships to underlying intrinsic aging processes, is the extent to which they may be secondary consequences of specific disease processes. (This difficulty is, of course, not unique to the kidney.) The fact that longitudinal studies of renal function have identified subsets of individuals who do not exhibit decrements of function with clinical testing, and who, in fact, appear to exhibit improvements of renal function, suggests to some workers that the alterations may, at least in part, be related to common age-related diseases.[103, 106]

With respect to the common geriatric problem of urinary incontinence, it is certainly the case that intercurrent pathology of various types, when managed properly, can reverse the incontinence.[107] We need more research, however, on such questions as the possible underlying contribution of intrinsic aging of the urinary bladder smooth muscle and in its neural innervation.

Why Do Human Females Generally Outlive Their Spouses?

In the United States, the longevity differential between males and females, based on life expectancy at birth, is currently about 7 years.[1,108] This female advantage is true in all of the developed countries. Is it related to an intrinsic biological advantage of the female or to differential life styles? There is no definite answer to this question.[108] We know that the human female is a somatic mosaic with respect to genes on the X chromosome; in some cells, she is operating on genetic information from the mother's X chromosome, while in others, the X chromosome inherited from the father may be active. This could theoretically provide an advantage, in terms of the buffering of deleterious effects from certain classes of X-linked recessive genes and in terms of a potentially more flexible metabolic repertoire. There is no hard evidence, however, that the female longevity advantage is a general property of mammalian species. In contrast to the present uncertainty as regards genetic contributions to the longevity differential, we have plenty of evidence of a role for life style differences, such as smoking behavior (although, for that particular example, there have been recent dramatic shifts in behavior in many cultures for both males and females).

Those interested in fuller discussions of this sociologically important issue should consult the recent monographs by Ory and Warner[109] and Smith.[1]

References

1. Smith DW: *Human Longevity,* New York, Oxford University Press, 1993.
2. Bhat PN: Changing demography of elderly in India. *Curr Sci* 1992;63:440–448.
3. Leopold AC: The biological significance of death in plants, in Behnke JA, Finch CE, Moment GB (eds.): *The Biology of Aging.* New York, Plenum Press, 1978, pp. 101–114.
4. Diamond JM: Big-bang reproduction and ageing in male marsupial mice. *Nature* 1982;298:115–116.
5. Curtsinger JW, Fukui HH, Townsend DR, Vaupel JW: Demography of genotypes: Failure of the limited life-span paradigm in *Drosophila melanogaster. Science* 1992;258:461–463.
6. Carey JR, Liedo P, Orozco D, Vaupel JW: Slowing of mortality rates at older ages in large medfly cohorts. *Science* 1992;258:457–461.
7. Manton KG, Stallard E, Woodbury MA, Dowd JE: Time-varying covariates in models of human mortality and aging: Multidimensional generalizations of the Gompertz. *J Gerontol* 1994;49:B169–B190.
8. Schachter F, Faure Delanef L, Gu'enot F, Rouger H, Froguel P, Lesueur-Ginot L, Cohen D: Genetic associations with human longevity at the APOE and ACE loci. *Nat Genet* 1994;6:29–32.
9. Fundale RH, Surani MA: Experimental analysis of genetic imprinting in mouse development. *Dev Genet* 1994;15: 515–522.
10. Rose MR: The evolution of animal senescence. *Can J Zool* 1984;62:1661–1667.
11. Kirkwood TBL: Comparative and evolutionary aspects of longevity, in Finch CE, Schneider EL (eds.): *Handbook of the Biology of Aging,* ed. 2. New York, Van Nostrand Reinhold, Co., 1985, pp. 27–44.
12. Williams GC: Pleiotropy, natural selection, and the evolution of senescence. *Evolution* 1957;11:398–411.
13. Medawar DB: *The Uniqueness of the Individual.* London, Methuen, 1957, pp. 17–70.
14. Rose MR, Graves JL: Evolution of aging, in Rothstein M (ed.): *Review of Biological Research in Aging.* Vol. 4. New York, Alan R. Liss, 1989.
15. Rose MR: Laboratory evolution of postponed senescence in *Drosophila melanogaster.* Evolution 1984;38:1004–1010.
16. Luckinbill LS, Arking R, Clare MJ, Cirocco WC, Buck SA: Selection for delayed senescence in *Drosophila melanogaster. Evolution* 1984;38:996–1003.
17. Luckinbill LS, Graves JL, Reed AH, Koetsawang S: Localizing genes that deter senescence in *Drosophila melanogaster. Heredity* 1988;60:367–374.
18. Martin GM, Turker MS: Minireview: Model systems for the genetic analysis of mechanisms of aging. *J. Gerontol* 1988;43:B33–B39.
19. Martin GM: Genetic modulation of the senescent phenotype in *Homo sapiens. Genome* 1989;31:390–397.
20. Altman PL, Dittmer DS: Life spans: Mammals, in *Growth: Biological Handbook.* Washington, DC, Federation of American Societies for Experimental Biology, 1962, pp. 445–550.
21. Cutler RG: Evolution of human longevity and the genetic complexity governing aging rate. *Proc Natl Acad Sci USA* 1975;72:4664–4668.
22. Sacher GA: Maturation and longevity in relation to cranial capacity in hominid evolution, in Tuttle R (ed.) Proceedings of the International Congress Anthropological and Ethnological Sciences, IXth. Published as *Antecedents of Man and After, Vol 1. Primates: Functional Morphology and Evolution.* The Hague, Mouton, 1975, pp. 417–441.
23. Wilson AC, White TJ, Carlson SS, Cherry LM: Molecular evolution and cytogenetic evolution, in Sparkes RS, Comings DE, Fox CF (eds.): *Molecular Human Cytogenetics, ICN–UCLA Symposia on Molecular and Cell Biology,* Vol. 7. New York, Academic Press, pp. 375–393.

24. Martin GM: Genetic syndromes in man with potential relevance to the pathobiology of aging, in Bergsma D, Harrison DE (eds.): *Genetic Effects on Aging, Birth Defects: Original Article Series,* Vol 14, No. 1. New York, Alan R. Liss, 1978, pp. 5–39.

25. Salk D, Fujiwara Y, Martin GM (eds.): Werner's Syndrome and Human Aging. Advances in Experimental Medicine and Biology, Vol 190. New York, Plenum Press, 1985.

26. Warner HR, Butler RN, Sprott RL, Schneider EL (eds.): *Modern Biological Theories of Aging.* Aging, Vol 31. New York, Raven Press, 1987.

27. Harman D: Aging: A theory based on free radical and radiation chemistry. *J. Gerontol* 1956;11:298–300.

28. Harman D: Free radical theory of aging: Role of free radicals in the origination and evolution of life, aging, and disease processes, in Johnson JE Jr, Walford R, Harman D, Miquel J (eds.): *Free Radicals, Aging, and Degenerative Diseases.* New York, Alan R. Liss, 1986, pp. 3–49.

29. Fridovich I: The biology of oxygen radicals. *Science* 1978;201:875–880.

30. Tappel AL: Vitamin E and free radical peroxidation of lipids. *Ann NY Acad Sci* 1972;203:12–28.

31. Martin GM: Interactions of aging and environmental agents: The gerontological perspective, in Baker SR, Rogul M (eds.): *Environmental Toxicity and the Aging Processes.* New York, Alan R. Liss, Progress in Clinical and Biological Research Monograph No. 228.

32. Martin GM: Cellular aging—Postreplicative cells: A review (Part II). *Am J Pathol* 1977;89:513–530.

33. Nakano M, Mizuno T, Gotoh S: Accumulation of cardiac lilpofuscin in mammals: Correlation between sexual maturation and the first appearance of lipofuscin. *Mech Ageing Dev* 1990;52:93–106.

34. Balin AK: Testing the free radical theory of aging, in Adelman RC, Roth GS (eds.): *Testing the Theories of Aging.* Boca Raton, FL, CRC Press, 1982, pp. 137–182.

35. Orr WC, Sohal RS: Extension of life-span by overexpression of superoxide dismutase and catalase in *Drosophila melanogaster. Science* 1994;263:1128–1130.

36. Halliwell B, Gutteridge JMC: *Free Radicals in Biology and Medicine,* ed. 2. Clarendon Press, Oxford, 1989.

37. Weindruch R, Walford RL: *The Retardation of Aging and Disease by Dietary Restriction.* Springfield, IL, Charles C. Thomas, 1988.

38. Masoro EJ, Yu BP, Bertrand HA: Action of food restriction in delaying the aging process. *Proc Natl Acad Sci USA* 1982;79:4239–4241.

39. McCarter R, Masoro EJ, Yu BP: Does food restriction retard aging by reducing the metabolic rate? *Am J Physiol* 1985;248:E488–E490.

40. Roth GS, Ingram DK, Cutler RG: Caloric restriction in non-human primates: A progress report. *Aging* 1991;3:391–392.

41. Austad SN: FRAR course on laboratory approaches to aging. *The Comparative Perspective and Choice of Animal Models in Aging Research. Aging,* Vol. 5, 1993, pp. 259–267.

42. Martin GM, Fry M, Loeb LA: Somatic mutation and aging in mammalian cells, In Sohal RS, Birnbaum LS, Cutler RG (eds.): *Molecular Biology of Aging: Gene Stability and Gene Expression.* New York, Raven Press, 1985, pp. 7–21.

43. Reid TM, Loeb LA: Tandem double CC → TT mutations are produced by reactive oxygen species. *Proc Natl Acad Sci USA* 1993;90:3904–3907.

44. Tkeshelashvili LK, Reid TM, McBride TJ, Loeb LA: Nickel induces a signature mutation for oxygen free radical damage. *Cancer Res* 1993;53:4172–4174.

45. Trainor KJ, Wigmore DJ, Chrysostomou A, Dempsey JL, Seshadri R, Morley AA: Mutation frequency in human lymphocytes increases with age. *Mech Ageing Dev* 1984;27:83–86.

46. Horn PL, Turker MS, Ogburn CE, Disteche CM, Martin, GM: A cloning assay for 6-thioguanine resistance provides evidence against certain somatic mutational theories of aging. *J Cell Physiol* 1984;121:309–315.

47. Martin GM, Smith AC, Ketterer DJ, Ogburn CE, Disteche CM: Increased chromosomal aberrations in first metaphases of cells isolated from the kidneys of aged mice. *Isr J Med Sci* 1985;21:296–301.

48. Schimke RT, Sherwood SW, Hill AB, Johnston RN: Overreplication and recombination of DNA in higher eukaryotes: Potential consequences and biological implications. *Proc Natl Acad Sci USA* 1986;83:2157–2161.

49. Esposito D, Fassina G, Szabo P, De Angelis P, Rodgers L, Weksler M, Siniscalco M: Chromosomes of older humans are more prone to aminopterine-induced breakage. *Proc Natl Acad Sci USA* 1989;86:1302–1306.

50. Salk D, Au K, Hoehn H, Martin GM: Cytogenetics of Werner's syndrome cultured skin fibroblasts: Variegated translocation mosaicism. *Cytogenet Cell Genet* 1981;30:92–107.

51. Fukuchi K, Martin GM, Monnat, RJ Jr: The mutator phenotype of Werner syndrome is characterized by extensive deletions. *Proc. Natl. Acad. Sci. USA* 1989;86:5893–5897.

52. Rünger TM, Bauer C, Dekant B, Müller K, Sobotta P, Czerny C, Poot M, Martin GM: Hypermutable ligation of plasmid DNA ends in cells from patients with Werner syndrome. *J Invest Dermatol* 1994;102:45–48.

53. Maynard Smith J: Theories of aging, in Krohn PL (ed.): *Topics in the Biology of Aging.* New York, John Wiley & Sons, 1965, pp. 1–35.

54. Clark AM, Rubin MA: The modification by X-irradiation of the life span of haploids and diploids of the wasp, *Habrobracon* SP. *Radiat Res* 1961;15:244–253.

55. Rothstein M. Evidence for and against the error catastrophe hypothesis, in Warner HR, Butler RN, Sprott RL, Schneider EL (eds.): *Modern Biological Theories of Aging*. Aging, Vol 31. New York, Raven Press, 1987, pp. 139–154.

56. Orgel LE: The maintenance of the accuracy of protein synthesis and its relevance to ageing. *Proc Natl Acad Sci USA* 1963;49:517–521.

57. Orgel LE: The maintenance of the accuracy of protein synthesis and its relevance to ageing: A correction. *Proc Natl Acad Sci USA* 1970;67:1476.

58. Adelman RC, Dekker EE (eds.): *Modification of Proteins During Aging*. Modern Aging Research. Vol. 7. New York, Alan R. Liss, 1985.

59. Watkins NG, Thorpe SR, Baynes JW: Glycation of amino groups in protein: Studies on the specificity of modification of RNase by glucose. *J Biol Chem* 1985;260:10629–10636.

60. Gallop PM: Biological mechanisms in aging: Post-translational changes in cells and tissues, in *Biological Mechanisms in Aging: Conference Proceedings, June 1980*. National Institutes of Health Publication No. 81-2194. Washington, DC, United States Government Printing Office, 1981, pp. 397–453.

61. Cerami A, Vlassara H, Brownlee M: Glucose and aging. *Sci Am* 1987;256:90–96.

62. Lee AT, Cerami A: Elevated glucose 6-phosphate levels are associated with plasmid mutations in vivo. *Proc Natl Acad Sci USA* 1987;84:8311–8314.

63. Masoro EJ, Katz MS, McMahan CA: Evidence for the glycation hypothesis of aging from the food-restricted rodent model. *J Gerontol* 1989;44:B20–B22.

64. Martin GM, Sprague CA, Norwood TH, Pendergrass WR, Bornstein P, Hoehn H, Arend WP: Do hyperplastoid cell lines "differentiate themselves to death"?, In Cristofalo VJ, Holečková E (eds.): Cell impairment in aging and development. New York, Plenum Press, Advances in Experimental Medicine and Biology, Vol. 53. 1975, pp. 67–90.

65. Hayflick L, Moorhead PS, The serial cultivation of human diploid cell strains. *Exp Cell Res* 1961;25:585–621.

66. Martin GM: Proliferative homeostasis and its age-related aberrations. *Mech Ageing Dev* 1979;9:385–391.

67. Rohme D: Evidence for a relationship between longevity of mammalian species and life-spans of normal fibroblasts *in vitro* and erythrocytes *in vivo*. *Proc Natl Acad Sci USA* 1981;78:5009–5013.

68. Martin GM, Sprague CA, Epstein CJ: Replicative life-span of cultivated human cells: Effects of donor's age, tissue and genotype. *Lab Invest* 1970;23:86–92.

69. Schneider EL, Mitsui Y: The relationship between *in vitro* cellular aging and *in vivo* human age. *Proc Natl Acad Sci USA* 1976;73:3584–3588.

70. Martin GM, Sprague CA, Norwood TH, Pendergrass WR: Clonal selection, attenuation and differentation in an in vitro model of hyperplasia. *Am J Pathol* 1974;137–153.

71. Smith JR, Whitney RG: Intraclonal variation in proliferative potential of human diploid fibroblasts: Stochastic mechanisms for cellular aging. *Science* 1980;207:82–84.

72. Pereira-Smith OM, Smith JR: Genetic analysis of indefinite division in human cells: Identification of four complementation groups. *Proc Natl Acad Sci USA* 1988;85:6042–6046.

73. Ryan PA, Maher VM, McCormick JJ: Failure of infinite life span human cells from different immortality complementation groups to yield finite life span hybrids. *J Cell Physiol* 1994;159:151–160.

74. Lumpkin CK Jr, McClung JK, Pereira-Smith OM, Smith JR: Existence of high abundance antiproliferative mRNA's in senescent human diploid fibroblasts. *Science* 1986;232:393–395.

75. Pereira-Smith OM, Fisher SF, Smith JR: Senescent and quiescent cell inhibitors of DNA synthesis. Membrane-associated proteins. *Exp Cell Res* 1985;160:297–306.

76. Stein GH, Atkins L: Membrane-associated inhibitor of DNA synthesis in senescent human diploid fibroblasts: Characterization and comparison to quiescent cell inhibitor. *Proc Natl Acad Sci USA* 1986;83:9030–9034.

77. Rittling SR, Brooks KM, Cristofalo VJ, Baserga R: Expression of cell cycle-dependent genes in young and senescent WI-38 fibroblasts. *Proc Natl Acad Sci USA* 1986;83:3316–3320.

78. Gorman SD, Cristofalo VJ: Reinitiation of cellular DNA synthesis in BrdU-selected nondividing senescent WI-38 cells by simian virus 40 infection. *J Cell Physiol* 1985;125:122–126.

79. de Lange T: Activation of telomerase in a human tumor. *Proc Natl Acad Sci USA* 1994;91:2882–2885.

80. Martin GM: Genetic modulation of telomeric terminal restriction-fragment length: relevance for clonal aging and late-life disease. *Am J Hum Genet* 1994;55:866–869.

81. Wright WE, Shay JW: The two-stage mechanism controlling cellular senescence and immortalization. *Exp Gerontol* 1992;27:383–389.

82. Denckla WD: Role of the pituitary and thyroid glands in the decline of minimal O_2 consumption with age. *J Clin Invest* 1974;53:572–581.

83. Dilman JM: Age associated elevation of hypothalamic threshold to feedback control, and its role in development, aging, and disease. *Lancet* 1971;1:1211–1219.

84. Finch CE: The regulation of physiological changes during mammalian aging. *Q Rev Biol* 1976;51:49–83.

85. Hazzard WR, Bierman EL, Blass JP, Ettinger WH Jr, Halter JB, Andres R (eds.): *Principles of Geriatric Medicine and Gerontology,* ed 3. McGraw-Hill, New York, 1994.

86. Harman SM, Talbert GB: Reproductive aging, in Finch CE, Schneider EL (eds.): *Handbook of the Biology of Aging,* ed. 2, New York, Van Nostrand Reinhold, 1985, pp. 457–510.

87. Gosden RG: *Biology of Menopause: The Causes and Consequences of Ovarian Ageing.* London, Academic Press, 1985.

88. Block E: Quantitative morphological investigations of the follicular system in women: Variations at different ages. *Acta Anat* 1952;14:108–123.

89. Snowdon DA, Kane RL, Beeson WL, Burke GL, Sprafka JM, Potter J, Iso H, Jacobs DR, Phillips RL: Is early natural menopause a biologic marker of health and aging? *Am J Public Health* 1989;79:709–714.

90. Wise PM, Weiland NG, Scarbrough K, Sortino MA, Cohen IR, Larson GH: Changing hypothalamopituitary function: Its role in aging of the female reproductive system. *Horm Res* 1989;31:39–44.

91. Finch CE, Felicio LS, Mobbs CV, Nelson JF: Ovarian and steroidal influences on neuroendocrine aging processes in female rodents. *Endocrine Rev* 1984;5:467–497.

92. Mobbs CV, Gee DM, Finch CE: Reproductive senescence in female C57BL/6J mice: Ovarian impairments and neuroendocrine impairments that are partially reversible and delayable by ovariectomy. *Endocrinology* 1984;115: 1653–1662.

93. Swaab DF, Fisser B, Kamphorst W, Troost D: The human suprachiasmatic nucleus; neuropeptide changes in senium and Alzheimer's disease. *Bas Appl Histochem* 1988;32:43–54.

94. Morimatsu M, Hirai S, Muramatsu A, Yoshikawa M: Senile degenerative brain lesions and dementia. *J Am Geriatr Soc* 1975;390–406.

95. Henderson VW, Paganini-Hill A, Emanuel CK, Dunn ME, Buckwalter JG: Estrogen replacement therapy in older women. Comparisons between Alzheimer's disease cases and nondemented control subjects. *Arch Neurol* 1994;51: 896–900.

96. Paganini-Hill A, Henderson VW: Estrogen deficiency and risk of Alzheimer's disease in women. *Am J Epidemiol* 1994;140:256–261.

97. Brenner DE, Kukull WA, Stergachis A, van Belle G, Bowen JD, McCormick WC, Teri L, Larson EB: Postmenopausal estrogen replacement therapy and the risk of Alzheimer's Disease: A population-based case-control study. *Am J Epidemiol* 1994;140:262–267.

98. Corso JF: *Aging Sensory Systems and Perception.* New York, Praeger, 1981.

99. Lakatta EG: Diminished beta-adrenergic modulation of cardiovascular function in advanced age. *Cardiol Clin* 1986;4:185–200.

100. Lakatta EG: Hemodynamic adaptations to stress with advancing age. *Acta Med Scand Suppl* 1986;711:39–52.

101. Levitzky MG: Effects of aging on the respiratory system. *Physiologist* 1984;27:102–107.

102. Brandstetter RD, Kazemi H: Aging and the respiratory system. *Med Clin North Am* 1983;67:419–431.

103. Lindeman RD, Goldman R: Anatomic and physiologic age changes in the kidney. *Exp Gerontol* 1986;21:379–406.

104. Davies I: Ageing in the hypothalamo-neurohypophysial-renal system. *Compr Gerontol* 1987;1:12–23.

105. Meyer BR: Renal function in aging. *J Am Geriatr Soc* 1989;37:791–860.

106. Shock NW, Andres R, Norris AH, Tobin JD: Patterns of longitudinal changes in renal function, in Orimo H, Shimada K, Iriki M, Maeda D (eds.): *Recent Advances in Gerontology, XI International Congress of Gerontology.* Amsterdam, Excerpta Medica, 1979, pp. 384–386.

107. Resnick NM, Yalla SV: Aging and its effect on the bladder. *Seminars Urol* 1987;5:82–86.

108. Smith DWE, Warner HR: Does genotypic sex have a direct effect on longevity? *Exp Gerontol* 1989;24:277–288.

109. Ory MG, Warner HR (eds.): *Gender, Health and Longevity: Multidisciplinary Perspectives.* New York, Springer, 1990.

Chapter 4

Alterations of Host-Defense Mechanisms and the Susceptibility to Infection and Other Diseases

Gurkamal S. Chatta, MD and *David C. Dale, MD*

Introduction

Immunosenescence is often accompanied by an increased incidence of neoplasia, autoimmune diseases, and infections. With the burgeoning geriatric population in the United States, there is heightened interest in the illnesses of the elderly and the economic implications thereof. Infectious diseases are among the most important clinical problems in the elderly, with bacterial pneumonias and influenza ranking as the fourth leading cause of death in the population over 65 years of age.[1-4]

Despite extensive research on immunosenescence, as yet there are no simple immunological explanations for the patterns of infections seen in the elderly. In addition to immune deficits, aging is also associated with decrements in organ structure and function and an increased incidence of degenerative diseases, which independently effect host-defense mechanisms. Superimposed on this are environmental changes, that is, increasing institutionalization, social isolation, and neglect. It is the interaction of all these factors that leads to the pattern of clinical illnesses seen.[3, 5]

In this chapter, we discuss (1) the epidemiology of infectious diseases in the elderly, (2) normal host-defense mechanisms, (3) immune defects with aging, (4) age-related decrements in organ structure and function, (5) increased incidence of underlying diseases, (6) the impact of altered environmental factors, (7) specific infections in the elderly, and (8) prevention and treatment of infections in the elderly.

Epidemiology

Although only 12% of the U.S. population is over 65 years old, 30% of beds in acute care facilities and 90% in chronic care facilities are occupied by the elderly. In economic terms this translates into 35% of total health care costs.[3,6,7] A significant proportion of this is accounted for by infectious diseases. On the basis of current data, it is difficult to differentiate the physiological effects of aging from the effects of accumulated insults and underlying chronic diseases. Nevertheless, there is ample clinical evidence for an age-related increase in certain infections, and a number of general statements[2,3] can be made:

1. Regardless of setting, there is an increased incidence of bacterial pneumonias, associated bacteremias, and resultant morbidity in the elderly.[2] Finklestein and coworkers[8] have demonstrated that in a study of pneumococcal bacteremia 75% of the patients were over 60 years old, 50% had an atypical presentation, and 60% had polymicrobial sputum cultures. Despite antibiotic treatment, there was 40% mortality and the hospital stay was uniformly protracted in the survivors. A 1981 National Health Survey of cases with pneumonia (Table 4.1) clearly shows the increased morbidity and mortality in the elderly.[9]

2. Bacteremia, irrespective of source, occurs more often in the elderly. A retrospective study of 500 patients with positive blood cultures revealed that 60% of these occurred in the elderly. On multivariate analysis, age held up as an independent predictor for increased mortality.[10] Afebrile bacteremia occurred almost exclusively in the elderly.[11]

3. Asymptomatic bacteriuria and symptomatic urinary tract infections are more prevalent in the elderly. Up to 15% of ambulant elderly women and 50% of the elderly in nursing homes are bacteriuric.[12] There is also an increased incidence of bacteremia following urinary tract infections. In one study of hospitalized women with nonobstructive pyelonephritis, 12 of 18 elderly women (median age 75 years) developed urosepsis as opposed to 0 of 7 young women (median age 27 years).[13]

4. Intra-abdominal infections, that is, cholangitis, liver abscess, and diverticulitis, are more prevalent in the elderly with a uniformly poorer prognosis than for younger patients.

5. Nosocomial infections of all types, that is, urinary tract infections, pneumonia, bacteremia, and wound infections, occur with a three- to five-fold increased frequency in the 70- to 90-year-old age group. One third of all hospitalizations from a nursing home are infection-related.[14–16]

6. The incidence of tuberculosis and the reactivation of the varicella-zoster virus is age-related and linked to a decline in cell-mediated immunity with aging.

7. Bacterial endocarditis is becoming primarily a geriatric disease. It is usually not associated with rheumatic heart disease, often has an atypical presentation, and has a 20% to 50% mortality.

Another characteristic of infections in the elderly is the extreme variability in clinical presentation. Localizing symptoms and signs are often absent; the only presenting features may be anorexia, malaise, dehydration, a change in mental status, or even frank delirium. A high index of suspicion is necessary to recognize serious infections of the elderly in a timely way. Not only is the febrile response to infection blunted,[16] but also the usual neutrophilia in response to infection may be absent.[17] Thus, there is often a delay in diagnosis and appropriate treatment, further compounding the already high morbidity and mortality to which the elderly are prone. The absence of fever in response to infection in the elderly is ominous, but even when it is present, it forebodes a serious illness. In a prospective study Keating and coworkers[18] of 1202 ambulatory patients presenting

Table 4.1 Pneumonia in the Elderly

	> 65 Yr	< 65 Yr
1. Hospitalization for acute pneumonia (per 1000 population/yr)	11.5	2.0
2. Length of stay (days per 100 hospital discharges)	10.3	7.5
3. Mortality (deaths per 100 hospital discharges)	12.8	1.5

Data from the National Health Survey, 1981.[9]

Table 4.2 Outcome of Fever in Adults Without Underlying Disease

	17–39 yr (%)	40–59 yr (%)	60–79 yr (%)	>80 yr (%)
Not hospitalized	79%	46%	23%	6%
Hospitalized, but no life-threatening disease	20%	46%	60%	73%
Life-threatening disease	1%	7%	16%	16%
Mortality	0%	1%	1%	4%

Data from Keating and Coworkers, 1984.[18]

with a temperature of 101°F or more, advancing age was significantly associated with more serious disease, a higher rate of hospitalization, and a poorer outcome (Table 4.2). In this study, a viral syndrome was thought responsible for the fever in 60% of those under 40 years old, 20% of those 40 to 60, and only 4% of those over 60. This again underscores the importance of a complete workup for a febrile illness in the elderly.

Normal Host-Defense Mechanisms

Host-defense mechanisms[5,19,20] are often subdivided into *nonspecific* and *specific* (Table 4.3). The nonspecific mechanisms provide defense against all types of microbes. The specific defenses reflect enhanced responsiveness due to previous exposure or immunization.

To gain access to the body, an invading organism or foreign antigen must breach the mucocutaneous barrier. The intact skin not only acts as a physical barrier, but also produces secretions that are microbicidal and has flora that prevent colonization by other microorganisms. The mucosal layer prevents microbial invasion by ciliary action, secretion of mucus, and production of several protective proteins, including surface immunoglobulin A(IgA). Having traversed the mucocutaneous barrier, the invading organism usually releases toxins that cause local tissue injury and increased vascular permeability. Exudation of plasma proteins, including the complement proteins, follows. Complement is activated by interaction with many foreign surfaces and bacterial products. Complement components from this activation serve as chemoattractants for neutrophils and as opsonins to facilitate phagocytosis. Neutrophils (polymorphonuclear neutrophila [PMNs]) are rapidly deployed to the site of insult, where they kill most common types of bacteria and limit infection. The involvement of tissue macrophages also aids the phagocytic process and results in the secretion of numerous pro-inflammatory cytokines, that is, interleukin-1 (IL-1), IL-7, IL-12, tumor necrosis factor (TNF), transforming growth factor beta (TGF-β), and so forth. These cytokines further augment the inflammatory response.[21,22]

Table 4.3 Host Defenses

Nonspecific	Specific
Skin and mucosa	B lymphocytes (humoral immunity)
Monocytes-macrophages	T lymphocytes (cell-mediated immunity)
Polymorphonuclear leukocytes	Natural killer cells (NK cells)
Complement	

As part of the acute inflammatory response (Figure 4.1), foreign proteins are processed by antigen presenting cells, that is, macrophages, dendritic cells, and B lymphocytes, and are presented to T lymphocytes in association with proteins of the major histocompatibility complex (MHC).[23] Thus CD4+ T cells see antigen compexed to MHC class II molecules and CD8+ T cells recognize antigen associated with class I MHC. Under the influence of cytokines, activation and expansion of T cells takes place. The activated T cells elaborate IL-2 and other lymphokines that cause clonal expansion of T cells and activation and differentiation of B cells. The latter, after maturing to plasma cells, secrete antigen-specific antibodies of different isotypes, that is, IgM, IgG, IgA, IgD, and IgE. The antibodies assist in host defense by fixing complement, opsonizing organisms, and neutralizing toxins. A primary antibody response (first exposure to antigen) involves secretion of IgM and a secondary antibody response involves secretion of IgG. The switch in isotype from IgM to IgG requires the help of T cells. Hence, the presence of antigen-specific IgG antibodies also implies the existence of T-cell immunity to that antigen.

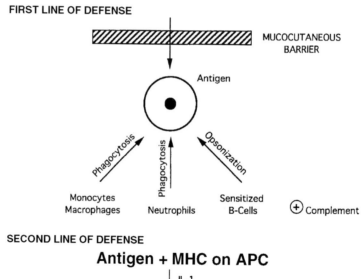

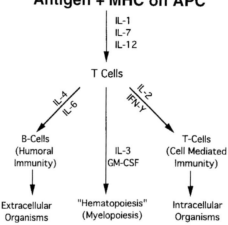

Figure 4.1. Host defense mechanisms. *MHC,* Major histocompatibility complex; *APC,* acetylsalicylic acid, phenacetin, and caffeine; *IL,* interleukin; *IFN-Y,* interferon Y; *GM-CSF,* granulocyte-macrophage–colony-stimulating factor.

T cells constitute 80% of circulating lymphocytes, are pivotal in coordinating the immune response, and are the effectors of cell-mediated immunity.[21-23] CD4+ T cells secrete multiple cytokines and are thought to be composed of at least two different subsets with different cytokine secretion profiles. They kill intracellular organisms, mediate delayed hypersensitivity reactions, and modulate immune responses. CD8+ T cells mediate their effects by lysing cells/targets following prior sensitization. Natural killer cells directly lyse their target cells without any prior exposure to antigen. It is important to understand that all the limbs of the immune network function in concert, with many of the steps occurring simultaneously. Cytokines are polypeptide products of activated lymphocytes and antigen-presenting cells that participate in a variety of cellular responses. They are produced by diverse cell types and have wide-ranging biological effects (Table 4.4).

Immune Defects with Aging

Aging has many important effects on the immune system, but in a number of areas the data are conflicting.[5,24,25] This is due to heterogeneity in the aging process and difficulty in separating the effects of age per se from the effects of occult diseases. It is also recognized that different components of the immune system age at differential rates, adding further complexity.

The effects of age on the immune system are summarized in the following sections.

Neutrophils

Neutrophils constitute the first line of defense against invading microorganisms.[5,20] Neutrophils leave the circulation by adhering to endothelial cells via a combination of adhesion molecules and

Table 4.4. The Major Lymphokines and Their Biological Effects

Lymphokine	Major Biological Properties
IL-1	Activates resting T cells; induces fever; activates endothelial cells and macrophages
IL-2	Growth factor for activated T cells; synthesis of other lymphokines
IL-3	Supports growth of multilineage bone-marrow stem cells
IL-4	B-cell and mast cell growth factor
IL-6	B-cell growth factor
IL-7	B-cell and T-cell growth factor
IL-12	Differentiation of naive CD4 T cells to the Th 1 subset
Granulocyte-macrophage colony-stimulating factor (GM-CSF)	Promotes growth of neutrophilic, eosinophilic and macrophagic cells
Granulocyte CSF (G-CSF)	Promotes growth of neutrophilic cells
Macrophage CSF (M-CSF)	Promotes growth of monocytes and macrophagic cells
Alpha and beta interferon	Antiviral activity
Gamma interferon	Induces class I, class II (DR) antigens on the surface of cells; antiviral activity
Tumor necrosis factor (TNF)	A cytotoxin; induces fever and acute phase responses

IL, Interleukin.

then migrate to the site of infection (chemotaxis). They ingest (by phagocytosis) and then kill microorganisms by (1) an oxidative pathway, involving the intracellular generation of hydrogen peroxide and superoxide and (2) a nonoxidative pathway, involving the intracellular release of neutrophil polypeptides (released by degranulation) that possess antimicrobial activity. There have been several studies that have evaluated different aspects of neutrophil function with aging, that is, adherence, chemotaxis, phagocytosis microbicidal capability, and response to cytokines. Although the data are somewhat conflicting, neutrophil functions at the level of the individual cells are not significantly altered with aging.[26-28] However, the total supply of neutrophils available to fight infections may be reduced in the elderly.[29] Neutropenia in the face of infection occurs more often in the elderly and is associated uniformly with a poor outcome. This suboptimal neutrophilic response to infection is thought to be secondary to a defect in neutrophil production and/or regulation.[30,31] However, at least in the healthy elderly, both neutrophil production and function can be upregulated to levels comparable to young adults with the exogenous administration of granulocyte-specific growth factor, that is, granulocyte colony-stimulating factor (G-CSF).[28]

Monocytes and Macrophages

Monocytes are also produced in the bone marrow. The circulating monocytes are transformed into tissue macrophages and are the principle cells for processing antigens. They elaborate a number of regulatory cytokines, including IL-1.[23] It is thought that their function is not significantly affected by the aging process.[32,33] Although the elderly have a blunted febrile response to infection, the production of IL-1—one of the mediators of the febrile response—is not effected by the aging process.[34]

T Cells

T cells account for 80% of circulating lymphocytes in the blood and are effectors of cell-mediated immunity. Their precursor cells are bone-marrow derived and these, in turn, migrate to the thymus, undergo a process of maturation, and subsequently circulate in the blood as either helper T cells, that is, the T4 subset, or cytotoxic T cells, that is, the T8 subset. The specificity of T cells is determined by clonotypic cell surface receptors (the CD3–T-cell receptor complex).[5,20] The increased predisposition to infections with intracellular organisms, that is, tuberculosis, listeria, legionella, and reactivation of varicella-zoster virus suggests a decline in cell-mediated immunity with aging. The diminished ability in the elderly to mount cutaneous delayed hypersensitivity reactions to skin test antigens also suggests a T-cell abnormality.[5,24,25,35-37] Extensive research in the field of T-cell aging is summarized in the following sections.

Thymus and Thymic Hormones

Thymic involution commences at sexual maturity and is complete by age 50. There is also a concomitant decline in thymic hormone concentrations. There is decreased transit of immature cells from the bone marrow to the thymus and also an increase in immature cells within the thymus.[5,24,36] Animal models of immune reconstitution have revealed partial correction of T-cell defects with thymic extract in aged mice.[38]

Blood Lymphocyte Counts

These counts may be either normal or reduced with aging. Most studies showing reduced counts indicate that all T-cell subsets are affected equally.[5,24] According to one longitudinal study by

Bender and coworkers[39] done over a 16-year period, a low blood lymphocyte count is an important marker for mortality from any cause within 3 years. Flow cytometric analysis reveals an increase in circulating immature cells with aging. According to some studies, there is also a decrease in number and/or function of cytotoxic T cells.

T-Cell Function

The consensus favors a decrease in T-cell proliferative responses with aging. Changes at the cellular level that contribute to this are (1) decreased synthesis of IL-2 receptors, (2) decreased binding of ligand to the CD3–T-cell receptor complex on the surface of T cells and, (3) defects in the activation of the protein kinase C system. Other studies of T-cell function reveal decreased production of IL-2, TNF, and gamma interferon. There also tends to be increased susceptibility of ultraviolet radiation–induced damage and a decrease in levels of DNA repair enzymes in T cells of older subjects.[5,24,36]

B Cells

Lymphocytes of the B-cell lineage are effectors of humoral immunity; they do this by elaborating antibodies to foreign antigens, microorganisms, or toxins. B cells are bone-marrow–derived and undergo their maturation in the bone marrow. The process of maturation involves acquiring surface immunoglobulin receptors. Antibody specificity to a wide variety of antigens is a result of immunoglobulin gene rearrangements. To a large measure, B-cell responses are regulated by T-cell subsets and their lymphokines.[5,20] Derangements in B-cell–mediated immunity with aging are suggested by the following:

1. Reduced antibody responses to T-cell–dependent and T-cell–independent antigens.

2. Lower antibody levels with vaccination (ie, for hepatitis B, influenza, and pneumococcal pneumonia) in the elderly.[5,24,40]

3. Age-dependent decrease in isoagglutinins.[5,24]

4. A rising incidence of autoantibodies and monoclonal gammopathies (3% over the age of 70) with aging.[41] It is of note, however, that there is little or no age-related change in the levels of serum immunoglobulins, and no study to date has incontrovertibly documented intrinsic B-cell defects with aging. The suboptimal antibody response to vaccination has been reported to be partially circumvented with a higher challenge dose of the vaccine, and it is thought to reflect a T-cell, rather than a B-cell, effect of the aging process.[42]

NK Cells

Most studies report either a decrease in or no change in NK cell functions.[5,24]

Complement

Complement is a complex of 20 or more proteins in the blood. Neither total complement levels nor complement function is impaired by the aging process.[5,24]

Age-Related Changes in Organ Structure and Function

Aging causes widespread changes in essentially all organ systems.[3,5] The changes that impact on the body's ability to fight infection are briefly summarized here.

Skin

Aging effects all the layers of the skin, that is, the epidermis, dermis, and subcutaneous tissue, along with its organelles. Changes in collagen and elastic tissue can be attributed to aging per se and are characterized by progressive cross-linking of collagen and increased fragmentation of elastic tissue. The net result is a generalized thinning of the integument, an increased propensity to dehiscence, and reduced skin vascularity. Hence, the skin is easily breached, with an attendant risk of skin and soft tissue infections. Furthermore, healing also tends to be delayed in the elderly, and the strength of the healed skin is decreased.

Respiratory System

Senescence of the respiratory tract results in (1) decreased mucociliary clearance of inhaled antigens and (2) increasing collapse of the alveoli and reduction in vital capacity as a result of fragmentation of elastic tissue. These changes are further exacerbated by a decrease in respiratory muscle strength, reduced chest wall compliance, and smoke and dust related pulmonary insults. Thus, not only is pneumonia more likely to occur, but it also tends to be more often bronchopneumonic in distribution.

Gastrointestinal System

The two most significant age-related changes occur in the esophagus and the stomach. In the former there is decreased peristalsis, reduced lower esophageal sphincter tone, and thus increased likelihood of aspiration. Gastric acidity declines significantly, leading to survival of bacteria in ingested foods and more frequent bacterial colonization of the stomach and small intestines. Of people over 60 years of age, 30% are thought to be achlorhydric, a change associated with increased respiratory infections with enteric organisms.

Genitourinary System

Both symptomatic and asymptomatic bacteriuria increases with aging. In the female, weakening of the pelvic floor leads to incomplete bladder emptying and resultant accumulation of residual urine. Atrophic vaginitis contributes to bladder infections from alterations in surface-bacteria flora and increased colonization by enteric organisms.

Increased Incidence of Underlying Diseases

The changes described in the preceding section are thought to be invariable concomitants of aging. The diseases mentioned in this section are more prevalent in the elderly. They are responsible for some of the defects in immune response, delayed wound healing, and the propensity to infection observed in a general population of older persons.[1-3]

Atherosclerosis is by far the most significant contributor to infection-related morbidity and mortality in the elderly. Its salient clinical expressions tend to be: (1) *Peripheral vascular disease,* which predisposes to skin and soft tissue infection, intractable ulcers, and occasionally osteomyelitis. It also contributes to delayed wound healing. (2) *Congestive heart failure,* which may contribute to the development of pneumonia and, because of poor tissue perfusion, slow healing of wounds. Peripheral edema also predisposes to lower extremity cellulitis. (3) *Cerebrovascular disease,* which is primarily a geriatric problem. The associated neurologic deficits often cause loss of mobility, falls, altered mental status, and aspiration pneumonia. Incontinence and urinary tract infection also occur frequently.

The prevalence of diabetes also increases with aging, that is, 15% to 17% in those over 60 years old.[3] It compounds the effects of atherosclerosis, causes neutrophil dysfunction, and contributes to delayed wound healing. Similarly, the age-related increase in chronic obstructive pulmonary disease contributes to the increased incidence of pulmonary infection.

Changes in Environment

It cannot be overemphasized that all aspects of care of the elderly must be planned in the context of their biopsychosocial milieu. Old age is often associated with loneliness, economic deprivation, and social isolation. Multiple sensory deficits, immobility, malnutrition and self-neglect also take their toll. All these factors contribute to both atypical presentations of infection as well as delay in care of the elderly.[3,43]

Of persons over 65 years of age, 25% require assistance with their activities of daily living; of those over 85 years of age, 50% do. Five percent of persons over 65 years of age are in nursing homes and require frequent hospitalizations. These environmental changes, that is, immobility and institutionalization, are known to promote colonization with gram-negative organisms and to foster nosocomial infections.[44] Nutrition in the elderly has been the focus of recent interest. Estimates of protein calorie malnutrition in the elderly range between 15% and 50%, with lower prevalence rates occurring in the ambulant elderly and higher prevalence rates in the institutionalized elderly.[3,45,46] Malnutrition is thought to impact adversely on multiple components of the immune system.

Specific Infections

Aging is associated with an increased incidence of certain infections and the presentation for many of these illnesses often differs substantially in older versus younger adults. For instance, fever and the neutrophil response to infection may be absent. Bacteremic episodes (irrespective of source) and the resultant morbidity and mortality are also higher in the elderly. The more common infections include those listed in the following sections.

Pneumonia

Pneumonias[1,2,17,47] are predominantly bacterial in origin, and the etiologic organisms depend on the clinical setting, that is, community-acquired or nosocomial (Table 4.5).

Table 4.5 Etiological Organisms in Pneumonia*

Community (%)		Hospital (%)		Nursing Home (%)	
S. Pneumoniae	40–60	Gram-negative organisms	45	Gram-negative organisms	29
Gram-negative organisms	6–40	S. Pneumoniae	10–20	S. Pneumoniae	26
H. Influenzae	2–20	Legionella	0–15	H. Influenzae	20
S. aureus	2–10	S. aureus	3–11	S. aureus	8
Legionella	0–20				

*See Ref. 47.

Pneumonia usually occurs because of aspiration of oropharyngeal bacteria. Aspiration is more likely in patients with strokes, dementia, and esophageal dysfunction. In many instances, bacterial pneumonia follows influenza, because this viral infection damages the bronchial mucosa and impairs ciliary function. The treatment of patients with suspected pneumonia should be dictated by gram stain of the sputum. However, in the elderly examination of the sputum is often inconclusive because of a weak cough, dehydration, or other problems. In this situation, empirical treatment must be instituted. In moderately ill patients, a single drug—for example, a second-generation cephalosporin or ampicillin and sulbactam (Unisyn)—is usually adequate. Sicker patients and those with nosocomial infections require the addition of coverage for gram-negative organisms, that is an aminoglycoside or aztreonam. Postinfluenzal pneumonia requires adequate coverage for *Staphylococlus aureus* (Table 4.6).

Urinary Tract Infection

The prevalence of bacteriuria increases with aging and ranges anywhere between 10% and 40%, causing urinary tract infections.[1,2,48] The sex differential of urinary tract infections also decreases considerably with aging. The etiologic organisms include enterococci, and a variety of gram-negative organisms, that is *Escherichia coli*, *Klebsiella*, and *Enterobacter*. Organisms other than

Table 4.6 Common Infections, Etiological Organisms, Empirical Treatment*

Infection	Organisms	Antibiotic choices
Pneumonia		
Community-acquired[†]	*S. Pneumoniae*, Gram-negative organisms, *H. Influenzae*, *S. aureus*, *Legionella*	Erythromycin **or** azithromycin Trimethoprim-sulfamethoxazole Augmentin Second generation cephalosporin[‡]
Nursing Home–acquired	Gram-negative organisms, *S. Pneumoniae*, *H. Influenzae*, *S. aureus*	Above and coverage for gram-negative rods with Ciprofloxacin, **or** aminoglycoside[§], **or** aztreonam
Postinfluenzal	*S. aureus*	Naficillin
Urinary tract		
Clinically stable	*E. coli*	Trimethoprim-sulfamethoxazole
Urosepsis	*Proteus, Klebsiella, Enterococcus, E. coli, Enterobacter*	Ampicillin[‡] or second generation cephalosporin and aminoglycoside
Cellulitis		
Uncomplicated	*S. aureus,* group A streptococci	Naficillin
Complicated	Anaerobes and gram-negative rods	Clindamycin and aminoglycoside

[†] Intravenous erythromycin should be initiated at the outset in suspected *Legionella*.
[§] In general, for sicker patients, aminoglycosides should be used as initial therapy and discontinued if unneeded, based on culture results.
[¶] Ampicillin must be used to cover enterococcus. In the event of penicillin allergy, vancomycin may be substituted.
[‡] Second generation cephalosporin: cefoxitin, cefuroxine.
* (See Refs. 1, 2, 47, 48).

E. coli are encountered more frequently in the elderly. Catheter-associated bacteriuria, which can be present in up to 80% of the elderly in nursing homes, is another major concern. Over 50% of nursing home occupants are incontinent, and more than half of them have catheters. The catheters are invariably colonized and attempts to eradicate bacteriuria with antibiotics are not only futile but also select for resistant organisms. Treatment should only be instituted if there is a change in the clinical status of the patient and after appropriate cultures have been taken. It is usually best to change the patient's catheter before the sample for urine culture is taken. Chronic asymptomatic bacteriuria in the absence of chronic catheterization should only be treated if the patient's clinical status warrants it (Table 4.6).

Skin and Soft Tissue Infections

The major problems associated with skin and soft tissue infections[2,49,50] are cellulitis and infected decubitus ulcers. Cellulitis can either be uncomplicated or occur in the setting of venous insufficiency, peripheral vascular disease, and diabetes. If uncomplicated, the etiologic organism is usually either Group A streptococcus or *S. aureus*. In the presence of diabetes or vascular disease the cellulitis tends to be a mixed infection, with anaerobes and gram-negative rods being the causative organisms.

Decubitus ulcers or "pressure sores" are invariably colonized and occasionally give rise to episodes of sepsis or osteomyelitis. Debridement of necrotic areas and the use of frequent wet-to-dry saline dressings to stimulate the growth of granulation tissue remain the mainstay of therapy. It is important to avoid occlusive dressings and topical agents that inhibit granulation. A course of systemic antibiotics should be instituted in the event of suspected sepsis (Table 4.6). In caring for the elderly, the single most important factor both for preventing and treating decubiti is keeping the pressure off susceptible areas, that is, the sacrococcyx, the greater trochanter, and the heels.

Tuberculosis

The elderly have become the single largest group of patients with active tuberculosis.[1,2,51,52] Although the majority of cases represent reactivation of past disease, in one study 17% of newly diagnosed cases were reported as representing a primary infection.[53]

Pulmonary tuberculosis in the elderly is often characterized by a paucity of localizing symptoms, nonspecific manifestations, and cutaneous anergy in up to 30% of patients with active disease. Sputum for staining is often negative and the chest radiograph may be noncontributory, revealing only old apical fibrosis. In this setting, bronchial washings obtained at bronchoscopy may greatly increase diagnostic yield. In the presence of a pleural effusion, a pleural biopsy has an over 80% diagnostic yield. Epidemics of tuberculosis in nursing home patients are an emerging problem, and miliary tuberculosis is also predominantly a geriatric problem. The latter, because of its insidious presentation, is often difficult to diagnose antemortem. Pulmonary tuberculosis is usually treated with isoniazid (INH) and rifampin for 9 to 12 months, and drug-resistant tuberculosis is not yet a problem in the elderly.

Skin testing for tuberculosis should be done as a two-step procedure in the elderly, that is, two intradermal injections of 5 tuberculin units of purified protein derivative (PPD) separated by a week, to distinguish between the booster effect and true conversion. Chemoprophylaxis is not generally recommended in elderly tuberculin reactors with a normal chest radiograph because of the higher risk of age-related INH hepatotoxicity. The strongest indication for INH chemoprophylaxis is in recent skin convertors, that is, new responders to a two-step PPD with more than 15 mm induration, because of the high risk of active tuberculosis in these individuals. INH prophylaxis for a period of 9 to 12 months with regular monitoring of liver function is recommended.

Intra-Abdominal Infection

Of people in their eighth decade of life, 30% have gallstones and 50% have diverticulosis. Not infrequently, complications such as cholecystitis, diverticulitis, and even frank sepsis develop.[1,2,54] At other times, the initial process is insidious, and the only presenting features may be nonspecific gastrointestinal symptoms, including "failure to thrive." In this setting, a liver abscess must be suspected and diagnosis pursued aggressively. A computed tomography (CT) scan with contrast is particularly helpful in this regard. When liver abscesses are present, they are often multiple. Drainage under CT guidance or ultrasonography is the mainstay of treatment. Antibiotic treatment should adequately cover gram-negative rods and anaerobes. In the case of a biliary source, initial coverage should include enterococci as well (Table 4.7).

Infective Endocarditis

Over the last two decades, infective endocarditis[1,2,55] has become a geriatric disease, with over 50% of the cases occurring in patients over 60 years old. Contributory factors include increased life expectancy, proliferation in the use of endovascular devices, and the higher incidence of bacteremia in the elderly. Diagnosis requires a high index of suspicion and still depends on positive blood cultures and, to some extent, on echocardiography. Mortality rates are between 20% and 50%. Staphylococcal endocarditis carries the worst prognosis. The organisms isolated most often are streptococci (ie, *Streptococcus viridans, S. bovis,* and *S. fecalis*) and staphylococci (ie, *S. aureus* and *S. epidermidis*). *S. bovis* should prompt a search for an underlying colonic cancer, and *S. fecalis* usually points to the urinary tract as the source of infection. *S. epidermidis* is most frequently associated with endovascular devices (ie, valves, shunts, and intravenous catheters). Less frequently,

Table 4.7 Intra-Abdominal Infections: Common Organisms and Empirical Treatment*

Source	Aerobes	Anaerobes	Antibiotics
Biliary tract	*E. coli, Klebsiella, Enterococcus*	*Clostridium*	Ampicillin and clindamycin and aminoglycoside **or** ampicillin and cefoxitin
Colon (ie, severe diverticulitis)[†]	*E. coli, Proteus, Klebsiella*	*Bacteroides, Peptostreptococcus*	Aminoglycoside[‡] and clindmycin **or** cefoxitin **or** metronidazole
Liver abscess	*E. coli, Streptococcus, Proteus, Klebsiella*	*Bacteroides, Peptostreptococcus, Fusobacterium, Clostridium*	Aminoglycoside and metronidazole **or** clindamycin **or** cefoperazone

[†] The efficacy of antimicrobial treatment in mild diverticulitis is not established.
[‡] In general, for sicker patients, aminoglycosides should be used as initial therapy and discontinued if unneeded, based on culture results.
*See Ref. 2.54.

endocarditis secondary to gram-negative organisms or candida occurs, invariably in a nosocomial setting.

In general, antimicrobial treatment for endocarditis should be given intravenously for 4 to 6 weeks. Streptococcal endocarditis is treated with high doses of penicillin G and an aminoglycoside (for the first 2 weeks) for synergism. For staphylococcal endocarditis, intravenous naficillin is used; vancomycin is required for *S. epidermidis* infections. Renal function should be monitored throughout the course of the treatment and the dosage tailored appropriately. Refractory heart failure and persistently positive blood cultures are indications for proceeding to surgery with prosthetic valve endocarditis.

Meningitis

A high index of suspicion is required to diagnose meningitis[1,2] in the elderly. The only presenting sign may be a change in mental status. In addition to the usual etiological organisms (meningococci and pneumococci), one must consider and rule out *Listeria* and *Cryptococcus*.

Herpes Zoster

This represents a reactivation of the varicella-zoster virus,[3,56–58] which usually lies dormant in sensory ganglia following chicken pox in childhood. The age-related decline in cell-mediated immunity correlates with the increasing incidence of herpes zoster. Immunosuppression, either disease- or drug-induced, also causes a recrudescence of the virus. Clinically, there is usually a sudden onset of burning or lancinating dermatomal pain (usually thoracic and invariably unilateral), followed 3 to 4 days later by a macular eruption in the same dermatomal distributio... Involvement of the trigeminal ganglion and facial nerve can cause keratitis and deafness. In the severely immunocompromised host, encephalitis, myelitis, and dissemination of the virus can occur. These complications are infrequent in the elderly in the absence of immunosuppressive drugs, hematologic malignancies, or other factors severely altering host-defense mechanisms. The most common complication in the elderly is postherpetic neuralgia, and it can last for months.

The goals of treatment are symptomatic relief (ie, with wet compresses and analgesics) in the acute phase and prevention of postherpetic neuralgia. A short course of prednisone (60 mg/day for 10 to 14 days) is thought to decrease the severity and duration of postherpetic neuralgia but is not of proven benefit. In the severely immunocompromised host, a 7-day course of acyclovir is given during the acute stage to prevent dissemination of the virus. Acyclovir is also indicated in documented cases of herpetic keratitis. A vaccine for the varicella-zoster virus is currently undergoing clinical trials.

Prevention and Treatment

In this section, the general principles of treatment are stressed and the subject of prophylaxis examined in greater detail. Prevention of infection may be achieved either by immunoprophylaxis or chemoprophylaxis.

Immunoprophylaxis[59,60]

In the elderly, vaccination is currently recommended for influenza, pneumococcus, and tetanus.

Influenza

Influenza and postinfluenzal pneumonia cause great morbidity and mortality in the geriatric population. During influenza epidemics, the attack rate in closed communities (ie, nursing homes) can approach 35%. Despite a suboptimal antibody response to vaccination in the elderly, overall vaccine efficacy is in the 70% range. Even if influenza occurs in vaccinated populations, it is less severe. In closed communities, vaccination also reduces morbidity in the nonvaccinated by inducing "herd immunity."[53,61] Yearly vaccination is recommended for the following: people over 65 years of age, inmates of chronic care facilities, patients with chronic cardiopulmonary problems, and patients with diabetes and chronic renal failure. Both the inactivated whole-virus vaccine as well as the subunit vaccine are in current use, and either of these can be administered concurrently with the pneumococcal vaccine—at different sites. Side effects are minimal, and the only contraindication is an allergy to chicken eggs, which are used in preparing the vaccine. Initial trials with a new liposome-based virsome influenza vaccine[62] in the elderly also look promising. Several studies have validated the effectiveness and the cost-benefit of the influenza vaccine, and recently the influenza vaccination was added to the list of services covered by Medicare.[53] During epidemics of influenza A, the drugs amantadine or rimantadine can be used for chemoprophylaxis of influenza A in nonvaccinated or recently vaccinated (ie, less than 2 weeks) subjects. However, these drugs have greater central nervous system toxicity in the elderly and should be used cautiously.

Pneumococcus

Vaccination for pneumococcus[63-67] has been the subject of intense debate. Although the older vaccine contained 14 serotypes, the vaccine in current use contains 23 serotypes. Several studies have looked at its efficacy (Table 4.8), and despite methodological differences, varying attack rates in these studies, and different outcome measures, it was concluded that the efficacy of the vaccine correlated directly with one's ability to mount an antibody response. The consensus at present[68,69] favors immunizing all asplenic individuals and everyone over 65 years of age with the 23-valent vaccine. People vaccinated more than 6 years ago with the 14-valent vaccine should also receive the 23-valent vaccine. The antibody response elicited by the vaccine is known to wane with time, and the risk of hypersensitivity reactions with a booster more than 6 years after the primary vaccine is low. However, revaccination in the elderly is not currently recommended.

Table 4.8 Studies on the Efficacy of Pneumovax*

Study	Design	Comments
Gaillat et al. (1985)	Prospective randomized[†]	Healthy, elderly subjects: 77% efficacy
Simberkoff et al. (VA Coop Study) (1986)	Prospective randomized[‡]	Elderly with chronic illnesses: No efficacy
Forrester et al. (1987)	Retrospective case control	Elderly with chronic illness: No efficacy
Sims et al. (1988)	Retrospective case control	Healthy elderly: 70% eficacy
Shapiro et al. (1991)	Retrospective case control	Healthy and hospitalized elderly: 60% efficacy

*See Refs. 63–67.
[†] The 14 serotype vaccine was used in these studies.

Tetanus

Although low in incidence, tetanus now occurs primarily in the elderly, with 60% of new cases being diagnosed in those over 60 years old.[70,71] Mortality is also disproportionately high in the elderly. Immunity to tetanus declines with aging, with a drop in the levels of circulating antitoxin. However, the booster response to the adult tetanus—diptheria (Td) toxoid preparation is known to be excellent even in intervals of 20 to 25 years after the primary series. Although initial recommendations called for a booster of Td every 10 years after the age of 65, there is increasing evidence that a single Td booster at age 60 years is sufficient and more cost-effective. In the absence of previous immunization or an unclear history thereof, a primary series is recommended. The recommendations for wound prophylaxis remain unchanged.

Chemoprophylaxis[1,2,72,73]

In brief, any invasive procedure in the presence of foreign prostheses, prosthetic heart valves, surgically constructed shunts, valvular heart disease, or a previous history of infective endocarditis is the basis for recommending chemoprophylaxis. In particular, dental manipulations and gastrointestinal and genitourinary procedures have a high incidence of bacteremia. Antibiotic prophylaxis in these settings should cover the local microbial flora associated with these tissues. Surgical prophylaxis in the absence of heart disease aims to prevent wound infection, infection at the operative site, and bacteremia. Chemoprophylaxis is currently recommended for colorectal surgery, vaginal hysterectomy, biliary tract surgery, cardiac surgery, hip operations, and urologic procedures. Antibiotics are usually administered preoperatively and up to 24 to 48 hours postoperatively and cover regional microbial flora and staphylococci (in the case of bone surgery).

Summary

Aging is associated with an increased frequency and severity of many types of illnesses, including infectious diseases. Specific changes in host-defense mechanisms account for only part of this increased susceptibility to infections. Good health care for the elderly requires an appreciation for the more subtle presentation of infections, for example, a blunted febrile response, occult signs of inflammation, and more frequent nonspecific signs, for example, altered mental status, immobility, and anorexia. When fever is present or the suspicion of infection is high, antibiotic intervention should be prompt. Initial treatment is often empirical and is based on recognized patterns of infection in the elderly, since smears and cultures may neither be available nor helpful. Preventive measures, including vaccinations and chemoprophylaxis, maintenance of nutritional status, and physical stamina are very important for prevention of infection in elderly individuals.

References

1. Yoshikawa TT, Norman DC: *Aging and Clinical Practice: Infectious Diseases—Diagnosis and Treatment,* ed 1. New York, Igaku-Shoin, 1987.
2. Yoshikawa TT (ed.): Clinics in Geriatric Medicine: Infectious Diseases in the Elderly, WB Saunders, No. 8, Philadelphia, 1992, pp. 701–947.
3. Kane RL, Ouslander JG, Abrass IB: *Essentials of Clinical Geriatrics,* ed 3. New York, McGraw-Hill, 1994.
4. Berk SL, Smith JR: Infectious diseases in the elderly. *Med Clin North Am* 1983;67:273–293.
5. Ben-Yehuda A, Weksler ME. *Host Resistance and the Immune System,* Clinics in Geriatric Medicine, No. 8, Philadelphia, WB Saunders, Nov. 1992, pp. 701–711.

6. Fredman L, Haynes SG: An epidemiologic profile of the elderly, in Phillips HG, Gaylord SA (eds.): Aging and Public Health. New York, Springer, 1985, pp. 1–41.

7. Hodgson TA, Ropstein AN. *Health Care Expenditures for Major Diseases.* Health and prevention profile, United States. Hyattsville, MD, USDHS, Public Health Service, National Center for Health Statistics, 1983, pp. 79–84.

8. Finklestein MS, Petkun WM, Freedman ML: Pneumococcal bacteremia in adults: Age dependent difference in presentation and in outcome. *J Am Geriatr Soc* 1983;31:19–27.

9. Current estimates from the National Health Interview Survey: United States, 1982. Data from the National Health Survey, Series 10, No. 150 (DHHS Publication No. PHS 85-1578). Hyattsville, MD: National Center for Health Statistics, 1985.

10. Weinstein MP, Murphy JR, Reller LB: The clinical significance of positive blood cultures: A comprehensive analysis of 500 episodes of bacteremia and fungemia in adults. II. Clinical observations with special reference to factors influencing prognosis. *Rev Infect Dis* 1983;5:54–70.

11. Gleckman R, Hilbert D: Afebrile bacteremia: A phenomenon in geriatric patients. *JAMA* 1981;248:1478–1481.

12. Yoshikawa TT: Unique aspects of urinary tract infection in the geriatric population. *Gerontology* 1984;30:339–344.

13. Gleckman RA, Bradley PJ, Roth RM: Bacteremic urosepsis. A phenomenon unique to elderly women. *J Urol* 1985;133:174–175.

14. Setia U, Serventi I, Lorenz P: Bacteremia in a longterm care facility. Spectrum and mortality. *Arch Intern Med* 1984;144:1633–1635.

15. Finnegan TP, Austin TW, Cape RDT: A 12 month fever surveillance study in a Veterans' long-stay institution. *J Am Geriatr Soc* 1985;30:590–594.

16. Norman DC, Grahn D, Yoshikawa TT: Fever and aging. *J Am Geriatr Soc* 1985;33:859–863.

17. Murphy TF, Fine BC: Bacteremic pneumococcal pneumonia in the elderly. *Am J Med Sci* 1984;288:114–118.

18. Keating HJ, Klimek JJ, Levine DS, et al: Aging and the clinical significance of fever in ambulatory adult patients. *J Am Geriatr Soc* 1984;32:282–287.

19. Nossal GJV: The basic components of the immune system. *N Engl J Med* 1987;316:1320–1325.

20. Abbas AK, Lichtman AH, Pober JS: *Cellular and Molecular Immunology,* ed 2. Philadelphia, WB Saunders, 1994.

21. Paul WE, Seder RA: Lymphocyte responses and cytokines. *Cell* 1994;76:241–.

22. Janeway CA, Bottomly K: Signals and signs for lymphocyte responses. *Cell* 1994;76:275–.

23. Germain RN: MHC-dependent antigen processing and peptide presentation: Providing ligands for T lymphocyte activation. *Cell* 1994;76:287–.

24. Saltzman RI, Peterson PF: Immunodeficiency of the elderly. *Rev Infect Dis* 1987;9:1127–1139.

25. Weksler ME, Schwab R: The immunogenetics of immune senescence. *Exp Clin Immunogenet* 1992;199:182–.

26. Corberand J, Nygen F, Laharrague P: Polymorphonuclear functions and aging in humans. *J Am Geriatr Soc* 1981;29:391–397.

27. McGregor R, Shalit M: Neutrophil function in healthy elderly subjects. *J Gerontol* 1990;45:M55–M.

28. Chatta GS, Price TH, Allen RC, Dale DC: The effects of in vivo rhG-CSF on the neutrophil response in healthy young and elderly volunteers. *Blood* 1994; (In press).

29. Timaffy M: A comparative study of bone marrow function in young and old individuals. *Gerontol Clin* 1962;4:13–18.

30. Baldwin JG: Hematopoietic function in the elderly. *Arch Intern Med* 1988;148:2544–2546.

31. Chatta GS, Andrews RG, Hammond WP, Dale DC: Hematopoietic progenitors and aging. *J Gerontol* 1993;48:M207–M.

32. Gardner ID, Lim TH, Lawton JWM: Monocyte function in aging humans. *Mech Ageing Dev* 1981;16:233–239.

33. Ding A, Hwang S, Schwab R: Effect of age on murine macrophages. *J Immunol* 1994;153:2146–2152.

34. Jones PG, Kauffman CA, Bergman AG, Cannon JG: Fever in the elderly. Production of leukocytic pyrogen by monocytes from elderly persons. *Gerontology* 1984;30:182–187.

35. Miller RA: The cell biology of aging: Immunological models. *J. Gerontol* 1989;44:B4–B8.

36. Makinodan T, Lubinski J, Fong TC: Cellular, biochemical and molecular basis of T-cell senescence. *Arch Pathol Lab Med* 1987;111:910–914.

37. Phair JP, Kauffman CA, Bjornson A, Hess EV: Host defenses in the aged: evaluation of components of the inflammatory and immune responses. *J Infect Dis* 1978;138:67–73.

38. Gravenstein S, Duthie EH, Miller BA, Roecker E, Ershler WB: Augmentation of influenza antibody response in elderly men by thymosin alpha one. A double-blind placebo-controlled clinical study. *Clin Invest* 1989;37:1–8.

39. Bender BS, Nagel JE, Adler WH, Andres R: Absolute periphereal blood lymphocyte count and subsequent mortality of elderly men. The Baltimore Longitudinal Study of Aging. *J Am Geriatr Soc* 1986;34:649–654.

40. Ammann AJ, Schiffman G, Austrian R: The antibody responses to pneumococcal capsular polysaccharides in aged individuals. *Proc Soc Exp Biol Med* 1980;164:312–316.

41. Radl J: Age-related monoclonal gammopathies. *Immunol Today* 1990;11:234–236.

42. Bender BS: B lymphocyte function in aging. *Rev Biol Res Aging* 1985;2:143–154.

43. Katz S: Functional assessment. *J Am Geriatr Soc* 1983;31:721–726.
44. Garibaldi RA, Brodine S, Matsumiya S: Infections among patients in nursing homes. *N Engl J Med* 1981;305:731–735.
45. Chandra RK: Nutrition immunity and infection: Present knowledge and future direction. *Lancet* 1983;1:688–691.
46. Corman LC: The relationship between nutrition, infection and immunity. *Med Clin North Am* 1985;69:519–531.
47. Bentley DW: Bacterial pneumonia in the elderly: Clinical features, diagnosis, etiology, and treatment. *Gerontology* 1984;30:297–307.
48. Nordenstam GR, Brandberg CA, Oden AS: Bacteriuria and mortality in an elderly population. *N Engl J Med* 1986;314:1152–1156.
49. Reuler JB, Cooney TG: The pressure sore: Pathophysiology and principles of management. *Ann Intern Med* 1981;94: 661–666.
50. Smith DM, Winsemius DK, Besdine RW: Pressure sores in the elderly. *J Gen Int Med* 1991;6:81–93.
51. Dutt AK, and Stead WW: Tuberculosis in the elderly. *Med Clin North Am* 1993;77:1353–1368.
52. Pust RE: Tuberculosis in the 1990's: Resurgence, regimens and resources. *South Med J* 1992;85:584–593.
53. Monto AS: Influenza vaccines for the elderly. *N Engl J Med* 1994;331:807–808.
54. Nichols RL: Intraabdominal infections: An overview. *Rev Infect Dis* 1985;7(Suppl.):709–715.
55. Wilson WR, Danielson GH, Guiliane ER: Prosthetic valve endocarditis. *Mayo Clin Proc* 1982;57:155–161.
56. Hope-Simpson RE: The nature of Herpes zoster: A long-term study and a new hypothesis. *Proc Roy Soc Med* 1965;58:9–13.
57. Weller TH: Varicella and herpes zoster. Changing concepts of the natural history, control, and importance of a not-so benign virus. *N Engl J Med* 1983;309:1363–1368.
58. Balfour HH: Current management of varicella-zoster virus infections. *J Med Virol* 1993; Suppl. 1 pgs. 74–81.
59. Gardner P, Schaffner W: Immunization of adults. *N Engl J Med* 1993;328:1252–1258.
60. Adult Immunizations 1994. Task Force on Adult Immunization: American College of Physicians, Infectious Diseases Society of America, and Centers for Disease Control and Prevention. *Ann Int Med* 1994;121:540–595.
61. Patriarca PA, Arden NH, HopIan JP, Goodman RA: Prevention and control of type A influenza infections in nursing homes. *Ann Intern Med* 1987;107:732–740.
62. Gluck R, Mischler R, Finkel B, Cryz SJ: Immunogenicity of a new virosome influenza vaccine in elderly people. *Lancet* 1994;344:160–163.
63. Shapiro ED, Clemens JD: A controlled evaluation of the protective efficacy of pneumococcal vaccine for patients at high risk of serious pneumococcal infection. *Ann Intern Med* 1984;101:325–332.
64. Simberkoff MS, Cross AP, Al-Ibrahim M: Efficacy of pneumococcal vaccine in high risk patients. *N Engl J Med* 1986;315:1316–1327.
65. Forrester HL, Jahnigen DW, LaForce FM: Inefficacy of pneumonococcal vaccine in a high-risk population. *Am J Med* 1987;83:425–430.
66. Sims RV, Steinmann WC, McConville JH, King LR, Zwick WC, Schwartz JS: The clinical effectiveness of the pneumococcal vaccine in the elderly. *Ann Intern Med* 1988;108:653–657.
67. Shapiro ED, Austrian R, Adair RK, Clemens JD: The protective efficacy of polyvalent pneumococcal polysaccharide vaccine. *N Eng J Med* 1991:325;1453–1460.
68. Broome CV, Breman RF: Pneumococcal vaccine: Past, present and future. *N Eng J Med* 1991;325:1506–1508.
69. Butler JC, Breiman RF, Campbell JF, Facklam RR: Pneumococcal polysaccharide vaccine efficacy. An evaluation of current recommendations. *JAMA* 1993;270:1826–1831.
70. Weiss BP, Strassburg MA, Feeley JC: Tetanus and diphtheria immunity in an elderly population in Los Angeles County. *Am J Public Health* 1983;145:802–804.
71. LaForce FM: Routine tetanus immunizations for adults: Once is enough. *J Gen Int Med* 1993;8:459–460.
72. Guglielmo BJ, Hohn DC, Hoo PJ: Antibiotic prophylaxis in surgical procedures. *Arch Surg* 1983;118:943–955.
73. Shulman ST, Amren DP, Bisno Al, et al: Prevention of bacterial endocarditis. A statement for health professionals by the Committee on Rheumatic Fever and Infective Endocarditis of the Counsel on Cardiovascular Disease in the Young. *Circulation* 1984;70;1123A–1127A.

Chapter 5

Nutrition and Aging

Lauren Nathan, MD, and Roy M. Pitkin, MD

Introduction

Throughout her life, a woman undergoes various physiologic changes that alter her nutritional requirements. Aging changes, coupled with the cessation of ovarian function at menopause and any accompanying disease states, bring about a distinct set of physiological, psychological, and social events that, perhaps more than at any period since early infancy, place a woman at risk for malnutrition. Age-related changes can affect nutritional status and many of the diseases of the elderly lead to alterations in nutrient requirements and metabolism. Certain medications may predispose to malnutrition due to drug effects on metabolism, absorption, appetite, and drug–nutrient interactions.

Immobility may increase the risk for osteoporotic fractures due to lack of exercise and inadequate exposure to sunlight. Depression and alcohol abuse, commonly encountered among the elderly, can also predispose to nutritional deficiency states. Socioeconomic factors can limit an elderly person's access to essential food items, as well as to proper health care. Death of a spouse may also jeopardize intake, not only due to depression-associated anorexia, but also by removing the incentive to prepare tasteful and nutritious meals.

The gynecologist, as the primary health care provider for a large segment of the female population, is uniquely suited to influence the nutritional aspects of women's health. In order to facilitate a better understanding of nutritional considerations in the elderly woman, this review highlights certain relevant biological aspects of nutrition and metabolism in the aged, as well as the impact of psychosocial factors in the development of malnutrition in the aging female population.

Background

Energy Balance

Population surveys indicate that energy intake tends to decrease progressively after the third decade. Depending on socioeconomic status, physical activity, and mental status, a woman's energy intake may be adequate, excessive, or deficient. Evaluation of energy status includes assessment of dietary intake, usual weight and height, recent weight changes, concurrent illness, and drug use. Physical examination should ascertain general body habitus, current body mass index (BMI) (weight in kg/height in m²; normal range in females is from 19.8 to 26 kg/m²), mid-arm circumference (average value in normal females is 23.2 cm), and tricep skinfold thickness (average value in normal females is 16.5 mm).[1]

Table 5.1 Body Mass Index (BMI)

Category	BMI (kg/m²)
Underweight	<19.8
Normal	19.8–26.0
Overweight	26.1–29.0
Obese	>29.0

Adapted from Lewis EF, Bell SJ; Nutritional assessment, in Morley JE, Glick Z, Rubenstein LZ (eds.): *Geriatric Nutrition, A Comprehensive Review*, New York, Raven Press, 1990, pp. 73–87.

Body weight or tricept skinfold thickness greater than 115% of ideal indicates positive energy balance in the past. BMI above 26.0 (Table 5.1) is another indicator of excessive prior energy intake.[2] Weight less than 80% of ideal (ideal body weight equal 45 kg for the first 152 cm in height and 0.9 kg for each centimeter over 152 cm) (Table 5.2), BMI less than 19.8, tricep skinfold thickness less than 80% of ideal, or loss of more than 10% of body weight, all suggest past energy deficiency.[1,2] Measurement of skinfold thickness may be subject to imprecision because of increased skin flaccidity and the lack of adequate standards for the elderly.

To obtain a more precise assessment of energy intake, the Harris-Benedict equation can provide an estimate of basal energy expenditure (BEE). For women, BEE = 665 + [9.6 × weight (kg)] + [1.7 × height (cm)] − [4.7 × age (yr)].[2] Caloric needs are then adjusted for activity level and disease states. The BEE is multiplied by 1.3 for moderate activity, 1.1 for a postoperative state, and 1.3 to 1.6 for the presence of severe infection.[2] The Recommended Dietary Allowance (RDA) for energy is not age-adjusted after 50, when it is 1,700 kcal (Table 5.3).

Protein

Studies of protein metabolism and requirements in the elderly are conflicting. This uncertainty probably reflects the lack of sensitivity and reproducibility of nitrogen balance studies, a result at

Table 5.2 Ideal Body Weight (IBW) in Elderly Persons

Height (ft/in)	Average IBW of women (lb)
4 9	100
4 10	103
4 11	106
5 0	109
5 1	112
5 2	116
5 3	120
5 4	124
5 5	128
5 6	132
5 7	136
5 8	140
5 9	144
5 10	148

Adapted from Metropolitan Life Insurance Company, 1983, Height and Weight Table. New York, 1990, pp. 73–87.

Table 5.3 Recommended Dietary Allowances, 1989

Nutrients	Females 51 years and over
Energy (kcal)	1,900
Protein (g)	50
Vitamins:	
Vitamin A (µg Retinol equivalents)	800
Vitamin D (µg)	5
Vitamin E (mg α-tocopherol equivalents)	8
Vitamin K	65
Vitamin C (mg)	60
Thiamin (mg)	1.0
Riboflavin (mg)	1.2
Niacin (mg NE)	13
Vitamin B_6 (mg)	1.6
Folacin (µg)	180
Vitamin B_{12} (µg)	2.0
Minerals:	
Calcium (mg)	800
Phosphorus (mg)	800
Magnesium (mg)	280
Iron (mg)	10
Zinc (mg)	12
Iodine (µg)	150
Selenium (µg)	55

Food and Nutrition Board, National Research Council: *Recommended Dietary Allowances,* ed 10. Washington, DC, National Academy Press, 1989.

least in part of to failure to control for cutaneous and respiratory nitrogen losses.[3] The confusion surrounding protein metabolism is compounded further by the inextricable metabolic interrelationships between energy and protein, such that optimal protein utilization requires a basal level of energy intake. Nevertheless, several age-related changes in protein metabolism are well recognized. Protein stores diminish with aging, largely as a result of the decline in lean body mass.[4] Total body protein synthesis is decreased in older persons; however, when calculated on the basis of body cell mass, protein synthesis in older individuals may be no different from, or actually slightly higher than, that in younger adults. Serum albumin levels decline with aging, and protein tolerance decreases as a result of declining renal function.[2] It is unclear whether declining renal function with age represents an unavoidable part of the aging process or an effect of long-standing excessive protein intake leading to progressive renal damage. The fact that usual protein intake by American adults exceeds the Recommended Dietary Allowance (RDA) by 1.5 times supports the latter postulate and has led to recommendations that protein intake be reduced in the American diet.[2]

Because protein metabolism in elderly humans is poorly understood, many unanswered questions remain regarding appropriate protein intake in this population. Nevertheless, since elderly individuals are at increased risk for developing problems that may affect their protein needs and since decreased energy intake may impair protein utilization, it has been recommended that elderly individuals consume 12% to 14% of calories as protein.[4] Alternatively, because energy intake varies and may be low, others have advised intake of 0.9 to 1.0 g/kg per day of protein to assure appropriate nitrogen balance.[5] Larger amounts may be needed in certain illnesses, undernutrition, and other stresses that may increase protein loss.

Lipids

Both serum cholesterol and amount of body fat increase in aging women.[4] The increase in serum cholesterol may be mediated by altered responses of low density lipoprotein (LDL) receptors to hormonal stimulation that then lead to increased endogenous cholesterol synthesis.[4] Studies in rats have demonstrated decreased cholesterol turnover with advancing age, but comparable investigations have not been performed in humans.[4]

Although the process of atherosclerotic plaque accumulation begins early in life, the impact of this process is frequently not evident until much later and, therefore, atherosclerosis represents an important health issue in the elderly population. Furthermore, in elderly females, its complications appear to be exacerbated by the estrogen-deficient state resulting from ovarian failure. Administration of estrogens postmenopausally appears to decrease, at least to some extent, the risk of sequelae from hyperlipidemia.

The role of dietary lipid modification among the elderly remains unclear. Restriction of fat and cholesterol in elderly persons has not been shown unequivocally to influence mortality from coronary artery disease. Furthermore, there appears to be less correlation between lipid levels and cardiovascular disease with advancing age; in one study of individuals over the age of 70 the prevalence of atherosclerotic coronary disease was very high, yet virtually no males and only one fourth of the females had hyperlipidemia.[6] Thus, while restriction of dietary fats by the elderly may be advisable to prevent obesity and its sequelae, it may be relatively unimportant in reducing the risk of cardiovascular disease. The need for dietary modification and the role of estrogens in women with hypercholesterolemia need further evaluation. For females 51 years of age and over, it is currently recommended that fat be limited to 30% of total calories and that cholesterol intake not exceed 300 mg/day.[5]

Carbohydrates

Plasma glucose levels and the incidence of type II diabetes mellitus increase with advancing age, reflecting changes in insulin action and metabolism as well as impaired insulin release in response to glucose challenges.[4] Increased body fat with advancing age may also be an important factor in the development of altered glucose metabolism, since studies of primitive cultures in which obesity does not exist show no age-associated increase in glucose levels.[4]

The average diet consists of 45% to 50% of calories as carbohydrate. Carbohydrates can be simple (mono- and disaccharides) or complex (polysaccharides with more than 10 monomeric units). Because many foods containing complex carbohydrates also contain large amounts of vitamins and minerals and produce less of a glycemic response,[7] it is recommended that elderly individuals consume a larger proportion of complex carbohydrates (55% to 60%) to increase nutrient density.[5]

Factors Associated with Nutritional Deficiencies

Altered Physiology

The aging process brings about a distinct set of physiological changes that can alter nutritional needs. Some of these changes are discussed below.

Changing Energy Requirements

Age-related changes in body composition, which probably reflect a complex interaction of the aging process itself, nutrition, and lifestyle factors include primarily loss of lean body mass and its replacement with adipose tissue.[8] Lean body mass diminishes progressively from a maximum in early adulthood, the rate of loss averaging 2% to 3% per decade.[8] Substitution of fat for muscle means that more metabolically active tissue is replaced with less metabolically active tissue, thus resting energy expenditure or basal metabolic rate falls proportionately. Furthermore, physical activity tends to decline with aging, accentuating declining energy needs.

If caloric intake is not decreased in the face of this change in requirement, obesity may result. If caloric intake is reduced appropriately without a concomitant increase in consumption of nutrient-dense foods, undernourishment can result because the requirements for nutrients other than energy do not decrease with advancing age.[9] When counseling elderly individuals about diet, it is therefore important to emphasize consumption of foods with increased nutrient density such as lean meats, fish, certain beans, iron-enriched cereals, and whole grain products.

Altered Threshold for Sodium and Water

With advancing age, there is a decrease in the ability of the kidneys to conserve sodium in response to low sodium intake. This decrease is due in part to declining renin production, leading to decreased activity of the renin–angiotensin–aldosterone system. In one nursing home study of elderly men, certain individuals required 2 grams of sodium per day to maintain serum sodium concentrations in the normal range.[10] The daily requirement for sodium in the elderly may therefore be higher than previously thought.

The aging kidney also loses centrating ability because of a decreased sensitivity to antidiuretic hormone.[2] The aging kidney also has reduced diluting abilities, and elderly individuals are more susceptible to both dehydration and overhydration.[2] Thus, in the elderly the requirement for water is higher but the maximal tolerable amount of water is lower, in comparison with younger individuals.

Altered Drive for Food and Water

Changes in the hypothalamus with aging may be partially responsible for the anorexia and decreased thirst found in many older individuals.[2] The normal opioid stimulus of the hunger center in the hypothalamus in the aged may be less robust, leading to anorexia.[2] Additionally, there is an augmentation of the release of cholecystokinin, which drives the satiety center,[2] further enhancing the propensity toward decreased food intake in the elderly. Neurotransmitter abnormalities such as reduced levels of neuropeptide Y and norepinephrine that occur with dementia may also lead to a decreased drive for food intake in the aged.[4]

The center for water homeostasis is also altered in the aged. In young individuals, this center is normally activated by hyperosmolarity and responds by stimulating the sensation of thirst, increased water intake, and increased antidiuretic hormone secretion. In the elderly, there is a partial blunting of the response such that there is a decrease in the sensation of thirst and drive for drinking.[2] The elderly are therefore placed at further risk for dehydration.

Gastrointestinal Changes

Due to atrophic changes in the gut with aging, there can be decreased secretion of hydrochloric acid, pepsin, and intrinsic factor, leading to impaired absorption of vitamin B_{12}, folate, and nonheme iron.[2] The requirements for these nutrients may therefore increase with aging. Hypochlorhydria may also impair absorption of certain calcium preparations, necessitating alteration of the specific type of calcium supplement prescribed. In general, calcium citrate is the preferred preparation in the elderly since it is more soluble in the presence of hypochlorhydria.[11]

Changes in structures responsible for taste may lead to increases in the threshold for perceiving food odors and flavors, thereby decreasing the pleasure associated with eating and thus the desire to eat. The ability and therefore desire to eat may be further diminished by poor dentition and ill-fitting dentures.

Altered Calcium Metabolism

Aging is associated with declining 1,25-dihydroxy-vitamin D levels, probably as a result of deficient diet, lack of sun exposure, and reduced capacity of the aging kidney to synthesize this vitamin.[2,12] The lower 1,25-dihydroxy-vitamin D levels lead to decreased intestinal absorption of calcium that, in turn, stimulates parathyroid hormone secretion, causing calcium resorption from bone.[12] Gastrointestinal changes encountered with aging (see above) may also impair calcium absorption from the intestine. Estrogen deficiency may exacerbate these age-related changes by decreasing intestinal receptors for 1,25-dihydroxy-vitamin D and thereby further impairing calcium absorption from the gut.[13] Estrogen deficiency may also increase renal calcium loss through a primary renal calcium leak.[14] All of these changes may increase the need for calcium or vitamin D, or both.

Chronic Diseases

Specific diseases common in the elderly are frequently associated with malnutrition. Gastrointestinal bleeding, commonly encountered in the elderly from a number of causes, leads to iron-deficiency anemia. Organic brain syndromes may result in a variety of nutritional deficiencies, including protein-calorie undernutrition. Chronic obstructive pulmonary disease, end-stage renal disease, chronic congestive heart failure, and neoplastic disease also result in protein-calorie undernutrition. In these latter situations, attempts to supplement nutritionally may fail because of an associated generalized impairment in metabolic and endocrinologic processes.[2]

Drugs

Drugs can influence nutritional status by affecting appetite, causing side effects such as intestinal bleeding, and by altering absorption, excretion, or synthesis of nutrients. Table 5.4 lists drugs commonly used in the elderly that can lead to nutritional deficiencies.

Psychosocial Factors

Nutrition is a biologic phenomenon, but eating has profound social and psychosocial implications as well. It is axiomatic in nutritional counseling that an individual's personal preferences, aversions, family and cultural background, and religion need to be acknowledged and considered when dietary advise is given.

Anorexia is commonly observed in the elderly, particularly the frail elderly in institutions and nursing homes. This may reflect the quality of food preparation or age-related deterioration in smell and taste, or both. Anorexia is also a particularly common symptom of depression, and any suggestion of anorexia, including unexplained weight loss, should prompt a thorough evaluation of mental status.

A substantial proportion of the elderly live alone, in many cases after years of living with a mate. Food preparation for oneself is not likely to be approached in the same way as when meals are shared with others. Unfortunately, a large proportion of elderly live in poverty, and others have physical disabilities that restrict shopping and meal preparation. All of this can influence nutritional status.

Table 5.4 Potential Drug–Nutrient Interactions in Some Commonly Used Drugs

Drug	Nutrient Lost	Mechanism
Aluminum hydroxide	Phosphorus Calcium	Binding of phosphorus calcium
Antacids	Thiamin	Decreased absorption due to altered gastrointestinal pH
Anticoagulants	Vitamin K	Vitamin K antagonist
Antihistamines		Appetite stimulation
Amphetamines		Appetite suppression, weight loss
Aspirin and other anti-inflammatoriers	iron, fat, and water soluble vitamins	Bleeding, malabsorption
Cathartics	Calcium	Impaired gastrointestinal motility
	Potassium	Impaired gastrointestinal motility
Cholestyramine	Vitamins A, D, E, K, folate	Malabsorption
Clofibrate	Carbohydrate	Enzyme inactivation
	Vitamin B^{12}	Decreased absorption
	Carotene	Decreased absorption
	Iron	Decreased absorption
Colchicine	Vitamin B^{12}	Decreased absorption due to damaged intestinal mucosa
	Carotene	
	Magnesium	
Corticosteroids	Zinc	Damage to intestinal mucosa
	Calcium	Gastrointestinal loss
	Potassium	
Digitalis	Protein/energy	Anorexia
	Zinc	Renal loss
	Magnesium	
Ethacrynic acid	Sodium	Depletion
Furosemide	Calcium	Depletion
	Potassium	
	Sodium	
Gentamicin	Potassium	Depletion
	Sodium	
Isoniazid	Pyridoxine	Pyridoxine antagonist
Levodopa	Protein	Competition for absorption
Methotrexate	Folate	Folate antagonist
Mineral oil	Fat, fat-soluble vitamins	Malabsorption
Neomycin	Fat	Decreases pancreatic lipase and binds bile salts and interferes with absorption
	Protein	
	Sodium	
	Potassium	
	Calcium	
	Iron	
	Vitamin B^{12}	
Penicillamine	Zinc	Altered nutrient excretion
	Vitamin B^6	
	Sodium	
Phenobarbital	Vitamin D	Impaired metabolism and utilization
	Folate	
Phenytoin	Vitamin D	Impaired metabolism and utilization
	Folate	
Steroids	Sodium	Depletion in adrenally suppressed patients
Sulfa drugs	Vitamin K	Deficiency
Tetracycline	Protein	Impaired uptake and utilization
	Iron	General malabsorption
	Vitamin K	Inhibits vitamin K synthesis
Tricyclic antidepressants		Weight gain due to appetite stimulation
Trimethoprim	Folate	Folate antagonist

Nutritional Problems

Obesity

Energy intake in excess of requirements, when continued over long periods of time, leads to excessive fat accumulation. This is a particular risk in the elderly because of the combination of lowered basal energy requirements and decreased physical activity. Management of the overweight person (ie, BMI more than 26, weight-for-height more than 120% of standard) is a complex therapeutic process that generally includes strong psychological and social components, along with induction of a moderate degree of negative energy balance. In essence, it represents a combination of exercise, behavior modification, and a diet that allows weight loss of 1 to 2 pounds per week.[2]

Substantial and diverse evidence from animal studies suggests that chronic energy restriction may prolong life span.[4] The mechanism by which this occurs is unclear, but it may involve decreased free radical formation or altered gene expression.[4] The risks and benefits of severe energy restriction in humans have yet to be clarified, and it is therefore not currently advised.

Weight control and exercise are recommended for all age groups. However, information about rigorous exercise and diet control in the elderly are lacking. Furthermore, while excessive adipose tissue has been purported to play a role in the etiology of certain disease states, in the elderly it may actually be beneficial by acting as a reserve of energy in the event of illness or other stress. Therefore, prior to recommending strict dietary interventions for weight loss, the precise role of adipose tissue in the elderly must be defined more clearly.

Protein-Calorie Undernutrition

Protein-calorie undernutrition is characterized by loss of both lean body mass and adipose tissue from insufficient intake of protein and energy. Primary energy deficiency presents with loss of lean body mass and adipose tissue without edema.[2] Primary protein deficiency presents with edema, hypoalbuminemia, fatty liver, and minimal loss of adipose tissue.[2] In the elderly, the most common presentation of protein-calorie undernutrition is a mix of these findings.[2] One definition of a mixed picture of protein-calorie undernutrition is weight loss of more than 10%, or body weight less than 80% of ideal, with serum albumin less than 3.5 g/dl.[2]

Protein-calorie undernutrition remains a major form of malnutrition in the homebound and institutionalized elderly. This disorder can be either primary or secondary. Primary causes of protein-calorie undernutrition include situations leading to inadequate access to food, such as poverty, social isolation, and failure to identify patients with organic brain syndromes who cannot obtain food themselves. Secondary causes include situations where the ability to utilize nutrition is impaired, such as in chronic disease states.

The diagnosis of protein-calorie undernutrition is made by the presence of decreasing mid-arm muscle circumference, creatinine–height index, serum cholesterol, and serum albumin.[2] Body weight and skinfold thickness may be normal, particularly if there was preceding obesity. Protein-calorie undernutrition places elderly persons at increased risk for pneumonia, immune dysfunction, skin breakdown, and other adverse sequelae of immobility.[2] Hypoalbuminemia may also have important implications for drug prescribing practices, especially with agents that bind strongly to plasma albumin. Since lower plasma albumin levels lead to increased concentrations of free drug, there is greater potential for toxicity and more rapid renal clearance.

Ideally, protein-calorie undernutrition should be prevented. Preventive strategies include frequent assessment of nutritional risk factors, frequent measurement of body weight, and at least yearly measurement of serum cholesterol and albumin. Once this disorder has developed, correctional strategies depend on the clinical setting. Providing home-delivered meals, treating depression, eliminating drugs that decrease appetite, and providing nutritional supplements are simple maneuvers to correct this problem. For patients who are neurologically impaired, providing eating assistance may be all that is required. Severely incapacitated or chronically ill patients with functional gastrointestinal tracts may require enteral nutrition.

Muscle Weakness

The decline in muscle mass and strength frequently encountered in the elderly individual may be due to a variety of factors, and undernutrition has been proposed as one of the reversible factors. Vitamin and energy deficiency has been associated with diminishing muscle function in both young and old subjects.[15,16] Furthermore, nutritional repletion in the form of vitamins or calories, or both, has been shown to improve muscle function at all ages.[15,16] However, exercise training may be equally, if not more, important than nutrition in the maintenance of muscle mass. In a randomized controlled trial Fiatrone and coworkers[17] compared progressive resistance exercise training, multinutrient supplementation, both interventions, and neither intervention in a group of frail nursing-home residents over a 10-week period. The authors found that all measures of muscle strength improved significantly in the subjects who exercised and were unchanged in those who had multinutrient supplementation without exercise. Thus, addition of exercise to nutrient supplementation may be indicated in older women with significant muscle weakness.

Micronutrient Deficiencies

Vitamins

Vitamin deficiencies are common in elderly individuals, typically reflecting decrease in food intake without simultaneous increase in nutrient density. Other factors that contribute to vitamin deficiency include atrophic gastritis, lack of exposure to sunlight, use of certain medications, pernicious anemia, and alcohol use. Elderly people commonly become deficient in vitamins, including vitamin B_{12}, folate, and vitamin D. Because fat-soluble vitamins are stored in various tissues and because conventional diets are rarely deficient in these nutrients, fat-soluble vitamin deficiency is rare.

Vitamin B_{12} deficiency affects 5% to 10% of elderly patients.[4] Its manifestations include macrocytic anemia, weakness, ataxia, diarrhea, and anorexia. The diagnosis is made by measuring serum B_{12} levels. Abnormal levels require further investigation to determine the precise cause of the deficiency. Treatment depends on the cause, but oral supplementation is generally adequate unless there is true pernicious anemia. The RDA for vitamin B_{12} for healthy individuals is 2 µg (see Table 5.3).

Low serum folate levels are frequently encountered in older persons. Folate deficiency may be caused by poor oral intake, poor absorption due to gastric atrophy, use of certain drugs, and alcohol abuse. The signs and symptoms of folate deficiency include anemia, dementia, stomatitis, and diarrhea. When folate and vitamin B_{12} deficiency coexist, folate supplementation may correct the anemia but could exacerbate the neurologic condition[2]; thus, it is essential that the cause of megaloblastic anemia be identified before treatment is instituted. The RDA for folate in healthy individuals is 200 µg (see Table 5.3).

Due to lack of exposure to sunlight, poor nutrition, and declining renal function, vitamin D deficiency is also common among the elderly. The etiology and sequelae of vitamin D deficiency are discussed more fully in the section on calcium. The RDA for vitamin D in elderly patients is 5 µg or 400 IU/day (see Table 5.3). Higher doses may be required in the face of renal insufficiency.

Determining adequacy of nutritional intake has traditionally been based on the presence or absence of well-defined deficiency or toxicity states. However, more recent evidence suggests that supplementation of certain vitamins and minerals may provide beneficial effects in addition to those that are strictly nutritional. For example, consumption of large amounts of vitamins C, E, and beta carotene reportedly has been associated with lower rates of coronary artery disease.[18–21] This protective effect is presumably due to the antioxidant properties of these vitamins.[18] Supplementation with large doses of vitamin E has been shown to favorably alter parameters of immune function in the elderly.[22] Niacin prescribed in large doses has been shown to reduce hypercholesterolemia.[4] Other beneficial effects from megadoses of various vitamins and minerals have been reported, but many of these benefits have not been proven scientifically. Regardless, serious consideration should be given to the proven benefits and potential toxicities of vitamin megadosing prior to recommending increasing dosages of vitamins and minerals beyond the recommended daily allowances.

Trace Elements

Zinc deficiency has been linked to several abnormalities, including anorexia, taste abnormalities, T-cell dysfunction, macular degeneration, and poor wound healing in elderly persons.[4] Zinc intake by most elderly individuals fails to meet the RDA of 12 mg (see Table 5.3). Individuals at risk for developing borderline zinc status include those who have diabetes mellitus, those taking diuretics, and those abusing alcohol. Zinc malabsorption occurs more commonly in elderly people.

Zinc is necessary for normal T-cell function. Deficiency has been associated with anergy, and zinc levels have been correlated with postimmunization antibody titers to influenza vaccine.[4] Zinc replacement has also been shown to improve mitogen responsiveness in patients with type II diabetes mellitus.[4] An association of zinc deficiency with anorexia has been demonstrated in animal studies. Although zinc replacement does not reverse the taste abnormalities seen with aging, studies have shown that zinc deficiency interferes with the opioid feeding drive and that the opioid feeding drive diminishes with advancing age.[4] Zinc also appears to play a role in the resolution of peripheral vascular ulcers and may slow the rate of vision loss associated with macular degeneration.[4] Previously, zinc deficiency was thought to play a role in the hyperglycemia of aging, but current evidence fails to support any such relationship.

Chromium has also been purported to play a role in the hyperglycemia of aging, because chromium levels decline with age and chromium deficiency in rats is associated with hyperglycemia, hypercholesterolemia, and corneal opacities.[4] However, the role of chromium in aging and hyperglycemia remains controversial.

Selenium deficiency has been linked to certain diseases commonly encountered in the aging population, including cancer, coronary artery disease, and immune dysfunction.[4] Selenium concentrations have also been found to decline with advancing age. A potential role of selenium in the pathogenesis of cancer comes from studies reporting a higher prevalence of cancer in areas with lower concentrations of selenium in forage crops.[4] Animal studies have shown that diets high in selenium prevent the development of cancer.[4] Furthermore, selenium and vitamin E have been shown to reduce radiation damage in irradiated cells.[4] While a role for selenium in the development of cardiovascular disease has been suggested, evidence for such a relationship is sparse. Suppressed cellular and humoral immunity may be related to selenium deficiency, since in animals selenium deficiency has been associated with an inadequate immune response to candidiasis.[4] However, studies of the role of selenium deficiency in immune function in the elderly have not been carried out.

The recommended daily intake of selenium is 50 to 200 μg (see Table 5.3). Selenium toxicity has been reported with intake above 350 to 700 μg/day and can be identified by the presence of a garlic odor on the breath, peripheral neuropathy, and fingernail changes.[4]

Iron deficiency is the most common cause of nutritional anemia in the elderly. Although blood loss from menstruation ceases to be a source of iron-deficiency anemia in elderly women, blood loss form other sources is the most common cause of iron deficiency in the geriatric population.[23] Major causes of blood loss include duodenal ulcers, hemorrhoids and postmenopausal bleeding. More subtle, chronic blood loss may also arise from colonic (especially caecal) carcinoma, chronic aspirin ingestion, diverticuli, and internal hemorrhoids. In a healthy elderly individual, adequate iron is usually available for red blood cell production. However, nutritional factors can lead to or exacerbate iron deficiency in the elderly. Elderly patients tend to consume diets that do not contain the 10 mg per day of iron necessary to absorb the 1 mg needed daily.[23] Furthermore, iron absorption may be compromised in the aged from excessive tea consumption, deficient vitamin C intake,[24] and achlorhydria that inhibits absorption of the ferric form of iron.[23] Thus, in addition to early identification of sources of blood loss as a cause of iron deficiency anemia, it is imperative to ensure that intake of iron is at least 10 mg per day and absorption is optimized (see Table 5.3).

Calcium and Vitamin D

Osteoporosis is one of the more common problems of aging. Estrogen replacement therapy is currently the mainstay of prevention of postmenopausal osteoporosis. However, calcium supplementation, either alone or in conjunction with estrogen replacement therapy, may also be important. To achieve a positive calcium balance, women on estrogen replacement therapy need 1,000 to 1,500 mg/day of calcium.[25] The average woman consumes 500 mg/day of dietary calcium. Dairy foods represent the major dietary source of calcium, so intakes above this level require either substantial ingestion of milk (1,200 mg calcium per quart) or milk products, or calcium supplements.

One of the barriers to adequate calcium dietary intake is lactose intolerance. The intestinal enzyme lactase breaks lactose into its component monosaccharides, glucose and galactose. With lactase deficiency, this does not occur and the disaccharides and other metabolites cause flatulence, cramping, and diarrhea, eventually leading to avoidance of calcium-rich dairy products. Rather than eliminating dairy products from the diet, however, decreasing lactose-containing foods by 20% to 30% can lessen symptoms of lactose intolerance.[5] Although milk contains substantial amounts of lactose, a number of other dairy products (eg, yogurt, cottage cheese, most cheeses) do not. Since calcium supplementation is not without side effects, optimizing calcium intake with diet is preferable.

It is generally believed that calcium supplementation alone probably cannot substitute completely for estrogen replacement therapy in preventing osteoporosis. Calcium is not very well absorbed and has little effect on trabecular bone. However, a recent study of a group of healthy, ambulatory postmenopausal women found that supplementation with calcium and vitamin D_3 reduced the risk of hip fracture by 43% and of other nonvertebral fractures by 32%.[26] While this reduction in fracture rate is less than that seen with estrogen replacement therapy, it is substantial, highlighting the importance of calcium supplementation in the elderly female.

In women who are hesitant to initiate hormone replacement therapy, who already have osteoporosis, or who have contraindications to estrogen replacement therapy, assessment of osteoporosis risk may be useful in guiding therapeutic decisions. Certain demographic characteristics correlate with increased risk of osteoporosis: a family history of the condition, smoking, and slim body build (obese women have less risk for osteoporosis, probably because of estrone production by aromatization of adrenal androgens in adipose tissue). Biochemically, calcium status can be assessed by measuring serum calcium, phosphate, alkaline phosphatase, and serum albumin. The urinary calcium–creatinine ratio following an overnight fast is a good index of the rate of bone resorption.[12] Bone densitometry studies have also been utilized to identify women at unusual risk of developing osteoporosis and who are therefore more likely to benefit from estrogen therapy and calcium supplementation. Estimation of calcium absorption from 24-hour urinary calcium excretion may provide useful information by allowing identification of individuals who may require vitamin D supplementation.[12] Calcium excretion studies may also allow identification of hypercalciuria, a condition that would be exacerbated by aggressive calcium–vitamin D supplementation.[12]

Nutritional Abuses

Alcohol abuse affects 1% to 10% of the elderly and is a frequently overlooked problem in the geriatric population.[27] Age-related changes may compound the elderly person's risk for nutritional complications of chronic alcohol use. Due to alterations in body composition, which alter the distribution of alcohol in the body, higher peak blood levels of alcohol are achieved in an older person, when compared with a younger person for a given amount of alcohol intake.[28] This places the person at risk for profound cognitive and physical impairment that can have significant long-term impact on nutritional status. Alcohol use is generally associated with low intake of vitamins and minerals, further compromising what is frequently a nutritionally inadequate diet. The more common vitamin deficiencies encountered in an alcoholic are thiamine and niacin deficiency, which present with peripheral neuropathy. Osteoporosis is also a complication of chronic alcohol abuse due to the inhibitory effect of alcohol on osteoblast proliferation and synthesis of bone matrix.[12] Alcohol abuse can also affect drug–nutrient interactions.[28] Although the incidence of physical and social problems related to alcohol use declines with age,[27] alcohol abuse remains a significant source of morbidity among the elderly and should be considered early on as a source of nutritional deficiency in this population.

Oral vitamin and mineral supplements are commonly taken by the elderly, with or without physician advice. Given the low risk of vitamin supplementation at RDA levels and the appreciable incidence of micronutrient deficiency in the older person whose nutritional status is marginal, a rationale exists for such therapy. On the other hand, with the prevalent beliefs regarding the beneficial effects of megadoses of vitamins, vitamin abuse and overload may be greater problems than inadequacy among the elderly in this country. Toxic effects from vitamins A, D, E, and C, niacin, and B-complex vitamins have been reported. Reports of the protective effect of vitamin A against lung cancer have led to some overdosing, resulting in toxic effects such as anorexia, dryness of the skin, resorption of calcium from bone with consequent hypercalcemia, and increased intracranial pressure.[4] This tendency to overdose via behavioral means may be exacerbated by the physiological changes of aging, such as decreased clearance of vitamin A,[29] which can increase vitamin A stores in the elderly. Excessive ingestion of vitamin D following reports that vitamin D at 5 to 10 times the RDA builds stronger bones has led to nausea, headache, decreased appetite, fatigue, interference with vitamin K absorption, and soft tissue calcium deposits.[4] Despite the lack of information on its role in human nutrition, vitamin E has been ingested in excessive amounts due to claims that it improves sexual performance and prevents cardiovascular disease and cancer.[4] Vitamin E toxicity, although rare, may result in thrombophlebitis, decreased wound healing, and gastrointestinal distress and may also interfere with vitamin K metabolism.[4]

While toxicity from excessive ingestion of water soluble vitamins is rare, harmful effects have been reported. Large doses of vitamin C can cause diarrhea, urinary oxalate stones, and malabsorption of vitamin B_{12}. Megadoses of vitamin C can also cause diarrhea, urinary oxalate stones, and malabsorption of vitamin B_{12}. Megadoses of vitamin C can also cause false-negative Hemoccult® results and can interfere with the measurement of urinary glucose and certain laboratory tests that require an autoanalyzer.[4] Megadoses of thiamine and niacin have caused liver damage and worsening of peptic ulcers. Vitamin B_6 megadosing has also caused nervous system and liver damage.

Screening

Various screening modalities have been proposed to identify patients at risk for undernutrition. These include diet histories, food records, anthropometric measures such as skinfold thickness, BMI, and biochemical markers. However, none has been validated as a good screening tool for use in the general elderly population.[30] Nevertheless, it is imperative that the practitioner make an attempt to assess nutritional status through history of food intake, periodic measurement of weight and height, evaluation of loss of subcutaneous fat, muscle wasting, edema and ascites, and possibly measurement of cholesterol, complete blood count, and albumin. For women at higher risk for osteoporosis, or for women who are not responding to traditional osteoporosis preventive measures, evaluation of calcium balance may also be useful.

Summary

Assessment of nutritional status and dietary advice based on that assessment represent important parts of primary health care. Factors of particular importance in aging women include the decline in energy needs, which must be accompanied by decreased caloric intake if obesity is to be prevented, and bone loss due to estrogen deficiency. Weight should be maintained in the normal range and dietary advise should follow the guidelines provided by the RDA. Regular exercise helps in weight regulation and has other physical and psychological benefits. Multivitamin supplements may be helpful in assuring adequate intakes, but megadoses should be avoided. A nutritional program should take into account the psychosocial situation of the geriatric patient as well as her own individual concerns.

References

1. Hazzard WR, Burton JR: Health problems of the elderly, in Martin JB, Fauci AS (eds.): *Harrison's Principles of Internal Medicine,* ed. 11. New York, McGraw Hill, 1987, pp. 450–554.
2. Rudman D, Cohan ME: Nutrition in the elderly, in Calkins E, Ford AM, Katz PR (eds.): *Practice of Geriatrics.* ed. 2. Philadelphia, WB Saunders, 1992, pp. 19–32.
3. Fukagawa NK, Young VR: *Protein and Amino Acid Metabolism and Requirements in Older Persons.* Clinics in Geriatric Medicine, Vol. 3. 1987, pp. 329–341.
4. Morley JE, Mooradian AD, Silver AJ, Heber D, Alfin-Slater RB: Nutrition in the elderly. *Ann Intern Med* 1988;109:890–904.
5. Bidlack WR: Nutritional requirements of the elderly, in Morley JE, Glick Z, Rubenstien LZ (eds.): *Geriatric Nutrition, A Comprehensive Review.* New York, Raven Press, 1990, pp. 41–72.
6. Bierman EL: Disorders of the Vascular System, in Martin JB, Fauci AS (eds.): *Harrison's Principles of Internal Medicine,* ed. 11. New York, McGraw Hill, 1987, pp. 1014–1024.
7. Asp NG: Nutritional classification and analysis of food carbohydrate. *Am J Clin Nutr* 1994;59(suppl):679S–681S.
8. National Research Council: *Recommended Dietary Allowances,* ed. 10. Washington, DC, National Academy Press, 1989, pp. 24–38.
9. Lipschitz DA, Chernoff R: Gastrointestinal metabolic and endocrine diseases, in Schrier RW, ed.: *Geriatric Medicine,* ed. 1. Philadelphia, WB Saunders, 1990, pp. 424–433.
10. Rudman D, Racette D, Rudman IW, Mattson DE, Erve PR: Hyponatremia in tube-fed elderly men. *J Chronic Dis* 1986;39(2):73–80.
11. Baylink DJ: Osteomalacia, in Hazzard WR, Andres R, Bierman EL, Blass JP (eds.): *Principles of Geriatric Medicine and Gerontology,* ed. 2, New York, McGraw-Hill, 1990, p. 826.
12. Jennings J, Perkel V, Baylink DJ: Osteoporosis, in Calkins E, Ford AM, Katz PR (eds.): *Practice of Geriatrics,* ed. 2, Philadelphia, WB Saunders, 1992, pp. 363–377.
13. Chan SDH, Chiu DKH, Atkins D: Oophorectomy leads to a selective decrease in 1,25-dihydroxycholecalciferol receptors in rat jejunal villous cells. *Clin Sci (Colch)* 1984;66:745–748.

14. Nordin BEC, Need AG, Morris HA, Horowitz M, Robertson WG: Evidence for a renal calcium leak in postmenopausal women. *J Clin Endocrinol Metab* 1991;72:401–407.
15. Brocklehurst JC, Griffiths LL, Taylor GF, Marks J, Scott DL, Blackley J: The clinical features of chronic vitamin deficiency. A therapeutic trial in geriatric hospital patients. *Gerontol Clin* 1968;10:309–320.
16. Hansen-Smith FM, Picou D, Golden MH: Growth of muscle fibres during recovery from severe malnutrition in Jamacian infants. *British J Nutr* 1979;41:275–282.
17. Fiatrone MA, O'Neill EF, Ryan ND, Clements KM, Solares GR, Nelson ME, Roberts SB, Kehayias JJ, Lipsitz LA, Evans WJ: Exercise training and nutritional supplementation for physical frailty in very elderly people. *New Engl J Med* 1994;330:1769–1775.
18. Ulbricht TLV, Southgate DAT: Coronary heart disease: Seven dietary factors. *Lancet* 1991;338:985–992.
19. Enstrom JE, Kanim, LE, Klein MA: Vitamin C intake and mortality among a sample of the United States population. *Epidemiology* 1992;3:194–202.
20. Stampfer MJ, Hennekens CH, Manson JE, Colditz GA, Rosner B, Willett WC: Vitamin E consumption and the risk of coronary disease in women. *N Engl J Med,* 1993;328:1444–1449.
21. Gaziano JM, Manson JE, Ridker PM, Buring JE, Hennekens CH: Beta carotene therapy for chronic stable angina. *Circulation* 1990;82(4)(suppl III):201 (Abstract).
22. Meydani SN, Barklund MP, Liu S, Meydani M, Miller RA, Cannon JG, Morrow FD, Rocklin R, Blumberg JB: Vitamin E supplementation enhances cell-mediated immunity in healthy elderly subjects. *Am J Clin Nutr* 1990;52:557–563.
23. Seligman PA: Hematologic and oncologic problems, in Schrier RW (ed.): *Geriatric Medicine.* Philadelphia, WB Saunders, 1990, pp. 399–416.
24. Roe DA: Nutritional deficiencies, in *Geriatric Nutrition,* ed. 3. Englewood Cliffs, NJ, Prentice-Hall, 1992, pp. 147–165.
25. Speroff L, Glass RH, Kass NG: *Clinical Gynecologic Endocrinology and Infertility,* ed. 4. Williams and Wilkins, 1989, pp. 121–164.
26. Chapuy MC, Arlot ME, Duboeuf F, Brun J, Crouzet B, Arnaud S, Delmas PD, Neunier PJ: Vitamin D_3 and calcium to prevent hip fractures in elderly women. *N Engl J Med* 1992;327:1637–1642.
27. Steiner JF, Kauvar AJ: Preventive medicine, in Schrier RW (ed.): *Geriatric Medicine.* Philadelphia, WB Saunders, 1990, pp. 32–45.
28. Roe DA: Drugs and nutrition in the elderly, in *Geriatric Nutrition,* ed. 3. Englewood Cliffs, NJ, Prentice-Hall, 1992, pp. 182–207.
29. Krasinski SD, Cohn JS, Schaefer EJ, Russell RM: Postprandial plasma retinyl ester response is greater in older subjects compared with younger subjects. *J Clin Invest* 1990;85:883–892.
30. Reuben DB, Greendale GA, Harrison GG: Nutrition screening in elderly persons: A review of current instruments and directions for future research. *J Am Geriatr Soc,* accepted for publication.

Chapter 6

Exercise and Aging: Physical Fitness

M. Elaine Cress, PhD and Felicity A. Green, OT

Traditionally we think of a woman's life in three phases—virgin, mother, and wise woman. In the virgin phase, a young woman is like a young plant, full of potential. In motherhood, she is in a period of flowering and producing. In the last phase, she is like fine aged wine, as this is a time when a woman can harvest wisdom from her experiences. Our youth-oriented society offers a whole host of products and attitudes to avoid even the appearance of age or aging and, more importantly, the work and wonder in the years beyond 50.

In this chapter we address an approach to the practice of exercise as it relates to health issues for the older woman. We discuss the benefits of exercise and how women can get started in various types of programs as well as integrating several types of exercise and relaxation techniques into a program. We define physical reserve as the energy over and above the energy needed to complete the required daily activities. This energy can be termed *discretionary energy*. In the later years, remaining independent requires not only ample strength and endurance to manage the demands of one's home, but having enough energy over and above the minimum for home maintenance (functional demand) to enjoy recreational and social interests.

As a mother, a woman's desires are often secondary to the family's needs. The postmenopausal years are a time when the concerns of raising her family are behind her, giving her time to reflect on her life experiences. This time may be a woman's first opportunity to experience herself as an individual separate from her children and husband. The postmenopausal years are a time of reflection and a time of challenge, often a physical challenge. The physical challenge begins as hot flashes and emotional fluctuations that may be reminiscent of adolescence. The following two decades, between 50 and 70 years of age, are a time of gradual but constant loss of bone, muscle mass, and muscle strength. The gift of youth, our physical fitness, must now be tended to daily, if it is to be maintained. The choices a woman makes about exercise, nutrition, and hormone replacement therapy will impact her quality of life for the remaining years. Women can use the postmenopausal years to harvest wisdom, weeding out the dictates of society and the habitual thinking that may have been important for the work of her earlier years but which no longer serve her.

So, how does a woman best approach a sweeping re-evaluation of her exercise and health needs in her menopausal and postmenopausal years? With the passing of the generous blessings of youth, the skin is less supple, strength begins to wane, and endurance abates. In general, muscles in all systems change similarly; as the legs get weaker, so does the upper body, the bladder control muscles, and the cardiovascular system. Most of the health issues for the older woman are chronic, resulting in a slow, insidious decline of the physical reserve. Without attention to maintaining physical capacity, soon one will notice that routine activities, such as the laundry or grocery shopping, use the day's energy reserve. An older deconditioned person must allocate the energy carefully, planning only one major activity a day. The thought of adding exercise to a day when there is barely enough energy to cover the necessities seems absurd! The important information to understand, however, is that by investing energy into an exercise program the returns are great. The investment comes back in the form of increased energy reserve and, therefore, decreased fatigue, decreased effort at routine activities, and increased discretionary time and energy to enjoy life. Conveying the benefits of exercise is a key factor in getting a person to start and sustain a regular exercise program. The best time to begin exercise training is before functional capacity deteriorates to the level that is required to meet the functional demands of daily life. The woman who invests time and energy in an exercise program, now, will receive returns in functional energy reserves for discretionary and social needs.

Taking Care of Herself

In evaluating a health and fitness plan for the second half of life, a woman should think about life holistically. As life's demands press into the schedule, she should maintain the commitment to a regimen of exercise, healthy eating, and relaxation. The woman in her fifties may find herself sandwiched between the demands of a career, teenagers, and aging parents. She must reinvest some of that energy in herself to meet sustained demands. For the older woman in her seventies, normal household activities take longer, minimizing the energy and time to exercise. Feeling overwhelmed, she may think that she could never meet all her obligations and exercise, as well. To maintain a discretionary energy reserve she, too, must reinvest some energy in her exercise to preserve her quality of life. Ultimately, the commitment is to oneself, recognizing that exercise is not an optional activity; it carries the same mandate for health as sleeping and eating, albeit the consequences of neglect are not as immediate. No one can exercise for another; the benefit comes from making the effort oneself. Johann Wolfgang Von Goethe wisely and eloquently stated the universal truth about making a commitment:

> Until one is committed, there is hesitancy, the chance to draw back, always ineffectiveness, concerning all acts of initiative (and creation). There is one elementary truth the ignorance of which kills countless ideas and splendid plans: that the moment one definitely commits oneself, then Providence moves too. All sorts of things occur to help one that would never otherwise have occurred. A whole stream of events issues from the decision, raising in one's favor all manner of unforeseen incidents and meetings and material assistance which no man could have dreamed would have come his way. Whatever you can do or dream you can, begin it. Boldness has genius, power and magic in it. Begin it now.

Benefits of Regular Exercise Training

Exercise training is the regular practice of physical exercise that is outside that level required for routine functioning and social activity. Physical activity, on the other hand, is the act of moving about while engaging in one's normal pattern of activity as dictated by social roles. From an epidemiological perspective, the most sedentary people (in the lowest quintile) of the population for physical activity have an increased risk of death from all causes. In other words, low physical activity is an independent risk factor for increased mortality. The exercise response is systemic, with marked benefits in several systems—musculoskeletal, cardiovascular, neuromuscular, immune, neuroendocrine—as well as mental and emotional well-being. In many cases, the ultimate outcome is in improved function and quality of life. Exercise benefits may be manifested in a number of ways, depending on the health status. Exercise benefits are expressed in relationship to the disease (physiological) or to the individual (symptom relief, functional improvement). Exercise may stop or reverse the progression of a disease or process, reduce symptoms with no change in the disease, or improve function with no change in the disease. Because the benefits can be approached from different perspectives, confusion exists in the literature and popular press about the efficacy of exercise. The loss of muscle mass and stamina with aging can be reduced or reversed, depending on the intensity of the exercise prescription. In conjunction with diet, exercise can halt the progression of adult-onset diabetes and obesity. In diseases such as emphysema and chronic obstructive pulmonary disease (COPD), although pulmonary function tests are not altered, with physical training symptoms of dyspnea and fatigue are ameliorated and functional ability is increased. In rheumatoid arthritis and osteoarthritis, improvement in pain-free function has been demonstrated. Compliance and, therefore, efficacy are often dependent on the level of instruction in techniques and expected benefits. Research on exercise efficacy, as seen through improved function, decreased symptoms, and reversed disease processes has been compiled into Table 6.1. (+ indicates the form of exercise recommended for a given disease or physical condition). Endurance training is categorized as weight-bearing walking, jogging, stair-climbing, cross-country skiing, aerobic dance, and non–weight-bearing swimming, rowing, and upper and lower body cycle ergometers. Resistance training is divided into low intensity (12 to 15 repetitions set at 40% to 60% of 1 repetition maximum (1 RM)[1] and high intensity (8 to 12 repetitions at 70% to 85% of 1 RM). Balance training includes static and dynamic exercises, including semitandem and tandem walking, balance beams, and posture training. Integrated exercise includes disciplines that integrate several modes of exercise training and require the individual to integrate the mind and body in the performance of the exercise. Hatha yoga integrates strength, flexibility, balance training, weight-bearing exercise, education, and relaxation. Tai chi chuan integrates balance, weight-bearing exercise, and relaxation. In these instances, weight-bearing exercise is included for bone health, rather than as an endurance training mode for cardiovascular health. The column headed "Instruction and Education" is included to indicate those programs in which compliance is particularly dependent on proper instruction. For example, instruction in: proper technique as in pelvic muscle training, balancing symptoms of pain and exercise load in arthritis patients, the rationale and expected benefits of exercise to improve compliance, and resistance-training technique to reduce injury. Diseases or conditions included in Table 6.1 are those most commonly reported by elderly women. Cancer, an important disease of aging, is not listed because of insufficient research into the benefits of exercise in cancer patients.

Endurance Training

Importance of Endurance Training

The Fick equation defines cardiovascular endurance as the product of cardiac output (heart rate * stroke volume) and oxygen extraction at the muscle. Cardiovascular endurance decreases with age at a rate of approximately one milliliter of oxygen per kilogram of body weight measured for one minute (VO_2ml/kg×min) each year. Between the ages of 50 and 80 the average loss in VO_2max may be between 25 and 35 ml/kg×min. Maximum heart rate decreases with age at an average rate of one beat per year. As this loss is relatively free of the influences of physical training, there is an expected age-related drop in maximal cardiac output because of the lower maximal heart rate. Muscle mass decreases with age, even in those who remain very active throughout life, but much

---

[1] 1 RM is the maximum amount of weight that can be lifted through one full repetition with good form. 1 RM can be estimated from a 4 RM, or the maximum amount of weight that can be lifted through four repetitions with good form.

Table 6.1 Recommended Exercise for Specific Health Issues

Health issue	Endurance training		Resistance training			Integrated exercise				
	Weight-bearing	Non–weight bearing	Low intensity	High Intensity	Muscle specific	Balance training	Range of motion	Hatha yoga	Tai chi chuan	Instruction and education
Osteoporosis	+			Back muscles		+				+
Arthritis	+	+	+				+	+	+	+
Falls	+			+	Ankle	+		+	+	+
Hypertension		+	+					+	+	
Coronary artery disease	+									
Peripheral vascular disease		+					+	+	+	+
Diabetes	+									
COPD or Emphysema	+		+		Breathing exercises		+	+		+
Depression	+		+	+				+		
Sleep disorders	+						+	+		+
Immune system function	+									
Obesity	+		+	+						
Incontinence	+				Pelvic muscle					+
Muscle mass	+			+				+		
Stamina	+		+							

+, Recommended form of exercise; *COPD*, chronic obstructive pulmonary disease.

more markedly in the sedentary. Disuse has a greater effect on stroke volume than on peripheral extraction of oxygen; therefore, the decrease in VO_2max with aging are synergistic as the losses in maximum heart rate (aging), stroke volume (disuse), and muscle mass are multiplied. The Fick equation provides an objective explanation of the rapid loss in fitness that seems disproportional to the time of inactivity. We all have heard an older family member who had gone on a cruise for a few weeks and then is shocked at the sudden decline in fitness, often explaining it away as overeating. The good news is that the turnaround can be almost as striking. Stroke volume is very responsive to physical training, as in the peripheral musculature. These training adaptations are multiplied together to give a relatively rapid augmentation of fitness. In addition, these benefits have not been shown to be limited by age.

Getting Started on Endurance Training

Endurance training is defined as the rhythmic contraction of large muscle groups at a specified heart rate for a specified duration. Endurance training can be either weight-bearing or non–weight-bearing. Weight-bearing exercise, most often in endurance-type activities, can have beneficial effects on bone mass in the lower lumbar and leg bone regions. On the other hand, weight-bearing exercises may exacerbate certain musculoskeletal problems of the lower body, hip, knee, and ankle. The type of exercise recommended for endurance training is dependent on preferences and capabilities of the individual doing the exercise. What is she capable of doing? What does she prefer or enjoy doing for exercise? Are there musculoskeletal limitations—eg, arthritic knee or range-of-motion limitations of the shoulder—to be considered? Convenience, time, and financial considerations are the most often cited barriers to initiating an exercise program. Consulting with a certified exercise professional* can optimize compliance, safety, and exercise efficacy. The fitness professional will program progression of duration and intensity to optimize balance between safety and improvement and will instruct the client on appropriate methods of monitoring exercise intensity. This exercise professional gives the client a resource for updating the program and for encouragement as well. Exercise is behavior, and behavior is hard to change!

Benefits of Endurance Training

Endurance training improves cardiovascular conditioning as measured by VO_2max. Training studies indicate that regardless of age, cardiovascular endurance can be improved. The improvement ranges from 10% to 30%, depending on the intensity of training (the target heart rate during training) and the mode of training (eg, involving more muscle groups, such as in cross-country skiing, is a more intense training stimulus). The minimum recommendations for endurance training from the American College of Sports Medicine are to get 30 minutes cumulative exercise per day, on at least 3 days each week. This bare minimum of exercise can help to get someone out of the lowest quintile of the population where most of the ill effects of inactivity are seen. This recommendation does not take into account the time needed to strength train, balance train, or any of the other forms of activity necessary to maintain proper function. The most salient benefits of exercise are manifest in submaximal work. Work physiologists expect that healthy young individuals can perform physical work at 50% of their maximal capacity for 8 hours with appropriate rest breaks.

---

*American College of Sports Medicine Fitness Instructor, American Council on Exercise (ACE) certified personal trainer, Aerobics Fitness Association of America, National Strength and Conditioning Association.

Reduced symptoms of fatigue are the principal benefits of exercise training on submaximal work. By comparing the same workload before and after training, one can see reduced heart rate, reduced ventilatory frequency, lower rate of perceived exertion, and lower systolic blood pressure. It then follows that for any given submaximal heart rate a person can do more work after training. As stated earlier, maximal heart rate is a product of age rather than training. Resting heart rate, however, is lowered by endurance training. An example of how endurance training improves the ability to perform work submaximally can be simply illustrated by the benefit of a lower resting heart rate with training. For a 75-year-old woman the estimated maximal heart rate is 145 beats per minute (220–75). Her pretraining resting heart rate is 80 beats/min. Before training, walking up one flight of stairs increases heart rate by 30 beats/min. The working heart rate is then 110 beats/min (80 resting heart rate +30). This is 75% of her maximal heart rate (110/145). After training, her resting heart rate is reduced to 60 beats/min and her weight is still the same as before training. Climbing the same set of stairs, her heart rate is increased only 25 beats/min. The working heart rate is now 85 beat/min (60 resting heart rate +25). The posttraining working heart rate is approximately 60% of her maximal heart rate (85/145). The working heart rate is lower for two reasons. First, the resting heart rate is lower and, second, because endurance training increases the stroke volume of each beat, the beating frequency can be lower to accomplish the same cardiac output. Therefore, with endurance training the same work output has gone from 75% to less than 60% of maximal heart rate. Perceived exertion at 75% of maximum is "hard" on the Borg Rate of Perceived Exertion scale, whereas 60% is considered to be "somewhat hard." The overall result is reduction in symptoms of fatigue, shortness of breath, and, possibly, muscle soreness. This is not the only mechanism for reduced symptoms of fatigue with endurance training, but it is one that can be easily demonstrated and understood by the patient.

Resistance Training

Importance of Resistance Training

The relationship between strength and the cross-sectional area of the muscle is well documented. The muscle itself is comprised of two general types of muscle fiber, slow twitch and fast twitch. Fast-twitch muscle fibers are designed for rapid and powerful movements; for instance, a fast-pitch throw or bench-pressing a multiple of one's body weight. Humans have a mix of these muscle fibers at birth that is a reflection of the genetic inheritance. This is really of importance only to the performance of the elite athlete in either endurance or power sport. For the population in general, how these muscle fibers contribute to our daily life is a result of our patterns of regular activity. Infants and young children have a cross-sectional area of the fast-twitch fiber that is 1.5 times that of the slow twitch. With age, the cross-sectional area of the slow-twitch fiber remains relatively stable, yet the fast-twitch fiber area declines consistently; in the twenties, fifties, and seventies the ratios shift from 1.0, to 0.85, to 0.7. A more detailed review of structure and function of muscle is detailed in Cress and Schultz. Cress and colleagues (1991) showed nearly a 26% decrease in the fast-twitch fiber was seen in a 1-year study of older women who did not participate in regular exercise as compared with a 29% gain in women who participated in a program that combined aerobic and strength training. Despite the decline in the fast-twitch fibers and strength, the aerobic fitness was maintained; these data indicate that in these women strength was more likely to be lost than aerobic capacity. This may indicate that in a sedentary life style, strength losses precede losses in cardiovascular fitness. The common explanation for the preservation of the slow-twitch fiber with age is that we all engage in endurance activity as a matter of course in our activities of daily living. The activities that preserve fast-twitch muscle, however, are dependent on motivation—the motivation to move quickly, to life more, and generally to elicit a perceived exertion in the range of hard to very hard. Therefore, the loss of fast-twitch fiber and hence muscle strength is directly influenced by the choice to remain sedentary or to work at low intensities. In the past the choice may have been made, in part, out of fear of injury, undue stress to the heart, or the belief that weight-lifting would create unsightly bulky arm muscle. These myths and excuses have been debunked, as weight-lifting is now prescribed successfully for cardiac patients and 90-year-olds.

Getting Started on Resistance Training

How does a woman, particularly an older woman, unfamiliar with the weight-room environment get started lifting weights? First, she should make the commitment to resistance-train for at least 3 months. This is enough time to overcome barriers of insufficient time and inconvenience. In 3 months one can expect to experience the results in improved body habitus, strength, and awareness of improved ease of functioning in most activities. Again, commitment to making a life-style change is the key to success. "Whatever you can do or dream you can, begin it. Boldness has genius, power and magic in it. Begin it now." (Goethe)

Many women of various sizes and shapes are in the gym lifting weights. Programs are available for women experiencing weight-lifting for the first time. With programs such as "Women on Weights," called WOW, the weight-room is exclusively for women, and trainers are available to answer questions and assist with programming. In the absence of such program that are free with the membership, one may need to employ a certified personal trainer, preferably a woman. This may cost around $200 ($25 to $35 per session). One can consider hiring a personal trainer in conjunction with a trainer partner, saving some money and gaining a workout buddy. The personal trainer will set up the program based on the desired goals and past experience of the individual. Six to 8 weeks (2 training sessions per week) should ensure adequate instruction on form and setting up the equipment. Follow-up sessions at 1 month, 6 weeks, and then every 3 months will reduce the cost, ensure adherence to good form, and provide means of updating the program so as to avoid boredom with the regimen. The personal trainer will provide an entry for the client who may otherwise feel uncomfortable in this atmosphere by being a model of good form, teaching weight-room etiquette, and providing a resource for questions about the program and concern over injury.

Benefits of Resistance Training

Resistance training increases both the maximal weight one can lift and the ability to sustain the submaximal contraction. For example, a person that can lift a maximum of 25 pounds through one full repetition (1 RM), is not able to sustain that contraction for longer than the time it takes to move the weight through the full range of motion (3 to 4 seconds). With progressive resistance training, the 1 RM can be increased to 50 pounds, and the length of time a person can hold 25 pounds is lengthened. In general, within injury-free boundaries, there is a dose-response effect with strength training; higher intensity training (75% to 85% of 1 RM) evokes greater gains in muscle strength and hypertrophy. The immediate benefits of resistance training include increased recruitment of muscle fibers in performance of the task one has trained toward. Long-term benefits include increased muscle mass, increased energy consumption at rest, improved functional strength, and decreased perceived effort when lifting the same amount of weight after training compared with before training. In addition, strength training has been found to be efficacious in addressing depressive symptoms. Training specific muscle groups to improve strength is necessary for certain diseases, for example, pelvic muscles for incontinence, diaphragmatic and chest wall muscles for COPD and emphysema patients, and ankle muscles for balance problems. Low-intensity resistance training may be used as an entry exercise before introducing progression to weight-bearing, endurance training, or high-intensity training.

Posture and Balance Training

Importance of Posture and Balance Training

Posture is our signature. Someone approaching from a distance can be identified long before you actually see the details of the face. Many older women have straight backs and good posture. The classic pathological posture of an old woman is flexion at the ankle, knees, hips, and elbows, a flattened lumbar region and dorsal kyphosis. In part, this posture is a consequence of a lifetime movement pattern in which most of the time is spent with the forward body in flexion. When sitting flexor muscles of the lower body are at approximately 90 degrees. During periods of activity the flexor muscles are again engaged, when lifting or carrying something with the arms, the elbows and shoulders in flexion. In walking and climbing stairs the ankles, knees, and hips are primarily in flexion.

Everyone is taller in the morning when they get out of bed than in the evening after gravity compresses the vertebral disks with upright posture. Spinal degeneration is a narrowing of vertebral disk space, formation of osteophytes, and sclerosis of the vertebral end plates. Scoliosis is the most prevalent spinal abnormality in the older population and contributes to increased postural sway. A flexible and properly aligned axial spine surrounded by well-toned muscles can be the first line of defense against balance problems in aging. Senile disequilibrium is associated with loss of mechanoreceptors (type I and type II) of the spinal apophyseal joints. The loss was of mechanoreceptors due to inflammation, injury, and abnormal mechanical stresses (poor posture and lifting habits) are related to decreased disk space. Type I mechanoreceptors are instrumental to static posture, and type II receptors found deeper in the capsule integrate with type I to produce fluid, phasic movement. Going to bed takes the compressive stress off the bones and joints, but it does not actually counteract the compressive effect. One can actively stretch the spine, release the hips and shoulders, and maintain space for the nerves, muscles, and blood vessels. Lower back pain is often a result of an imbalance between the strength of the muscles and the tightness of the attachments on the front and back of the pelvis. In a standing posture, a weak iliopsoas muscle and shortened hamstrings result in a flat lower back, lacking the normal lower lumbar curve. Sit-ups can strengthen the abdominal muscles, most particularly the rectus abdomonis, and not strengthen the iliopsoas. Lower back pain can also result from the shortening of the hip flexor muscle, pulling the anterior pelvis forward and down and creating a strain on the L1–L5 region of the vertebrae. Balance of strength and flexibility between the muscles of the upper and lower back region is a general prescription for good back health. In dorsal kyphosis foreshortened pectoralis muscles from moving the sternum bone down and posteriorly results in stiffness across the chest. The tissue between the head of the humerus and the pectoralis major results in a protruding clavicle and concave shoulder chest area. Consequently, the scapula becomes abducted, overstretching the rhomboid muscles. The rhomboid muscles then have overstretch weakness, as the muscle contractile proteins do not overlap optimally for strength. In the kyphotic posture, the center of gravity is moved forward, making the anterior–posterior posture more unstable. The elbows tend to flex and often extend posteriorly to act as a compensatory counterbalance. To lift something or move the arm forward means the person must rely on plantarflexor strength to maintain her balance. These muscles also are often weak. A woman with this posture has very limited range of sway, putting her at increased risk for falling. The seeds of this classic dowager's posture can be seen in many teenage girls. A conscious effort is required to correct this posture. The posture can be partially corrected by actively strengthening the rhomboid muscles through a rowing resistance exercise. Corrective action can be accelerated by increasing the flexibility across the front of the chest. Additional treatment includes lying in a prone position on a hard surface such as a floor and slightly supporting the head so that the chin is perpendicular to the floor, working actively to adduct the scapula, and moving the humerus bone to the floor. Placing light sandbags on each arm will help to lengthen the pectoralis muscles. This prone position will also increase the flexibility of the connective tissue between the ribs. The ribs are like bucket handles that become tightly woven together when a person is always in kyphotic posture. This corrective action is anatomically beneficial for lung function. The neck is another area that needs corrective action in a person with a kyphotic posture. The muscles on the back of the neck are shortened and the muscles on the front of the neck are weak. The lifting of the sternum and clavicle region will move the scapula into a position where it is more perpendicular to the floor, allowing the back–neck to lengthen and the chin to become parallel to the floor. The muscles along the spine (the erector spinae) can be strengthened with exercise. They can then act to create length in the spine even in a standing position against gravity. The body is continually adapting to the changes in its environment. By strengthening the muscles around the spine, the internal organs have more room within the thoracic cavity and the muscle pull on the vertebral bones is in a direction to counter the wedging effect of gravity on the anterior vertebrae of the thoracic region.

Posture control and maintaining balance in the face of perturbing events is a result of the successful integration of several systems: the sensory systems (visual, vestibular, proprioceptive), motor control, central nervous system, and musculoskeletal systems (range of motion, strength). Deciphering the mechanism of failure is particularly difficult in integrated systems because the decline in one system is compensated by adaptation of the other systems. Researcher's imply stress the nervous system to delineate postural incompetence in elderly subjects. In general, for elderly individuals: the muscles of the ankle react slowly; therefore, they activate the antagonist muscles of the ankle that results in a stiffening of the joints in order to compensate for lack of balance control. They are more apt to use the muscles of the hips to correct imbalance due to ankle weakness. This may lead to an overcompensation and erratic postural responses, increasing the risk of falling. Elderly people have a higher amplitude of response within muscle groups; this can lead to a jerking response and enhance the risk of falling. They lose their balance more quickly than younger subjects when given inappropriate visual or somatosensory cues, indicating that the elderly have a higher risk of falls in dim lighting. However, on repeat trial elderly people improved quickly, indicating that balance can be improved with training under conditions of sensory deprivation and conflict. Balance problems may not be a normal course of aging but may be a result of comorbid conditions. Elderly subjects with the greatest pathology (cardiovascular, neurolgic, and musculoskeletal comorbidity) had the poorest postural response pattern.

Integrating Posture and Balance Training

Endurance training is primarily for the cardiovascular system; strength training is primarily for the musculoskeletal system; balance training is for the neuromuscular system. Balance training can be broken into static and dynamic components. Static exercise includes balancing the center of gravity while remaining in the same spot. To make the balance training progressively more difficult, the exercises are performed with a progressively narrower base of support by moving from a wide double-legged support, to semitandem, to tandem, to single-legged support, and to static bipedal toe raises. In addition, sit-to-stand movement, cervical spine rotations or twists and side bending, and scapular retraction and elevation all address problems of posture and balance. Dynamic balance is maintaining balance during movement and can be made progressively more difficult by narrowing the base of support, side steps, crossover steps forward and backward, high steps, heel-to-toe walking, and toe tapping (dorsifexion). These exercises can be incorporated into a strength training program while waiting for a machine or between weight-lifting sets when working muscles of the upper body. In endurance training these exercises can be included as part of the warm-up and cool-down periods. Hatha yoga incorporates all these balance training techniques as a part of the regular practice.

Range of Motion

Range of motion is used as a gentle form of exercise to maintain joint mobility. Range of motion or the ROM dance is a poem set to music that systematically leads the participant through all joints in a soothing and relaxing pace. Range of motion is also maintained by strength training those muscles around a joint. For example, performing dips for the triceps can help to maintain shoulder extension.

Upper Body Weight-Bearing Postures

Most of our exercise and daily activities are done with an upright posture. Very rarely are we required to have our head in a position lower than our heart. Bone formation is facilitated by weight-bearing exercise. Loss of bone mass in the upper body, principally the thoracic region, is a good reason to shift weight onto our hands and upper body. Benefits of postures in which the head is lower than the torso may include: (1) strengthening the arm and trunk muscles of the upper body; (2) reversing the gravitational pull on the bones of the upper back; (3) increasing the blood flow to the upper body and the head and neck region.

Much has been written about the decline of muscle and bone mass with age, the loss of height, the increase in fat, and so forth. Bone responds to the stresses put on it. Gradually increasing the amount of weight on the bones of the upper body may have beneficial effects on the bone mass of the arms and vertebrae of the upper back. This piezoelectric effect, first described by Wolf in the 1800s, explains how bone responds to mechanical stress. The effects of mechanical stress are easily seen by the lines of trabecular bone in the head of the femur. The weaving of trabecular bone is particularly strong and light; therefore, it is the principal bone structure of the vertebrae, the head of the femur, and the lining of the canal of the long bones. Bone screening was originally done with single photon absorptiometry of the wrist until technology was developed that allowed for the measurement of spine bone density with dual photoabsorptiometry (DPA). Prior to developing the DPA, predictions of axial or spinal bone density were made from appendicular or arm bone measurements of bone mineral content (BMC). Later, the prediction of spinal bone mineral content from wrist bone mineral measurements were found to be erroneous. At this time, vertebral BMC is assessed at the lumbar (L2–L5) region due to the interference of the sternum and ribs when trying to measure the BMC of the thoracic vertebrae. The thoracic vertebrae, however, are clearly where the most wedging is seen on X-ray examination, and the anatomical deformity is most evident. Yet, the measurement taken at L2–L5 are used to predict the outcome of interventions geared to change the bone mineral content of the thoracic region. At this time, mechanical stress is the only effective means of stimulating new bone growth, and bone density is a product of local mechanical stress. The effects of gravity on bone through weight-bearing activity are much greater than those that can be produced by simple weight-lifting. Studies relating the cross-sectional area of the back muscle to bone density indicate a positive correlation; however in longitudinal studies by Sinaki and coworkers[3] using exercise to strengthen the back extensor muscles, does not show an increase in vertebral bone density. Gravitational forces on bone are much greater than those that can be exerted by the pull of the muscle alone. Using the two in combination would then, logically, provide the greatest protective effect against losing bone mass in the axial spine. One of the authors, Felicity Green, illustrates the positions. The positions shown in Figures 6.1A and 6.1B are the progressive increase of weight on the arms and upper back area. By starting with a position as shown in Figure 6.1A, a person can increase the strength and other adaptive responses to the position before moving to the position shown in Figure 6.1B. Figures 6.2A and 6.2B illustrate a method of learning to do handstands in a doorway. The handstand should follow after someone is fully comfortable with doing the positions in Figure 6.1B. These four figures illustrate a method of progressively increasing the gravitational effect of weight on the upper spine. Twisting exercises, when done properly with attention to length in the spine, can increase the strength of the muscle surrounding the vertebrae. This not only increases the muscle tone (erector spinae muscles) but acts on the bone of the vertebrae as well. The twisting action balances the length of the muscle and connective tissue across the chest and back region, a necessary component to improved upright posture. Figure 6.3 shows a method of spinal rotation or twisting on a chair. The legs are well-grounded and firm, and the right hand is used to open the front right chest area and create the rotation around the spine. This should be done for both sides of the body. In persons with a single-curve scoliosis, the twist should be done away from the concave side of the spine.

Another possible effect of having the head in a lower position than the heart may be to increase the strength of the capillary walls in the upper body. The body is changing with age and adapting to the environment from the moment of birth. In a study by Williamson and colleagues to evaluate the effect of age and hydrostatic pressure on the basement membrane of skeletal muscle, infants (less than 6 months of age), children (3 to 5 years), and adults (25 to 75 years) were evaluated. The samples were taken from pectoralis, rectus abdominus, quadriceps femoris, and gastrocnemius muscles. In comparing the muscles within each group, in the infants no difference in the average basement membrane thickness was found. In the children, the basement membrane wall thickness of the gastrocnemius had increased by one third over that of the muscles positioned higher in the body. In the adults, the basement membrane wall thickness of the gastrocnemius was approximately twice that in the pectoralis muscle, with the quadriceps muscle being one third thicker than those located in the pectoralis muscle. These data suggest that there is a progressive thickening of the basement membrane of capillaries in response to the higher hydrostatic pressures in location farther below the heart. When these mean basement membrane wall thicknesses are compared across age groups, the adults have twice the thickness at the chest level when compared with infants, whereas the basement membrane at the calf level is approximately 3.5-fold greater than in the infants. This cross-sectional comparison suggests that a doubling of the wall thickness is a result of hydrostatic pressure, and the other 1.5-fold increase may be due to age. Many factors can cause vessel wall weakness, including disease and genetic influences. The adaptation to hydrostatic pressure may depend on the strength of the capillary walls. If hydrostatic pressure were gradually increased in the head and neck area with exercises that position the head at varying levels below the torso, the increased basement membrane walls might act to strengthen vessel walls in later life. As with any exercise, postures with the head in a lower position should be begun gradually, and the earlier in life they are the more readily the body can adapt. Although there are no data on the effect of positions with the head below the center of gravity, conservative precautions should be taken in patients with high blood pressure, COPD, corpulmonale, congestive heart failure, pulmonary hypertension, left ventricular dysfunction, angina, and cardiac arrhythmia. Persons with arthritis of the hand area should progress downward gradually from higher surfaces. There are very few positions in weight training or endurance training that call for the head to be lower than the heart.

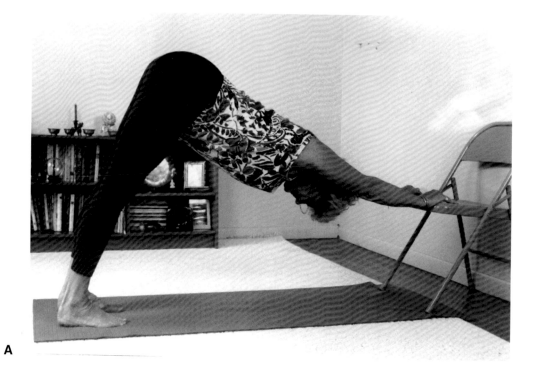

A

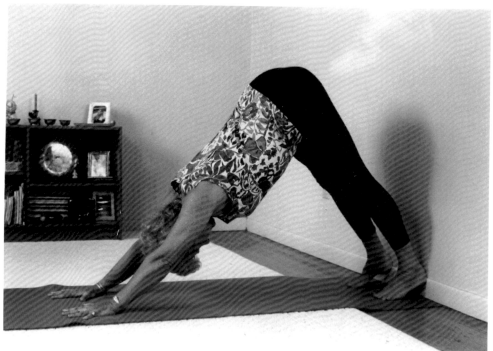

B

Figure 6.1 Progressive weight-bearing for the upper body. **(A)** Posture 1. **(B)** Posture 2.

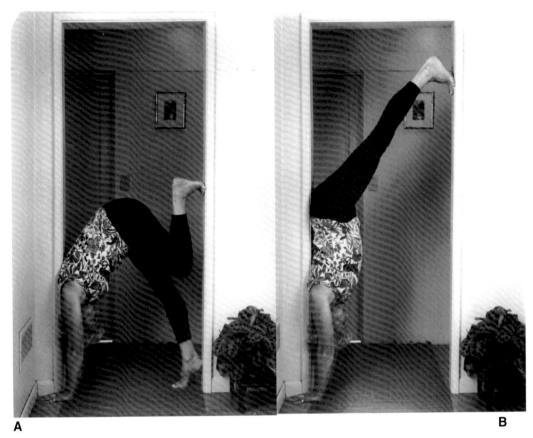

Figure 6.2 (A) Partial handstand in doorway. **(B)** Full handstand in doorway.

In Figures 6.1*A*, 6.1*B*, 6.2*A*, and 6.2*B*, the torso weight is on her hands and her head is lower than her heart. This is a way to gradually increase the hydrostatic pressure in the head and neck region.

Exercise Programming

In the words of singer Bonnie Raitt, "Time is more precious, when we have less of it to waste." Most women do not want to or have time to spend hours in the gym trying to recoup the vim, vigor, and slim figure of their youth. The form of exercise programming depends on the goal. The recommendations in Table 6.1 indicate the mode of exercise training most likely to be efficacious in reducing symptoms and improving function. A well-balanced program of endurance, strength, and flexibility training is the most reasonable approach to a lifetime benefit from exercise. This can be accomplished in several ways. In Table 6.2 a 3-, 4-, and 5-day-a-week schedule of combined exercise programming is suggested to integrate endurance, strength, and flexibility. Until a woman has adequate information to work on her own, she has several options. She can join a gym, health club, or YWCA that has classes in weight training and get an exercise prescription from an exercise professional for endurance training. Formal classes in flexibility are important to learn proper body alignment and postural awareness. These may be offered as flexibility classes or yoga classes. Another method of instruction is for one or two people to hire a personal trainer. A female trainer is a good role model and resource for older women.

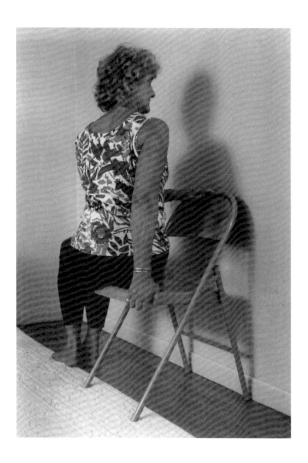

Figure 6.3 Twisting posture.

The importance of specific instruction on the exercise technique, progression of training, and the benefits of exercise is often overlooked. If exercise is ineffective, it is generally because it was not done, that is, noncompliance. To hand a person a pamphlet on exercise and expect that the responsibility for prescribing exercise is met is absurd. In order to expect exercise compliance, a person is entitled to a proper prescription, instruction, and encouragement.

Conscious Relaxation

What is conscious relaxation? After a day of normal activity, our muscles and connective tissue have stored energy. The muscle bonds require adenosine triphosphate (ATP), the common currency of energy exchange, to break to bond. Going to bed relieves the stress of gravity on the body, but without actively commanding the body to stop the brain's activity and relax the muscles, there is

Table 6.2 Sample Exercise for Integrating Endurance, Strength and Flexibility

Days/week	Endurance	Strength	Flexibility
5	3 days (30 min)	2 days (30–45 min)	1 day (30–45 min)
4	3 days (30 min)	1 day (60 min)	3 (30 min—combine with endurance)
3	3 days (30 min)	3 days (20 min)	3 days (20 min)

residual tension in the muscles and thoughts in the brain. Elderly people frequently have difficulty getting adequate rest and sleeping through the night. As with so many of the problems of geriatric patients, the cause is multifocal; however, attention to relaxation is a piece of the puzzle. Among the aspects of poor sleep, older people have a blunted amplitude in slow wave sleep patterns and temperature excursions of the body. Daily conscious relaxation coupled with vigorous exercise during each day may provide the contrast to activity that helps in overall body and mind health and rest. Conscious relaxation does not have to be done at bed time; it is often practiced in the early morning to provide a time when the mind and the body are both quiet. Many techniques have been described, and audiotapes are available on guided relaxation. A simple, effective relaxation technique of approximately 20 minutes is described here and, like everything in life, it gets better with practice.

> Lie down, preferably on the floor or a firm surface, support the head, close the eyes, and have a light cover for warmth during the full relaxation period. Draw the thoughts, like tendrils, in away from the external world and pay attention to the feelings in the body. Allow the body to feel heavy and let it be fully supported by the floor. Breathing evenly through the nose as deeply as comfortable, lengthen the exhalation slightly relative to the inhalation. This will help to facilitate the relaxation. Continue this for 10 to 20 minutes without interruption.

Notice that this is much more refreshing than a nap. This technique may help with sleep if practiced right before bedtime.

Acknowledgment

The authors acknowledge with appreciation Dr. Ilse Riegel, University of Wisconsin, McArdle Cancer Institute, for her expertise in editing this manuscript.

Resources

Books

1. Corbin DE, Metal-Corbin J: *Reach for it! A Handbook of Health, Exercise and Dance Activities for Older Adults.* Dubuque, IA, Eddie Bowers Publishing, 1990.
2. Iyengar GS: *YOGA: A Gem for Women.* New Deli, India, Allied Publishers, 1983.
3. Mehta, S, Mehta M, Mehta S: *Yoga, The Iyengar Way.* New York, Alfred A. Knopf, 1990.
4. Minton SC: *Body and Self.* Champaign, IL, Human Kinetics Publishers, 1989.
5. Scaravelli V: *Awakening the Spine.* San Francisco, Harper, 1991.

Video

1. Catalog: "The Complete Guide to Exercise Videos," Video Specialties, Inc., 1-800-433-6769.
2. Harlow D, Yu P: "The ROM Dance: A Range of Motion Exercise Relaxation Program." Madison, WI: WHA Television, 1993. Also a version adapted for chair exercisers.

References

1. *Guidelines for Exercise Testing and Prescription,* Pate RR, Blair SN, Durstine JL, Eddy DO, Hanson P, Painter P, Smith LK, Wolfe LA (eds.). Philadelphia, London, Lea & Febiger, 1991.
2. *Menopausal Years the Wise Woman Way,* Weed SS: New York, Ash Tree Publishing, 1992, pp. 19–38.
3. *Light on Yoga,* Inyengar BKS: Revised ed. New York, Schocken Books, 1979.
4. Tilz GP, Domej W, Diez-Ruiz A, Weiss G, Brezinschek R, Brezinschek HP, Huttl E, Pristautz H, Wachter H, Fuchs D: *Immunobiology,* 1993;188:194.

5. Edinger JD, Morey MC, Sullivan RJ, Higginbotham MB, Marsh GR, Dailey DS, McCall WV: *Sleep*, 1993;16:351.
6. Belza BL, Henke CJ, Yelin EH, Epstein WV, Gilliss CL: *Nurs. Res* 1993;42:93.
7. Fujimoto S, Kurihara N, Hirata K, Ota K, Matsushita H, Wakayama K, Nishimoto K, Kanao K, Kobayashi S, Otani M, et al: *Nippon Nyobu Shikkan Gakkai Zasshi (Japanese J Thorac Dis)* 1992;30:1449.
8. Lyngberg KK, Ramsing BU, Nawrocki A, Harreby M, Danneskiold-Samsoe B. *Arthritis Rheum* 1994;37:623.
9. Ytterberg SR, Mahowald ML, Krug HE: *Baillieres Clin Rheumatol* 1994;8:161.
10. Neuberger GB, Smith KV, Black SO, Hassanein R: *Arthritis Care Res* 1993;6:141.
11. Hoenig H, Groff G, Pratt K, Goldberg E, Franck W: *J. Rheumatol* 1993;20:785.
12. Hansen TM, Hansen G, Langgaard AM, Rasmussen JO: *Scand. J Rheumatol* 1993;26:107.
13. Galloway MT, Jokl P: *Bull. Rheum Dis* 42:1.
14. Kirsteins AE, Dietz F, Hwang SM: *Am J Phys Med Rehabil* 70:136.
15. Liemohn W. *Rheum Dis Clin North Am* 1990;16;945.
16. McCubbin JA: *Rheum Dis Clin North Am* 1990;16:931.
17. Perlman SG, Connell KJ, Clark A, Robinson MS, Conlon P, Gecht M, Caldron P, Sinacore JM: *Arthritis Care Res* (1990);3:29.
18. North TC, McCullagh P, Tran ZV, KB Pandolf KB, and Holloszy JO (eds.) in *Exercise and Sport Sciences Reviews*, "Effect of Exercise on Depression" Baltimore, Hong Kong, London, Sydney, Williams & Wilkins, 1990, pp. 379–415.
19. Risch SV, Norvell NK, Pollock ML, Risch ED, Langer H, Fulton M, Graves JE, Leggett SH: *Spine.* 1993;18:232.
20. Smith, Jr. CW: *Prim Care* 1991;18:271.
21. Vorhies D, Riley BE: *Clinc Geriat Med* 1993;9:745.
22. Vale F, Reardon JZ, ZuWallack RL. *Chest* 1993;103:42.
23. Gardner AW: *J Gerontol* 1993;48:M231.
24. Ciaccia JM: *J Vasc Nurs* 1993;11:1.
25. Dougherty M, Bishop K, Mooney R, Gimotty P, Williams B: *J Reprod Med* 1993;38:684.
26. Buchner DM, Coleman EA: *Phys Med Rehabil Clin North Am* 1994;5:357.
27. Shephard RJ: *Geriatrics* 1993;48:61.
28. Gallagher W: *The Atlantic Monthly,* 1993;51.
29. Cress ME, Schultz E: *Top Geriatr Rehabil* 1985;1:14.
30. Cress ME: *Top Geriatr Rehabil* 1993;8:22.
31. Cress ME, Thomas DP, Johnson J, Kasch FW, Cassens RG, Smith EL, Agre JC: *Med Sci Sports Exerc* 1991;23:752.
32. Dalsky GP, Stocke KS, Ehsani AA, Slatopolsky E, Lee WC, Birge SJ: *Ann Int Med* 1988;108:824.
33. Sinaki M, Offord K: *Arch Phys Med Rehab* 1988;69:277.
34. Sinaki M, McPhee MC, Hodgson SF, Offord KP: *Mayo Clin Proc* 1986;61:116.
35. Pogrund H, Bloom RA, Weinberg H: *ACTA Orthop Scand* 1986;57:208.
36. Borg G: *Scand J Rehab Med* 1970;2:92.
37. Karvonen MJ: *Ann Med Exper Biol Fenn* 1957;35:507.
38. Wolff J. Das Gesetz der Transformation der Knochen. *Quarto.* Berlin, 1892.
39. Williamson JR, Vogler NJ, Kilo C: *Am J Pathol* 1971;63:359.

Chapter 7

Aging and Pharmacotherapeutics

George N. Aagaard, MD

Chemistry and pharmacology have ushered physicians into an era of great promise. An endless stream of new drugs goes through the stages of development and clinical trials. Many are proved safe and effective and are added to the drug therapy armamentarium. The optimal use of this armamentarium in the prevention and treatment of illness in older women is an opportunity and a challenge to physicians.

The challenge of safe and effective use of drugs in older patients exists for several reasons. First, older patients have more diseases. More diseases usually mean that more drugs are prescribed. More drugs mean the possibility of more adverse drug reactions and a greater chance of significant drug–drug interactions. Branch found that 15% of an elderly population took two or more prescription medications daily.[1] Law and Chalmers reported that 87% of patients 75 years of age and older were receiving drug therapy regularly and 34% of these took three or four drugs per day.[2]

Second, apart from the greater exposure to drugs associated with an increased burden of chronic disease, there may be an increased vulnerability to drugs, which is related to the aging process. A drug may be handled differently (pharmacokinetics) in older patients, or a drug may act differently (pharmacodynamics) in older patients.

Third, the aging process may cause changes that make it more difficult to obtain compliance from older patients. Hearing loss may make it difficult to understand spoken explanations or instructions. Visual changes may impair the ability to understand written instructions or to read labels on drug containers. Loss of memory or confusion may make it difficult to comprehend or follow instructions regarding medications.

The considerations noted above explain why the idea prevails that drug therapy in elders should be approached with caution because elders are more vulnerable to adverse reactions. Certainly it is true that elders are more likely to have postural hypotension even without drugs. Therefore, they are more likely to have a significant postural drop in blood pressure with any drug that may cause this significant and dangerous response. However, elders show a wide range of responses to drugs, and this requires that physicians prescribe thoughtfully for these patients and follow them closely.

Pharmacokinetic Effects of Aging

Drug Absorption

Since most prescribed drugs are given by mouth this discussion will be limited to changes with aging in the gastrointestinal tract and their effect on the absorption of drugs. There are a number of aspects of gastrointestinal function that might change with aging which could influence the absorption of a drug. These include (1) gastric fluid pH; (2) gastric emptying time; (3) intestinal motility; (4) gastrointestinal fluid secretion: volume and composition; (5) gastrointestinal blood flow; and (6) gastrointestinal disease and the general health of the patient. However, there is little or no evidence that changes related to aging influence drug absorption significantly. Changes in the pH of the gastric fluid are offered as an example.

The pH of gastric fluid tends to increase with age and to a greater degree in women than in men. This could influence both the rate at which a drug goes into solution and the rate at which it is absorbed from the stomach. The dissolution rate of alkaline drugs could theoretically be impaired by achlorhydria, or a significant decrease in gastric acidity. This would suggest that drugs might be prescribed in solution instead of as pills to avoid the process of dissolution in the stomach. Alkalinity of the gastric juice might also reduce the rate of absorption of alkaline drugs in the stomach. However, despite well-established evidence that changes in gastric acidity occur with advanced age, there is no good evidence of reduced drug absorption. Changes in drug absorption do, however, occur as a result of drug interactions. (See below.)

Drug Distribution

When a drug is absorbed into the blood it becomes available to all the tissues and organs to which blood circulates. The drug shifts from the blood to receptor sites, to storage depots, and to sites where it may be metabolized or excreted. The rate and extent of movement of a drug depend on the concentration of the drug and the affinity of the drug for receptors and storage tissues. Drugs tend to move from sites of higher concentration to sites of lower concentration.

Drugs in the plasma are present in two forms, free drug and plasma protein–bound drug. The amount of drug that is bound to plasma proteins is dependent on the affinity of the drug for the plasma protein. Most protein-bound drug is bound to plasma albumen. In a sense, plasma protein–bound drug serves as a readily available store of drug that is called on when free drug is removed from plasma.

It is free drug that acts by binding to receptors. It is free drug that is also metabolized by hepatic enzymes or excreted by the kidney. When free drug is removed from the plasma for either of these purposes it is replaced by plasma protein–bound drug. If free drug is increased by the administration of a larger dose of drug, more drug will become bound to plasma protein, but an additional amount of drug will be available at sites where it may activate a receptor or be metabolized or excreted.

With aging, bodily changes occur that can influence the distribution of drugs. Total body water and blood volume tend to decrease. Lean body mass (muscle tissue) tends to decrease. There is a relative increase in body fat. Novak compared body fat in young adults with those 65 to 85 years of age.[3] Body fat increased from 18% to 36% of total body weight in men and from 33% to 45% in women. This means that drugs which are readily soluble in fat are more readily stored in older patients and to a greater extent in women than in men. Such a drug would have a greater volume of distribution and when a single dose is administered would have a lower plasma volume than would be attained if the drug were relatively insoluble in fat.

Drug Metabolism

Liver size decreases with age. Liver blood flow also decreases with age. It is logical to assume that drugs which are metabolized by the liver would have reduced clearance and a prolonged plasma half-life. However, studies to determine the site and rate of metabolism of a drug are difficult to design, conduct, and interpret.

O'Malley and coworkers found that the plasma half-life of antipyrine and phenylbutazone were increased 45% and 29% respectively, in aged patients as compared with young adults.[4] The increase for the antipyrine half-life was even greater for women (78%). In a large study, Vestal and coworkers found that there was a great variation between individual subjects and that only a small part of the reduced clearance could be ascribed to the influence of age alone.[5] Vestal and Wood also showed that smoking had less effect in inducing enzymatic metabolism in the aged.[6]

Renal Excretion

Kidney function decreases with age, with the result that drugs which are eliminated chiefly by the kidney show an increased plasma half-life and a decreased clearance rate. Beginning in the fourth decade of life changes in renal blood flow, renal mass, glomerular filtration rate, and active tubular secretion and resorption occur.[7] The decrease in renal blood flow is greater than would be explained by the decrease in cardiac output that occurs with aging.

The reduced capacity to excrete drugs may not be adequately reflected by the serum creatinine concentration, which may be normal in an elderly patient while the creatinine clearance is definitely abnormal. The serum creatinine concentration may be in the normal range because of reduced production of creatinine due to a reduced muscle mass in the older patient. Therefore, it is best to use creatinine clearance to estimate renal function in prescribing a drug that is eliminated largely by excretion by the kidney. A rough estimate of creatinine clearance can be obtained with this formula:

$$\frac{(140 - \text{age}) \times \text{wgt (kg)}}{72 \times \text{creatinine (mg/dl)}}$$

For women use 75%.

Pharmacodynamics in Aging

Pharmacodynamics deals with the response that a drug elicits in a patient. Is that response greater or smaller than the "usual" response? The idea is widely held that the aged are more "sensitive" or more responsive to drugs than are younger adults. This is true in some instances, but it is not universally true. It takes significantly more isoproterenol to produce an increase of 25 beats per minute in aged subjects than is required in younger subjects.[8] The same study reported that the response to the beta-adrenergic blocker, propranolol, was reduced in older patients. Vestal's findings suggest that the affinity of beta-receptors for both agonists and antagonists may decrease with age. Another explanation is that the sensitivity of aged patients to drugs that act on beta receptors is decreased.

Increased sensitivity to drugs with aging is suggested by several studies. Reidenberg and coworkers showed that the dose of diazepam which caused depression was inversely related to age.[9] In addition, the drug plasma level at which depression occurred was inversely related to age.

Increased sensitivity to a single 10-mg dose of nitrazepam was found in older as compared with young patients.[10] Older patients made more mistakes in a psychomotor test, despite similar plasma concentrations and half-lives in the two groups.

Cook and coworkers studied the response to intravenous diazepam in patients being prepared for dental or endoscopic procedures.[11] He found that patients age 80 years of age required an average dose of 10 mg compared with 30 mg for patients aged 20. The plasma levels required for sedation at age 20 were two to three times those required at age 80.

Older patients also appear to be more sensitive to warfarin. In both humans and rats, Shepard and coworkers found that older subjects had a greater anticoagulant response even though they received a smaller weight-related dose.[12] The authors also found that at the same plasma level of warfarin there was a greater inhibition of vitamin K clotting factor synthesis in the older group. They found no significant differences in pharmacokinetics between the two age groups.

In summary, older patients may be more or less sensitive to drugs. The opiates, benzodiazepines, barbiturates, and anticoagulants may elicit an increased response. For other drugs such as isoproterenol and beta blockers the response may be reduced. Drug treatment must be individualized, and the response of the patient must be closely followed.

Adverse Effects of Drugs

In prescribing any drug a physician must consider and balance three major factors: (1) the natural history of the disease: What are the hazards to life and health if the disease is left untreated? (2) the effectiveness of the drug in the disease as now presented in the patient, and (3) the hazards of the drug in a patient with a similar clinical picture. In a mild, self-limited illness it would be unwise to prescribe a drug that may cause serious adverse effects in a significant number of patients. However, the possibility of adverse effects should not deter the use of that particular drug in a life-threatening illness. In any discussion of adverse drug effects it must be acknowledged that it may be difficult to reach agreement on a definition. Karch and Lasagna have suggested that an adverse drug reaction is "any response to a drug that is noxious and unintended and that occurs at doses used in man for prophylaxis, diagnosis, or therapy, excluding failure to accomplish the intended purpose."[13] Even with agreement on a definition it may be difficult to obtain agreement of experienced clinicians on the classification of specific symptoms or signs in a patient. The differentiation between signs of adverse drug effects and the symptoms and signs of an illness may be challenging.

Many studies of adverse drug effects suffer from a lack of controls. Reidenberg and Lowenthal compared healthy students and hospital staff who were taking no medications with a group who were receiving medications.[14] They found that many symptoms commonly considered adverse drug effects were complained of by their healthy subjects. Prominent among these symptoms were fatigue, inability to concentrate, irritability, and insomnia.

Despite the difficulties mentioned above, there is good reason to suggest that adverse drug effects are more frequent and more severe in older patients. Seidl and coworkers found an adverse drug reaction in 9.9% of patients 21 to 30 years of age and in 24% percent of patients 81 years of age and older.[15] Castleden and Pickles reviewed spontaneous reports of adverse drug reactions (ADRs) received by the Committee on Safety of Medicines in the United Kingdom.[16] They found a correlation between the use of drugs and the number of reports of ADRs. This was true for two nonsteroidal anti-inflammatory drugs (NSAIDs). The authors also found that the ADR was more likely to be serious or fatal in elders. The most common ADRs caused by the two NSAIDs in the elderly affected the gastrointestinal and hemopoietic systems. The drug suspected of causing a gastrointestinal ADR was an NSAID in 75% of the reports and 91% of fatal reports of gastrointestinal bleeds and perforations were in patients over 60 years of age.

Of equal importance to drugs as a cause of life-threatening ADRs is the unfavorable effect they may exert on the quality of life of patients. It is important to determine if a drug disturbs the ability to function socially, decreases initiative, impairs memory, impairs sexual function, disturbs sleep patterns, or increases fatigue.

A host of drugs can cause psychiatric symptoms, ranging from mania and hallucinations to confusion, disorientation, and depression.[17] Mental confusion, especially in the elderly, has been reported with cimetidine.[18]

In the past when sulfonamides were available but penicillin was not, pneumonia was often treated with a sulfonamide. Acute psychoses were reported that would clear when the drug was discontinued. Lamy[19] has estimated that 40 drugs or groups of drugs may cause delirium.

Cognitive impairment due to an ADR was found in 35 of 308 patients being evaluated for Alzheimer-type dementia. The drugs most often involved were minor tranquilizers, antihypertensives, and major tranquilizers.[20]

Sexual dysfunction may be an ADR from antihypertensive drugs. Central sympatholytics, beta-adrenergic blockers, and alpha-adrenergic blockers are frequent offenders; even the thiazide diuretics can cause problems, especially if hypokalemia is present.[21] Psychotropic drugs can also cause sexual dysfunction. Major tranquilizers, antidepressants, and the benzodiazepines all have this potential. Cimetidine and metoclopramide may both cause increased prolactin levels, which may be associated with decreased libido and later with impotence. Anticholinergic drugs may also be associated with sexual dysfunction. These include atropine, antispasmodics, antiparkinson agents, antihistamines, muscle relaxants, and antiarrhythmics. Not all of the drugs in these classes will cause sexual dysfunction, but the potential is present and should be ruled out in those patients who complain of impairment.

In older patients a significant problem is drug-induced Parkinsonism (DIP).[22] Major tranquilizers, antiemetics, methyldopa, reserpine, and diazepam have all been implicated.

Many ADRs are dose-related. Either the daily dose is too large or the drug is given for too long, with toxicity that occurs over time. In some instances it may be possible to eliminate the ADR by reducing the dose or temporarily stopping the drug.

Drug–Drug Interactions as a Cause of Adverse Drug Reactions

Since older patients take more medications they are more vulnerable to drug–drug interactions. A patient who is taking one or more different drugs has the potential for a drug–drug interaction if an additional drug is prescribed. Similarly, the patient who is taking two or more drugs could be at risk if one drug is discontinued. Space does not permit a full discussion of this subject, but examples are given of clinically significant interactions that have been reported.

It is important to emphasize that drugs may influence the manner in which the body handles or responds to another drug.

1. A drug may change the rate of absorption and hence the bioavailability of another drug
2. A drug may increase the rate of metabolism, **or**
3. A drug may decrease the rate of metabolism, **or**
4. A drug may decrease the rate of excretion of another drug.
5. A drug may also influence the protein-binding of another drug.

Drug absorption may be changed by another drug by the following mechanisms:

1. Drug binding in the gastrointestinal (GI) tract;
2. Changes in GI pH;

3. Changes in GI motility;

4. Changes in intestinal flora;

5. Changes in drug metabolism within the wall of the intestine.

Iron salts may reduce the absorption of tetracyclines by binding it in the stomach.[23] Binding resins such as cholestyramine may reduce the absorption of thyroxin, warfarin, and thiazides.[24–26]

Dissolution of a drug and its absorption may be changed by drugs that alter the pH of the stomach. Drug absorption and bioavailability of cefpodoxime may be reduced by antacids or H2 blockers. Both the peak plasma concentration and the area under the concentration–time curve were reduced by giving Maalox.[27]

Change in GI motility may influence the rate of drug absorption. Since most drugs are absorbed in the intestine, delay in gastric emptying may slow absorption. As an example the absorption of acetaminophen may be slowed when Probanthine® is given. On the other hand, metoclopramide, which increases the speed of gastric emptying, may shorten the time required for acetaminophen to reach the intestine.[28]

Most bacterial growth is in the colon, and most drug absorption occurs proximal to the colon. However, in about 10% of patients digoxin is deactivated by bacterial metabolism to a significant degree. In such patients, elevated digoxin plasma levels may result from initiating antibiotic therapy with an agent such as erythromycin.[29]

It is possible to avoid some of the drug interactions that occur through binding of a drug or by change of pH by properly timing administration of the drug.

The drugs that induce enzyme activity include phenobarbital, glutethimide, rifampin, and the anticonvulsants, carbamazepine, phenytoin, and primidone. Phenobarbital will induce the enzyme that metabolizes warfarin and thus shorten its plasma half-life and reduce its anticoagulant effect.[30]

Drugs that inhibit enzyme activity are found in many different groups and include allopurinol, cimetidine, diltiazem, erythromycin, isoniazid, omeprazole, and verapamil. This is only a partial list, and it is growing constantly. Enzyme inhibition results in delayed clearance and the possibility of higher plasma levels and toxicity. Omeprazole inhibits the metabolism of diazepam and phenytoin.[31]

Drugs may decrease the renal elimination of drugs by altering active tubular secretion or passive tubular reabsorption. In past times, this capability has been utilized to reduce the dose of expensive drugs or drugs that had been available in limited supply. When penicillin was tightly restricted, probenecid was given because it competes with penicillin for tubular secretion, and higher plasma levels of penicillin could be achieved if the patient was receiving probenecid. By the same token, probenecid may reduce tubular secretion of methotrexate and cause serious toxicity.[32] Similarly, clofibrate has been reported to enhance the hypoglycemic action of sulfonylureas.[33]

A decrease in binding of a drug that is highly bound to plasma proteins will result in an increase in free drug available to the drug receptors and could cause an increased response or even toxicity. However, the increased amount of free drug is also available for metabolism or excretion. Hence, the level of free drug in the plasma should gradually return to normal. Warfarin is highly bound to plasma proteins. If a patient who is taking warfarin is given chloral hydrate, a primary metabolite of chloral hydrate is formed, trichloroacetic acid, which displaces warfarin from its binding sites. The result is an increase in prothrombin time that may last for a week, until the free warfarin level returns to the previous level.[34]

Because older patients take more drugs, they are theoretically at greater risk of drug–drug interactions. Fortunately, clinically significant adverse reactions are much less frequent than the theoretical possibilities. Nonetheless, it is important to look for a change in pharmacokinetics whenever a new drug is prescribed or a drug is discontinued.

It is also important to recognize that the time course of drug interactions may vary considerably, depending on the type of interaction, the doses of the interaction drugs, and the condition of the patient.

Practical Suggestions for Optimal Drug Therapy in Older Women

1. Take a careful drug history including all drugs currently being taken, both prescription and nonprescription. Ask the patient to bring all drugs currently being taken to the office for the first visit. Ask what was the response to each drug. A prolonged response to a modest dose of diazepam given in preparation for a procedure suggests caution when considering the use of a benzodiazepine. Learn about past adverse effects. Ask if there have been compliance problems. If so, why? Inquire about the use of cigarettes, alcohol, beverages containing caffeine, laxatives, aspirin, Tylenol, antacids, and sleeping preparations.

2. Prescribe a drug only if there is a clear need and if the chances of benefit clearly outweigh the costs in adverse effects and dollars.

3. Enlist the patient's continuing participation in the drug therapy program. Explain the need for and the goals of the therapy. Describe how the medication should be administered. Ask for feedback on the response to the drug, with emphasis on any adverse affects. Include a family member or other observer in the instructions and in the arrangements for feedback.

     Request information regarding the time and degree of a favorable response. A prompt favorable response to a low dose or to a few doses suggests that the patient may develop toxicity to the drug over a relatively short time.

4. Evaluate the patient frequently and carefully for the desired response and for adverse effects. After any change in the drug therapy program (any addition or deletion), follow the patient closely for any possible drug–drug interaction.

5. Always consider the drug therapy program as a possible cause for any unfavorable change in the patient. If it is possible that a drug may be the cause, discontinue it and observe the patient closely.

6. Prescribe a low dose initially. If the dosage must be increased, make the increments smaller and at longer intervals than you would use in younger patients. If a patient has any difficulty in swallowing tablets, try to obtain a liquid preparation.

7. Give the patient written instructions regarding medications. Keep instructions up-to-date. Make certain that the patient can read and understand the instructions. Review the instructions with the patient and have all the medications available.

8. Be certain that the patient can open the drug containers and can read the labels. Help the patient to identify each drug and to differentiate between tablets of similar appearance. Highlight those drugs that need special attention, for example, those to be taken at least one hour before meals, or before bedtime.

9. Whenever possible use once-a-day dosing of drugs.

10. Help the patient to develop or acquire a system that will help her to be confident that she has taken all of the drugs which had been advised. Insofar as possible, try to fit the drug treatment program into the patient's daily schedule.

11. For a patient in hospital, be certain that all drugs which will be taken after discharge are reviewed and written instructions given. If possible, have a family member present.

12. Ask the patient to bring all medications with her at each office visit. Review these at each visit to see if any might be discontinued.

13. When appropriate, use plasma drug levels for guidance in drug dosage and the interval between doses.

References

1. Branch LG: *Understanding the Health and Social Service People over age 65.* Washington, DC, United States Department of Health, Education, and Welfare. A report submitted the Administration on Aging, 1977, p. 77.
2. Law R, Chalmers C: Medicines and elderly people: A general practice survey. *Brit Med J* 1976;1:565–8.
3. Novak LP: Aging, total body potassium, fat-free mass and cell mass in males and females between ages 18 and 85 years. *J Gerontology* 1972;27:438–443.
4. O'Malley K, Crooks J., Duke E: Effect of age and sex on human drug metabolism. *Brit Med J* 1971;3:607–609.
5. Vestal RE, Norris AH, Tobin JD: Antipyrine metabolism in man: Influence of age, alcohol, caffeine, and smoking. *Clin Pharmacol & Ther.* 1975;18:425–432.
6. Vestal RE, Wood AJJ: Influence of age and smoking on drug kinetics in man: Studies using model compounds. *Clin Pharmacokinetics* 1980;5:309–319.
7. Hollenberg NK, Adams DF, Solomon HS: Senescence and the renal vasculature in normal man. *Circ Res.* 1974;34:309–316.
8. Vestal RE, Wood AJ, Shand DG: Reduced beta-adrenoreceptor sensitivity in the elderly. *Clin Pharmacol Ther.* 1979;26:181–186.
9. Reidenberg MM, Levy M, Warner H: The relationship between diazepam dose, plasma level, age and central nervous system depression in adults. *Clin Pharmacol Ther.* 1978;23:371.
10. Castleden, CM, George CF, Marcer D: Increased sensitivity to nitrazepam in old age. *Brit Med J* 1977;1:10–12.
11. Cook PJ, Flanagan R, James IM: Diazepam tolerance: Effect of age, regular sedation and alcohol. *Brit Med J* 1984;289:351–353.
12. Shepard AMM, Hewick OS, Moreland TA. Age as a determinant of sensitivity to warfarin. *Brit J Clin Pharmacol* 1977;4:315–320.
13. Karch FE, Lasagna L: Toward the operational identification of adverse drug reactions. *Clin Pharmacol Ther* 1977;21:247–254.
14. Reidenberg, MM, Lowenthal DT: Adverse nondrug reactions. *N Engl J Med* 1968;279:678–679.
15. Seidl LG, Thornton GF, Smith JW: Studies on the epidemiology of adverse drug reactions. III. Reactions in patients on a general medical service. *Johns Hopkins Hosp Bull* 1966;119:299–315.
16. Castleden CM, Pickles H: Suspected adverse drug reactions in elderly patients reported to the Committee on Safety of Medicines. Brit J Clin Pharm 1988;26:347–353.
17. Medical Letter: Drugs that cause psychiatric symptoms. 1984;26:75–78.
18. Medical Letter: Cimetidine (Tagamet): Update on adverse effects. 1978;20:77–78.
19. Lamy P: Adverse Drug Effects. *Clin Geriatr Med* 1990;6:293–307.
20. Larson EB, KuKull WA, Buchner D: Adverse drug reactions associated with global cognitive impairment in elderly persons. *Ann Intern Med* 1987;107:169–173.
21. Medical Letter: Drugs that cause sexual dysfunction. 1983;25:73–76.
22. Wilson JA, Maclennan WJ: Review: Drug-induced Parkinsonism in elderly patients. *Age Ageing* 1989;18:208–210.
23. Neuvonen PJ, Turakka H: Inhibitory effects of various iron salts on the absorption of tetracycline in man. *Eur J Clin Pharmacol* 1974;7:357–360.
24. Northcutt RC, Stiel JN, Hollifield JW: The influence of cholestyramine on thyroxine absorption. *JAMA* 1969;208:1857–1861.
25. Jahnchen E, Meinertz T., Gilfrich HJ. Enhanced elimination of warfarin during treatment with cholestyramine. *Br J Clin Pharmacol* 1978;5:437–440.
26. Hunninghake DB, King S, LaCroix K: The effect of cholestyramine and colestipol on the absorption of hydrochlorothiazide. *Int J Clin Pharmacol Ther Toxicol* 1982;20:151–154.
27. Saathoff N, Lode H., Neider K. Pharmacokinetics of cefpodoxime proxetil and interactions with an antacid and an H2 receptor antagonist. *Antimicrob Agents Chemother* 1992;36:796–800.
28. Nimmo J, Heading RC, Tothill P: Pharmacological modification of gastric emptying effects of propantheline and metoclopramide on paracetamol absorption. *Br Med J* 1973;1:587–589.
29. Lindenbaum J, Rund DG, Butler VP, Jr.: Inactivation of digoxin by the gastrointestinal tract flora: reversal by antibiotic therapy. *N Engl J Med* 1981;305:789–794.

30. Orme M, Breckenridge A: Enantiomers of warfarin and phenobarbital. *N Engl J Med* 1976;295:1482–1483.
31. Gugler R, Jensen JC: Omeprazole inhibits oxidative drug metabolism: studies with diazepam and phenytoin in vivo and 7-ethoxycoumarin in vitro. *Gastroenterology* 1985;89:1235–1241.
32. Lilly MB, Omura GA: Clinical pharmacology of oral intermediate-dose methotrexate with or without probenecid. *Cancer Chemother Pharmacol* 1985;15:220–222.
33. Daubresse JC, Daigneux D, BruiWier M: Clofibrate and diabetes control in patients treated with oral hypogycemic agents. *Br J Clin Pharmacol* 1979;7:599–603.
34. Udall JA: Warfarin-chloral hydrate interaction: Pharmacological activity and clinical significance. *Ann Intern Med* 1974;81:341–344.

Chapter 8

Hormone Replacement Therapy

Donald E. Moore, MD

Introduction

Soon after conjugated equine estrogens (CEE) were approved in the United States by the Food and Drug Administration in 1942, they were promoted as the fountain of youth for women in their forties, fifties, and sixties. Skin would not lose its elasticity, wrinkles would not appear, and the woman would feel young again. Then, in the mid-1970s, a cancer scare arose. An increased risk of endometrial cancer was recognized in estrogen users, and the number of users dropped 50% over the next 5 years. The number of users began to increase in the late 1980s. In the 1980s, prevention of osteoporosis became apparent, followed in the late 1980s by a number of studies suggesting that estrogen replacement therapy (ERT) may reduce the risk of cardiovascular disease. Now in the 1990s, investigators are trying to better understand an apparently small increased risk of breast cancer, to shore up an understanding of all of these relationships, to fine tune them, and to attempt to clarify the benefits versus risks for hypoestrogenic postmenopausal women.

Causes of Hypoestrogenicity in the Older Woman

At the time of menopause a shift to a state of hypoestrogenicity accelerates. The ovaries of women between the ages of 40 and 58 (average age of menopause is 51) become depleted of oocytes as well as their complementary granulosa cells, the estrogen- and progesterone-producing cells of the ovary. After menopause much of the major source of estrogen, primarily estrone, arises from the aromatization of androstenedione in body fat; the amount of aromatization of androstenedione to estrone and testosterone to estradiol more than doubles in postmenopausal women and relates directly to the amount of body fat. Follicle-stimulating hormone (FSH) and luteinizing hormone (LH) levels rise steadily during the first 12 months after menopause, and then they either level off or decrease. The stromata of the ovaries continue to produce androgens throughout life (Figure 8.1). Because the ovaries are still active after menopause, perhaps a better term for *ovarian failure* would be *ovarian shift*.

Although the depletion of estrogen- and progesterone-producing cells is a gradual 40- to 50-year-long process, the last menstrual period can be abrupt in a small percentage of women. In most women, however, the menopause is preceded by irregular or oligomenorrheic menstrual cycles. The last 2 years before natural menopause may consequently be associated with the symptoms of menopause or climacteric; this perimenopausal interval prior to menopause (Figure 8.2) can be a time of rising FSH levels, rising and falling estradiol levels, and vasomotor symptoms.

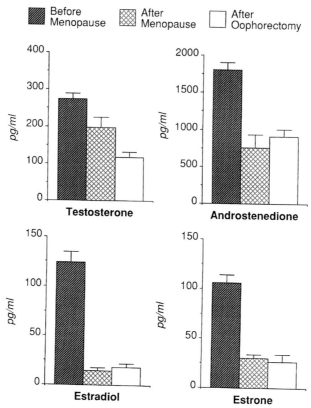

Figure 8.1 The mean (± standard error) serum androgen and estrogen levels in women with endometrial cancer before (n = 5) and after menopause (n = 16) and 6 to 8 weeks after oophorectomy (n = 16). These levels were not significantly different from those without endometrial cancer. (Modified with permission from Judd HL: Hormonal dynamics associated with menopause. *Clin Obstet Gynecol* 1976;19:775–778.)

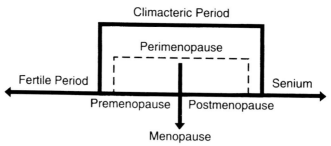

Figure 8.2 The climacteric period. (Redrawn from Jaszmann LJB: Epidemiology of the climacteric syndrome, in Campbell S (ed.): *The Management of the Menopause and Post-menopausal Years.* Baltimore, University Park Press, 1976 pp. 11–23. Used by permission of the author.)

An effective treatment for these symptoms is the use of a low-dose combination oral contraceptive (COC), perhaps one containing 20 µg of ethinyl estradiol. The change to estrogen replacement therapy (ERT) could be done once the FSH is elevated, which could be identified by discontinuing the COC for 1 month when age 51 is reached and measuring serum FSH. If normal, COCs could be reinstituted and FSH again rechecked every year.

About one third of women will undergo a surgical menopause in the United States (Figure 8.3). This creates two changes in women that are not seen with other hypoestrogenic states. First, the hormonal changes are immediate and therefore so are the symptoms. Second, the stromata of the ovary, which again are active throughout life, are no longer available to produce androgens, particularly testosterone. It is probable that testosterone plays some role in female libido.

Should Ovaries be Removed at Hysterectomy?

Approximately 1 in 50,000 women over the age of 40 years will develop ovarian cancer each year. However, there is some question whether bilateral oophorectomy will protect a woman from developing ovarian cancer because a similar cancer of the peritoneal surfaces can develop despite bilateral oophorectomy.[1] Furthermore, surgical extirpation of both ovaries before menopause increases the risks of cardiovascular disease and osteoporosis more than if the ovaries are left intact, although premenopausal women undergoing hysterectomy and ovarian conservation still develop vasomotor symptoms (VMS) according to Oldenhave and coworkers.[2] The benefits of ovarian conservation prior to menopause probably outweigh the risks of ovarian cancer. The benefits of ovarian conservation after menopause are unknown, but again the ovary does continue to produce testosterone after natural menopause.

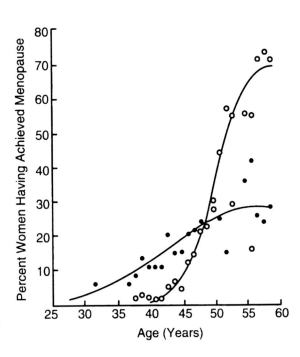

Figure 8.3 Observed and fitted percentages of the study respondents having achieved operative (•) or natural (.) menopause as a function of age. (Redrawn from Krailo MD. Pike MC: Estimation of the distribution of age at natural menopause from prevalence data. *Am J Epidemiol* 1983; 117:357; with permission.)

Symptoms and Signs of Postmenopausal Hypoestrogenisity

Physiology and Treatment of Hot Flashes

Seventy-five percent of women report vasomotor symptoms at menopause.[3] These symptoms are severe in about 15%. The prevalence of vasomotor symptoms tapers to 25% at 5 years after menopause and 15% at 16 years after menopause.[4] Some women in their seventies and eighties still report hot flashes. Women with surgically induced menopause tend to have a higher prevalence and severity of hot flashes, at least initially. Erlik, Meldrum, and Judd[5] found significantly lower levels of estradiol and estrone in women with vasomotor symptoms.

Cultural differences may effect the reporting of hot flashes. Postmenopausal women from Western societies report far more frequent hot flashes than their counterparts in Japan and Indonesia or Mayan women in Yucatan, Mexico. Of note, Martin and coworkers[6] found that the Mayan Indians also have a low prevalence of osteoporotic fractures, despite low serum levels of estradiol and estrone.

Usually, hot flashes occur spontaneously, but stress, emotional responses, external heat, a confining space, caffeine, or alcohol may trigger hot flashes.[4] The external temperature can modulate hot flashes; there is significant reduction in both frequency and intensity of hot flashes during the day and in a cool as compared with a warm room.

A hot flash is commonly 1 to 5 minutes in duration but ranges from seconds to 15 minutes or more.[4] Hot flashes are described as waves of heat, drenching sweats, anxiety, and palpitations. Women report a sense of impending hot flash before the flash actually starts. There is an apparent resetting of the body's thermostat or temperature set point in the hypothalamus that the body perceives as a need to eliminate heat. The resultant response in the skin apparently results in the objective and symptomatic changes. The heart rate and skin blood flow increase, particularly in the hands and fingers. There is a rapid drop in skin resistance and an increase in skin conductance. Finger and toe temperatures rise 7°F, and perspiration commences. As a result of the vasodilation and perspiration, there is heat loss and a drop in internal temperature of 1°F. Shivering may occur and facilitate the return of body temperature to normal.

During a hot flash there is an episodic release of LH and presumably gonadotropin-releasing hormone (GnRH) (Figure 8.4). However, the release of LH and GnRH is thought only to be a

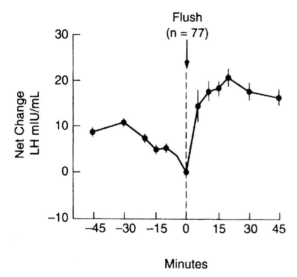

Figure 8.4 Mean (= standard error of the mean) serum luteinizing hormone (LH) concentration during 77 flush episodes expressed as a net change in milli-international units per milliliter from the onset of the flush at 0 on the x-axis. This graph incorporates 5-minute sampling from 20 minutes before to 20 minutes after each flush episode. It can be seen that the flush onset is coincident with a rise in serum LH levels. (Redrawn from Casper R, Yen SSC: The menopause and perimenopausal period, in Yen SSC, Jaffee RD (eds.): *Reproductive Endocrinology—Physiology, Pathophysiology, and Clinical Management*, ed 2. Philadelphia, WB Saunders, 1986, p 411. Used by permission of Robert F. Casper.)

secondary response to a neurotransmitter from higher centers of the brain. Epinephrine has been shown to increase, while norepinephrine decreases during hot flashes. There is also some increase in β-endorphin, β-lipotropin, and adrenocorticotropic hormone (ACTH) concentrations during hot flashes. Cortisol, dehydroepiandrosterone (DHEA), and androstenedione levels also increase. (Meldrum and coworkers)[7]

Clinical risk factors for vasomotor symptoms include an ectomorphic body structure; a strong family history of osteoporosis; a low calcium intake; inactivity, cigarette smoking, and alcohol abuse; and early hypoestrogenicity caused genetically, by early or surgical menopause, by hypothalamic pituitary failure, by excessive exercise, or by certain hormonal excesses such as glucocorticoid excess or thyrotoxicosis.

Even men, after orchiectomy, can experience vasomotor symptoms.

Some women develop insomnia if the vasomotor symptoms are severe enough at night. The lack of sleep compounded by an age-related decrease in rapid eye movement (REM) sleep can lead to depression, irritability, a loss of sense of worth, and memory loss. From the Netherlands, Oldenhave and coworkers[8] report more "atypical" symptoms in postmenopausal women who have more severe VMS. These atypical symptoms consist of tenseness, fatigue, palpitations, irritability, pins-and-needles sensations, restless legs, dizziness, tiredness on waking, depression, forgetfulness, reduced energy, shortness of breath, muscle and joint pain, lack of self-confidence, headache, migraine, burning micturition, itching labia, vagina discharge, and urine loss. As a group, however, postmenopausal women do not experience more clinical depression than premenopausal women do. Because there is a correlation between the severity of the climacteric symptoms and the rate of bone loss Oldenhave and coworkers[8] hypothesize that "the severity may prove to be a marker of the rate of climacteric bone loss."

Since hot flashes are the consequence of estrogen withdrawal, estrogen is the standard against which all other treatments must be compared. Several double-blind, crossover, placebo-controlled studies have demonstrated the efficacy of estrogen over placebo in treating hot flashes. A prototype of this study was performed by Coope[9] in 1976. (Figure 8.5) A double-blind crossover study of 30 menopausal women was performed by using conjugated equine estrogens (CEE) versus placebo. For the first 3 months the two groups were randomly allocated to either CEE therapy or placebo. The conjugated estrogen (Premarin®)-treated group ingested 1.25 mg daily 21 out of 28 days, with a 7-day gap between each course. The placebo group was given lactose tablets identical in taste and appearance to Premarin. After 3 months each group crossed over to the opposite medication (Figure 8.5). The group initiated with estrogen had a 90% decrease in the average number of hot flashes that returned to baseline when crossed over to placebo. The group initiated with placebo had a 50% reduction that decreased almost 100% when crossed over to Premarin.

One treatment, that of clonidine, does not decrease the number of objective signs of hot flashes but does decrease the perception of hot flashes.[10]

Place and coworkers[11] found in a multicenter, double-blind, randomized, parallel-group clinical trial comparing Premarin to transdermal estradiol showed a similar efficacy with estradiol (Estraderm) and Premarin for hot flashes. Side effects were similar. Medroxyprogesterone acetate[12] megestrol acetate (20 mg twice a day),[13] ethinyl estradiol, and norgestrel[14] also reduce the incidence of hot flashes. In general, estrogen-containing medications are more effective in treating VMS.

Estrogen therapy may have other beneficial effects that are not readily apparent but which patients will relate as "feeling better." Ditkoff and coworkers[15] found an improvement in an income management scale and in the Beck Depression Inventory after Premarin compared with pretreatment testing.

Stress may also be improved. Lindheim and coworkers[16] found that transdermal estrogen therapy blunted the biophysical stress responses to mathematics and speech tasks; it also blunted the

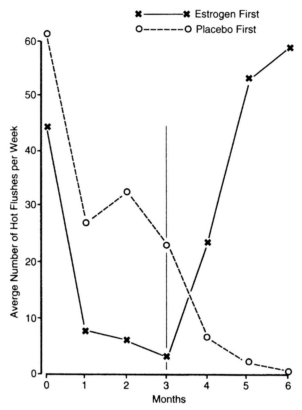

Figure 8.5 Prevalence of hot flushes in 30 postmenopausal women randomly assigned to either placebo or conjugated equine estrogens (CEE) treatment for 3 months and then crossed over to the opposite medication for an additional 3 months in a double-blind clinical trial. (Redrawn from Coope J: Double-blind cross-over study of estrogen replacement therapy, in Campbell S (ed.): *The Management of the Menopause and Post-menopausal Years.* Baltimore, University Park Press. 1976, pp 159–168. Used by permission of the author.)

increases in plasma corticotrophin, cortisol, androstenedione, and norephinephrine compared with placebo and nontreatment baseline. This stress-blunting effect of estrogen may have a protective effect on the cardiovascular system.

Genitourinary Atrophy

Those genitourinary tissues that are embryonically estrogen-dependent remain so for life.[17] Upon estrogen withdrawal, these tissues atrophy. The thick, stratified squamous epithelium of the vaginal mucosa of the reproductive-aged woman regresses to two- to three-cell thickness in the estrogen-deprived postmenopausal woman. Vaginal dryness and atrophy can result and lead to atrophic vaginitis, irritation, and dyspareuria in 20% to 38% of postmenopausal women.[18]

The same happens to the urethral mucosa, with a consequent 30% reduction in urethral closure pressure.[19] The trigone of the bladder attenuates due to atrophy; urinary urgency and frequency can result. The supportive tissues of the pelvic organs weaken and result in a loss of support to the base of the bladder and urethra. The urethrovesical junction may prolapse, thereby removing itself from the abdominal cavity. The vulva, cervix, and uterus decrease in size. The cervix may become flush with the back of the vagina. These changes increase the likelihood of urinary incontinence and inadequate control of urination.

The symptoms of dyspareunia and urinary incontinence need to be explored routinely, aggressively, and empathetically with the patient by the physician. Otherwise, the problems may not be identified because many women feel embarrassed by them.

Most of these changes can be treated by estrogen replacement therapy (ERT).[17,20,21] With ERT the vaginal mucosa thickens, the pH of the vagina decreases, and there is a decrease in vaginal dryness. Estrogen therapy can be delivered either vaginally or orally with the same efficacy. A dosage of 0.3 mg/day of CEE, orally or vaginally, produces a satisfactory therapeutic result in most women with vaginal mucosal atrophy; 0.1 to 0.2 mg of estradiol in a vaginal cream also is effective.[22] Handa and coworkers[23] found that 0.3 mg of CEE 3 times a week was also effective and caused no change in the preexisting atrophic state of the endometrium.

Similarly, ERT has a beneficial effect on the estrogen-dependent tissues of the urinary tract. The urethral mucosa thickens, and the proximal portion of the urethra becomes less prolapsed and returns to the abdominal cavity. Upon return of the proximal part of the urethra to the abdomen, the pelvic diaphragm becomes more effective in preventing the loss of urine with coughing, sneezing, or making any other Valsalva maneuver.[21] Furthermore, once the proximal portion of the urethra becomes more of an abdominal organ, the intra-abdominal pressure is transmitted equally to both the bladder and the urethra[20]. Therefore, a postmenopausal woman with urinary incontinence may benefit from a trial of ERT[19,24]. Approximately 50% will show improvement[21].

In a randomized, double-blind, placebo-controlled, clinical trial of 93 postmenopausal women with recurrent urinary tract infections, by Raz and coworkers[25] the number of urinary tract infections were 0.5 in the estriol-treated group compared with 5.9 episodes per patient-year in the control group (p < 0.001). Lactobacilli bacteria appeared in the vaginas of the treated group but not in the vaginas of the control group.

Skin Changes

The skin after menopause undergos some degree of atrophy and loss of collagen[26-28]. In hypoestrogenic animals the epidermis undergoes atrophy, the number of capillaries decreases, and collagen fibers fragment. In women, skin collagen content declines in relation to menopausal age but not chronological age. Skin thickness tends to decrease at the rate of about 1.2% per year and collagen at the rate of 2.1% per year in early menopause. Estrogen therapy helps the skin of postmenopausal women look healthier. Estrogen decreases the fragmentation in the dermis of estrogen-deficient women and increases the capillaries. The skin thickens, and the skin collagen and water content increases. Brincat and Studd[26] compared a group of postmenopausal women with and without ERT and found that the ERT group had more collagen in their skin than the untreated group. Maheux and coworkers,[27] in a randomized, double-blind, placebo-controlled, 12-month clinical trial found that the Premarin-treated (0.625 mg) group by ultrasonography and biopsy had significant increases in the thickness of the skin and dermis. ERT seems to effect a return of skin thickness and collagen even in late postmenopause and acts prophylactically in early postmenopause. Brincat and Studd[26] suggest that the behavior of the connective tissue element in skin may reflect similar changes in the organic matrix in bone.

Estrogens and Cholecystectomy

ERT doubles the risk of cholecystectomy. In the Nurses' Health Study the risk increased with increasing duration and dosage.[28] The risk continued after discontinuation of ERT: Relative risk (RR) (RR, 1.3; 95% Confidence interval[CI] 1.1–1.6) for postmenopausal women who had stopped taking ERT for 5 or more years. "Estrogen administration decreases bile acid concentration, increases biliary cholesterol and raises the cholesterol saturation of the bile." From the number of cases and women-years of use in the Nurses' Health Study, a crude incidence of 4.0 per 1,000 per year for nonusers and 6.4 per 1,000 per year for users can be calculated.

Cardiovascular Disease

Women have a 31% lifetime chance of dying from coronary artery heart disease (CAHD), 2.8% from breast cancer, 2.8% from an osteoporotic fracture, and 0.7% from endometrial cancer[29]. Therefore any consideration of estrogen's impact on a woman's life must take into account the much greater impact that CAHD has on mortality and quality of life.[30]

Although women live longer than men and their onset of cardiovascular disease (CVD) is 10 to 20 years later than men, more women die from CVD than from cancer, particularly after age 70. If indeed a woman's own endogenous estrogens are cardioprotective until the menopause, then ERT makes rational sense after the menopause (whether natural or surgical).

The published data supports an increased risk of cardiovascular disease after premature ovarian failure and after surgical menopause.[31] The risk is not so clear after natural menopause, perhaps because the age of menopause varies so widely—from age 40 to 58—and the hormonal changes occur over the course of several years.

A review of all relevant major epidemiological studies by Grodstein and Stampfer[32] found a protective effect of exogenous estrogens (mainly Premarin) on CVD.[33] By meta-analysis the overall relative risk for coronary artery disease was 0.65 (95% CI, 0.60–0.70) for women who had ever taken ERT and 0.49 (95% CI, 0.43–0.56) for women currently taking ERT (Figure 8.6). There is evidence to suggest that this protective effect is reduced after discontinuation of the ERT. The largest study to date, the Nurses' Health Study,[34] reported an RR of 0.56 (95% CI, 0.40–0.80) for current users but 0.83 (95% CI, 0.65–1.05) for past users. This protective effect did not seem to be related to duration of use, independent of age. These observations suggest less of a protective effect on a long-term process such as atherosclerosis. However, Bush and coworkers[35] do have

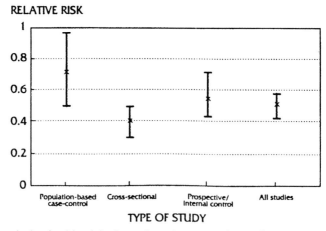

Figure 8.6 Meta-analysis of epidemiologic studies of coronary heart disease and the use of estrogen, current use Relative risk (RR) ± 95% confidence interval (CI). (From Grodstein F, Stampfer M. Estrogen replacement therapy and cardiovascular disease. *Am J Med*, in press; with permission.)

evidence that up to 30% of the protective effect is related to the beneficial effect estrogens have on lipoproteins. The effect that estrogens have on women over the age of 70 is less clear. Krumholtz and coworkers[36] found no correlation between CAHD and total cholesterol (TC) or high-density lipoprotein–cholesterol (HDL-C) in women over 70 years of age.

Estrogens do have a beneficial impact on lipoproteins. Lobo and colleagues[37] at the University of Southern California found that after 1 year of daily Premarin use (0.625 mg), high-density lipoprotein–cholesterol (HDL-C) increased by 13.5% (primarily due to an increase in HDL_2-C), low-density lipoprotein–cholesterol (LDL-C) decreased by 16%, and total cholesterol decreased by 6%. In other studies, apolipoprotein B decreased in most studies, while apolipoprotein A and very low–density lipoproteins–cholesterol (VLDL-C) increased.

Estrogens may have a direct effect on the coronary artery intima that is independent of their effects on lipoproteins. Clarkson, Adams, and colleagues[38-40] at Bowman Gray School of Medicine have been studying the effects of sex hormones on the coronary arteries of cynomolgus monkeys being fed atherogenic diets. Not only did the group treated with estrogen have coronary artery atherosclerotic plaque size half that of the untreated monkeys (Figure 8.7), but in another study the group treated with estrogen had less accumulation of LDL and products of LDL degradation in the intima of the coronary arteries by more than 70%. Mügge and coworkers[41] present some in vitro evidence that estrogens relax *human* coronary artery rings as well.

Some of the estrogen protective effect was demonstrated by Haarbo and coworkers[42] at the University of Copenhagen. They randomized 62 early postmenopausal women to placebo or estradiol valerate combined with a progestin and continued the study for two years. They found that the estrogen–progestin therapy prevented the increase of abdominal fat seen after menopause ($p < 0.05$) (a waist-to-hip ratio of more than 0.8 is a risk factor for coronary heart disease). This effect was independent of the effect on serum lipids and lipoproteins.

Sullivan and coworkers[43] found that the risk of coronary artery disease identified by coronary

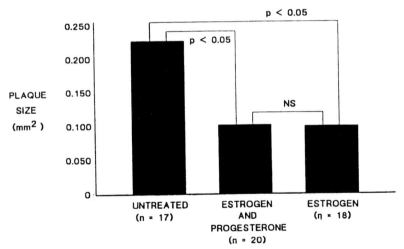

Figure 8.7 Effect of hormone replacement therapy on coronary artery atherosclerosis extent (mm²) in ovariectomized cynomolgus macaques fed a moderately atherogenic diet. Both hormone therapy groups had half the plaque extent of the untreated group. (Adapted from Adams MR: Arterial changes: Estrogen deficiency and effects of hormone replacement, in Lobo RA (ed.): *Treatment of the Post-Menopausal Woman: Basic and Clinical Aspects.* Raven Press, New York, 1994; with permission.) 243–250

arteriography in women using ERT compared to nonusers was 0.44 (95% CI, 0.29–0.67) after adjustment for age, smoking, diabetes, cholesterol level, and hypertension. The authors[44] also found that women with *normal* coronary arteries *did not* benefit from ERT in the 10 years after the catheterization. In contrast, in women with more than 70% coronary artery stenosis in at least one coronary artery or a 50% or greater stenosis of the left main coronary artery, those who had ever taken ERT had a much higher 10-year survival (97%) than those who had never taken ERT (60%) (p < 0.007) (Figure 8.8). Coronary arteriography provides a more accurate measure of coronary artery disease than does history; for example, more than 50% of women with angina pectoris have normal coronary arteries (syndrome x).

Cerebrovascular Disease

According to Grodstein and Stampfer's[32] review of the literature, little impact of estrogens on cerebrovascular disease was demonstrated in the Nurses' Health Study. However, in the Leisure World Study[45] there was a 70% reduction in mortality due to stroke in current users. Finucane and coworkers[46] also found a 70% reduction in stroke mortality.

Progestins

Most studies of ERT to date have too few patients who took progestins along with estrogens to analyze. Psaty and coworkers[47] point out that just as with ERT and CVD, there are no *large* clinical trials (randomized, placebo-controlled, blinded, long-term) for hormone replacement therapy (HRT) and that few studies reported on dosage or duration of use. Such clinical trials would require an extremely large numbers of patients and would extend for 1 to 2 decades.

However, 5 or 10 mg of medroxyprogesterone acetate (Provera®) might have a detrimental effect on the cardiovascular system as it has an adverse effect on lipids. Lobo in a review[37] states that although LDL-C decreases to a degree similar to that seen with Premarin alone, the increase seen in HDL-C levels may be attenuated in women taking continuous Premarin plus Provera.

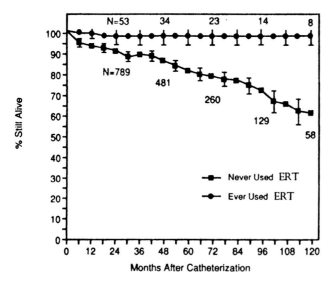

Figure 8.8 Ten-year cumulative survival (actuarial methods) of women with left main coronary stenosis of 50% or greater or other stenosis of 70% or greater. (From Sullivan JM, Vander Zuaag R, Hughes JP, et al: Estrogen replacement and coronary artery disease: Effect on survival in postmenopausal women. *Arch Intern Med* 1990; 140:2557; with permission.)

However, progestins may reverse the increased risk of thrombosis seen with higher doses of estrogens, as might be seen in oral contraceptives, and therefore may be protective. The International Consensus Conference on Postmenopausal Hormone Therapy and the Cardiovascular System[48] concludes that there may be some diminution of the beneficial effects of estrogen on the cardiovascular system with added progestins.

Effect of Varying Dosage, Type, and Delivery of Estrogens

High doses of Premarin (2.5 and 5.0 mg) given to male survivors of myocardial infarctions in the National Cooperative Coronary Drug Project[49,50] in the late 1960s and early 1970s resulted in an excess number of events of nonfatal myocardial infarction, pulmonary embolism, and thrombophlebitis compared with the placebo group. In postmenopausal women the evidence is less clear. The Nurses' Health Study[34] reported an "increase in the risk of coronary disease among women taking more than 1.25 mg/day (RR, 2.8%; 95% CI, 0.9–8.2)." The thrombogenic effects of higher dosages may offset the athero-and direct cardio-protective effect of lower dosages.

Although an "estrogen is an estrogen," conjugated equine estrogens, or Premarin, contain estrogens that are present for months in the circulation. Furthermore, all of the large US epidemiological studies have only been able to analyze the effects of Premarin on the cardiovascular system, as other estrogens have been used so infrequently in the past. We therefore must make judgments based on biochemical data and short-term studies.

Other oral estrogens, such as estradiol, seem to have a similar positive impact on lipoproteins. Transdermal estradiol, on the other hand, seems to have the same effect on LDL-C and total cholesterol as does Premarin, but not on HDL-C. HDL-C and its subfraction HDL_2-C may be more important, at least in women. For example, if a woman has a sustained HDL-C serum level of 55 mg/dl or more, the risk of coronary heart disease is very low, independent of the LDL-C or total cholesterol levels.[51]

Osteoporosis

Without preventive therapy women, as they become hypoestrogenic at menopause, will lose cortical bone at the rate of 1% to 3% per year and trabecular bone at the rate of 2% to 5% per year.[52] After a few years the rate of bone loss decreases, although bone loss continues. As a result osteopenia and osteoporosis can develop, and after 10 to 30 years fractures can result. Osteoporosis leads to fractures in 25% to 40% of women by the age of 70. The life-long risks for wrist fractures is 15%. By the age of 80, 16% of women will have had a hip fracture, a severely debilitating and life-threatening event in the healthy woman over 65.[53] Up to 50% of these older women will die of complications during the first year after a hip fracture, and up to 30% of the survivors may become totally disabled.

Vertebral fractures are twice as common as hip fractures; 20% to 35% of ambulant women over the age of 60 on roentgenograms show evidence of asymptomatic vertebral fractures. Vertebral fractures result in loss of height, pain, and—if severe—deformity and disability.

Bone mass peaks by the mid thirties and then begins to decline (Figure 8.9). Although the hypoestrogenicity of menopause accelerates the rate of bone loss, the rate of hip fractures in the United States begins to rise before menopause, in the early forties. Thin, white women (particularly Scandinavian) and Asian women are at higher risk. Those women with more initial bone mass will have thicker bones that are resistant to fracture later in life. Therefore, healthy living patterns throughout life are

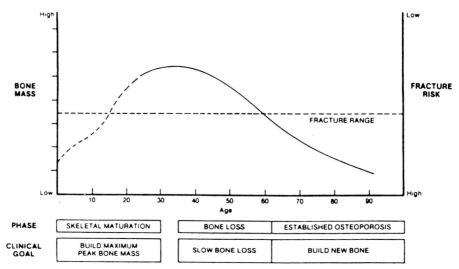

Figure 8.9 The process of bone gain and loss throughout lifetime. Bone mass peaks in early adulthood, and it is lost progressively thereafter. During the first 10 years after menopause, the process of bone loss is accelerated. (From Bilezikian JP, Silverberg SJ: Osteoporosis: A practical approach to the perimenopausal woman. *J Women's Health* 1992; 1:21–27, with permission.)

beneficial to bone: a good calcium intake (1,000 to 1,500 mg every day), a good weight-bearing exercise experience, and avoidance of excess alcohol and cigarette smoking.

Remodeling of bone takes place constantly. Osteoclasts break bone down and osteoblasts rebuild. A balanced state is dependent on the net calcium balance which in turn is dependent on availability of calcium, parathyroid hormone regulated intestinal absorption and renal excretion of calcium, weight-bearing stress on the bone and sex hormones (estrogen in the female and testosterone in the male). Collagen and other factors are also involved in bone metabolism. Alcohol and smoking, as mentioned above, can adversely effect this balance as well. Genetics and family history are not as potent nor as predictive as the above personal living styles.

Prevention of Bone Loss and Fractures by Estrogen Replacement Therapy

Both estrogens and progestins help to maintain calcium and bone dynamic balance and therefore prevent osteoporosis and fractures. This estrogen can be delivered orally in any type or transdermally and have a net positive effect. Most studies show about a 50% reduction of osteoporosis or fractures in current users of ERT. Since most women who choose ERT use it only for 2 to 3 years the effect is probably more a delaying action on the risk of fractures by the number of years of ingestion.[54] For example, Christensen and coworkers[55] found a positive bone mineral balance in women who ingested a combination estrogen–progestin pill for 2 years (Figure 8.10). The placebo group was in negative balance during these 2 years. After crossover, the former users entered negative balance on placebo and the former placebo users entered positive balance on the treatment. This study and others even suggest a favorable impact on the age-related steady loss of bone density experienced by women after their mid-thirties; however, there are no large long-term prospective studies to address this question in perimenopausal women.

The longer ERT is used the longer the persistence of a protective effect, as long as the requisite calcium intake is maintained. Also, Ettinger and coworkers[56] found a suggestion of a dose-response

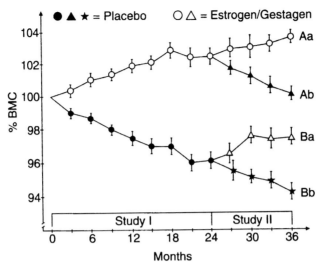

Figure 8.10 Bone mineral content (BMC) as a function of time and treatment in women who had passed through natural menopause 6 months to 3 years before. The estrogen was a combination of estradiol, 4 mg, and estriol, 2 mg, and norethindrone acetate 1 mg or placebo. (Redrawn from Christensen C, Christensen MS, Transboel IB. Bone mass in postmenopausal woman after withdrawal of oestrogen/gestagen replacement therapy. *Lancet* 1981;2:459. Used by permission of C. Christensen.)

effect; subjects ingested at least 1,500 mg of calcium and oral estradiol or placebo (Figure 8.11). Women with intact uteri were given medroxyprotesterone acetate. "In the placebo group spinal trabecular bone density decreased 4.9% annually (P < 0.001)," while there was an increase in spinal trabecular bone density seen in the 0.5 mg 17β-estradiol group, which was significantly different from the placebo group (P < 0.001), suggesting efficacy even with such a low dose. Previous studies with Premarin suggest that one must use a dose of 0.625 mg or higher for full efficacy[57].

Who Should Receive Estrogen Replacement Therapy?

Do the bones of menstruating perimenopausal women benefit from ERT? Gambacciani and coworkers found that they do in the subgroup with oligomenorrhea but not in normal cycling women. The authors used low-dose oral contraceptives (20 μg ethinyl estradiol plus 150 μg desogestrel) in a 2-year follow-up study. Elders and coworkers[59] found that calcium supplementation alone with 1,000 mg and 2,000 mg elemental calcium a day in perimenopausal women reduces the loss of lumbar bone to 1.3% and 0.7%, respectively, the first year, compared with 3.5% for the untreated control group, but that bone turnover balance was still negative.

Very few studies have been done in women over the age of 65. Using markers of bone formation, Prestwood and coworkers[60] found that in 11 women (mean age of 77 years) given Premarin (0.625 mg for 6 weeks) bone turnover was reduced.

Postmenopausal women should increase their calcium intake, according to Reid and coworkers.[61] The mean calcium intake in women 19 to 34 years of age is 670 mg/day, and in women 35 to 50 it is 550 mg/day, far lower than the recommended 1,000–1,500 mg daily.

In a 2-year study of 122 women ingesting an average of 750 mg/day of calcium at least 3 years after the menopause, Reid and coworkers[61] found a 43% lower rate of total-body bone mineral

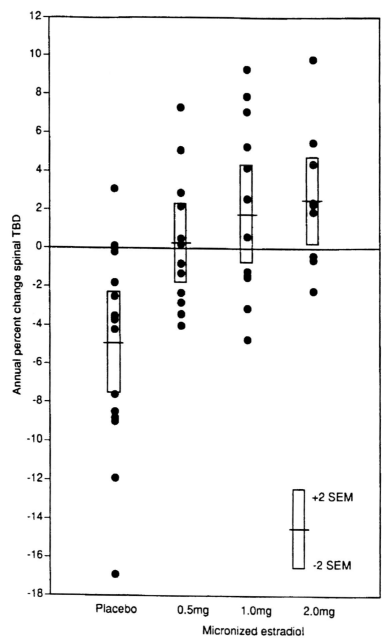

Figure 8.11 Changes in mean (± 2 standard error of the mean) annual percentage and each subject's spinal trabecular bone density (total bone density TBD) in 46 postmenopausal women given micronized estradiol (phase1). All subjects received calcium supplements. (From Ettinger B, Genant HK, Steiger P, Madvig P: Low-dosage micronized 17β-estradiol prevents bone loss in postmenopausal women. *Am J Obstet Gynecol* 1992;166:479–488; with permission.)

density loss in the women given a 1,000-mg supplement of calcium compared with the placebo group.

However, calcium is not enough for women at high risk of osteoporosis. Who is at high risk? Although genetic and family history of osteoporosis are slightly helpful, other personal health-style practices and body mass index (BMI) as discussed earlier are more important. Grisso and coworkers[62] also found that "among black women, thinness, previous stroke, use of aids in walking, and alcohol consumption are associated with an increased risk of hip fracture." "Postmenopausal estrogen therapy for 1 year or more was protective for women under 75 years of age (odds ratio, 0.1; 95% CI, < 0.1 to 0.5)." How cost-effective is screening high-risk women using bone mineral density studies, such as dual energy X-ray absorptiometry, remains to be evaluated.

ERT and Endometrial Cancer

Endometrium, exposed to estrogen without any progestin, over the course of years may undergo hyperplasia that can progress to adenomatous hyperplasia, atypical hyperplasia, and finally in situ carcinoma. These pathological changes will progress to frank endometrial cancer 1%, 27%, 81%, and 100% of the time, respectively, if no intervention occurs.[63] They also will regress if treated with progestins 100%, 100%, 70%, and less than 50% of the time, respectively. Progestins control the endometrial gland cell mitoses induced by estrogen.

Women at risk for endometrial carcinoma are those that are overweight, diabetic, hirsute, or amenorrheic: those conditions that are associated with endogenous estrogens or androgens unopposed with progesterone. Term pregnancy, high cholesterol levels, smoking[64] and combination birth control pills, on the other hand, are protective.

In the United States endometrial carcinoma is reported in 33,000 women each year, resulting in 5,500 deaths. About 1 woman in 36 will develop endometrial cancer in her lifetime and after the age of 50, 1 per 1,000 white women will develop endometrial cancer per year.

Estrogen therapy enjoyed three decades (1942–1975) without any recognized serious side effects. Then, in 1975, large case-control studies began reporting an increased risk of endometrial cancer in users. These risks were not affected by whether the estrogen was taken intermittently, cyclically, or continuously, but did show a dose response and an increase with duration of use (Figure 8.12). The RR ranged from 1.7 to 20, depending on the duration of use. Many women stopped ERT.

Chu and coworkers[65] reported a better 4-year survival rate in women with endometrial cancer who were using estrogens compared with those who were not (Figure 8.13). The explanation lay in the low level of malignancy in most of the estrogen-related cancers; estrogen seems to induce endometrial cancers of low stage and grade, although the risk of more advanced endometrial carcinoma is also increased. In general, a routine pretreatment endometrial biopsy in an asymptomatic woman who plans to take estrogen without a progestin need not be performed since the prevalence of endometrial cancer in asymptomatic women is so low (less than 1 per 1,000). However, in women taking unopposed estrogens the risk of endometrial cancer increases sevenfold after 10 years of use. Furthermore, after at least one year of use 20% to 30% will have developed endometrial hyperplasia. Therefore, yearly vaginal ultrasonography to evaluate endometrial thickness or endometrial biopsies might be considered. How aggressively one should monitor the endometrium is also influenced by the observation that 75% to 90% of all women who develop early-stage endometrial cancer do become symptomatic; that is, they have abnormal bleeding.

Estrogen-induced endometrial tumors can be completely prevented by the addition of at least 13 days of a progestin per month. The protective effect of a progestin seems to be more related to the duration of ingestion than the dosage or whether or not withdrawal bleeding occurs. Moyer

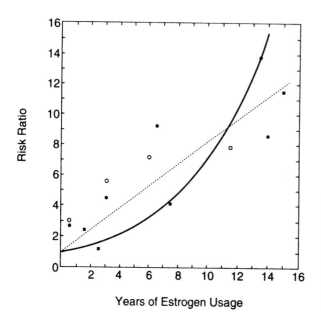

Figure 8.12 Dose response between the risk ratio for endometrial cancer and the length of estrogen usage: linear fit (*dotted line*) vs. exponential fit (*solid line.*) (Redrawn from Cramer DW, Knapp RC: Review of epidemiologic studies of endometrial cancer and exogenous estrogen. *Obstet Gynecol* 1979;54:521–526.

and coworkers[66] found that a low dosage of an estrogen plus at least 9 days of a progestin per month prevented bleeding *and* reduced to almost zero the mitotic activity of the endometrium. Therefore, the goal of HRT is to induce amenorrhea for patient satisfaction and convert the endometrium to a atrophic state to prevent endometrial adenocarcinoma. Unfortunately, just as the protective effect of oral contraceptives lasts 5 to 10 years after discontinuation, so does the adverse effect of unopposed estrogens on the endometrium last at least 6 years after discontinuation.

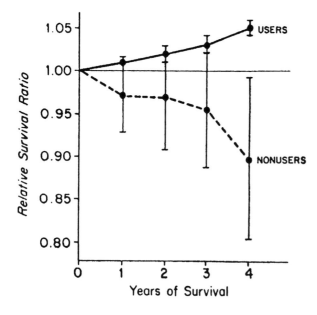

Figure 8.13 Annual relative survival ratio with 95% confidence intervals. (From Chu J, Schweid AI, Weiss NS: Survival among women with endometrial cancer: A comparison of estrogen users and nonusers. *Am J Obstet Gynecol*, 1982;143:569–573 with permission.)

Estrogens and Breast Cancer

Breast cancer is hormonally responsive and probably hormonally induced. The presence of estrogen and progesterone receptors (both dependent on estrogen) are predictive of the cancer's response to palliative hormonal therapy. Tamoxifen, an antiestrogen, has a life-prolonging effect on women with breast cancer. Pregnancy, a hormonally rich event, has a long-term preventive effect in contrast to an induced abortion, which increases the risk of breast cancer. Breast cells and their oncogenic potential seem responsive to these different hormonal milieu; however, the exact role that estrogen and progesterone play in the induction of breast cancer has not been clarified. The question germane to this discussion is: Does low-dose estrogen therapy increase the risk for breast cancer, and what effect do progestins have?

Epidemiology

Breast cancer is the most important and common cancer in women who do not smoke, with a mortality approaching 25%.[67] About 1 in 9 women will eventually get breast cancer, and about 2.8% of all women will die from it. The attack rate is 2 to 3 per 1,000 per year after the age of 50. Although the risk of breast cancer increases with age, some women die from breast cancer at a young age. In the United States, 175,000 new cases are diagnosed each year, and there are 44,500 deaths.

Risk of Breast Cancer: Those Treated with Estrogen Replacement Therapy

Colditz and other investigators in the Nurses' Health Study[68] report in their meta-analysis of 1993 a 40% increase risk of breast cancer (RR, 1.40; 95% CI, 1.20–1.63) in current users. Former users and women with fewer than 5 years of ERT had no increased risk; the risk associated with current use seems to disappear after 2 years. However, an increase of 20% to 30% was found in women who had taken ERT for 10 to 15 years or more, respectively. A family history of breast cancer or benign breast tumors or bilateral oophorectomy had no apparent effect on these relationships.

The authors point out that they "cannot rule out some detection bias contributing to this elevated risk" since women who elect ERT are more likely to see a physician more often and thereby be screened for breast cancer more often. Therefore their breast cancers would be discovered earlier, inflating the number of cancers in the user group. The theoretical advantage of this earlier discovery, of course, is a better survival rate in users, which has been reported, albeit inconclusively.

The use of progestins in combination with ERT in the meta-analysis above lowered the risk to 1.13, although it was not significantly elevated (95% CI 0.78–1.64).

Not all of the other five meta-analyses through 1993 agree; three found no increased risk. This may be partly explained by the lack of distinction between current and past ERT.

Any increase risk for breast cancer, of course, is of great concern to women who must decide whether or not to take estrogens. However, again, if the risk is real, it is low; it is not present until after 5 years of use, it diminishes rapidly after discontinuation; and users have a better survival rate. There also is the concern that since there is such a large heterogeneity in the studies used in the meta-analyses a low risk may not ever be able to be accurately evaluated.

Benefits versus Risks

There are two reasons postmenopausal women may wish to consider ERT: treatment and prevention.[69,70] ERT is effective in reducing vasomotor symptoms and insomnia and in improving general well-being, dyspareunia due to vaginal dryness, and urinary tract infections.

A healthy, 50-year-old woman has a life expectancy of 83 years. Would she benefit from 25 years of ERT? She has a 46% chance of getting heart disease and a 31% chance of dying of it (Table 8.1). She also has a 15% chance of getting a hip fracture and a 2.8% chance of dying of it. To date, the data suggest that those risks could be cut in half with only a small increased risk of breast and endometrial cancer. From both a personal and public health view it makes sense for her to take ERT for 25 or more years (although no study has such long-term data to confirm this). Gorsky and coworkers[71] also point to a gain of "3951 quality-adjusted life years" for 10,000 women taking estrogens for 25 years compared with women not using estrogens. Of note is the observation that the preventive use of ERT is beneficial only *while* she is currently taking the medication. Therefore, she must continue the ERT as long as she wishes to take advantage of the protective effect.

On the other hand, if she is in good health, has no medical diseases—such as diabetes or hypertension—does not smoke, eats only 25% of total calories as fat that is mostly unsaturated, avoids partially hydrogenated vegetable oils, exercises, has a gynoid waist-to-hip ratio less than 0.8, has an HDL cholesterol 60 or greater, has no history of coronary artery disease, and has normal bone-density studies she probably would not benefit from long-term ERT.

The woman who smokes would benefit from stopping; ERT probably would be of benefit (possibly in higher doses). The woman with heart disease or osteoporosis would benefit from ERT in preventing further deterioration.

Fear of Estrogens

So if on balance it appears that estrogen has a net beneficial effect why aren't more than 5% to 10% of postmenopausal women currently taking estrogens? Some women have a general fear of all medications and shy away from traditional medicine. They might say that estrogens taken by mouth and acted on by the gastrointestinal tract and liver are not really the same as the more natural ovarian production of estrogens. Some women are so afraid of cancer that even a small increased risk of breast or endometrial cancer may loom large. Other women are fearful of the side effects—nausea, bloating, painful breasts, and bleeding—and now that they are into the menopause really do not want to go back and experience those hormonal effects again. Since less than 10% of women take ERT, few of their friends take ERT. There may be a fear of commitment; that is, once started the medications must be continued for decades to be effective. There can be a fear of dependency. Bewley and Bewley report that "oestrogens are psychoactive: they lift mood, can be given by injection, and their use has powerful psychological effects." Some women can get into a cycle of increasing dosages with tolerance and withdrawal symptoms.

Physicians may be concerned about prescribing estrogens for several reasons. It has been felt from animal experiments, that estrogens increase the risk of breast cancer, even before the epidemiological data became available in humans. The coronary drug project at Framingham[49,50] suggested that male survivors of myocardial infarctions (MIs) do poorly on ERT, particularly in the higher doses of 2.5 and 5.0 mg CEE per day. If estrogens increase the adverse effects in male survivors of MIs, are estrogens really safe in women? Birth control pills at the higher doses used in the 1960s increased the risk of myocardial infarction in women who were over the age of 35 and who smoked. Therefore, if birth control pills can increase the risk of myocardial infarction, why would not ERT do the same? Part of the answer is that birth control pills have a much higher potency, probably 2 to 5 times higher than ERT. The higher doses may indeed increase the risk for coagulation and cardiovascular disease, while current lower doses do not. Also, smoking has profound effects and probably has a synergistic adverse effect on the cardiovascular system when used with oral contraceptives. This does not seem to be the case with the less potent ERT preparations.

Table 8.1 Risks versus Benefits of Estrogen Replacement Therapy

	Annual no. of new cases	Annual no. of hospitalizations (1988)	Annual no. of deaths	Annual rate of new cases per 1000 (increases with age)	Lifetime risk of getting the disease (%)	Lifetime risk of dying from the disease (%)	Theoretical additional cases prevented (+) or caused (−) by ERT annually*	Theoretical additional deaths prevented (+) or caused (−) by ERT annually*
Coronary artery disease	400,000†	250,000‡	200,000‡	8–10	46	31	+200,000	+100,000
Osteoporosis-related fractures	1,300,000	204,000	40,000	1–30 (hip)	15 (hip)	2.8 (hip)	+650,000	+20,000
Endometrial cancer	33,000	34,000	5,500	1	3	0.7	−99,000	−16,650
Breast cancer	175,000	161,000	44,500	2–5	9	2.8	−52,500	−13,350
Total							+698,500	+90,000

*Based on relative risk (RR) 0.5, 0.5, 4.0, and 1.3, respectively.

Assuming *all* postmenopausal women would take 0.625 mg conjugated equine estrogens (CEE) daily with no progestogen.

†Manson JE et al: The primary prevention of myocardial infarction. *N Engl J Med* 1992;326:1406–1416; *Arch Intern Med* 1989;149:2445–2448; *Am J Obstet Gynecol* 1991;164:165–174; and Paganini-Hill A: (chpt title) in Lobo RA (ed.): Morbidity and Mortality changes with estrogen replacement therapy. *Treatment of the Postmenopausal Woman: Basic and Clinical Aspects*. New York, Raven Press, 1994.

‡Estimated from *MMWR* July 31, 1992, Trends in ischemic heart disease mortality—United States, 1980–1988; Vol 41(30):548–556.

Estrogen, Progestin, and Other Pharmaceutical Preparations

Premarin in daily oral doses of 0.625 mg is the gold standard with which all other estrogen preparations must be compared, at least in the United States. Most of the epidemiological studies on which we draw our conclusions are based on Premarin, since it has been the major source of estrogen usage in the United States for many years. Because these data sets are large and of long duration, we can generally conclude that 0.625 mg/day is more effective than 0.3 mg/day and safer than 1.25 mg/day. Little can be said about other estrogens from an epidemiologic point of view, since the numbers of patients treated are so much smaller. Unfortunately, most US studies also cannot say much about the progestins and their effects on the coronary arteries and breast because of the small number of users. Most of our understanding of other estrogens and of the progestins come from smaller data bases, indirect biochemical surrogates, and inferences. According to the 1994 Physicians' Desk Reference, Premarin is currently an extraction of "sodium salts of water-soluble estrogen sulfates blended to represent the average composition of material derived from pregnant mares' urine. It contains estrone, equilin, and 17α-dihydroequilin, together with smaller amounts of 17β-estradiol, equilenin and 17α-dihydoequilenin as salts of their sulfate esters." The source of the Premarin that the epidemiologic studies were based on was pregnant mares' urine. Equilin and equilenin do not occur naturally in the circulation of the human female. One of equilin's metabolites, 17β-equilin sulfate, is extremely potent and its unconjugated form, 17β-equilin, has a high affinity for endometrial estrogen receptors. Therefore, according to Bhavnani Cecutli,[73] "the major *in vivo* activity of equilin sulfate present in conjugated equine estrogen preparations is expressed via its metabolites 17β-dihydroequilin sulfate and 17β-dihydroequilin." Another example of a difference is the half-life. Although estrone and estradiol are cleared from the body in a matter of days, equilin is still measurable in the serum 13 weeks after the last tablet (at 144 pg/ml in one study).[74]

Comparing other estrogens with Premarin therefore is difficult. We are interested in identifying those estrogens and dosages that have the same protective effects as 0.625 mg/day Premarin on coronary artery disease and osteoporosis, while keeping the risks for breast cancer, endometrial cancer, and endometrial bleeding as low as possible.

Mashchak and coworkers[75] used serum FSH changes and liver globulin production to get some sense of relative potency among four oral preparations. Although there were some inconsistencies in the data, the lowest dosages they identified as having no undesirable impact on the liver were 1.25 mg of estropipate (Ogen®), 1.0 mg of micronized estradiol (Estrace®), and 0.3 mg of conjugated estrogens. Ethinyl estradiol (Estinyl®) was difficult to access due to lack of parallelism, but from its relative effect on serum angiotensinogen the equivalent dose would be about 5 µg of ethinyl estradiol.

Although the addition of a progestin to the estrogen regimen has a protective effect on the endometrium, its effect on bone and the cardiovascular system has only been studied on a limited scale. Lufkin and coworkers[70] randomly assigned postmenopausal women with one or more vertebral fractures to either a 0.1-mg transdermal estradiol patch (Estraderm®) designed to cause the absorption of 100 µg of estradiol into the circulation each day and 11 days per month of 10 mg medroxyprogesterone acetate (MPA), or a placebo. Compared with 39 women assigned to placebo, the 36 women assigned to the Estraderm and MPA had a lower vertebral fracture rate (RR, 0.39; 95% CI, 0.16–0.95).

The effect of progestins on lipoproteins may be adverse to or may counter the beneficial effects observed with estrogen alone. Luciano and coworkers[116] found that the addition—to 0.625 mg of CEE—of a low-dose progestin (MPA 2.5 mg or 5.0 mg daily for 12 days of each 25-day treatment cycle or 5.0 mg/day, continuously) resulted in an increase in HDL-C and decreases in LDL-C and total cholesterol, all favorable changes. However, in a review Lobo[77] points out that MPA attenuates the beneficial effects on lipoproteins in a dose-related reduction, and even a dosage of MPA as low as 5 mg/day attenuates some of the increases in estrogen-induced HDL-C. Other 19-nortestosterone derived progestins may have even a greater adverse impact. Crook and coworkers[78], for example, found a *decrease* in HDL-C when 150 µg cyclic dl-norgestrel was added to CEE 0.625 mg/day or norethindrone acetate 250 µg/day was added to the 50 µg/day transdermal estradiol patch, despite a favorable effect on total-C and LDL-C (both decreased). These studies suggest a low enough dosage of progestin (such as MPA 2.5 mg/day or micronized progesterone) might be found that will have beneficial effects on the endometrium without adverse effects on the bone or coronary arteries. More studies are needed. For the present, higher dosages or more potent progestins should be avoided, if possible.

Wiklund and coworkers[79] from Sweden randomized 242 women to the 50 µg/day estradiol transdermal patch or placebo. They measured quality of life changes and found a marked improvement in both groups, but more so in the estrogen-treated group, particularly health-related quality of life (P = 0.0003) and well-being (P = 0.003).

When a progestin is added to reduce the risk of endometrial cancer it also increases the occurrence of bleeding. Hillard and coworkers[80] in London used a protocol of continuous daily combined 0.625 mg CEE/5mg MPA or 350 µg norethindrone acetate for 78 weeks in 79 postmenopausal women. They were switched over from a previous sequential estrogen–protestogen treatment. Although the endometrium of most of the women was atrophic, 67% of the women had withdrawn from the study mainly because of chronic irregular bleeding, while about 70% of those still continuing had developed amenorrhea. The authors concluded that "women with persistent early bleeding should probably revert to sequential treatment"; at least the bleeding then would be predictable and 85% will have regular uterine bleeding. An alternative was presented by Spaulding.[81] Those women taking 0.625 mg Premarin plus 2.5 mg/day Provera who bled were first switched to 5.0 mg/day Provera. In the 13% who continued to bleed, endometrial ablation was successfully performed.

In a one-year, double-blind, multicenter study Archer and Pickar[82] randomized 1,724 postmenopausal women to 0.625 mg/day Premarin plus 2.5 or 5.0 mg/day MPA, 5.0 or 10.0 mg MPA sequentially or placebo. Breakthrough bleeding or spotting occurred in 27% to 38% of the cycles on continuous combined therapy, in 17% to 19% of the cycles on sequential therapy; and in 24% of the cycles on Premarin with placebo (Figure 8.14). Breakthrough bleeding tended to increase with time in the estrogen-alone group, decrease in the continuous group, and slightly decrease or stabilize early in the sequential groups (Table 8.2). Cycles with no bleeding at all occurred in 61% to 73% of the combined continuous group, 16% to 19% of the sequential groups, and in 76% of the estrogen-alone group. Withdrawal bleeding or spotting occurred in 77% to 81% of the cycles of the combined continuous group.

Another alternative is to give the progestin for 2 weeks every 3 months, with the endometrium being evaluated annually. In a 4-year study, Williams and coworkers[83] found hyperplasia at 2 years in 2 of 50 women who took 2 to 4 weeks of 10 mg MPA every 3 months along with CEE 0.625 mg/day. An elevation of HDL-lipoprotein cholesterol that was seen prior to MPA returned to baseline immediately after MPA. There were fewer days of bleeding in the women given the progestin for 14 days every 3 months compared with women given the progestin every month. According to Ettinger and coworkers,[84] in a similar study, "women preferred the quarterly regimen by nearly four to one."

Why Not Give Estrogens Alone, Without Progestins?

This would result in much fewer problems with bleeding, the number one reason why women stop using HRT. Any postmenopausal woman without a uterus and on ERT need not take progestins.

Table 8.2 Number of Cycles with Breakthrough Bleeding (Excludes Cycles with Breakthrough Spotting Only)

| | Continuous treatment group | | Sequential group | | Estrogen alone |
Cycle	CEE + 2.5 MPA	CEE + 5 MPA	CEE + 5MPA	CEE + 10 MPA	CEE + placebo
2	107 (34%)	71 (23%)	36 (11%)	33 (10%)	26 (8%)
5	63 (21%)	32 (11%)	32 (11%)	23 (8%)	46 (16%)
8	54 (19%)	23 (8%)	20 (7%)	18 (6%)	37 (14%)
11	36 (13%)	16 (6%)	22 (8%)	22 (8%)	45 (18%)
Total no. of cycles	844 (22%)	475 (13%)	307 (8%)	311 (8%)	532 (15%)

CEE, Conjugated equine estrogens; MPA, medroxyprogesterone acetate.

In women with a uterus the decision is not so clear. Since progestins are not necesssary for ERT's prevention of osteoporosis and since they may even have a detrimental effect on coronary artery disease, the net gain to life expectancy by giving estrogens alone probably would be a positive one, particularly if more women would find ERT acceptable. Each individual patient and her physician must struggle with this issue until a clearer consensus is reached.

Estradiol

Estradiol, the naturally occurring and most potent estrogen in the human female, can be given orally, vaginally, transdermally, or intramuscularly. Oral preparations of estradiol are micronized and provided in 1-, 2-, or 4-mg (1,000 to 4,000 μg) tablets. One or two 1-mg tablets are usually enough to treat the vasomotor symptoms of most women: however, sometimes as much as 4 mg of estradiol must be used orally per day[85]. Approximately 90% of the estradiol is converted by the gastrointestinal tract and liver to estrone and estrone sulfate, and only 10% of the unconjugated estrogens in the serum remain as estradiol.[86] This is in contrast to parenterally administered estradiol in which the serum levels of estradiol are the dominate form of the absorbed unconjugated estrogens and there is much less impact on liver globulins.

Vaginal estradiol is provided as a cream in a calibrated applicator. One gram of preparation contains 100 μg of estradiol, which results in peak blood levels of 50 to 100 pg/ml of estradiol 2 to 12 hours after insertion. One hundred to 200 μg of vaginal estradiol is usually effective in controlling vasomotor symptoms; titration can be accomplished by adjusting the nightly dose of vaginal estradiol to her symptoms. Vaginal estradiol and transdermal estradiol are particularly effective in women who do not respond well to oral CEEs.

Transdermal Estradiol

Estradiol transdermal patches are supplied in two different dosages. Estraderm 0.05 has a contact surface of 10 cm^2 and contains 4 mg of estradiol. The 0.05 refers to the number of milligrams of estradiol delivered per day to the circulation. The second dosage is Estraderm 0.1, which has a 20-cm^2 contact surface, contains 8 mg of estradiol, and delivers 0.1 mg of 100 μg of estradiol to the circulation per day. One or two patches are used at one time and are changed twice a week. Mild skin irritation occurs in about 30% of patients.

Injectable Estradiols

Estradiol valerate or estradiol cypionate are injectable estradiols and are given once a month. For example, 1 mg of estradiol valerate can be given intramuscularly once a month. The serum levels of estradiol are initially quite elevated, rapidly fall over the course of 2 weeks, and taper off by 4 weeks. Other methods, because of their more steady serum levels, are preferable.

Progestins

Regular monthly bleeding is the major side effect of the addition of progestins to ERT. Other side effects include breast tenderness, bloating, edema, abdominal cramps, anxiety, irritability, depression, and a premenstrual tension–like syndrome. Prior and coworkers,[87] however, found no more symptoms with low-dose medroxyprogesterone acetate than with placebo. A small percentage of patients cannot take progestins at all because of the side effects. The C-19 nortestosterone derivatives, norgestrel, norethindrone, and norethindrone acetate tend to be androgenic and associated with acne and greasy skin and hair, although in low dosage this effect tends to disappear. The C-21 derivative medroxyprogesterone acetate is associated with depression and anxiety. Oral micronized progesterone requires high dosages and multiple divided ingestions because of a short half-life and causes drowsiness in a number of patients. Transdermal norethindrone acetate in preliminary trials shows some promise. To reduce side effects, reduce the dosage or use an alternative progestin with lower potency. Oral norethindrone, 0.35 mg/day, is an alternative to Provera, but it has a greater detrimental effect of lipoproteins.

The incidence of withdrawal bleeding with each cycle of unopposed estrogen regimens is approximately 25%. When progestins are added, about 85% of women will have regular monthly withdrawal bleeding.

Androgens

The ovaries continue to produce androgens after menopause (albeit somewhat less). Therefore, there probably would be little benefit in adding androgens to ERT for women with intact ovaries. In women with both ovaries removed, the efficacy, safety, and dosage of androgens have not been determined. Sherwin and coworkers[88] at McGill University in Montreal have found that androgens enhance the intensity of sexual desire and arousal and the frequency of sexual fantasies, but not sexual activity per se in oophorectomized women. The measurement of serum levels of testosterone may be helpful as well. If androgen therapy is to be used, natural testosterone would be preferable, particularly if titrated to a level not only of improved symptomatology but also to physiological blood levels of testosterone. Just as there may be detrimental effects on the cardiovascular system with high dosages of estrogen, so might there be disadvantages with supraphysiological dosages of androgens.

Calcium Supplements

It is recommended that women take 1,000 to 1,500 mg/day of calcium from the teen years throughout their lives. Retail sales of calcium supplements totaled more than $77 million in 1987.[23] There are some 40 different calcium supplements available. There appears to be no difference in the amount of calcium absorbed from the various calcium salts in the commercial supplements, milk, and calcium-fortified orange juice. Therefore, the main basis for comparison is the cost. According to Hegarty and Stewart,[23] the cost per year of the various sources of calcium that would provide 800 mg/day of calcium ranged, in January 1988 in Houston, from $11 to $412 per year. Milk, which has other benefits as well, was $175 to $266. A practical approach is to ingest one calcium carbonate tablet (such as Tum's® or Rolaids®) with each meal as a supplement. Each Tum's tablet contains 200 mg of elemental calcium; a Rolaids tablet contains 165 mg of elemental calcium.

Other Therapeutic Approaches

Tamoxifen has been shown to be effective in a pilot trial of tamoxifen versus placebo. Powles observed a reduction in LDL cholesterol and apolipoprotein B with tamoxifen.[89] There is some evidence that postmenopausal bone loss may be reduced by tamoxifen and that tamoxifen is estrogenic rather than antiestrogenic on the female genital tract.[90,91] Bellergal has also been used for symptomatic relief.

Transdermal Clonidine

A randomized, prospective, double-blind, placebo-controlled study of transdermal clonidine demonstrated a highly significant reduction in the number of perceived hot flashes, few side effects, and no significant effect on blood pressure[10,92].

References

1. Tobacman JK, Tucker MA, Kase R, Greene MH, Costa J, Fraumeni JLJ. Intraabdominal carcinomatosis after prophylactic oophorectomy in ovarian cancer prone families. Lancet 1982;ii:795.
2. Oldenhave A, Jaszmann LJB, Everaerd WTAM, Haspels AA. Hysterectomized women with ovarian conservation report more severe climacteric complaints than do normal climacteric women of similar age. Am J Obstet Gynecol 1993;168(3):765-71.
3. Dewhurst CJ. Campbell S, (ed.): Frequency and severity of menopausal symptoms. In: The Management of the Menopause and Post-menopausal Years. (University Park Press: Baltimore), 1976: 25–27.
4. Kronenberg F. Hot Flashes. In: Lobo RA, (ed.): Treatment of the Postmenopausal Woman: Basic and Clinical Aspects. New York: Raven Press, 1994, pp. 97–117.
5. Erlik Y, Meldrum DR, Judd HL. Estrogen levels in postmenopausal women with hot flashes. Obstet Gynecol 1982; 59(4):403–07.
6. Martin MC, Block JE, Sanchez SD, Arnaud CD, Beyene Y. Menopause without symptoms: The endocrinology of menopause among rural Mayan Indians. Am J Obstet Gynecol 1993;168:1839–45.
7. Meldrum DR, Tataryn IV, Frumar AM, Erlik Y, Lu KL, Judd HL. Gonadotropins, estrogens, and adrenal steroids during the menopausal hot flash. J Clin Endocrinol Metab 1980;50:685–689.
8. Oldenhave A, Jaszmann LJB, Haspels AA, Everaerd WTAM. Impact of climacteric on well-being. Am J Obstet Gynecol 1993;168(3):772–80.
9. Coope J. Double-blind cross-over study of estrogen replacement therapy. In: Campbell S, ed. The Management of the Menopause and Post-menopausal Years. Baltimore: University Park Press, 1976: 159–168.
10. Laufer LR, Erlik Y, Meldrum DR, et al: Obstet Gynecol 1982; 60:583.
11. Place VA, Powers M, Darley PE, Schenkel L, Good WR. A double-blind comparative study of Estraderm and Premarin in the amelioration of postmenopausal symptoms. Am J Obstet Gynecol 1985;152:1092–9.
12. Bullock JL, Massey FM, Gambrell RD Jr. Use of medroxyprogesterone acetate to prevent menopausal symptoms. Obstet Gynecol 1975; 46:165–8.
13. Loprinzi CL, Michalak JC, Quella SK, et al. Megestrol acetate for the prevention of hot flashes. N Engl J Med 1994;331(6):347–352.
14. Dennerstein L, Burrows GD, Hyman G, Wood C. Menopausal hot flushes: A double blind comparison of placebo, ethinyl oestradiol and norgestrel. Br J Obstet Gynaecol 1978;85(11):852–56.
15. Ditkoff EC, Crary WG, Cristo M, Lobo RA. Estrogen improves psychological function in asymptomatic postmenopausal women. Obstet Gynecol 1991;78(6):991–95.
16. Lindheim SR, Legro RS, Bernstein L, et al. Behavioral stress responses in premenopausal and postmenopausal women and the effects of estrogen. Am J Obstet Gynecol 1992;167:1831–6.
17. Bergman A, Brenner PF. Beneficial effects of pharmacologic agents—genitourinary. In: Mishell DR Jr., ed. Menopause: Physiology and Pharmacology. Chicago: Yearbook Medical Publishers, Inc., 1987, pp 151–164.
18. Bachmann GA. Vulvovaginal complaints. In: Lobo RA, ed. Treatment of the Postmenopausal Woman: Basic and Clinical Aspects. New York: Raven Press, 1994, pp. 137–42.
19. Reed T. Urethral pressure profile in continent women from childbirth to old age. Acta Obstet Gynecol Scand 1980;59:331.
20. Bergman A, Brenner PF. Alterations in the urogenital system. In: Mishell DR Jr., ed. Menopause: Physiology and Pharmacology. Chicago: Yearbook Medical Publishers, Inc., 1987, pp. 67–75.
21. Hilton P. The use of intravaginal oestrogen cream in genuine stress incontinence. Br J Obstet Gynaecol 1983;90:940–944.
22. Gordon WE, Hermann HW, Hunter DC. Safety and efficacy of micronized estradiol vaginal cream. South Med J 1979;72:1252–1258.

23. Hegarty V, Stewart B. The cost of calcium supplements. *N Engl J Med*, Letter 1988;319:449.

24. Fantl JA, Cardozo L, McClish DK, and the Hormones and Urogenital Therapy Committee. Estrogen therapy in the management of urinary incontinence in postmenopausal women: A meta-analysis. First report of the Hormones and Urogenital Therapy Committee. *Obstet Gynecol* 1994;83(1):12–18.

25. Raz R, Stamm WE. A controlled trail of intravaginal estriol in postmenopausal women with recurrent urinary tract infections. *N Engl J Med* 1993;329(11):753–56.

26. Brincat M, Studd J. Skin and the menopause. In: Mishell DR Jr., ed. Menopause: Physiology and Pharmacology. Chicago: Yearbook Medical Publishers, Inc., 1987, pp. 103–114.

27. Castelo-Branco C, Duran M, Gonzalez-Merlo J. Skin collagen changes related to age and hormone replacement therapy. *Maturitas* 1992;15:113–19.

28. Maheux R, Naud F, Rioux M, et al. A randomized, double-blind, placebo-controlled study on the effect of conjugated estrogens on skin thickness. *Am J Obstet Gynecol* 1994;170(2):642–649.

29. Formosa M, Brincat MP, Cardozo LD, Studd JWW. Collagen: The significance in skin, bones, and bladder. In: Lobo RA, ed. Treatment of the Postmenopausal Woman: Basic and Clinical Aspects. New York: Raven Press, 1994, pp. 143–151.

30. Grodstein F, Colditz GA, Stampfer MJ. Postmenopausal hormone use and cholecystectomy in a large prospective study. *Obstet Gynecol* 1994;83(1):5–11.

31. Lobo RA. *Treatment of the Postmenopausal Women: Where We are Today*. In: Lobo RA, ed. Treatment of the Postmenopausal Woman: Basic and Clinical Aspects. New York: Raven Press, 1994, pp. 427–32.

32. Paganini-Hill A. Morbidity and mortality changes with estrogen replacement therapy. In: Lobo RA, ed. Treatment of the Postmenopausal Woman: Basic and Clinical Aspects. New York: Raven Press, 1994: 399–404.

33. Rosenberg L, Hennekens CH, Rosner B, et al: Am J Obstet Gynecol 1981;139:47–51.

34. Grodstein F, Stampfer MJ: Menopausal Medicine. A Newsletter of the American Fertility Society 1994;2.

35. Stampfer MJ, Grodstein F. Role of hormone replacement in cardiovascular disease. In: Lobo RA, ed. *Treatment of the Postmenopausal Woman: Basic and Clinical Aspects*. New York: Raven Press, 1994, pp. 223–233.

36. Stampfer MJ, Colditz GA, Willett WC, et al. Postmenopausal estrogen therapy and cardiovascular disease. *N Engl J Med* 1991;325(11):756–762.

37. Bush TL, Barrett-Connor E, Cowan LD, et al. Cardiovascular mortality and noncontraceptive use of estrogen in women: Results from the Lipid Research Clinics Program Follow-up Study. Circulation 1987;75(6):1102–09.

38. Krumholz HM, Seeman TE, Merrill SS, et al. Lack of association between cholesterol and coronary heart disease mortality and morbidity and all-cause mortality in persons older than 70 years. *JAMA* 1994;272(17):1335–40.

39. Lobo RA. Effects of hormonal replacement on lipids and lipoproteins in postmenopausal women. *J Clin Endocrinol Metab* 1991;73(5):925–30.

40. Adams MR, Kaplan JR, Manuck SB, et al. Inhibition of coronary artery atherosclerosis by 17-beta estradiol in ovariectomized monkeys: Lack of an effect of added progesterone. *Arteriosclerosis* 1990;10:1051–57.

41. Adams MR, Washburn SA, Wagner JD, Williams JK, Clarkson TB. Arterial changes: Estrogen deficiency and effects of hormone replacement. In: Lobo RA, ed. *Treatment of the Postmenopausal Woman: Basic and Clinical Aspects*. New York: Raven Press, 1994, pp. 243–50.

42. Clarkson TB, Shively CA, Morgan TM, Koritnik DR, Adams MR, Kaplan JR. Oral contraceptives and coronary artery atherosclerosis of Cynomolgus monkeys. *Obstet Gynecol* 1990;75:217.

43. Mugge A, Riedel M, Barton M, Kuhn M, Lichtlen P. Endothelium independent relaxation of human coronary arteries by 17β-oestradiol in vitro. *Cardiovascular Research* 1993;27:1939–1942.

44. Haarbo J, Marslew U, Gotfredsen A, Christiansen C. Postmenopausal hormone replacement therapy prevents central distribution of body fat after menopause. *Metabolism* 1991;40(12):1323–1326.

45. Sullivan JM, Zwaag RV, Lemp GF, et al. Postmenopausal estrogen use and coronary atherosclerosis. *Annals Intern Med* 1988;108:358–63.

46. Sullivan JM, Zqaag RV, Hughes JP, et al. Estrogen replacement and coronary artery disease. *Arch Intern Med* 1990;150(12):2557–2562.

47. Paganini-Hill A, Ross RK, Henderson BE. Postmenopausal oestrogen treatment and stroke: A prospective study. *Br Med J* 1988;297:519–522.

48. Not found

49. Psaty BM, Heckbert sR, Atkins D, et al. A review of the association of estrogens and progestins with cardiovascular disease in postmenopausal women. *Arch Intern Med* 1993;153(6):1421–27.

50. Lobo RA, Speroff L. International consensus conference on postmenopausal hormone therapy and the cardiovascular system. *Fertil Steril* 1994;61(4):592–95.

51. Coronary Drug Project Research Group, The Coronary Drug Project. Initial findings leading to modifications of its research protocol. *JAMA* 1970;214:1303–1313.

52. Finucane FF, Madans JH, Bush TL, Wolf PH, Kleinman JC. Decreased risk of stroke among postmenopausal hormone users. *Arch Intern Med* 1993;153(1):73–79.
53. Coronary Drug Project Research Group, The Coronary Drug Project. Findings leading to discontinuation of the 2.5mg/day estrogen group. *JAMA* 1973;226:652.
54. Gorodeski GI, Utian WH. Epidemiology and risk factors of cardiovascular disease in postmenopausal women. In: Lobo RA, ed. *Treatment of the Postmenopausal Woman: Basic and Clinical Aspects*. New York: Raven Press, 1994, pp. 199–221.
55. Christiansen C. Treatment of Osteoporosis. In: Lobo RA, ed. Treatment of the Postmenopausal Woman: Basic and Clinical Aspects. New York: Raven Press, 1994, pp. 183–95.
56. Cummings SR, Black DM, Rubin SM. Lifetime risks of hip, Colles', or vertebral fracture and coronary heart disease among white postmenopausal women. *Arch Intern Med* 1989;149:2445–48.
57. Weiss NS, Ure CL, Ballard JH, Williams AR, Daling JR. Decreased risk of fractures of the hip and lower forearm with postmenopausal use of estrogen. *N Engl J Med* 1980;303:1195–1198.
58. Christiansen C, Christensen M, Transbol I. Bone mass in postmenopausal women after withdrawal of oestrogen/gestagen replacement therapy. *Lancet* 1981;i:459–461.
59. Ettinger B, Genant HK, Steiger P, Madvig P. Low-dosage micronized 17β-estradiol prevents bone loss in postmenopausal women. *Am J Obstet Gynecol* 1992;166(2):479–88.
60. Lindsay R, Hart DM, Clark DM: Obstet Gynecol 1984;63:759–763.
61. Gambacciani M, Spinetti A, Taponeco F, Cappagli B, Piaggesi L, Fioretti P. Longitudinal evaluation of perimenopausal vertebral bone loss: Effects of a low-dose oral contraceptive preparation on bone mineral density and metabolism. *Obstet Gynecol* 1994;83:392–96.
62. Elders PJM, Netelenbos JC, Lips P, et al. Calcium supplementation reduces vertebral bone loss in perimenopausal women: A controlled trial in 248 women between 46 and 55 years of age. *J Clin Endocrinol Metab* 1991;73(3):533–40.
63. Prestwood KM, Pilbeam CC, Bruleson JA, et al. The short term effects of conjugated estrogens on bone turnover in older women. J Clin Endocrinol Metab 1994;79(2):366–71.
64. Reid IR, Ames RW, Evans MC, Gamble GD, Sharpe SJ. Effect of calcium supplementation on bone loss in postmenopausal women. *N Engl J Med* 1993;328(7):460–64.
65. Grisso JA, Kelsey JL, Strom BL, et al. Risk factors for hip fracture in black women. *N Engl J Med* 1994;330(22):1555–59.
66. de Lignieres B, Moyer DL. Influence of sex hormones on hyperplasia/carcinoma risks. In: Lobo RA, ed. *Treatment of the Postmenopausal Woman: Basic and Clinical Aspects*. New York: Raven Press, 1994, pp. 373–83.
67. Brinton LA, Hoover RN: Epidemiology of gynecologic cancers in eds Hoskins WJ, Perez CA, Young RC: Principles and Practice of Gynecologic Oncology, 1992, Philadelphia, p 8.
68. Chu J, Schweid AI, Weiss NS. Survival among women with endometrial cancer: A comparison of estrogen users and nonusers. *Am J Obstet Gynecol* 1982;143(5):569–73.
69. Moyer DL, deLignieres B, Driguez P, Pez JP. Prevention of endometrial hyperplasia by progesterone during long-term estradiol replacement: Influence of bleeding pattern and secretory changes. *Fertil Steril* 1993;59(5):992–997.
70. Spicer DV, Pike MC. Epidemiology of breast cancer. In: Lobo RA, ed. Treatment of the postmenopausal women: Basic and clinical aspects. New York: Raven Press, 1994, pp. 315–24.
71. Colditz GA, Egan KM, Stampfer MJ. Hormone replacement therapy and risk of breast cancer: Results from epidemiologic studies. *Am J Obstet Gynecol* 1993;168(5):1473–80.
72. American College of Physicians. Guidelines for counseling postmenopausal women about preventive hormone therapy. *Annals Intern Med* 1992;117(12):1038–1041.
73. Grady D, Rubin SM, Petitti dB, et al. Hormone therapy to prevent disease and prolong life in postmenopausal women. *Annals Intern Med* 1992;117(12):1016–1037.
74. Gorsky RD, Koplan JP, Peterson HB, Thacker SB. Relative risks and benefits of long-term estrogen replacement therapy: A decision analysis. *Obstet Gynecol* 1994;83(2):161–166.
75. Bewley S, Bewley TH. Drug dependence with oestrogen replacement therapy. *Lancet* 1992;339(2):290–91.
76. Bhavnani BR, Cecutti A. Pharmacokinetics of 17β-dihydroequilin sulfate and 17β-dihydroequilin in normal postmenopausal women. *J Clin Endocrinol Metab* 1994;78(1):197–204.
77. Whittaker PG, Morgan MRA, Dean PDG, Cameron EHD, Lind T. Serum equilin, oestrone, and oestradiol levels in postmenopausal women receiving conjugated equine oestrogens ("Premarin"). *Lancet i* 1980;:14–16.
78. Mashchak CA, Lobo RA, Donzono-TakanO R, et al. Comparison of pharmacodynamic properties of various estrogen formulations. *Am J Obstet Gynecol* 1982;144(5):511–18.
79. Lufkin EG, Wahner HW, O'Fallon WM, et al. Treatment of postmenopausal osteoporosis with transdermal estrogen. *Ann Intern Med* 1992;117(1):1–9.
80. Lobo RA. The role of progestin in hormone replacement therapy. *Am J Obstet Gynecol* 1992;166:1997–2004.
81. Crook D, Cust MP, Gangar KG, et al. Comparison of transdermal and oral estrogen-progestin replacement therapy: Effects on serum lipids and lipoproteins. *Am J Obstet Gynecol* 1992;166:950–955.

82. Wiklund I, Karlberg J, Mattsson LA. Quality of life of postmenopausal women on a regimen of transdermal estradio therapy: A double-blind placebo-controlled study. *Am J Obstet Gynecol* 1993;168(3):824–30.

83. Hillard TC, Siddle NC, Whitehead MI, Fraser DI, Pryse-Davies J. Continuous combined conjugated equine estrogen-progestogen therapy: Effects of medroxyprogesterone acetate and norethindrone acetate on bleeding patterns and endometrial histologic diagnosis. *Am J Obstet Gynecol* 1992;167(1):1–7.

84. Spaulding LB. Endometrial ablation for refractory postmenopausal bleeding with continuous hormone replacement therapy. *Fertil Steril* 1994;62(6):1181–85.

85. Archer DF, Pickar JH, Bottiglioni F. Bleeding patterns in postmenopausal women taking continuous combined or sequential regimens of conjugated estrogens with medroxyprogesterone acetate. *Obstet Gynecol* 1994;83(5):686–92.

86. Williams DB, Voigt BJ, Fu YS, Schoenfeld MJ, Judd HL. Assessment of less than monthly progestin therapy in postmenopausal women given estrogen replacement. *Obstet Gynecol* 1994;84(5):787–93.

87. Ettinger B, Selby J, Citron JT, Vangessel A, Ettinger VM, Hendrickson MR. Cyclic hormone replacement therapy using quarterly progestin. *Obstet Gynecol* 1994;83(5):693–700.

88. Callantine MR, Martin PL, Bolding OT, Warner PO, Greaney MD. Micronized 17β-estradiol for oral estrogen therapy in menopausal women. *Obstet Gynecol* 1975;46:37–41.

89. Yen SSC, Martin PL, Burnier AM, Czekala NM, Greaney JMD, Callantine R. Circulating estradiol, estrone and gonadotropin levels following the administration of orally active 17β-estradiol in postmenopausal women. *J. Clin Endocrinol Metab* 1975;40:518.

90. Prior JC, Alojado N, McKay DW, Vigna YM. No adverse effects of medroxyprogesterone treatment without estrogen in postmenopausal women: Double-blind, placebo-controlled, crossover trial. *Obstet Gynecol* 1994;83(1):24–28.

91. Sherwin BB, Gelfand MM, Brender W. Androgen enhances sexual motivation in females: A prospective, crossover study of sex steroid administration in the surgical menopause. *Psychosom Med* 1985;47:339–351.

92. Powles TJ: Lancet 1990; ii:48.

93. Boccardo F, Bruzzi P, Rubagotti A, Nicolo G, Rosso R: Oncology 1981;38:281

94. Neven P, DeMuylder X, van Belle Y, Vanderick G, DeMuylder E: Letter: Lancet 1989;1:375.

95. Nagamani M, Kelver M, Smith E. Treatment of menopausal hot flashes with transdermal administration of clonidine. *Am J Obstet Gynecol* 1987;156:561–565.

Chapter 9

Screening and Prevention

Linda Pinsky, MD, Wylie Burke, MD, PhD, and
Wendy H. Raskind MD, PhD

In contrast to conventional medical treatment of active symptoms, the goal of preventive health care is to maintain or improve future health. This goal has three components: (1) The prevention of disease when possible; (2) the early identification of treatable conditions; and (3) the preservation of independence and useful function. All of these should be considerations during a routine visit to a physician. History taking, physical examination, and screening tests each contribute to preventive health care. In addition, patient education is important. Patients vary in their awareness of preventive care and of current screening recommendations and often need to have the rationale and benefits of these activities explained.

Disease prevention is possible only when modifiable precursors of disease can be recognized early. Frequently, such efforts require patients to undertake changes in their life-style. Helping the patient to understand the importance of such changes is a key part of preventive care. For example, smoking cessation significantly reduces the risk of chronic obstructive pulmonary disease, coronary artery disease, stroke, lung cancer, and other cancers. Most smokers find quitting to be extremely difficult. Furthermore, if the patient gives up smoking, no guarantee can be given that the diseases associated with smoking will be fully prevented. These realities complicate the task of helping a patient to stop smoking. Specific information on the value of a preventive measure helps a patient to undertake changes in long-standing habits. Similarly, the physician's counseling efforts are made easier when patients can be given concrete suggestions to follow. Approaches to counseling patients on smoking cessation and other preventive life-style changes are discussed in more detail below.

Other true preventive measures include immunizations, control of elevated blood pressure, and periodic dental cleaning. Some measures thought of as preventive in nature are actually measures aimed at identifying disease in early, treatable stages. These include screening for colon, cervical, and breast cancer. Although not strictly preventive, such screening may make cure a possibility or significantly limit the morbidity of a disease process. Like life-style changes, effective screening often requires education of patients so that they can understand both the purpose and the limitations of screening procedures.[106,381]

The maintenance of useful function and independence involves a different kind of preventive care; in this area, potentially disabling conditions are identified in order to make interventions that preserve or improve an individual's functional state. For example, a hearing disorder may be ameliorated by use of a hearing aid, and an exercise program may offset some of the physical limitations imposed by arthritis. A variety of screening techniques are available to aid in reaching the goals of preventive health care. Issues of cost, efficacy, and convenience are important in evaluating these techniques. The individual patient's needs must also be considered because her risks depend to some extent on her age, past medical history, family medical history, and risk factor exposure.[106,331,379,381,384]

Cardiovascular Disease

Coronary Artery Disease

The most common cardiovascular disease, and the one for which screening is most effective, is coronary artery disease (CAD). Risk factors for CAD are well defined (Table 9.1), and many of these can be modified to reduce risk, through life-style changes and medical treatment.[2–4,7,9,11–12,14–15]

Each year, 2.5 million women are hospitalized in the United States for cardiovascular disease. There are 500,000 associated deaths of which half are attributed to CAD.[15] Despite this, most preventive, diagnostic, and therapeutic strategies for women are based on studies predominately or exclusively involving men.

CAD can present as anginal pain, or it may manifest initially as sudden death or a myocardial infarction (MI). For these reasons, it is worthwhile to detect and, when possible, reduce risk factors in asymptomatic adults. On average, clinical manifestations occur 10 years later and myocardial infarction 20 years later in women than in men. Additionally, there is a 6- to 7-year greater life expectancy of women compared with men, resulting in an elderly population that is predominantly female.[15] Misclassification of deaths as cardiac-related is more likely to happen in the elderly, especially those with concurrent illness. Some of the deaths attributed to CAD in women may actually represent multisystem failure in end-of-life disease. To date, the actual incidence of clinically significant heart disease in women has not been accurately ascertained.

The later onset and possibly lower rate of clinically important CAD needs to be considered in choosing risk-reduction programs for women. At the same time, there may be missed opportunities for preventive care, due in part to prior perception of CAD in women as a benign process. The initial analysis of Framingham data suggested that CAD in women had a more favorable outcome, in that the angina pectoris observed in the female cohort rarely progressed to MI. Angina was the first major coronary manifestation in 56% and 43% of Framingham women and men respectively. Only 14% of the women with angina progressed to MI within 5 years as compared with 25% of

Table 9.1 Risk Factors for Coronary Artery Disease

Positive Risk Factors

Cigarette smoking
Hypertension
Diabetes mellitus
Age (male 45 years and over, women 55 years and over or premature menopause without
    estrogen replacement)
Family history of premature coronary artery disease
HDL < 35 mg/dl
(Obesity and physical inactivity, although not listed as separate risk factors by NCEP, are
    considered areas for intervention.)

Negative Risk Factor

High HDL 60 mg/dl or more

---

the men. Later angiographic evaluation suggests that these differences reflect a larger proportion of noncardiac chest pain in women rather than a more benign prognosis for those with true angina.[15] For example, in the Coronary Artery Surgery Study (CASS), 50% of women but only 17% of men with chest pain had normal coronary arteries angiographically.[5] In the 26-year follow-up on Framingham, 40% of all coronary events occurred in women; retrospective review of the Framingham data demonstrates that older women with angina had the same adverse prognosis as did the men. This is consistent with the findings of the Cleveland Clinic study in which 90% of postmenopausal women with suspected severe angina undergoing angiography had significant CAD, as compared with only 50% of premenopausal women.[1]

Women who have myocardial infarction have a substantial increase in morbidity and mortality, an increased mortality with coronary artery bypass grafting (CABG), and notably lesser success with percutaneous transluminal coronary angioplasty (PTCA) than men. Poorer outcomes may be related in part to older age or use of urgent or emergent procedures. Symptomatic CHD results in more functional limitations, greater morbidity, and more severe impairment of quality of life in women than in men.

Stroke

Cerebrovascular disease is the second most common cardiovascular disease after CAD and the third leading cause of death in the United States, after heart disease and cancer.[6] Hypertension, smoking, and diabetes are the leading risk factors for stroke.[13,14] The presence of CAD also represents a risk factor for stroke.[8-10] Thus, attention to risk factors for CAD contributes to stroke prevention as well.

Hypertension

The prevalence of hypertension is equal in women and men, although there is a greater degree of uncontrolled hypertension in men but the benefits of treating hypertension are less well studied in women. Although some earlier studies failed to detect a treatment benefit in middle-aged hypertensive women, studies involving older women clearly demonstrated benefit of treatment. The Systolic Hypertension in the Elderly Program (SHEP)[41] found 36% fewer fatal and nonfatal strokes and 27% fatal and nonfatal MI in actively treated elderly persons as compared with a placebo-treated control group, with benefits across all age, race, gender, and blood pressure subgroups.[41] In regard to choice of medication, a study found no significant differences in the effects on quality of life in women using a beta blocker, angiotensin-converting enzyme (ACE) inhibitor, or calcium channel blocker.[20] At present, there are not sufficient data to confirm any gender difference in benefit or treatment approach to hypertension, although further study is indicated.[18]

Although often considered a disease in itself, hypertension is usually asymptomatic. The cutoff point between normal and elevated blood pressure is a matter of arbitrary definition, since blood pressure is a continuous trait. In general, blood pressures up to 140/90 mm Hg are considered normal in adults over the age of 50, because it is only at blood pressures above this range that marked increases in cardiovascular disease occur. In the elderly, elevated blood pressure is the most important risk factor for CAD, and for all ages, systolic blood pressures are more predictive of risk for CAD than diastolic blood pressures.[9,19] Blood pressure elevation is common, occurring in at least 15% to 20% of the adult US population. Because in developed countries, average blood pressure rises with age, the prevalence increases with each decade of life.[25,27] Isolated systolic hypertension is defined as a systolic pressure greater than 160 mm Hg and a diastolic pressure less than 90 mm Hg. A new system of categorizing hypertension has been devised (Table 9.2).[44]

Table 9.2 Classification of Blood Pressure for Adults Aged 18 Years and Older

Category	Systolic, mm Hg	Diastolic, mm Hg
Normal	<130	<85
High normal	130–139	85–89
Hypertension		
Stage 1 (mild)	140–159	90–99
Stage 2 (moderate)	160–179	100–109
Stage 3 (severe)	180–209	110–119
Stage 4 (very severe)	>210	>120

From the 5th report of the Joint National Comm. on Detection, Evaluation and Treatment of High Blood Pressure (JNCV) Arch - Intern - Med 1993; 153:154–83.

The risk of cardiovascular disease at any blood pressure is significantly increased if target organ disease is present. This includes hypertensive nephropathy or retinopathy (hemorrhages or exudate); a history of transient ischemia attack or stroke; peripheral vascular disease; and evidence of left ventricular hypertrophy by electrocardiogram or limited echocardiogram.[44]

Many individuals have labile blood pressure, with measurements varying between normal and hypertensive levels. Labile blood pressure is presumed to increase the risk both for fixed hypertension and for the complications of hypertension. However, the risk of disease appears to be lower than that conferred by continuous hypertension.[11] Some individuals have normal blood pressure at home and elevated pressure when under circumstances of anxiety—for example, when in a doctor's office ("white coat hypertension.") These individuals have lower risks of cardiovascular disease than would be expected from their high blood pressure readings in the doctor's office, and there is evidence that target organ disease correlates better with out-of-office measurements.[26,38]

These patterns of variation in blood pressure underscore the importance of having several blood pressure measurements taken before a patient is diagnosed to be hypertensive.[39] When an elevated reading is obtained, unless the level is dangerously high, the patient should be encouraged to have several readings taken outside the doctor's office. Community screening programs, fire stations, and some pharmacies provide this service. Patients should be informed of the importance of measuring blood pressure in a resting state (after at least 5 minutes of sitting).

Technique is also important. The cuff, appropriately sized for the patient's upper arm, should be inflated to at least 30 mm Hg above the systolic pressure determined by radial artery palpation. The cuff is deflated at a rate of 2 to 3 mm Hg/sec to record the systolic pressure (point at which the first Korotkoff sound is heard) and diastolic pressure (point at which the Korotkoff sounds disappear). Change in tone is not a reliable measure of the diastolic pressure. Falsely elevated pressures can be obtained if the patient clenches her fist, the cuff is too small (bladder less than 80% of arm), or the arm is below the level of the right atrium. If the patient purchases a home blood pressure apparatus, it should be calibrated against the doctor's office mercury sphygmomanometer. Office personnel responsible for blood pressure measurements should review instructions for accurate measurement on a regular basis.[42]

Control of hypertension markedly reduces cerebrovascular mortality and morbidity.[29] The effect of blood pressure lowering on CAD is less dramatic, possibly because some antihypertensive drugs introduce other risks for cardiac disease by lowering potassium or raising lipid levels.[29,30] These observations underline the importance of treating hypertension in the context of careful evaluation of other cardiac risk factors, and of minimizing the use of drug treatment when possible.

Treatment should usually be initiated with life-style changes. In general, patients with any degree of hypertension will benefit from dietary changes, weight loss, and regular exercise.[32,34,39,40] In some patients, blood pressure may be reduced by as much as 10 to 20 mm Hg with reduction of salt in the diet. Not all individuals are salt-sensitive, and there is no simple objective method to identify those hypertensive individuals who will benefit from salt reduction. However, limiting salt intake to moderate levels (1.5 to 2.5 g/day of sodium) is safe, and should be recommended as an initial measure to all patients with elevated blood pressure.[44] Other dietary changes that may contribute to blood pressure lowering include increased calcium, magnesium, and potassium intake, moderation in alcohol use, increased fiber, and decreased saturated fat.[24,27,28,31,35,39,44,47] Increased dietary potassium is also associated with a lowered risk of stroke-associated death, independent of its effect on blood pressure.[33] These dietary changes are best accomplished through changes in the kinds of foods eaten, rather than through the use of pharmacologic supplements. Some specific guidelines for dietary counseling are discussed below under Nutrition.

Obesity is associated with an increased risk for hypertension. For patients who are obese, even a modest weight loss of 5 to 10 pounds may be associated with some blood pressure lowering,[44] and hypertension may resolve in patients who reduce to their lean body mass. Weight loss should be undertaken by sensible alterations in diet and exercise patterns, because pounds lost during "crash" diets are almost always quickly regained. See further discussion of weight loss programs under Nutrition.

Exercise is helpful in both primary prevention of hypertension and in reduction of elevated blood pressure. Moderate exercise, such as brisk walking, reduces blood pressure and may prevent hypertension.[22] A program of regular, daily exercise is preferable to infrequent strenuous workouts. Stress is associated with acute rises in blood pressure and may contribute to chronic elevation; however, the effects of stress-reduction techniques on hypertension remains controversial at this time.[43-45] Rest in a quiet room, transcendental meditation, and biofeedback are among the relaxation techniques that may be helpful in the treatment of hypertension.[21] Patients generally benefit most from specific training in a particular technique by a skilled teacher.[16]

Patients whose blood pressures remain above 140/90 mm Hg despite hygienic measures may need pharmacological treatment. In patients with stage 1 hypertension, weight loss and other nondrug methods should be attempted for at least 3 to 6 months before instituting pharmacological treatment. The decision regarding the appropriate blood pressure level at which to begin a drug is made on an individual basis and must take into account the existence of other cardiovascular risk factors. Even if medications are used, life-style modifications should continue to be pursued, as they may reduce the number and dose of antihypertensive medications needed as well as decrease other cardiovascular risk factors. Drug therapy should be initiated cautiously, because untoward reactions are common if the blood pressure is reduced too rapidly. Decreased metabolism and delayed excretion of drugs are mechanisms that render the elderly particularly prone to develop orthostatic hypotension. The lowest dose available should be prescribed initially. Antihypertensive medications may cause many side effects.[23] These include hypokalemia, slowed heart rate, elevated plasma low-density lipoprotein (LDL) levels, lowered plasma high-density lipoprotein (HDL) levels, and reduced kidney or liver function. Patients taking blood pressure medicines have increased frequency of somatic complaints, including malaise and weakness, and may develop significant depression. The choice of medication for a patient also must be individualized, based on possible benefit for other existing conditions, drug interactions, and the likelihood that the patient will suffer side effects of the particular drug. Treatment of hypertension in the very old is controversial. The SHEP did not report the results for this subgroup separately.[41] In the European Working Party for High Blood Pressure in the Elderly, treating hypertension after age 80 was not found to be beneficial.[17] A Finnish study also suggests less aggressive treatment of hypertension after age 85; however the designs of these studies make these results questionable.[36] As present studies are inconclusive, caution should be used in treating this age group.

The benefits of hypertension treatment occur only if the treatment is sustained. Noncompliance with medication is common, particularly if the cost is high, multiple daily doses are required, or side effects occur. Compliance may be improved by continuity of care with a single health care provider.[37] Long-term therapy is usually required; therefore, cost of medication and frequency of dosing are important considerations.

Smoking

The cardiovascular health hazards of smoking are well documented. Approximately 30% to 40% of deaths from CAD can be attributed to smoking,[256,274] and smokers have an almost twofold higher risk of heart disease than nonsmokers. Two recent studies have explicitly addressed the effects of smoking cessation in the elderly. The risks for developing CAD and mortality from existing CAD were both shown to be reduced after cessation of smoking.[11,12] Smoking is harmful to health in numerous other ways as well, and for this reason smoking cessation should be a first step in any program to reduce cardiac risks. Health effects of smoking and guidelines for helping smokers to quit are discussed below.

Hypercholesterolemia

Epidemiological studies have demonstrated that the risk for CAD increases with serum cholesterol levels in both men and women. In older women, the association between total cholesterol and coronary heart disease (CHD) is present but less consistent than for other age–sex subgroups.[48,49,61] Although the demarcation between "normal" and "abnormal" cholesterol levels is arbitrary, as it is with blood pressure, demonstrable increases in CAD rate can be shown for levels of cholesterol above 200 mg/dl, and levels above 300 mg/dl are associated with a marked increase in CAD rate.[9] The cholesterol can be separated into HDL and LDL fractions; triglycerides can also be measured. The HDL fraction exerts a protective effect. HDL levels are higher in postpubertal women than in men, and remain so even after menopause.[64] The protective effect of HDL may contribute to the overall lower risk of CAD seen in women as compared with men. A low level of HDL is a significant risk factor in all age–sex categories; in older women, this association was seen in large observational studies, although it was weaker than in middle-aged counterparts. Although HDL does not decrease in the perimenopausal period, there is a continual increase in the LDL and total cholesterol to levels that, on average, exceed those of men of comparable age.[53] The LDL fraction is found to be most predictive of risk of early onset CAD overall;[48] this trend persists in older women, although the difference in relative risk is not statistically significant. Because cardiovascular disease is so prevalent in this age group, a small reduction in individual risk may be of benefit to the population. The role of triglycerides in CAD is uncertain, but it is suspected to be of increased importance in women.[61]

Several trials of cholesterol-lowering treatment in middle-aged men without previously identified CAD have demonstrated that mortality and morbidity from CAD can be reduced; the results of these trials have been widely cited as a rationale for aggressive screening and intervention programs.[52,54,60] However, the actual reduction in myocardial infarction or CAD death was small (1% to 2%) and the overall mortality was not reduced. Thus the risk-benefit ratio for the use of lipid-lowering medications is not clear, particularly in women whose a priori risk for CAD is significantly lower than in men.[51,55,56,59] The National Cholesterol Education Program (Adult Panel II)[62] has recently modified its guidelines accordingly, emphasizing different approaches to primary and secondary prevention, such that drug therapy is not routinely recommended in premenopausal women.[62,63] When considering drug therapy in postmenopausal women there are several factors that must be taken into account when the decision. As discussed above, CAD occurs at a later age in women than in men. Data on treatment of hypercholesterolemia in the elderly is contradictory. A recent study found no association in primary prevention between cholesterol levels and CAD mortality and morbidity in men and women older than 70[58] contradicting previous studies.[2,51,65] (1984) Participants in the negative study had a mean age of 79, greatly exceeding that of the other studies and suggesting there may be a difference in the importance of cholesterol between the young old and the very old. Second, although the correlation between LDL cholesterol and cardiovascular or total mortality persists in older women, it is much weaker than in men. Currently, there is limited data on the benefits of cholesterol lowering in women. Additionally, the higher levels of HDL cholesterol generally seen in women, even postmenopausally, may provide sufficient protection. Correspondingly, there exists some data suggesting that estrogen replacement therapy (ERT) may provide protection, as discussed below.

Who, then, should be screened? Panels of health officials in Canada and the United States have set different guidelines that are subject to frequent revision.[50,57,62] While some groups advocate universal screening of adults, it is most important to screen individuals with other identified CAD risk factors (Table 9.1).

Recent National Cholesterol Education Program (NCEP) recommendations suggest that screening laboratories include a HDL-cholesterol as well as a total cholesterol.[62,63] The HDL assay is less well standardized and is much less reproducible than the total serum cholesterol. It is important, therefore, to have it measured through a laboratory that participates in a reliable standardization program. If a persistently elevated cholesterol level or a depressed HDL cholesterol level is found on screening or if a person has known atherosclerotic disease, a full lipid profile should be obtained to determine the LDL fraction.[62]

In contrast to total cholesterol and HDL cholesterol, which are measured directly, LDL cholesterol is a more difficult laboratory measurement and is generally calculated as follows:

$$LDL = TC - HDL - \frac{TG}{5}$$ where TC is total cholesterol and TG is triglycerides.[64] Because triglycerides are affected by recent fat ingestion, LDL levels should be obtained after an overnight fast.

If the LDL cholesterol is reproducibly elevated, secondary causes of hyperlipidemia should be sought. Unless the LDL level is extremely high (over 180 mg/dl) and the HDL level proportionately low (less than 35 mg/dl), pharmacological treatment should be deferred until life-style measures have been tried (Table 9.3).[51,56,62]

As the data are inconclusive, caution must be applied in the treatment of hypercholesterolemia in older women. The emphasis should be on hygienic approaches. As with hypertension, a number of life-style changes can improve the serum cholesterol level. The most important of these is reduction in dietary cholesterol and fat. Weight control and exercise also play major roles in control of cholesterol levels. In the usual American diet, 36% or more of calories derive from fats, well above the 30% recommended for the general population by the American Heart Association. Much of the excess fat is contained in processed foods or in food preparation at restaurants, especially buffets or those serving "fast food." Older individuals, especially those living alone, may frequently eat in such restaurants, for reasons of budget and convenience, and may be unaware of the high fat and salt content of the food they are eating.

While asymptomatic elevations of cholesterol in the elderly are generally not treated, medication

Table 9.3 NCEP Adult Treatment Panel II Guidelines

Primary Prevention

Check total cholesterol and HDL cholesterol
Do lipoprotein analysis if:
HDL < 35 mg/dl
TOTAL CHOLESTEROL > 200 mg/dl AND TWO OR MORE RISK FACTORS
TOTAL CHOLESTEROL > 240 mg/dl

Begin dietary therapy if:
LDL > 130 mg//dl and TWO OR MORE RISK FACTORS   Goal < 130 mg/dl
LDL > 160 mg/dl   Goal < 160 mg/dl

Begin drug therapy if man over 35 years old, or postmenopausal women* and:
LDL > 160 mg/dl and TWO OR MORE RISK FACTORS   Goal < 130 mg/dl
LDL > 190 mg/dl   Goal < 160 mg/dl

Secondary Prevention

Do lipoprotein analysis
Start dietary therapy if LDL > 100 mg/dl   Goal < 100 mg/dl
Start drug therapy if LDL > 130 mg/dl   Goal < 100 mg/dl

HDL, High-density lipoprotein; LDL, low-density lipoprotein.
*Consider estrogen replacement therapy first.
From National Cholesterol Education Program: Second Report of the Expert Panel on Detection, Evaluation and Treatment of High Blood Cholesterol in Adults (Adult Treatment Panel II). Circulation 1994; 89: 1333–1445.

may be considered in older women with known CAD and elevated cholesterol or in those with extreme elevations of LDL-C (more than 250 mg/dl). Factors such as an increased sensitivity to medication side effects, limited life expectancy due to concurrent illness, and expense should be considered when contemplating medical therapy.

Estrogen Replacement Therapy (ERT) and Cardiovascular Disease

Evidence suggests that estrogen influences CAD via an increase in HDL and a decrease in LDL. Another lipid component, Lp(a), also a suspected risk factor for CAD, is probably decreased by estrogen while triglycerides are increased. Additionally, estrogen decreases LDL oxidation as well as lipid uptake into the vascular wall. Recent studies have demonstrated that estrogen reverses acetylcholine-induced vasoconstriction and reduces endothelin production.[66–68] The effects of concomitant progestin use is uncertain. Progestin tends to be antithrombotic; theoretically, it opposes the beneficial effect of estrogen on blood lipids although some recent observational studies suggest that the clinical effect may be positive.[74,78,81,82,87]

   A meta-analysis of 31 studies on estrogen use and cardiovascular disease was recently reported. (Stampfer, 1991)[84] The relative risk for all studies ranged from 0.16 to 4.25, with a summary estimated risk of 0.56; this summary represents a pooling of heterogenic studies. The summary relative risk of 15 prospective cohort studies with internal controls, the study design that provides the most accurate estimate, is 0.58. However, these studies can overestimate the effect of estrogen due to selection bias; women who use estrogen have been found to be leaner and healthier than nonusers; users tend to have a higher educational status and possibly be more compliant with health care instructions and medications.[67,85,86] These confounding factors, in the face of studies that show strong and consistent evidence of the effectiveness of estrogen, underscore the need for randomized intervention trials. The only existing intervention trial is small and had few cardiac events, so its positive results need further corroboration.[79,80]

Who then should receive ERT? Clearly its use must be individualized.[66,68,73,77] The apparent benefits in coronary artery disease reduction[83,86] (as well as protection from osteoporosis) must be balanced against the increased rate of gallbladder disease and the increased risk of cancer. The use of unopposed estrogen is definitely associated with increased endometrial cancer; the concomitant use of progestin appears to negate this risk,[76] but the effects of progestin on heart disease are still under investigation. The risk of breast cancer is more controversial. A Swedish study demonstrated that the prolonged use of ERT (for more than 10 yr) increased the relative risk of breast cancer.[69] A recent meta-analysis suggested a relative risk of 1.3 of breast cancer in women on ERT.[64,72,73] The absolute risk of heart disease is greater than that of breast cancer; this ratio is modified by a woman's family history of each disease as well as the presence of other risk factors for them. The decision to begin ERT must take into account each woman's risk of heart disease, cancer, and osteoporosis. Epidemiologically, the risk of breast cancer is greatest in the early menopause years, while an increased risk of CAD occurs in the later years. For some women, a small increased risk of breast cancer occurring at an earlier age may be less acceptable than a later risk of heart disease, emphasizing the importance of patient participation in decision about the use of ERT.[71]

Risk-benefit ratio is also influenced by how long the hormonal therapy is used. Studies confirm a greater protective benefit in current users over former users, but there has not yet been an adequate number of studies on which to base recommendations for duration of therapy.[70,84,85] Results of studies regarding efficacy by age have been contradictory, as have those comparing cause of menopause (surgical versus natural). Most, but not all, studies have observed greater protection in nonsmokers than in smokers.[66]

Diabetes

Diabetics are at increased risk for CAD and other vascular diseases, including both stroke and peripheral vascular disease. A diabetic patient should receive regular supervision by a physician experienced in the management of this condition. Some patients will receive preventive health care from a physician other than the one who supervises their diabetes. This is particularly likely to be the case if routine preventive health care is provided by a gynecologist, while an internist or family practitioner manages the diabetes. Under these circumstances, it is prudent to remind the patient of the importance of regular physician visits for management of the diabetes and of adhering to dietary restrictions.

Positive Family History

Family history of early coronary artery disease (age 55 or younger in men, age 60 or younger in women) is the strongest single risk factor for CAD.[90-93] Certain rare lipid disorders (eg, familial hypercholesterolemia; familial combined hyperlipidemia) account for a small proportion of families in which early CAD occurs. These families are characterized by a pattern of autosomal dominant transmission, in which the increased risk of CAD is inherited vertically from one generation to the next, and in which each child of an affected individual is at 50% risk to inherit the lipid disorder and associated increased risk for CAD.[88] In the majority of families with early CAD, the increased risk for CAD is a polygenic trait, with the additive effect of several genes each contributing in a small way to the overall risk. Polygenic inheritance of blood pressure and cholesterol levels accounts for the increased incidence of early heart disease in some of these families.[91–93] Shared environmental factors, such as smoking or high fat diets may also contribute to the familial incidence of early heart disease. However, even when other known risk factors are taken into account, a family history of early CAD confers an increased risk of heart disease.[92,93]

When a patient has a positive family history for early heart disease, modification of other cardiac risk factors becomes more important. Explaining the significance of the positive family history to the patient may help to motivate life-style changes, including smoking cessation, reduced dietary saturated fat, and increased exercise. Modification of other cardiac risk factors has been shown to reduce the incidence of CAD in individuals with a strong family history of heart disease.[89,90]

Sedentary Life-style

As part of a program to reduce the risk of CAD, all women should be advised to pursue a regular exercise program, unless they are physically unable to do so. While no studies have specifically assessed the cardiac benefits of exercise for older women, studies of male cohorts suggest that a sedentary life-style represents a risk factor of almost the same magnitude as cholesterol elevation for CAD.[97] Some studies have suggested that regular exercise may help to prevent the development of hypertension, diabetes, and obesity and to improve elevated blood pressure and cholesterol levels.[289] Exercise appears to be effective at lowering blood pressure and improving outcome even in the absence of weight loss. Benefits of exercise are discussed further under Lifestyle.

Obesity

Obesity has been implicated as an independent risk factor for cardiovascular disease in some but not all studies addressing this issue.[94,98] Obesity is associated with other risk factors, notably hypertension, diabetes, and a sedentary life-style, and it is difficult to determine the effect attributable to each separate factor. Recent data have suggested that a particular pattern of obesity—intra-abdominal fat deposition, identified by a high waist-to-hip ratio—is associated with increased cardiovascular risk.[96,99] Intra-abdominal fat deposition appears to be increased in smokers[95] and is also associated with lipid and insulin abnormalities[100] so questions about the interrelationship of obesity and other risk factors remain. In any case, women with central obesity benefit from improvement in other cardiac risk factors, especially smoking and may also benefit from weight loss.

Aspirin Use

The efficacy of aspirin in the secondary prevention of cardiovascular disease has been shown in both women and men in randomized trials.[101,106] The results in women were similar to those in men, although there was not sufficient statistical power to detect if any gender difference does exist.

Randomized trials of primary prevention have had conflicting results and involved only men. In the Physicians Health Study[111] of approximately 22,000 subjects, low doses of aspirin resulted in a significant (46%) reduction in risk of first MI. Effects on stroke and cardiovascular deaths were inconclusive due to the small number of these events.[111] In contrast, the smaller British Doctor's Trial[110] found no statistical benefit of aspirin; this may reflect a lack of statistical power.[110] Of note is that both studies showed a trend, albeit not a statistically significant one, toward a higher rate of hemorrhagic stroke in those taking aspirin.[110,111] As a result of these trials, the US Preventive Task Force[115] recommends aspirin for primary prevention of MI in men but makes no recommendation for women.

In the absence of randomized trials, observational trials attempt to define the use of aspirin in women. Two prospective studies have failed to show any benefit, although the designs of these studies have flaws.[105,108] A case control of 776 men and women showed that regular aspirin use resulted in a greater than 50% reduction in risk of first MI.[102] Prospective study of the Nurses' Health cohort of approximately 88,000 women with 475,000 person-years of follow-up demonstrated a reduction in first MI with the use of one to six aspirins per week.[107]

At this time, use of aspirin for primary prevention must be individualized; it should be considered in women whose risk of a first MI outweighs the potential consequences of its long-term use, including gastrointestinal bleeding. The use of aspirin in secondary prevention is more clearly established[103,104,109] but, again, it must be weighed against relative contraindications.

Cancer

Most cancer prevention strategies involve methods for early detection, either of cancer or of precancerous processes. Treatment can then be initiated sufficiently early to improve the likelihood of cure. Limitations in cancer prevention reflect the fact that methods for detection of presymptomatic disease or for effective early treatment are not uniformly available. For example, no accurate method of screening to detect stage I ovarian cancer is yet available, nor has screening via chest radiograph and/or cytology reduced mortality in lung cancer. For breast and cervical cancer, however, routine screening provides a significant benefit.

The incidence of most cancers increases with age, making cancer screening of particular importance for older women. The most common cancers affecting women are lung, breast, and colon cancer (Table 9.4). Methods for screening are available for two of these, breast and colon cancer, as discussed below.[113-115] Cervical cancer screening is also an important preventive health procedure for women, as discussed in Chapter 18 of this volume. For most other cancers, screening or early detection options are limited, and when available are appropriate primarily for individuals at increased risk.

Lung Cancer

Lung cancer in women has increased dramatically from the mid-1960s to the present.[116,117] Although the number of women diagnosed with lung cancer is only about half the number diagnosed with breast cancer, lung cancer causes more deaths. The poorer survival seen in lung cancer is due to the lack of effective means for early detection and treatment as described below. The increase

Table 9.4 Estimated Incidence of Cancer in American Women*

	Annual Incidence New Cases/yr	Deaths Deaths/100,000/yr
Lung cancer	70,000	23.0
Breast cancer	182,000	22.0
Colorectal cancer	7,000	12.0
Cervical cancer	13,500	2.7
Endometrial cancer	31,000	2.7
Ovarian cancer	22,000	8.0
Melanoma	15,000	
Leukemia/lymphoma	41,200	

Modified from Boring CC, Squires TS, Tong T: Cancer statistics, 1993. *CA Cancer J Clin* 1990;43:7–26.

correlates with the rising percentage of women smokers that began in the 1920s, and has only recently begun to decline. Of particular concern is an increase in smoking among young women noted in the 1980s. These smoking trends suggest that lung cancer will continue to be frequent among women for some time to come.[119] Although lung cancer represents a significant health problem, smoking cessation is the only preventive measure of proven value.[118,122]

Several clinical trials, including large-scale efforts at the Mayo Clinic[120] and The Johns Hopkins University,[121,123] have assessed the efficacy of annual chest radiographs, with and without periodic sputum cell examination in male smokers for identifying lung cancer in early, more treatable stages. Even in this high-risk group, no difference in mortality from lung cancer from regular screening could be demonstrated. Small differences in stages of cancers detected and in 5-year mortality rates among those with lung cancer could be shown in some trials. However, the lack of a difference in overall mortality rates suggests that such differences derived primarily from false-positive results in more intensively screened groups and from lead-time bias. Lead-time bias is the effect of *apparent* increased length of survival seen when a cancer is identified at an earlier stage by screening than it would have been by clinical symptoms. When no difference in ultimate mortality rate is found, as was the case in trials of lung cancer screening, it can be concluded that screening resulted in earlier diagnosis without additional benefit.

One cautionary note should be made, however. In the trials of chest X-ray screening for lung cancer, the control groups tended to have chest X-ray screening done relatively frequently as part of their regular health care, and many cancers were discovered incidentally. For example, in the Mayo Clinic Trial,[120] one third of the lung cancers detected in the study were found in chest radiographs done for purposes other than screening. Even when this effect is accounted for, as analyzed by Eddy,[118] there is no statistical evidence that chest X-ray screening identifies lung cancers at an early enough stage to change mortality outcome. These data do, however, underscore the importance of chest radiographs in the work-up of new or persistent respiratory symptoms in smokers.

Breast Cancer

Breast cancer is diagnosed annually in more than 180,000 women in the United States. The rate of breast cancer has risen over the past 2 decades and is only partially accounted for by increasing longevity and improved diagnostic methods. According to recent statistics from the National Cancer Institute, the average American woman has a 1 in 10 chance of developing breast cancer by age 80 and a 1 in 8 chance by age 95.[133] Major risk factors, producing more than a twofold increased risk for breast cancer, are shown in Table 9.5 and include age, family history of breast cancer, heavy radiation exposure, and prior history of breast cancer, carcinoma in situ, multiple breast biopsies, and the finding of atypical hyperplasia on biopsy.[117,125] Lesser risk is conferred by early menarche, late menopause, nulliparity, and late birth of the first child.[125] A number of other factors have been identified as possible contributors to breast cancer, including ERT, a high fat diet, obesity, moderate-to-heavy alcohol use, sedentary life-style, and a history of abortion before the first pregnancy.[127,135,143] However, known risk factors account for only about half of all breast cancers in women.

Breast cancer mortality is higher in black women than in white women.[129] Recent data from the Centers for Disease Control show that the death rate from breast cancer is 92 in 100,000 for white women over age 50 and 104 in 100,000 for black women; before age 50 the rates are 5.7 and 9.1 per 100,000 respectively. In a recent analysis of data from the National Cancer Institute, by Eley and coworkers,[120] the risk of dying from breast cancer was two times higher for blacks than whites, with stage at diagnosis a major contributor to the difference. Thus, preventive efforts

Table 9.5 Risk Factors for Breast Cancer

Major risk factors
    Age
    Family history of breast cancer or cancer-prone family
    Heavy radiation exposure
    Past history of
    Breast cancer
    Carcinoma in situ of the breast
    Atypical hyperplasia
    Multiple breast biopsies
Minor risk factors
Nulliparity or late first pregnancy
    Early menarche/late menopause
Possible risk factors
    Estrogen therapy
    High-fat diet
    Obesity
    Moderate-to-heavy alcohol use
    Sedentary lifestyle
    History of abortion before first pregnancy

are particularly important for black women. Both incidence and death rates are much lower for other ethnic groups.

Mammography provides an effective screening technique for the detection of early, treatable breast cancer. Current techniques involve only limited radiation exposure and have been shown to reduce mortality from breast cancer in women 50 years of age and older. For this reason, regular mammography screening is uniformly recommended in this age group.[128,130,136,137]

Controversy exists regarding the use of mammography screen before the age of 50.[130,131,136–142] Large-scale trials in Scandinavia[141] and Canada[139] have failed to demonstrate a reduction in cancer mortality for women screened in their forties. Study design and mammography techniques for these studies have been criticized, and some observers consider the issue unresolved.[142] It seems certain that any benefit of mammography screening must be significantly smaller in women under age 50 than in women over this age. The reduced efficacy in younger women is most likely accounted for by a lower frequency of disease and reduced sensitivity of mammography related to increased breast density. Breast cancers appear to develop more rapidly in younger women, and this may reduce the efficacy of annual screening as well. Another problem with mammography screening in younger women is the high rate of false-positive results. For example, Eddy[128] has estimated that false-positive results occur 20 time more frequently than true-positive cancer diagnoses in mammography studies of women in their mid-forties.[128]

Recommendations from various agencies reflect this controversy. The National Cancer Institute recently modified its guidelines and now recommends that routine mammography screening begin at age 50.[131] The American College of Physicians and the US Preventive Health Task Force similarly recommend mammography screening onset at age 50.[115,137] The lack of proven benefit for mammography before age 50 is the primary argument for these recommendations. The high risk of false-positive results also argues against routine screening in younger women. However, the American Cancer Society continues to recommend mammography at 1- to 2-year intervals between the ages of 40 and 50 on the grounds that some benefit from screening in this age group is theoretically likely.[114]

There is, however, uniformity regarding the recommendation that mammography should be done at younger ages in patients whose family history places them at increased risk for breast cancer.[128] In assessing the importance of family history, several factors are taken into consideration: number of affected relatives; age at which relatives were affected; and bilateral versus unilateral disease. The greater the number of relatives affected and the closer the biological relationship of the affected relatives, the more significant the family history.[126] Early age of onset is also an indicator of higher genetic risk. For example, a woman whose mother and sister both developed breast cancer before age 50 has a three- to fivefold increased risk above average for breast cancer, and she is likely to benefit from annual mammography screening beginning as early as age 30.[126] On the other hand, a woman with a family history of unilateral breast cancer in an aunt aged 60 has little, if any, increased risk for breast cancer above that of the general population. Claus and coworkers[117] have developed detailed charts of empirical risks based on the Cancer and Steroid Hormone Study, conducted by the Centers for Disease Control, for use in counseling women on their risk for breast cancer related to family history.[126]

The actual use of mammography in the United States is low, even in the over-50 age group.[124] Surveys indicate that only one half to two thirds of women over age 50 have ever had a mammogram, and far fewer have had mammography on an annual basis. In a case-control study of older women by Brown and Hulka,[124] those with breast cancer were found to have a lower likelihood of metastatic disease if they had undergone screening, as would be expected; but most surprisingly, only 6% of control women had ever had mammography. Screening rates are lower for blacks and economically disadvantaged women than for middle-class white women, accounting in part for the increased breast cancer mortality seen in black women.[129,134] Several studies have documented the importance of physician advice in motivating women to complete mammography screening.[131,134]

Although mammography has received the most attention in discussions of breast cancer prevention, physical examination is important as well. All agencies support the use of breast self-examination, and most also recommend an annual clinical examination of the breasts beginning at age 40. Breast self-examination has not been extensively studied, but anecdotal data identify it as a means of detecting early, treatable disease.[132] This simple procedure is readily learned by most women. Breast models help to teach standard techniques, and are useful in both patient education and medical training.[125]

Colorectal Cancer

Colorectal cancer is the third most frequent cancer in women, after lung and breast cancer.[112] The lifetime risk for colorectal cancer among North American women is 5%. It is believed that most colon cancers arise in the distal colon from adenomatous polyps. Such polyps occur in as many as 10% to 25% of the population and are readily visible on endoscopic examination of the colon.[147,153] Only a minority of adenomatous polyps will become cancerous, with the time course for development of cancer from a polyp estimated to be 5 to 10 years. Factors that increase the risk of colorectal cancer are shown in Table 9.6.

Two methods of screening for colorectal cancer are available. These are testing of stool for occult blood (which may be caused by polyps or cancer, or other benign conditions) and lower endoscopy (sigmoidoscopy or colonoscopy), which permits direct visualization of a polyp or cancer. Controversy exists regarding the cost and efficacy of each method.[144,150,152,153] However, data that have been emerging over the last few years have increasingly supported the use of both techniques as a means to reduce colon cancer mortality.[145,148,151]

The American Cancer Society currently recommends testing of stool for occult blood on an annual basis, beginning at age 50.[114] Not all polyps and cancers will bleed, and this method may fail to detect 50% of colon cancers. However, it offers the opportunity to detect early cancer or a precancerous polyp through use of a simple, noninvasive test. The American College of Physicians also recommends this test, however, the US Preventive Services Task Force recommends it only for those individuals with risk factors for colon cancer, as listed in Table 9.6.[113,115] The primary argument against the routine use of this test is the high false-positive rate; only 5% to 10% of occult blood reactions are due to cancer or precancerous lesions; the majority are due to benign conditions such as hemorrhoids and diverticulosis.[147,152] Bowel work-ups resulting from stool testing (usually a flexible sigmoidoscopy and a barium enema) involve a small risk of significant complications, including hemorrhage and bowel perforation, and a negative test may engender a false sense of security. Nevertheless, testing for occult blood in stool permits the identification of individuals at increased risk of colon cancer, with a test that is both inexpensive and noninvasive.

As with stool testing, there are differing recommendations regarding the use of endoscopic procedures for colon cancer screening. The flexible sigmoidoscope permits visualization of the colon to 60 cm. In addition to cancerous lesions, polyps can be located and biopsied. Colonoscopy is then performed if adenomatous polyps are found, to permit visualization of the entire colon and to remove the adenomatous polyp(s). The American Cancer Society recommends routine use of flexible sigmoidoscopy screening for all adults, beginning at age 50.[114] Two sequential annual examinations are recommended, with repeat testing every three years thereafter. The American College of Physicians also now recommends the use of flexible sigmoidoscopy, on a schedule of 3 to 5 years, starting at age 50; this recommendation is based on recent studies indicating benefit.[113] The US Preventive Services Task Force recommends this procedure only for individuals with increased risk for colon cancer.[115]

As with other cancer screening measures, there is concern regarding false-positive results and procedure risks from flexible sigmoidoscopy screening, as well as the significant cost attached to routine screening of all adults 50 and over.[115] Hyperplastic polyps, which are benign and not associated with colorectal cancer, are more common than adenomatous polyps, and their presence may lead to additional work-up and procedure risk. A negative result from flexible sigmoidoscopy examination may also create a sense of false security, as proximal polyps and cancers are not ruled out. These uncertainties make it impossible to argue for a specific approach to sigmoidoscopy screening at this time. It may be prudent to inform patients of the range of recommendations proposed by expert panels regarding colorectal cancer screening and to help patients to decide which screening program they prefer, taking into account the average lifetime risk of colorectal cancer, and the uncertainty, cost, and risk intrinsic to the screening procedures.

It is generally agreed that patients with high-risk family history should be routinely screened.[113–115] (see Table 9.6). These include individuals with a family history of polyposis coli, two or more first-degree relatives with colorectal cancer, or a history otherwise compatible with the family cancer syndrome (see below). Others at increased risk include individuals with ulcerative colitis, a past history of colon polyps, or a past history of colon, endometrial, ovarian, or breast cancer.

Table 9.6 Risk Factors for Colorectal Cancer

Factors that increase risk:
   First-degree relative with colon cancer
   History of colorectal, breast, endometrial, or ovarian cancer
   History of adenomatous polyp(s)
   Ulcerative colitis
Highest-risk group:
   Two or more first-degree relatives with colorectal cancer
   Family cancer syndrome
   Family of polyposis coli

Ovarian Cancer

Ovarian cancer is a relatively rare cancer, accounting for only 4% of cancer in women. Unfortunately, no screening technique has been shown to have high sensitivity for detection of early disease. Survival is poor for individuals with ovarian cancer, reflecting the fact that most cases are beyond stage 1 at the time of diagnosis.[154–157] Methods currently available for screening include pelvic examination, pelvic ultrasonography and the serum marker CA-125. All are poorly sensitive for the detection of early disease. In addition, pelvic ultrasonography and CA-125 have been shown to have high false-positive rates. Thus no method for routine screening can be recommended at this time.

Cancer-Prone Families

Familial clustering of cancer may occur either as a result of inherited factors or from shared environmental exposure. Family studies have provided strong evidence for inherited risk in many families showing clustering of colorectal, breast, ovarian, and endometrial cancer. Some families exhibit a single cancer type, while others include both colon and breast or breast and ovarian clusters. Often, cancers other than the predominant type occur in low frequency, and may reflect either the coincidental appearance of sporadic cancer cases unrelated to the inherited risk factor or a small effect of the inherited risk factor on other cancer types.

Research in molecular genetics has begun to identify the specific genes responsible for cancer predisposition in some high-risk families. For example, mutations in BRCA1, a gene on chromosome 17, appear to account for cancer predisposition in about half of high-risk breast cancer families and in the majority of families with breast and ovarian cancer.[158] Similarly, mutation in HNPCC genes on chromosomes 2 and 3 account for cancer predisposition in many colon cancer–prone families.[146,149]

A cancer-prone family is suggested by the presence of cancer in two or more first-degree relatives, or in a pattern suggestive of autosomal dominant inheritance, in which risk is passed on from one generation to the next and the number of affected individuals approaches 50% in each generation.[158–162] Typically, early onset of cancer and multiple primary tumors in one or more of the affected individuals are also seen. Genetic testing may soon have a role in testing unaffected individuals from such high-risk families to determine whether or not they have inherited the risk. When an inherited predisposition to cancer is identified, careful cancer screening can be offered. For example, for individuals from colon cancer–prone families, screening with both stool testing and endoscopy is recommended. Most experts recommend colonoscopy rather than sigmoidoscopy for screening in these high-risk individuals. For individuals with increased risk for breast cancer, mammography beginning at age 25–35 is usually recommended. Prophylactic mastectomy is also an option, but unfortunately no reliable data are available to quantify the degree of protection afforded by this surgery. No proven screening methods are available for woman with an inherited risk of ovarian cancer. Studies of the use of ultrasonography and the serum marker CA-125 are in process and may provide some benefit; however, a high false-positive rate, leading to unnecessary surgery, has occurred with this screening approach.[159]

Skin Cancer

Melanoma

The incidence of melanoma has doubled every 10 to 15 years since the 1930s.[168,169] The lifetime risk of melanoma for the average American is currently 0.6% and is estimated to rise to 1% by the year 2000.[168] Factors that increase the risk for melanoma include fair skin and hair color, positive family history for melanoma, large congenital nevi, and the presence of pigmented lesions meeting the criteria for dysplastic nevi.[164–167,170,171] A history of severe sunburn or blistering also appears to increase the risk for melanoma. For example, Green and coworkers[166] found that after controlling for other known risk factors, patients with six or more severe sunburns (pain lasting more than 48 hr) had a 2.4-fold increased risk of melanoma compared with those without a history of sunburns.

Congenital nevi of greater than 20-cm diameter have a 5% to 20% risk of degenerating into melanoma.[171] The risk from smaller congenital nevi has not been well quantified, but is assumed to be above that of the general population. Acquired nevi rarely exceed 5 or 6 mm, so that nevi larger than this merit careful review. Dysplastic nevi occur in 2% to 8% of the population and are defined by four characteristics: (1) macular and papular components, (2) irregular borders, (3) variegated pigmentation within the same lesion, and (4) diameter of 5 to 12 mm.[167] Congenital nevi or nevi with dysplastic characteristics should be referred for biopsy. When lesions with dysplastic characteristics are 1 cm or larger or show progressive increase in size or asymmetric growth, melanoma should be suspected.

An annual full skin examination is recommended for patients with dysplastic nevi, large congenital nevi, or a positive family history of melanoma.[163] Melanomas may occur de novo, without a prior suspicious nevus. A high index of suspicion toward new or changed pigmented lesions will help to prevent diagnostic delay. Patients with both dysplastic nevi and a positive family history are at a particularly increased risk. The lifetime risk of melanoma is estimated to be 100% when an individual has dysplastic nevi *and* two first-degree relatives (parents, siblings, or children) with melanoma.[167] Such individuals should be referred to a dermatologist for careful surveillance.

Other Skin Cancers

Sun exposure (both sunburn and accumulated lifetime exposure) is the major risk factor for other skin cancers.[165] Fair-haired and fair-skinned individuals are at greater risk and should be advised to use sun-protective skin preparations when exposed to bright sunlight. The most common skin cancer is the *basal cell* cancer. This is identifiable as a pearly papule often displaying prominent associated telangiectasia. As basal cell cancers grow, they may develop a central ulceration. Surgical removal is generally curative. *Squamous cell* cancers arise from areas of *actinic keratosis*. The latter are erythematous lesions 0.5 to 5 mm in size, with irregular adherent scale. On pathological examination they consist of dysplastic squamous cells confined to the epidermal layer of the skin. They can be readily treated with liquid nitrogen cryotherapy. As the dysplastic tissue extends into the dermal layer, the lesions increase in size and become indurated. Surgery is required at this stage to remove the cancerous process and, as with basal cell cancers, is curative.

Musculoskeletal Disease

Osteoarthritis

Osteoarthritis, often called degenerative joint disease (DJD), is the most frequent cause of disability in the elderly. In fact, autopsy studies have shown that even as early as 40 years of age some pathological abnormalities can be detected in the weight-bearing joints of almost all individuals.[176] By age 75, there is radiographic evidence for degenerative joint changes in 85% of patients[178] and, in contrast to osteoporosis, the disease occurs with similar frequency in all ethnic groups. The most frequently involved regions are the distal and proximal interphalangeal joints, knees, hips, and lower lumbar and cervical vertebrae.[177] The pattern of joint involvement suggests a genetic component. Although osteoarthritis often develops in joints previously damaged by trauma or affected by inflammatory arthritis, it also occurs without identified precipitating cause. With the exception of knee involvement, there is conflicting opinion regarding the role of obesity in etiology or exacerbation of DJD.[174,175]

The main symptom is pain, which is aching in nature and usually of moderate severity. Except with advanced disease, the pain is commonly increased with activity and relieved by rest. Although brief morning stiffness is frequently present, DJD usually is not characterized by the prolonged post/rest stiffness seen in inflammatory arthritis. Muscle spasms may contribute to the discomfort. Physical examination can reveal enlargement of joints, without the boggy synovial swelling of the inflammatory arthritides, pain on palpation, and crepitus with movement. Osteophyte growth and cartilage irregularities can result in limitation of movement, which can be disabling in severe cases with hip and knee involvement. Radiographic studies often show the specific changes of osteoarthritis and the diagnosis is usually made without difficulty.

Treatment should be conservative, as long as is possible, since the disease is chronic, slowly progressive, and rarely crippling. The patient should be reassured that the natural history of DJD usually does not necessitate aggressive intervention and that benign therapies often provide relief. It is reasonable to suggest a plan of weight reduction for the obese patient, especially those with involvement of weight-bearing joints. Warm baths or moist heat packs can decrease muscle spasm and joint stiffness. Physical therapy can maintain or improve range of motion and strengthen supporting musculature, but care must be taken to avoid repetitious movements that may accelerate joint degeneration. The provision of walking aids and large-handled appliances can simplify and improve the activities of daily living. The nonsteroidal anti-inflammatory drugs (NSAIDs) have become a mainstay of therapy for DJD. These drugs decrease the mild synovitis that may be present and provide good pain relief. Enteric coated aspirin is usually well tolerated, but the drug of choice for an individual patient is chosen empirically on the basis of patient compliance, frequency of dosing, side effects, and cost. It must be remembered that a major morbidity of aspirin and NSAIDs is upper gastrointestinal bleeding, especially in the elderly. In addition, NSAIDs may result in fluid retention and renal dysfunction. Recent studies suggest that acetaminophen may be as effective for symptomatic relief as NSAIDs given in analgesic or anti-inflammatory dosages.[172,173] Narcotics should be avoided; the disease is long-term, not "curable," and other pain-reducing measures are available. Narcotics have some very undesirable side effects for the geriatric population, including constipation and central nervous system depression. Surgical procedures are usually reserved for patients with intractable pain or progressive functional disability.

Osteoporosis

Osteoporosis results from a decrease in bone density, caused by increased bone resorption relative to bone formation. Beginning in the fourth decade of life there is a continuous slow decrease in bone density. In both men and women, the maximal bone density in young adulthood varies, which is at least in part a result of genetic factors. For instance, blacks have a greater maximal bone density than do whites and Asians.[212] However, in women, the decade immediately after menopause is marked by a more rapid loss of bone density.[202] An increased incidence of Colles' and vertebral fractures is seen soon after menopause, whereas hip fractures occur later in life.[212] As the density of bone decreases, the severity of the trauma sufficient to cause a fracture also decreases. To compound the situation, falls occur more frequently as people age, in part due to decreased vision, neurological impairment, dementia, arthritis, and the effects of medications.

Risk factors for osteoporosis are shown in Table 9.7.[182,202,207,209,212,220] Assessing these risk factors in individual women provides an opportunity for primary or secondary prevention. Patient history should include screening for family history of either known osteoporosis or symptoms suggestive of it (height loss, kyphosis, nontraumatic hip fractures); race; menopausal status; personal behaviors, such as activity and exercise history; alcohol intake; present or past cigarette smoking; medication use; and risk for falls. Dietary history may indicate inadequate calcium intake, a history of chronic dieting, lactose intolerance, or anorexia. Chronic disease may heighten the risk; for example, rheumatoid arthritis, with or without the use of steroids, is associated with increased risk for osteoporosis. Gastrointestinal diseases may adversely affect nutrition. Thyroid disease may also confer increased risk of osteoporosis. Due to the action of thyroxin, bone resorption is increased in patients with hyperthyroidism; this also occurs, to a lesser degree, in patients who are on thyroxin replacement therapy at doses sufficient to suppress thyroid-stimulating hormone (TSH). (This suppression may exist in the absence of any signs or symptoms of hyperthyroidism.) Some, but not all, studies of perimenopausal women with this level of replacement have demonstrated a decrease in bone density; none have shown evidence of an increased rate of fractures. Although overreplacement of thyroxin has only a small—if any—effect on the development of osteoporosis, it is advisable to maintain the TSH in the normal range when treating primary hypothyroidism.[216,218] By some estimates, one fifth of all women over 65 years of age have vertebral fractures, and one third of all women who reach very old age (over 85 years) will have suffered a fractured hip.[212] The morbidity of hip fracture is extremely high—as many as 20% of patients die within 1 year of complications directly related to this event, and approximately half of the survivors are no longer able to live independently. Although sometimes characterized by immediate, severe, localized back pain, vertebral fractures are often asymptomatic, detected only as loss of height or kyphosis. These fractures may also be diagnosed by chest radiograph ordered for another purpose.

Standard radiographs are not a good screen for osteopenia because at least 30% of bone density must be lost before osteopenia is detected on X-ray.[194,203,212] Currently available techniques for quantitation of vertebral and other bone density are expensive[203] and show overlap between the groups with and without osteoporosis.[194,207] Although low bone density is the strongest known risk factor for osteoporotic fractures, most women have some degree of osteoporosis by the age at which hip fractures occur and not all elderly women with decreased bone density suffer fractures.[188] Recent analyses have found it to be cost-effective to screen asymptomatic, perimenopausal white women for low bone mass to allow targeting of hormone replacement to the subset of women at highest risk.[186,219] However, the value of screening depends on whether the findings would influence

Table 9.7 Risk Factors for the Development of Osteoporosis

Sex (female > male)
Age
Positive family history
Race: White or Asian
Endocrine: hyperthyroidism, hyperparathyroidism
Prolonged use of glucocorticoids
Cigarette smoking
Alcohol abuse
Early oophorectomy
History of lactose intolerance
Sedentary life-style/immobilization
Body habitus: small, lean
Low calcium intake

a physician's or patient's decision regarding therapy. Because the evidence favors estrogen therapy in many postmenopausal women, large-scale screening is not currently indicated.[194] Rather, bone density assays should be reserved for patients with symptoms and those in high-risk groups who are reluctant to begin estrogen or who have relative contraindication to it. Use of glucorticoids, hyperparathyroidism, and radiographic osteopenia are other accepted indications for bone mineral density measurements. Site-specific dual photodensitometry should be used because the risk of fracture correlates specifically with the density at that site, that is, vertebral fractures with vertebral density and hip fractures with hip–femoral neck density; measurement at both sites is advocated.

The only approach to osteoporosis shown to be cost-effective is prevention. This can be achieved either through increasing peak bone mass or decreasing the rate of later bone loss. Several therapies have benefit in preventing or ameliorating osteoporosis. Peak premenopausal bone mass is related to the level of physical activity.[179] Studies have consistently demonstrated a direct relation between weight-bearing exercise and bone mass, in both pre- and postmenopausal women.[189] Exercise not only slows the rate of bone loss but can result in some bone gain.[200]

Additionally, exercise in postmenopausal women improves coordination and muscle strength, which may decrease the number of falls. For this and other reasons discussed herein, increased physical activity should be encouraged.[185] Conversely, cigarette smoking or the excess use of alcohol leads to decreased bone density. A recent study of female twins discordant for tobacco use reported that women who smoke one pack per day throughout adulthood will have a 5% to 10% decrease in bone density by the time of menopause.[196] Women who smoke begin menopause 1 to 2 years earlier, demonstrate more rapid bone loss in the initial postmenopausal years, and have a higher incidence of postmenopausal fractures than nonsmokers.[197] ERT, the most effective therapy currently known, is less effective in smokers than in nonsmokers. In one study, there was a 1.26 relative risk of hip fractures in women who smoked and took estrogen as compared with a 0.37 relative risk in nonsmoking estrogen users.[199] Clearly, patients should be counseled to discontinue smoking.

An attempt should be made to optimize a women's nutritional status. A decrease in vitamin D levels leads to decreased calcium absorption, especially after age 70.[184,213] Adequate intake is approximately 400 to 800 units/day, especially in winter. The St. Louis OASIS fall and hip fracture study showed that vitamin D supplementation and summer sunlight exposure of greater than 1 hr/day in women over the age of 75 conferred significant protection from hip fractures.[187] Similar protection was seen in elderly female nursing-home residents who received supplemental vitamin D and calcium.[184]

The average intake of calcium is less than two thirds the recommended daily allowance (RDA), currently set at 800 mg/day and substantially less than the 1,200 to 1,500 mg/day that may be needed to restore a positive calcium balance after menopause.[204] If dietary calcium is low, and there is no history of nephrolithiasis or hypercalcemia, supplementation at least up to the RDA should be attempted using low cost calcium carbonate tablets (each standard calcium carbonate tablet provides 200 mg of elemental calcium). A recent article demonstrated that calcium supplementation of 1,000 mg/day significantly slowed axial and appendicular bone loss in normal postmenopausal women.[209] A retrospective, population-based, case-controlled study found that women taking calcium had a relative risk of hip fractures of 0.75, with longer duration of supplemental calcium therapy associated with decreased risk.[198] Calcium balance is affected by other dietary components, such as sodium, protein, and caffeine. Heaney found that urinary calcium excretion is increased by 40 to 80 mg for each 2.3 g of sodium ingested. Protein has a similar but much smaller effect on urinary loss.[195] Consumption of large amounts of caffeine results in increased calcium excretion in the urine but the impact on bone density is negligible if calcium consumption is adequate.[181]

Calcium supplementation may have some beneficial effect on bone density, but postmenopausal estrogen replacement actually decreases the frequency of all types of fractures.[190,191,199,202] The most significant factor in the development of osteoporosis in women is the estrogen deficiency that accompanies menopause. The benefit of ERT has been supported by many studies. ERT has been shown to be most effective if started within 5 to 6 years of menopause, during the period of greatest bone loss.[193] ERT beginning at menopause prevents the acceleration of bone loss that otherwise occurs; if will result in a 3% to 5% bone gain during the first 12 months if started more than 6 years after menopause. Estrogen therapy is not entirely benign and the risk-benefit ratio should be considered when advising widespread use of these medications. When bone densitometry is used as the criterion for a woman who will take estrogen solely if she is at increased risk for osteoporosis, bone density more than one standard deviation below the mean for menopausal women would be a strong indication for initiating therapy. Women with intermediate values should have bone densitometry repeated in 2 to 5 years and should begin ERT if the estimated rate of bone loss is greater than average. There is general agreement that high-risk patients, especially those with surgically induced early menopause, should be strongly advised to use ERT. One study found that postmenopausal bone loss can be prevented by low-dose conjugated equine estrogen (0.3 mg/day) and calcium supplements[191] but the usual recommended dosage is 0.625 mg/day. The optimal duration of estrogen therapy is not known. Epidemiologically, the use of ERT declines as women enter their sixties, yet the rate of hip fractures doubles with each postmenopausal decade, and there is an increase in associated mortality in the elderly. A recent study concluded that at least 7 years of therapy is necessary for the long-term preservation of bone density, with the caveat that even this duration may have little residual effect by age 75.[192] It is widely recommended that ERT be given for 5 to 10 years. Although it is possible that more prolonged use would provide protection from fractures, at present the benefit of ERT to women over 75 years of age has not been adequately studied, and there is some evidence suggesting that an increased duration of ERT is associated with an increased risk of breast cancer. Long-term use of unopposed conjugated estrogens is associated with a persistent three- to fourfold increased risk of endometrial cancer.[214] However, this relatively common cancer is not a leading cause of cancer deaths[208] because it is usually diagnosed at an early stage when cure is still possible. The addition of a progestin (and reinstitution of cycling) for patients who have not had a hysterectomy probably decreases the risk of endometrial cancer,[175] but patients may be reluctant to accept this therapy. New regimens that combine low-dose continuous progestin with estrogen have been shown to prevent endometrial hypertrophy (and dysplastic changes) and decrease the incidence of withdrawal bleeding.[76,87]

Progestin therapy, however, may also be associated with negative side effects, including breast tenderness, depression, irritability, and decreased cardioprotective high-density lipoprotein levels.[70,74] Estrogens, on the other hand, cause increases in HDL levels. It is unclear whether the alteration in lipoprotein ratios that result from low-dose progestins will negate the beneficial effect of estrogens on cardiovascular disease. Recent studies have produced conflicting data about hormone replacement as a risk factor for breast cancer.[169] Resolution of these issues will require further studies. For now, decisions regarding ERT must be individualized. Absolute contraindications include acute or chronic liver disease, acute vascular thrombosis, and probably breast cancer. Relative contraindications, including gallbladder disease, migraine headaches, chronic thrombophlebitis, hypertension or a history of endometriosis, also must be considered. (For a more complete discussion of hormone replacement, refer to the section on cardiovascular disease in this chapter and Chapter 8.)

Some researchers foresee therapy with biphosphonates, analogues of pyrophosphate that act as potent inhibitors of bone resorption, replacing estrogen therapy as the primary method of prevention in the near future.[204] At present, ERT is clearly the first line of therapy for postmenopausal osteoporosis; for those having contraindications to hormonal therapy, calcitonin and the biphosphonate etidronate are the next options, currently used only for women with existing osteoporosis or who have a very high risk of developing it.

Studies of fluoridation of water supplies give conflicting results and the role of fluoride supplementation in the prevention and therapy of this disease is still unclear. Although fluoride increases bone mass, fluoride supplementation results in bone with abnormal structure and possibly increased fragility.[211,212] At present, however, fluoride is not recommended in the routine treatment of osteoporosis. Other medical therapies of moderate and severe osteoporosis are being evaluated in research settings; patients with complex problems should be referred to specialists for management.

Equally important in the management of osteoporosis is the prevention of falls that can lead to fractures. The lifetime risk of hip fracture in women age 50 is approximately 17%, increasing exponentially after age 70. Hip fracture repair, a major cause of morbidity and mortality, also represents a major economic burden, with US costs expected to increase from $7 billion in 1986 to $86 billion by the year 2020.[205,206,217] Exercise helps to optimize muscle strength and balance as well as increase bone density. Vision should be evaluated as well as the use of sedatives and other medications that impair concentration. Home evaluations for to assess the need for railings and proper lighting, for flooring and carpeting hazards, and for other potential risks should be done when indicated.

Direct trauma to the hip has been implicated in 60% to 99% of all hip fractures; energy absorption is a determinant of potential hip fracture.[183] This explains, in part, the reduced risk of hip fracture in overweight women; Obesity is also associated with decreased bone loss. In a recent controlled trial in Danish nursing homes, hip fractures were shown to be prevented by use of external hip protectors.[201]

Vision and Hearing

Impairments of the visual and auditory senses are common occurrences during aging that may reduce the quality of life and contribute to social isolation. Patients may assume that decreased senses are normal consequences of aging and, therefore, may not volunteer that they have a problem. Primary care providers should specifically inquire about changes in visions and hearing so that appropriate referrals can be made. The frequency of significant eye disease, including presbyopia, glaucoma, and cataracts, is low in the population under 40 years of age, but thereafter increases steadily.[222,233]

Glaucoma is a condition of increased intraocular pressure that results from a decrease in drainage of the aqueous humor from the eye. If untreated, the increased pressure leads to cupping and then atrophy of the optic disc and eventually to decreased visual fields and visual acuity.[237] Rare in childhood and early adulthood, glaucoma rises in prevalence with each decade after age 40. Approximately 0.4% to 1.6% of individuals older than 40 have some degree of visual impairment secondary to glaucoma.[222] As is the case for many conditions, patients with a positive family history of glaucoma are at increased risk to develop this condition. Timely intervention usually prevents loss of vision. Unfortunately, most patients with early glaucoma are asymptomatic; a significant loss of peripheral vision can occur before a patient is aware that there is a problem. The presence of glaucoma also places the patient at increased risk to develop cataracts.

A cataract is defined as an opacity in the lens. Congenital cataracts are stable defects, whereas presenile (occurring in late childhood and early adulthood) and senile cataracts (usually appearing after ages 30 to 40) usually progress and may cause severe visual impairment.[236] Cataract formation is a physiological change of aging so that, although they are "abnormal," some evidence of lens opacification can be detected by slit lamp examination in over 96% of people older than 60 years.[230] These common senile cataracts are usually characterized by very slow progression. Most never reach a size that causes significant visual deterioration. However, since the prevalence is so high, cataract formation is one of the most common causes of serious loss of vision, accounting for approximately 15% to 20% of cases of blindness.

There are factors besides aging that increase the likelihood that a person will develop cataracts. Many drugs, including ergotamines and systemic or ophthalmic corticosteroids are toxic to the lens. Prolonged use may result in cataracts. Diabetics tend to develop typical senile cataracts at an earlier age, and these cataracts enlarge more quickly than those occurring in the nondiabetic population. More rarely, diabetics may develop specific "diabetic cataracts," characterized by increased sorbitol, fructose, and glucose content in the lens.[230]

Genetic factors are involved in the predisposition to cataracts. In some families acquired cataract formation is transmitted as an autosomal dominant trait.[234] Finally, cataracts may form following trauma to the lens. Regardless of etiology, removal of the cataract is the only way to restore lost vision.

With aging, the nearest point at which an object can be brought into clear focus becomes more remote. This disturbance in accommodation for near vision is called presbyopia—literally "aged vision"—and results from decreases in lens elasticity and contractibility of ciliary muscles.[229] The latter change reduces the ability of the eyes to converge, and physical hardening of the lens prevents it from assuming a rounded shape, movements that are both necessary for close vision. The maximum degree of accommodation decreases with age from childhood to approximately age 75, with onset of clinically significant presbyopia at about 45 years. Presbyopia interferes most with reading, but convex reading glasses can substitute for the loss of accommodative power.

Since most eye impairments are remediable and if untreated may lead to substantial deterioration in quality of life, it is important to identify those persons who might benefit from an ocular evaluation. In addition, impaired vision is implicated in many falls and resultant hip fractures in the elderly. In general, persons who complain of visual disturbances should be promptly referred to an ophthalmologist. Decreased visual acuity, blurred vision, impaired night vision, and eye pain are examples of symptoms that may indicate serious eye pathology. Frequent routine screening eye examinations are no longer recommended for all asymptomatic individuals, since abnormalities are rarely found and the cost-benefit ratio is unfavorable. The American Academy of Ophthalmology recommends ophthalmologic evaluations every 2–4 years for asymptomatic individuals aged 40 and older and every 1–2 years for those 65 and over, primarily for the detection of presbyopia.[223] More intensive surveillance should be reserved for people who are at increased risk for eye diseases, such as those with diabetes, hypertension, or a family history of glaucoma or progressive blindness.

Hearing loss is a common finding in otherwise healthy persons and may decrease quality of life. If uncorrected, a moderate-to-severe hearing deficit can hinder the ability to live independently.[227,232] Two major factors in hearing loss are noise exposure and aging. The most common effect of presbycusis ("aged hearing") is progressive bilateral loss of the ability to detect high frequency tones.[226] The decrease in range of tone sensitivity is usually quite insidious, and the associated symptom of tinnitus may be the first hearing abnormality noticed by the patient. Approximately 5.2% of people aged 18 to 44 have some degree of hearing impairment, but the prevalence increases steadily to 13.6% at 45 to 64 years, 24.4% at 65 to 74 years, and 37.8% at or above age 75.[224] Although only a portion of older persons will have hearing loss severe enough to warrant intervention (recent data suggest that a handicapping hearing loss exists in 29% of people over age 65,[232] screening is worthwhile because inexpensive, easily performed tests are available. The gold standard hearing test is the pure-tone audiogram to identify the frequencies at which a signal is not heard. Recently, a portable otoscope containing an audiometer has become available. This instrument emits tones at four frequencies and three intensities and is appropriate for use by primary care physicians.[235,238] For purposes of screening, however, the most important parameter to study is the ability to discern normal spoken conversation, because this determines the degree to which the hearing impairment is a problem in daily life. For example, the patient may communicate without difficulty in a quiet examining room but not by telephone or in the presence of background noise.

Two maneuvers that are fairly sensitive in detecting hearing impairment are whispered voice for speech discrimination and the finger-rub test.[239] The first is performed by whispering a series of common one or two syllable words beginning at a distance of 6 inches from the test ear and gradually moving away. The distance at which the patient cannot correctly repeat at least 50% of the words is noted. Appropriate vocabulary lists are published.[221] Alternatively, after first positioning the examiner's hand close to the patient's ear, the examiner rubs his thumb and index finger together and slowly withdraws the hand until the patient can no longer hear the signal. Whispered voice should be correctly discerned to approximately 19 cm and finger rub should be heard at 8 cm from the external auditory canal.[239]

A simple, 15-question, self-administered test developed by the American Academy of Otolaryngology–Head and Neck Surgery (AAO-HNS)[225] can be given to the patient to score at home (Figure 9.1). A score of 10 or above indicates that the patient is significantly hearing impaired and audiological evaluation by an ear, nose, and throat (ENT) specialist should be urged. Scores between 6 and 9 suggest that the patient is at risk to develop future significant impairment. ENT evaluation can be recommended at this stage. Copies of this test can be purchased from the AAO-HNS.

One easily remedied contributory factor to impaired hearing at any age is cerumen impaction. There is a tendency for cerumen in older individuals to be dry and to inspissate. Once the external canal is cleared by gentle irrigation or wax dissolving drops, recurrent impaction can be avoided by weekly instillation of a few drops of baby oil.

Mouth

The American College of Physicians, The US Preventive Services Task Force, and the Canadian Task Force all recommend routine evaluation of the oral cavity in patients over age 65. A yearly dental examination is part of an optimal health maintenance program, however, some patients may see their dentists only infrequently, especially if the patient lacks dental insurance coverage. Physicians who provide primary care to geriatric patients should be aware of the relatively common oral conditions that occur in this population.[227] Periodontal disease is the most common cause of tooth loss in the elderly. Areas of dentin normally protected by a covering of gum become susceptible to development of caries that also contribute to loss of teeth. Good oral hygiene practices, including daily brushing and flossing, can prevent these dental problems.

Oral examination can also reveal precursors to oral cancer that are most often the result of tobacco and alcohol exposure, but that also occur in the presence of chronic irritation, such as might result from ill-fitting dentures. In contrast to candida (thrush), the white patches of leukoplakia are painless and cannot be scraped off. Most of these lesion are benign, but as many as 10% contain regions of dysplasia or carcinoma in situ. Erythroplakia are red lesions of mucosa that are much more frequently dysplastic or frankly malignant. Because early diagnosis increases the likelihood of curative surgery,[230] visual examination of the oral mucosa and tongue is reasonable in patients who are at higher than normal risk to develop oral squamous cell carcinoma, especially those patients who do not regularly receive dental checkups.

	Almost Always	Half the Time	Occasionally	Never
1. I have a problem hearing over the telephone.				
2. I have trouble following the conversation when two or more people are talking at the same time.				
3. People complain that I turn the TV volume too high.				
4. I have to strain to understand conversations.				
5. I miss hearing some common sounds like the phone or doorbell ringing.				
6. I have trouble hearing conversations in a noisy background, such as a party.				
7. I get confused about where sounds come from.				
8. I misunderstand some words in a sentence and need to ask people to repeat themselves.				
9. I especially have trouble understanding the speech of women and children.				
10. I have worked in noisy environments (assembly lines, jackhammers, jet engines, etc.).				
11. Many people I talk to seem to mumble (or don't speak clearly).				
12. People get annoyed because I misunderstand what they say.				
13. I misunderstand what others are saying and make inappropriate responses.				
14. I avoid social activities because I cannot hear well and fear I'll reply improperly.				
To be answered by family member or friend: 15. Do you think this person has a hearing loss?				

Scoring

To calculate your score, give yourself 3 points for every time you checked the "Almost always" column, 2 for every "Half the time," 1 for every "Occasionally," and 0 for every "Never." If you have a blood relative who has a hearing loss, add another 3 points. Then total your points.

- 0 to 5—Your hearing is fine. No action is recommended.
- 6 to 9—Ask your doctor about a hearing test.
- 10 and above—strongly recommend a hearing test.

Figure 9.1 Five-Minute Hearing Test (From American Academy of Otolaryngology—Head and Neck Surgery: Five-Minute Hearing Test, Washington, DC, 1989).

Depression and Dementia

Depression is a common disorder in later life.[240] Because no biological parameter is useful clinically to diagnose depression, recognition of this treatable disorder depends on a careful history. Diagnostic criteria for depression are listed in Table 9.8.[239] It is important to keep in mind that elderly patients may deny saddened mood even when depression is present. Instead, they may complain of somatic symptoms (eg, abdominal pain and headache) for which no anatomical or physiological explanation is apparent. A recent onset of this type of hypochondriacal behavior should prompt a careful search for the signs and symptoms of depression listed in Table 9.8.

Later life is a time of changes in life-style, and a time when the deaths of friends and relatives occur more frequently. Prolonged grief is not normal. If mourning lasts longer than is appropriate for a person's sociocultural peer group, the diagnosis of depression should be considered. Talking

Table 9.8 Criteria for the Diagnosis of Major Depression

A. At least 5 of the following symptoms present during the same 2-week period:
• Depressed mood most of day
• Markedly diminished interest or pleasure in all or most activities most of day
• Significant change in weight or appetite
• Insomnia or hypersomnia
• Psychomotor agitation or retardation (observable by others)
• Fatigue or loss of energy nearly every day
• Feelings of worthlessness or inappropriate guilt nearly every day
• Diminished ability to concentrate, or indecisiveness, nearly every day
• Recurrent thoughts of death or suicidal ideation
B. Symptoms cause significant distress or impairment
C. Symptoms are not due to direct effect of a substance or of a medical condition
D. Symptoms are not better accounted for by a bereavement

From *Diagnostic and Statistical Manual of Mental Disorders* ed. 4, American Psychiatric Association, 1994, Washington, DC

with a family member may help in making this judgment. The presence of an apparent environmental precipitant does not influence response to antidepressant medication.

Dementia is a syndrome of acquired deficits of memory and other cognitive abilities sufficiently severe to impair social or occupational functions.[239] In our aging society, dementia is a health problem of truly staggering proportion. Population studies suggest that approximately 5% of persons over age 65 and 20% of persons over age 80 have the dementia syndrome.[248] Although dementia is common, these studies demonstrate that such impairment is not a normal concomitant of the aging process and imply that the term "senility" should be abandoned. Dementia of the Alzheimer's type (DAT), which is usually a relentlessly progressive disease, is by far the most common cause of dementia in the elderly, accounting for at least 70% of cases. After DAT, the most frequent cause of dementia is vascular dementia, accounting for approximately 15% of cases. This dementing process potentially can be prevented by control of hypertension, but no treatment for the dementia itself is available. Ethanol is directly toxic to brain tissue and, with or without thiamine deficiency, can lead to alcoholic dementia,[247] comprising 5% of dementias in later life. This disorder often has a reversible component if the patient can be kept free of alcohol. Another 5% of dementias result from Parkinson's disease.[247] Among the causes of the remaining 5% of cases of dementia in later life are brain structural abnormalities, such as tumors, subdural hematomas, and normal pressure hydrocephalus; inherited neurodegenerative diseases; metabolic derangements; infectious processes including tertiary syphilis, encephalitides, and Creutzfeldt-Jakob disease and, ever more commonly, acquired immunodeficiency syndrome (AIDS).

Although the dementias that result from metabolic abnormalities are theoretically curable, by the time recognizable mental dysfunction is present, intervention rarely produces complete resolution of the impairment.[242,246] Therefore it may be reasonable to screen asymptomatic older persons for the more common of these diseases, including hypothyroidism and B_{12} deficiency (usually the result of pernicious anemia). Thyroid function tests and complete blood counts with indices and smear evaluation are usually sufficient to detect these disorders, although cognitive dysfunction has been reported in pernicious anemia before the development of anemia.[250]

Depression can mimic dementia. However, the apparent cognitive deficits in depression are more the result of poor concentration and motivation than of actual memory loss. Careful observing and interviewing should allow the physician to distinguish between the two diagnoses. For either depression or dementia a detailed drug history should be obtained. Sleeping pills, alcohol, beta blockers, antihistamines, and muscle relaxants are among the medications that can significantly affect mood and intellectual function. If dementia is suspected, a detailed neurological examination seeking localizing signs is important. The Mini Mental State Exam (MMSE) is a 10-minute, comprehensive, reliable instrument that evaluates memory, language, and praxis.[244] As part of the work-up of dementia, a VDRL test for syphilis is often obtained. However, tertiary syphilis is now a rare disease in women, and a screening VDRL test in the absence of dementia and with no history of syphilis exposure is not indicated.

Aging women will often have aging husbands who are also at risk to develop dementia. The simple question, "How is your husband?" may elicit the patient's worries regarding the cognitive functions of her spouse. The patient should then be advised to have her spouse evaluated. Although, in this case, the patient is not the one with the "disease," the burden of caring for a person with dementia is substantial—physically, psychologically, and financially. Unfortunately, there are currently no effective medical therapies for the neurodegeneration underlying DAT and many other etiologies of demential. There are, however, collaborative efforts in academia and industry to develop effective interventions. For instance, the cholinesterase inhibitor tacrine has recently been shown to symptomatically improve cognitive function in a subgroup of DAT patients.[245] Physicians need to be aware of community resources such as the Alzheimer's Association, a nationwide organization that can provide invaluable peer support and may offer information to concerned individuals about current research protocols and new therapies.

Lifestyle

A major component of preventive health care is the promotion of a healthy life-style. For most Americans, this requires a conscious effort to improve eating habits and increase levels of exercise. Smoking and excessive alcohol intake may also be issues. Patients should be reminded to use seat belts. The importance of life-style changes should not be underestimated. Time spent helping a patient to quit smoking or begin an exercise program may provide greater benefit than more conventional medical care, such as prescribing antihypertensive medications. Because the education and emotional support required by a patient who is making drastic changes in her life-style is time-consuming, it may be appropriate to refer the patient to a program or provider specializing in this area. However, advice from a physician carries special weight. Patients should always be told in simple, unambiguous terms of the health benefits derived from life-style changes.

Smoking

Smoking is responsible for 11% of deaths among women.[281] It is a causative factor in CAD, stroke, peripheral vascular disease, chronic obstructive pulmonary disease (COPD), and several cancers (Table 9.9). It is a contributing factor in other conditions, such as osteoporosis. Public awareness of the health consequences of smoking is increasing, but many still fail to appreciate the broad deleterious effects of smoking. Quitting should be a goal for all smokers.

Although the risk of smoking in middle age is well known, some people have argued that long-term smokers who survive into old age are somehow different. Recent studies, focusing explicitly on smoking in the elderly, demonstrate that smoking-associated mortality extends well into later life.[267] Current studies using female subjects confirm that women are at risk for all the problems caused by smoking that occur in men. The risk of disease has been shown to diminish when smoking has been discontinued. Persistent smokers have a 2.2-fold greater risk of dying from coronary heart disease and a 1.6-fold greater death rate than individuals who quit smoking.[259] A former smoker who remains without evidence of cardiovascular disease for 10 years after quitting

Table 9.9 Representative Disease Risks of Smoking

Disease	Relative risk[*]	Attributable risk (%)[†]
Coronary artery disease	1.7	30
Stroke	1.2–1.5	18
Subarachnoid hemorrhage	5.7	
Lung cancer	7.3	87
Oral, laryngeal, and esophageal cancer	2–27	62
Bladder cancer	2–3	31
Chronic obstructive pulmonary disease	30	82

[*]Relative risk of death for smokers compared to nonsmokers.
[†]Percent of deaths attributable to smoking.

will subsequently have minimal if any increased risk of heart disease compared with a nonsmoker,[279] and significant reduction in the risk of MI is seen within 2 to 3 years.[278,284] Studies of older smokers with CAD reveal that quitting reduces future risk of MI and mortality even after many years of accumulated risk. A cohort study of over 100,000 women, aged 30 to 55 at time of entry, demonstrated that the risk of a fatal or nonfatal coronary event in those who smoked at least 25 cigarettes a day was more than five times that of nonsmokers and with light smoking (1 to 4 cigarettes daily) the risk was more than doubled.[284] In the same population, cigarette smoking was also found to be a risk factor for ischemic and hemorrhagic stroke and smoking cessation decreased this risk, with maximal benefit beginning 2 to 4 years after quitting.[263–265] The residual risk for cancer diminishes more slowly—over about a 15 to 20 year period—but, as with cardiovascular disease, the risks of disease are lower for persons who quit smoking than they are for those who continue.[256] The overall mortality rate due to cigarette smoking decreases to almost that of those who never smoked in 10 to 14 years after quitting.

Even patients who have already developed smoking-related conditions benefit from quitting. Reduced re-infarction rates and slowed progressions of COPD, for example, can be documented when patients with CAD or COPD stop smoking.[256, 281] Abstention from smoking has been shown to increase cerebral perfusion in elderly patients[277] and is associated with improvement in symptoms from peripheral vascular disease.[246]

The physician plays an important role in motivating the smoker to quit. Brief physician counseling may result in quitting rates of 3% to 20%,[252,273] and repetitive counseling is likely to increase this rate. Key steps in helping a patient to quit include the following.[256,260,270,271,273]

1. Identify smoking as a medical problem for the patient.

2. Inform the patient of the risks of smoking and the benefits of quitting. The more specific and personalized the health advice, the more likely it is to have an effect.

3. Help the patient to formulate a concrete plan for quitting. This includes identifying alternatives to smoking, for example, exercise, social activities, and chewing gum.

4. Discuss the benefits of changing the social environment. For example, it may help the patient to socialize with friends who are nonsmokers or to coordinate her quitting efforts with those of friends. If the spouse is a smoker, cessation is much more likely to succeed if he tries to quit as well.

5. Provide continued follow-up. Ask the patient about progress on smoking each time she is seen.

When a patient is shown that she has smoking-related changes in pulmonary function and carbon monoxide levels, she is more likely to quit smoking.[276] Concern about weight gain is often cited as a reason for continued smoking in women and the use of the term *slim* in the names of many cigarette brands directed at women encourage this attitude.[275] The Nurses' Health Study showed, on average, a 1.4 to 2.8 kg greater weight gain over 8 years in persons who quit as compared with those who continued smoking, but the health risks of smoking by far exceed those of this minor weight gain.[7] Counseling about weight may help increase women's motivation to quit.

Additional interventions that may help a patient to quit smoking include the use of hypnosis, nicotine-containing gum and nicotine patches.[252,258,263] Recent research has shown that the use of transdermal nicotine patches for 6 to 8 weeks is an effective aid for smoking cessation with success rates ranging from 22% to 42% versus placebo patch rates of 5% to 28%.[251,255,262,266,269,282,283] The variation in rates appears to be related to the nature and intensity of concomitant counseling.[266] Nicotine patches reduce some aspects of nicotine withdrawal, specifically craving for cigarettes and negative moods, without affecting others, such as hunger and weight gain. The most frequent side effect is local skin irritation (1.5% to 3%). The theoretical risk that smoking while using the nicotine patch might increase the risk of MI has not been observed in practice.

It is not necessary for the primary physician to be actively involved in all aspects of the effort. New models for smoking counseling in the outpatient setting stress a multidisciplinary approach; referral to other providers for an active smoking cessation program should always be considered.[261–262] However, the interest of the primary provider in the patient's progress helps maintain the motivation to quit.

Exercise

A regular exercise program should be recommended to all women unless a specific medical or physical condition prevents it.[285,291] Sedentary individuals benefit from even modest increases in regular physical activity. Health benefits include a reduced risk of heart disease and hypertension, easier weight control, maintenance of muscle strength, improved glucose control in diabetics, and decreased risk of depression.[276] In a study of ambulatory elderly individuals, regular physical activity was associated with a lower overall risk of bone fracture.[287] Moderate exercise programs have been shown to contribute to prolonged longevity as well as improved health.[2,286]

Nevertheless, surveys suggest that less than 10% of individuals 65 and older exercise on a regular basis, despite data indicating that even modest levels of exercise provide health benefits.[2] An increased level of exercise has been identified as an important national health goal[288,291] and represents a method for improving health that is simple and accessible for most patients.

It is important to advise the patient to advance slowly above her usual level of physical activity. A patient who has been almost entirely sedentary will benefit from brief walks of a few minutes and should not attempt vigorous exercise.[285] For patients who are able to do so, the goal should be a program of moderate aerobic exercise, such as brisk walking, swimming, or using an exercise bicycle for 30 minutes, three or more times a week.[285,290] It may take several months to achieve this goal, especially for patients who are not currently exercising. Although significant cardiovascular conditioning can be maintained by exercising three times a week,[285] additional benefits are obtained if exercise is accomplished daily. Patients who are trying to lose weight, for example, will benefit from daily exercise. It may be easier for a patient to maintain a daily exercise program if she includes different activities: walking, swimming, and exercise bicycle. On busy days, even a brief walk is beneficial.

Table 9.10 National Cancer Institute Dietary Guidelines

Reduce fat intake to 30% or less of calories
Increase fiber intake to 20 to 30 g daily
Eat a variety of vegetables and fruits daily
Avoid obesity
Consume alcoholic beverages in moderation, if at all
Minimize consumption of salt-cured, salt-pickled, and smoked foods

From Butrum RR, Clifford CK, Lanza E. NCI dietary guidelines, *Am J Clin Nutr* 1988; 48:888–95

Nutrition

Most patients will benefit from some modifications in diet.[303] The National Cancer Institute Dietary Guidelines[294] (Table 9.10) can be translated into nutritional counseling using the USDA "Food Pyramid" with patients (Figure 9.2). Based on average patterns of food consumption in the United States,[301,312] the following guidelines should be provided:

1. *Fats and cholesterol.* Saturated fats and cholesterol should comprise 30% or less of total calorie intake. In the current average American diet, calories from fat make up 36% to 43% of the daily calorie intake,[300,312] so that for most persons some reduction in fat-containing foods is required to reach this goal. Food preparation methods that add fat (eg, frying) should be avoided.

2. *Fiber.* All individuals should be encouraged to increase intake of fiber and complex carbohydrates. The National Cancer Institute recommends 20 to 30 g/day of fiber, however, the current average intake in the American diet is 11 g/day.[294] Ideally, fiber-containing foods and whole grain or cereal products should be eaten at each meal. See Table 9.11 for food group equivalents to meet the minimum daily fiber recommendation.

3. *Sodium.* There is no evidence that high salt diets are harmful to individuals with normal blood pressure. Conversely, there is no benefit to a diet high in salt. The Surgeon General has recommended reduced salt intake as a nutritional goal for the general population.[311] This can

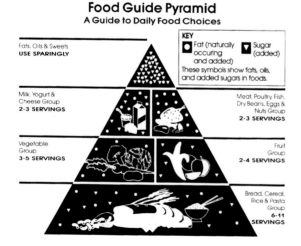

Figure 9.2 United States Department of Agriculture (USDA) Food Pyramid.

Table 9.11 Twenty Grams of Dietary Fiber per Day[*]

3 slices of whole wheat bread
1 serving of moderate fiber cereal
3 servings of vegetables (1 serving = ❖ cup)
2 servings of fruit (1 serving = 1 medium apple)

[*]*Approximate dietary fiber content.*

be accomplished by avoidance of foods high in salt (eg, potato chips and canned soup) and by limiting the use of salt in food preparation. For individuals without hypertension, an appropriate goal for sodium intake is 5 to 6 g/day.[296] For individuals with hypertension, a more limited intake of 1.5 to 2.5 g/day is recommended.

4. *Calcium.* The National Research Council's recommended calcium intake for women over age 24 is 800 mg/day, but the actual intake is on average only 500 to 600 mg/day.[298] Some experts recommend a higher calcium intake (eg, 1,000 mg/day before menopause and 1500 mg/day after menopause).[295,312] Calcium deficiency is an important contributor to the development of osteoporosis in postmenopausal women (see Osteoporosis). The best way to achieve adequate calcium intake is through consumption of calcium-rich foods, specifically dairy products. An 8-ounce glass of milk provides 250 to 300 mg of calcium, irrespective of the fat content of the milk.[295] Other foods rich in calcium include spinach, broccoli, sardines, salmon, and tofu.[296,299,305] Comparative calcium contents for these foods are shown in Table 9.12.

Patients unable or unwilling to obtain adequate calcium from foods in their diet can use calcium supplements. Absorption of calcium from supplements is low, averaging only about 30% and decreasing with age.[295] The most common side effects of calcium supplements are gastrointestinal discomfort and constipation. Different calcium salts do not appear to differ significantly in the production of side effects or in absorption.[295,312] Calcium supplements may interfere with iron absorption or cause depletion of phosphate, and intake of amounts higher than 3 to 4 g/day of elemental calcium causes hypercalcemia.[295] Calcium supplements are contraindicated in individuals with a history of calcium-containing urinary tract stones.

5. *Potassium.* Potassium contributes to blood pressure control in hypertensive individuals and is protective against stroke mortality. A diet providing approximately 75 mEq of potassium daily is optimal.[296] This can be accomplished by consuming the recommended five or more servings of a combination of fruits and vegetables per day, including green and yellow vegetables and citrus fruits. (A serving equals a half-cup portion or medium-sized piece of fruit). Dietary supplements are not recommended for the general population.[295]

Table 9.12 Calcium Content of Foods

	Calcium content (mg)
Skim milk, 1 cup	303
Sardine, 8 medium	354
Salmon, 3 oz. canned	167
Broccoli, 1 medium spear	205
Spinach, 1 cup cooked	245
Tofu, 1 piece (1″ × 2.5″ × 2.7″)	108

From Pennington JAT, Church HN: *Bowes and Church's Food Values of Portions Commonly Used*, 13 ed, New York 1980; and Calcium Supplements, Medical Letter 1989; 31:101–103.

6. *Vitamins*. Many elderly individuals are in the habit of consuming vitamin supplements, in the mistaken belief that they will provide "energy" and make up for waning appetites. In fact, vitamin supplements may not be required by individuals who eat a well-balanced diet, and they represent a needless expense for many elderly individuals on fixed incomes.[293] Further, overuse of vitamin pills may result in overdosing of fat-soluble vitamins (vitamins A, D, and E, in particular) because these are not readily excreted, or in toxicity from the water-soluble vitamin pyridoxine (B_6).

7. *Antioxidants*. Dietary antioxidants, such as vitamins A, E, and C and beta carotene, retard oxidative processes in the body. Epidemiologically, increased antioxidant intake is associated with less cardiovascular disease and a lower than average rate of cancer, particularly lung cancer. To date, this strong protective association with cancer has not been confirmed by intervention trials.[300] A recent Finnish study surprisingly found a higher incidence of lung cancer among those who received beta carotene than among those who did not.[310] Much of nutritional cardiovascular research focuses on the increased atherogenicity of oxidized LDL. Two major observational studies of primary prevention, one in women and one in men, found vitamin E supplementation to be associated with a reduced risk of coronary artery disease.[307,308] A prospective study of hyperlipidemic men found a similar association with high serum carotenoids.[304] Studies suggest the antioxidant effect is stronger in smokers than nonsmokers.[307]

In counseling patients, consumption of five or more servings of fruit and vegetables, especially green and yellow vegetables and citrus fruit, should be recommended. Population studies show a correlation between high intake of vegetables and fruits and a lower risk of cancer; this protective effect may be due to more than just the antioxidant components. Insufficient data exists at present to advocate the use of antioxidant supplements and too little is known about the long-term effect of pharmacological doses.[310] It is important to remember, however, that studies suggest that if there is a positive effect of dietary antioxidants, it appears to require levels that generally are not achieved by diet alone, but rather that require supplementation. Definitive recommendations await the results of several large trials now in progress.

Obesity and Weight Loss

In general, weight rises with age. For women, this may be due in part to reduced metabolism related to the cessation of menses; reduced physical activity is often a factor as well. Standard weight tables do not reflect this age-related increase and underestimate the "ideal" body weight for older people.[292] As shown in Figure 9.3, a weight gain of as much as 1 pound per year, or 10 pounds per decade, is acceptable and without an associated increase in mortality.

Women who are at or over 115% of ideal body weight, however, may experience excess morbidity and mortality, and appropriate counseling regarding weight loss should be offered. Similarly, central obesity is associated with increased risks for cardiovascular disease and breast cancer, as discussed above, and women with this pattern of weight gain may benefit from weight loss.[297] Women with hypertension and diabetes may also benefit from weight loss, even with mild degrees of obesity.[306] Of note, recent surveys of the US population show an increased prevalence of obesity in all age and gender groups, as compared with 30 years ago, most markedly over the last decade.[305]

Weight measurements should be taken on a regular basis, because rapid loss or gains may be significant. An involuntary weight loss of 10 pounds or greater over 1 year may be due to occult cancer, gastrointestinal or thyroid disease, diabetes or depression, and an appropriate work-up should be considered.

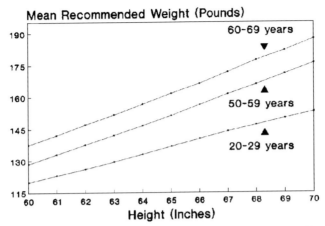

Figure 9.3 Mean recommended weights for women of different age groups. Based on the analysis of Andres.[283]

Similarly, rapid weight gain may be an indicator of hypothyroidism or, if an organic cause can be ruled out, suggests the need for counseling regarding food intake and exercise.

Diet Counseling

Safe and effective dieting can be accomplished by following simple guidelines. Most individuals who lose weight while dieting, however, will regain the weight subsequently, and patients should be encouraged to diet only when a specific medical indication is present. When plans to diet are made, the patient should be counseled as follows:

1. Weight loss should be slow and steady. The patient's goal should rarely exceed 2 to 4 pounds a month.

2. The patient should eat regular, fully balanced meals, with calorie reduction accomplished primarily by an increase in fruit and vegetable intake and a decrease in foods containing fat and sugar.

3. The patient should pursue moderate exercise on a daily basis.

4. The patient should not avoid favorite foods, even they are of relatively high caloric content. Portions should be reduced instead. The diet should be one that can be tolerated for long periods of time.

5. The patient needs to be seen on a regular basis—weekly or monthly—by a dietitian or other counselor to discuss meal plans and check weight. Community-based programs may serve this purpose and additionally provide the patient with valuable social support.

Bladder and Bowel Function

Urinary Incontinence

Loss of bladder control in the elderly is a common problem. It is estimated that 20% of community dwellers and 40% of those institutionalized are affected, and the problem is underreported. Older women are affected nearly twice as frequently as older men.[317] Age-related changes, such as larger urine volume (due to decreased concentrating ability of the kidney), decreased muscle tone, and slower reaction times or limited mobility predispose women to incontinence. A short urethral length and decreased urethral closure pressure seen with decreased estrogen levels increase the risk.[316] These factors alone or in concert with previous childbearing or current obesity or illnesses, acute or chronic (such as infection, stroke, and Parkinson's disease), can lead to loss of bladder control. Incontinence may result in decreased self-esteem, social isolation, and loss of independent care. Treatment, through exercise, behavior modification, and medication is usually effective and well tolerated. (See Chapter 16 for more thorough discussion.)

Fecal Incontinence

Fecal incontinence is a less common problem that is multifactorial in origin and nearly always associated with urinary incontinence. It often precludes independent living, reflected by a prevalence of less than 1% in the community but a higher prevalence (25% to 35%) in institutions.

Causes of fecal incontinence include colorectal diseases that cause diarrhea (infection, colorectal carcinoma, inflammatory bowel disease, ischemic colitis, diverticular disease, and medications); anorectal incontinence due to external and internal sphincter weakness combined with anal sensory impairment (idiopathic fecal incontinence); fecal impaction; neurological causes, such as stroke, impaired consciousness, and dementia; and immobility. Results of evaluation, including a rectal examination as an essential part of the physical examination, can help direct treatment at the cause of incontinence. Fecal impaction should be evacuated by enema or suppository and the underlying condition treated. Maintaining a firm stool helps the incontinence associated with anorectal incontinence. Dementia-associated incontinence responds well to planned evacuation.[313]

Constipation

Constipation is a common complaint in older patients. Despite an increase in these subjective complaints and an increase in habitual laxative use with aging, some epidemiological data suggests that there is not an increase in actual constipation in the elderly.[314,316] Sometimes this complaint derives from the mistaken idea that normal bowel function requires daily evacuation; for some people, it may be normal to have a bowel movement every 2 to 3 days. Constipation implies the less frequent and difficult evacuation of stool that is firm and hard. Patients will sometimes complain of having small "pellets" of stool. This is usually due to poor eating habits and lack of exercise. While low fiber intake is often cited as a causative factor, other data suggest that constipation in the older population correlates with caloric intake rather than fiber intake or other dietary factors. Laxative abuse may also be a factor. While there should always be concern for the possibility of a pathological cause (gastrointestinal, metabolic, endocrinological, and neurological disorders), particularly if the constipation represents a distinct change in bowel habits, most patients will benefit from a trial of increased fluid and fiber intake and increased exercise. Psychological distress may also result in slowed colonic transit time and should be evaluated as a possible etiology. Medications that may contribute to constipation include codeine and other narcotics, calcium supplements, diuretics, antihistamines, and antidepressants. Patients who have used laxatives frequently may require the use of periodic enemas over several weeks while a new bowel program is being established.

Fiber and Fluid

Fiber intake should be increased to 20 to 30 g/day. Ideally, fiber-rich foods or supplements should be taken with each meal. Wheat bran has been found to be the most effective form to increase stool weight; a tablespoon to a half-cup of bran can be added to cereal, salad, or other food each day. Bran muffins and bread are also helpful, but provide smaller quantities of bran. Other important sources of fiber are vegetables, fruits, beans, oats, and whole grain cereals. Large portions should be encouraged.[318] Psyllium, 1 teaspoon to 1 tablespoon, up to three times a day, is an alternative.

A fluid intake of 6 to 8 glasses (48 to 64 ounces) a day is recommended. Older patients will sometimes avoid fluid intake for social reasons, for example, to prevent stress incontinence or nocturia. When a bowel program is begun, the patient should be encouraged to keep a diary of fluid intake for several days to encourage adequate intake.[318]

Bowel evacuation is more likely to occur after a meal, as a result of the gastrocolic reflex. Patients should be advised to arrange their days so that they have time and adequate facilities for bowel evacuation after at least one of their daily meals. This may be particularly important while traveling. Arranging meals so that they occur at around the same time every day is also helpful.

Use of Medications

Older patients often use many medications, including prescription and over-the-counter preparations. People age 65 or older account for one third of all prescription drug use. A full list of all medications being used should be obtained on an annual basis. A recent 1-year cross-sectional survey of drug prescribing in over six thousand Americans age 65 or older living in the community found almost one quarter of them exposed to potentially hazardous prescription medications.[310] The medications investigated are those that have been found to be ineffective, more toxic than equally effective alternatives, or place the elderly at risk for subtle central nervous system dysfunction. These include benzodiazepenes and oral hypoglycemic agents with long half-lives, short-duration barbiturates, antidepressants with strong anticholinergic properties, less effective and less safe opioid analgesics, ineffective dementia treatments, dipyridamole, and selected NSAIDs, muscle relaxants, gastrointestinal antispasmodics, and antiemetics. The study may underestimate the actual incidence of inappropriate prescribing in that excessive drug dose and duration, medication interactions, and use of an otherwise appropriate medication prescribed inappropriately were not assessed.[321] The findings of this study are consistent with those of studies done previously in nursing homes residents, and in hospitalized or institutionalized older patients.

The physician should be alert to medications as a cause of otherwise unexplained symptoms. As discussed in Chapter 7, older patients may experience an increased incidence of side effects from medications. This risk is increased by the frequent use of polypharmacy, as interactions between different medications may occur. A few examples of specific problems related to over-the-counter medications are noted below:

1. *Antihistamines and decongestants.* Most over-the-counter cold preparations are combinations of antihistamines and decongestants. Antihistamines can cause drowsiness and anticholinergic side effects including dry mouth, urinary retention, and, in the extreme, confusion. Decongestants, the most common of which is pseudoephedrine, typically cause symptoms related to sympathetic stimulation, including irritability, increased pulse rate and blood pressure, and sleeplessness. The combination of these two medications in a single preparation can, understandably, cause a mixture of side effects. Patients may experience fewer side effects if combined

preparations are avoided. For example, pseudoephedrine may be taken during the day and an antihistamine at night, for control of nasal congestion. Doses lower than those recommended by the manufacturer are often sufficient to provide relief of symptoms.

2. *Nose drops.* Many effective nasal preparations for nasal congestion contain sympathomimetics, such as oxymatazoline. They are effective in resolving congestion, but should not be used for longer than 3 days. With prolonged use, patients experience reactive congestion on withdrawal of the medication.

3. *Sedatives.* Sedative use is common. The active ingredient in most over-the-counter sleeping medications is an antihistamine (eg, diphenhydramine) with side effects as noted above.

4. *Aspirin.* Many individuals take aspirin on a regular basis for headache, fever, and musculoskeletal pain. It may sometimes be prescribed for arthritis or to prevent stroke or myocardial infarction. Patients using aspirin should be informed about the potential for gastrointestinal side effects (bleeding, peptic symptoms) and the medication's effect on coagulation; elderly women, in particular, may be susceptible to the anticoagulant effect of aspirin, and should be instructed to report any easy bruising associated with use of the drug.

5. *Nonsteroidal anti-inflammatory drugs.* Over-the-counter availability of NSAIDs has benefitted patients because of lower cost for these medications, which aid in the management of arthritis, other musculoskeletal pain, menstrual pain, and headache. Despite labeling, however, patients are not always aware of side effects. These include esophageal reflux, gastrointestinal bleeding, and fluid retention.[319] These medications may also impair renal function; in patients using high doses of these medications chronically, renal function should be monitored on a regular basis.

6. *Acetaminophen.* Chronic use of acetaminophen may also have an adverse effect on renal function.[320] This medication is frequently used for headache, musculoskeletal pain, and fever. It is often recommended for patients who have had adverse gastrointestinal side effects from aspirin or NSAIDs, as a safer drug. Patients may thus underestimate the potential for side effects and may not report the regular use of this medication unless asked.

Laboratory Screening Tests

The development of automated instruments capable of simultaneously measuring blood levels of many components has dramatically altered many physicians' approaches to routine screening. Rather than requesting the measurement of one specific element, a panel of 6, 8, 12, or even 20 items is obtained. This is a situation in which more is not necessarily better than less. Each blood level is a continuous variable; there is no absolute demarcation between normal and abnormal. Therefore, the normal range cited for each variable is usually the mean value plus or minus 2 standard deviations calculated from a population of presumably normal individuals. By definition, for each test, 5% of normal individuals will have values that fall outside the "normal" range— 2.5% below and 2.5% above. As the size of the panel increases, the proportion of normal individuals having completely normal results decreases. A population of 8,651 randomly selected patients attending a routine health evaluation program were screened for 20 laboratory abnormalities. Whereas 74.1% of these patients had normal results for a subset panel of 8 components, only 45.1% had completely normal results for the entire set of 20 tests,[342] even in this population at low risk to have the illnesses suggested by the abnormal values. These results are consistent with the theoretical predictions of false-positive rates for panels of varying sizes.[333] Another observation of this study was that items found to be abnormal on the initial screen often reverted to normal on retesting.

One underlying premise of routine periodic screening is that earlier diagnosis of disease, before symptoms are recognized, will result in reduced morbidity or mortality. Unfortunately, for many illnesses detectable by such screening, early diagnosis usually does not change outcome. Another consideration of screening is that it should be cost-effective in both economic and human terms. Again, for multi-item biochemical screening this criterion is not met. The use of large batteries of tests increases the frequency of abnormal results, decreases the tests' practical significance, and leads to additional testing, additional office visits, and additional patient anxiety. A disease label may result in increased cost of or inability to obtain life or health insurance. After considering these and other factors, Canadian and American medical commissions recommended against the use of biochemical profiles as screening tools in asymptomatic individuals.[331,352] However, it is our opinion that screening tests for individual biochemical components is justified in some cases, depending on the physician's pretest level of suspicion that an abnormality might be found.

An abnormal test should always be repeated to ensure that the abnormality persists and is not the result of day-to-day variation. For each biochemical abnormality detected in a multiphasic profile there is a list of conditions that could be etiological. However, most of these conditions are uncommon and rarely present without symptoms or clinical signs. The less common the condition being considered, the more likely an abnormal value is a false positive. Markedly abnormal values are most likely to represent a disease process than are marginal abnormalities. The ordering of some specific laboratory tests should be considered when there is even a limited suspicion that the patient may have one of the more common diseases discussed below.

Diabetes Mellitus

Diabetes mellitus is a heterogeneous group of diseases, characterized by an inability to process glucose properly. Insulin-dependent diabetes (type I) results from a destruction of the pancreatic islet cells that produce insulin. Although the usual age of onset is in childhood to young adulthood, some patients develop this form of diabetes much later in life. Non–insulin-dependent diabetes (type II) in most cases is a disease of older adults, affecting approximately 3% of the US population.[343] The mechanism by which type II diabetes arises is not entirely understood. There is relative insulin and glucose insensitivity, impaired but not absent insulin release, and a relationship to obesity, such that increased weight increases the risk to develop the disease.[348] Genetic factors are important for development of both forms of the disease.[365] A substantial portion of overt diabetics will develop complications including cardiovascular disease, renal failure, neuropathy, and blindness. Many patients with either form of diabetes will complain of polyuria, polydipsia, and polyphagia, making the diagnosis in these patients relatively straightforward. However, older people with diabetes often do not develop this classic symptom triad. The most common presentation of diabetes in the elderly is insidious weight loss and fatigue; diabetes should always be considered in the differential diagnosis of these nonspecific complaints. Some patients with abnormal glucose metabolism are entirely without symptoms. Routine periodic testing for diabetes in the asymptomatic population became part of the standard health maintenance program when it was thought that initiation of treatment in the presymptomatic stage of diabetes was more effective than treatment begun at the onset of symptoms. As yet, studies have failed to document a benefit from early diagnosis of type II DM and overdiagnosis and therapy can be dangerous.[328,346] It seems reasonable to limit screening to patients at higher than average risk to develop diabetes, that is, obese persons, especially those with a family history of diabetes, and women with a history of gestational diabetes.[356] Although there may be no need to begin medications prior to development of symptoms, an overweight patient might be spurred to alter her diet and lose weight as an alternative to the prospect of medical therapy.

What test for glycemia should be employed? Urine testing, although simple and noninvasive, is insensitive. The renal threshold for glucose excretion in general is above 160 mg/dL, and varies both among patients and for a single patient over time.[353] The glucose tolerance test (GTT) will result in overdiagnosis of diabetes in the aging population, since there is a gradual increase in both fasting and postprandial glucose levels with age. Even with conservative standards set for the aged, nearly 50% of people over 60 years of age will have an abnormal GTT. The 2-hour postprandial glucose level normally rises by 5 to 10 mg/dL per decade over 50, whereas the fasting level changes much more modestly (1 to 2 mg/dL per decade over 50).[334] Therefore, the fasting plasma glucose measurement is a better screening tool for older persons. Both the National Diabetes Data Group[356] and the World Health Organization[339] would make a diagnosis of diabetes if the fasting plasma glucose concentration is at least 140 mg/dL on more than one occasion. A random plasma glucose level repeated 200 mg/dL or higher has also been accepted by consensus as diagnostic of diabetes.[355,356] The glycosylated hemoglobin level (HbA1C) provides a measure of the degree of hyperglycemia in the preceding 1 to 3 months.[355] Although HbA1C can be used to screen for diabetes,[341,365] more commonly it is used to assess the effectiveness of therapy.

One important caveat is that the majority of people with mild, asymptomatic glucose intolerance will not develop frank diabetes;[349,357] some revert to normal glycemia and others remain in the borderline range. Once a diagnosis of glucose intolerance is made, however, surveillance should be continued so that intervention can be started promptly once symptoms occur.

Thyroid Disease

Thyroid function does not naturally diminish with aging; thyroxine (T4) and thyroid stimulating hormone (TSH) levels remain normal. However, hypothyroidism is much more frequently seen in older than in younger populations. Most affected individuals present after age 50. Symptoms and signs of this condition include lethargy, constipation, dry skin, alopecia, memory impairment, and depression—complaints that may be attributed to the aging process and may not be investigated further. Some elderly patients may have none of the classic symptoms besides lethargy and weakness. Since untreated hypothyroidism can lead to irreversible dementia, physicians should be alert to symptoms that indicate this diagnostic possibility. In one study, 4% of patients at least 60 years old who were evaluated at the time of hospital admission were found to have previously unrecognized hypothyroidism.[325] In the healthy, nonhospitalized elderly population the prevalence of hypothyroidism has been estimated to be as high as 5%.[358]

There is no consensus on whether to screen routinely for hypothyroidism in the healthy asymptomatic elderly patient.[106,331,379,381] The American College of Physicians recommends screening of women over age 50 with nonspecific symptoms, while the US Preventive Task Force recommends screening of women greater than 60 years old; the Canadian Task Force does not recommend screening in this group. Some argue that such screening is not cost-effective, since the yield is low. On the other hand, the consequences of untreated hypothyroidism in the elderly can be severe and include dementia. Certainly, those patients at increased risk should be tested, including those with a history of neck irradiation or hyperthyroidism. Hypothyroidism can be a long-term complication of hyperthyroidism, especially when the patient has received radioactive iodine. Given the benign nature and low cost of thyroid testing, it may be reasonable to screen all older patients every 1 to 2 years. An elevated TSH level reflects the response of the hypothalamic-pituitary axis to decreased thyroid hormone levels and is sufficient as a screening test for thyroid gland failure.[362]

Unlike hypothyroidism, the elderly comprise only about 20% of patients affected by hyperthyroidism. Symptoms of hyperthyroidism include decreased energy, weight loss, and muscle weakness. Again, however, symptoms are more common in young patients than in older patients and mimic "normal" aging. Hyperthyroidism should be suspected in a patient who appears more nervous and agitated than normal, especially when tachycardia is present. The elderly patient may present with atrial fibrillation or congestive heart failure, complications of hyperthyroidism that are unusual in younger people.[335,354] The etiology of hyperthyroidism in the elderly is often nodular goiter and rarely Grave's disease, so ophthalmopathy is usually not seen. One subset of older hyperthyroid patients has depressed activity and mental functioning and may appear to be hypothyroid. The term "apathetic hyperthyroidism" has been applied to this condition.[369] Although TSH levels are suppressed in hyperthyroid states, an elevated free-T4 index (FTI), calculated from T4 and triiodotyronine resin uptake (T3RU), is sufficient for the diagnosis to be made in otherwise healthy patients.

Hyperparathyroidism

Primary hyperparathyroidism is characterized by excessive parathormone secretion, usually the result of parathyroid adenomas, that leads to elevated plasma calcium levels. Symptoms include fatigue, weakness, depression, bone and abdominal pain, and renal stones. In addition, 50% of those with hyperparathyroidism have hypertension, although hyperparathyroidism is responsible for less than 1% of the cases of hypertension.[336] Bone mineral loss can be significant, adding to the morbidity of osteoporosis that frequently coexists. Perhaps the most striking effect of multichannel autoanalyzers has been the dramatic increase in the diagnosis of primary hyperparathyroidism.[330] Once assumed to be a very rare disease, diagnosed only after onset of symptoms, primary hyperparathyroidism is now estimated to occur in 25 of 100,000 in the general population. The incidence of this disease is two times greater in women than in men and rises with age, so that approximately 188 of 100,000 women over age 60 are affected.[345]

There are several caveats to remember when interpreting an elevated random screening calcium: (1) As discussed, 2.5% of the normal population will have an elevated calcium on any one occasion—13 times the frequency of hyperparathyroidism in the segment of the population at highest risk. Therefore, an elevated calcium determination should be documented on at least three occasions prior to referral to a specialist. (2) The unbound ionized calcium fraction, on which the diagnosis rests, is dependent on the amount of binding to serum proteins. For this reason, the measured total calcium concentration obtained in a screening battery must be adjusted for the albumin level simultaneously obtained. For every 0.1 g/dl albumin above 4.0, 0.1 mg/dl should be subtracted from the calcium level. If the albumin level is below 4.0 g/dl, the correction factor is added to the calcium level. (3) Ionized calcium levels will rise in acidosis, such as might occur in blood pooling distal to a tourniquet. Repeat calcium determinations should be obtained with care to keep the tourniquet time to a minimum.

The diagnosis of hyperparathyroidism should be considered when calcium is persistently elevated in the presence of high normal, minimally elevated, or elevated intact parathyroid hormone (PTH). Hypercalcemia due to other causes, such as malignancy or sarcoidosis, suppress PTH. The presence of paraneoplastic PTH-related protein will not elevate intact PTH levels.[340]

There is an unresolved controversy regarding the appropriate therapy, medical versus surgical, during the asymptomatic stage of hyperparathyroidism, especially in the geriatric population.[329,336,370,372] A recent National Institutes of Health consensus panel established guidelines for medical versus surgical treatment of the condition.[336] Nonsurgical management is considered for those people with mild-elevations of calcium who have not had any episodes of life-threatening hypercalcemia and who have normal renal function and bone integrity. Conversely, surgery is recommended for anyone with calcium 1.0 to 1.6 ng/dl (0.25 to 0.4 mmol/L) above the accepted normal range; creatinine clearance reduced by 30% compared with age-matched patients; a 24-

hour urine calcium excretion that exceeds 400 mg; or a bone mass more than two standard deviations below the mean of age-gender—and race-matched controls. Surgery is also suggested for those who are unlikely to get follow-up, have co-existing illnesses that complicate management, or are less than 50 years old. Because of the complexity of the diagnosis and management of hyperparathyroidism, patients are generally followed in consultation with an endocrinologist.

Renal Disease

Even in the absence of diseases that directly affect the kidney, renal function changes dramatically in the process of normal aging. Beginning in young adulthood renal plasma flow decreases by 10% each decade, so that by 80 years of age there has been a 50% reduction.[371] In addition, gradual loss in the number of nephrons leads to a decline in glomerular filtration rate. (GFR)[360,361] These factors contribute to a fall in creatinine clearance that begins to be detectable at about age 35. A reciprocal rise in serum creatinine is not seen, however, since creatinine clearance depends on muscle mass, which also decreases with age.[360] The lower muscle mass of women results in approximately 20% lower creatinine clearance values than those in men. A creatinine value above 1.5 mg/dl is unlikely to be solely the result of normal aging and indicates that renal disease may be present. When prescribing drugs that are renally excreted, it should be remembered that the serum creatinine overestimates the glomerular filtration rate in older people and some measure of creatinine clearance should be obtained. A 24-hour urine collection for direct measurement of the creatinine excreted may be difficult for an older woman to provide. A useful estimate can be calculated from the patient's serum creatinine, age, and weight as follows:

$$\frac{(140 - \text{Age}) \times \text{Weight in kg}}{72 \times \text{Creatinine}}$$

Aside from diminished creatinine clearance, other renal changes with aging include decreased concentrating and sodium-conserving abilities.[316] However, maximal renal capacity far exceeds what is needed; so although renal function is markedly diminished with aging, under normal circumstances extracellular volume and osmolality are adequately regulated. Situations that perturb water and solute balance may overwhelm the kidneys of older persons and significant volume depletion may result. Examples of such stresses are febrile illnesses, strenuous exercise, and decreased fluid intake while on diuretics. Even in the absence of heart disease, volume overload may result from increased intake of solute and water either orally or in the form of radiologic contrast. Abnormal serum sodium concentrations, reflecting water excess or deficit may also result in these situations.

Creatinine and blood urea nitrogen (BUN) levels should be measured periodically in patients taking drugs that might have adverse effects on kidney function, such as NSAIDs and Tylenol, antihypertensive medications, and diuretics. Patients with diseases that might result in renal dysfunction, including hypertension and diabetes, should have these blood tests as well.

Complete Blood Count

The complete blood count (CBC) is a common component of screening batteries performed on asymptomatic ambulatory patients. However, there is evidence to suggest that this screening test rarely detects a serious underlying disorder and often leads to further, more expensive testing.[337,363] Patients with significant anemia almost always have symptoms, fatigue being the most common complaint. Although mild anemia is common in otherwise healthy elderly persons, most studies have not found this to be of clinical consequence unless it is associated with underlying illness. Certainly, a patient who has complaints suggestive of upper or lower gastrointestinal tract bleeding or unexplained fatigue deserves a hematocrit or hemoglobin measurement as part of the evaluation. There may also be merit in obtaining a screening hematocrit in women who have heavy menstrual bleeding, since the diet may not contain an adequate supply of iron, and iron supplementation may prevent the development of severe, symptomatic anemia. Red cell indices are helpful in the diagnosis of pernicious anemia, but the disease is not common and permanent complications in the absence of symptoms is extremely rare. The white cell count and differential are only helpful in the evaluation of suspected illnesses such as infections or malignancies. The values fluctuate too widely from day to day and abnormalities are too nonspecific to be of utility in screening.[348,363]

Urinalysis

Dipstick evaluation of urine samples is easy to perform and relatively inexpensive. Chemically impregnated strips are able to detect several urine components, including hemoglobin, protein, and the white cell enzyme leukocyte esterase.[350] As with other screening tests, there is a controversy regarding the utility of this practice,[346] since it is not clear that identification of minor abnormalities or diagnosis of urinary tract diseases in the presymptomatic phase is of benefit. Some researchers who oppose the ordering of urinalyses (UAs) in the absence of clear indications argue that a change in therapy is rarely made on the basis of urine results, even when an abnormality is present.[324] This does not seem to be a valid reason for discontinuing the screening process, but rather indicates that additional studies are necessary to define the long-term outcome of patients whose urine abnormalities went untreated.

The frequency of abnormalities found on urinalyses in any population is very high; in 6,000 women included in one study of mass screening of asymptomatic working adults, at least one abnormality was detected in 12%. The most frequent abnormal finding was hematuria, present in 8% of samples.[332] In contrast to gross hematuria, which requires full urologic work-up, asymptomatic microhematuria rarely implies serious pathology. No neoplasms were identified in females ascertained with asymptomatic microhematuria who were followed prospectively for 10 years.[326] After thorough evaluation of patients whose urinalysis was abnormal, hematuria was most often attributed to trigonitis or a related condition. However, hematuria may indicate the presence of renal calculi which, if untreated, can lead to decreased renal function. Papillary necrosis., often the result of analgesic abuse, may also cause microscopic hematuria. Use of offending medications should be discontinued to prevent progression of renal disease.

Pyuria, detected by a positive leukocyte esterase reaction on dipstick testing, may indicate bacterial cystitis or bladder colonization.[326,327,364] A recent cohort study and controlled clinical trial of the effect of antimicrobial treatment on asymptomatic bacteriuria in elderly women showed that urinary tract infection is not an independent risk factor for mortality and that antibiotic treatment did not decrease mortality.[322] On the other hand, symptomatic urinary tract infection should be treated with appropriate antibiotics. Sterile pyuria, once the hallmark of renal tuberculosis, is now most frequently the result of interstitial nephritis such as might result from analgesic abuse.

Proteinuria may reflect hematuria, urinary tract infection, or intrinsic renal disease, such as idiopathic nephrotic syndrome. However, protein may be excreted in the urine following strenuous exercise, fever, exposure to cold, or emotional stress.[323] If proteinuria is consistently present on a qualitative test, a measure of total daily protein excretion should be obtained accurately by 24-hour urine collection, if possible, or estimated from a single voided specimen.[343]

Published guidelines for periodic health examinations do not include urinalyses for asymptomatic persons.[106] Therefore, no firm recommendations can be made regarding the frequency with which

UAs should be obtained. Instances in which UA is indicated include hypertension, diabetes, history of chronic use of potentially toxic renal medications, and, of course, symptoms attributable to the urinary system. As with other laboratory tests, abnormalities found initially on UA often become normal on retesting. Only if the abnormality persists should the more labor-intensive microscopic evaluation be performed. Patients with confirmed abnormal findings for which a benign explanation is not readily apparent should be referred to a nephrologist.

Electrocardiogram and Chest X-Ray Examination

Both electrocardiogram and chest X-ray examination have been used as routine screening tests in the past. Analyses of their effectiveness suggest that they are not useful as screening tests in asymptomatic individuals.[367,368]

Screening for Human Immunodeficiency Virus (HIV)

There is a steady increase in the number of HIV-infected patients and patients with acquired immunodeficiency syndrome (AIDS) over the age of 60. Compared with younger patients with AIDS, a higher proportion of the affected elderly is female.[380] Exposure may occur as a result of sexual contact with homosexual or bisexual men. As there is decreased disclosure of sexual orientation among the elderly, women should be informed of the necessity for safe sex practices.[383] Elderly female partners of HIV-positive men are at greater risk than younger women for sexual transmission due to age-related thinning of vaginal mucosa (causing tissue disruption) as well as an age-related decrease in immune function. In addition, there is less use of condoms in this age group. Transfusion-related transmission is currently the most frequent etiology (64%) in patients over age 70; this frequency is likely to decline as a result of improved blood screening.[380]

Disease progression appears to be more rapid in the elderly, but this may represent a delay in diagnosis rather than shorter survival time. The resemblance of the nonspecific symptoms of HIV infection—fatigue, anorexia, weight loss, and decreased function—to the symptoms of other chronic illnesses that are common in the elderly may be responsible for this delay.[383]

Dementia may be an early manifestation of AIDS. AIDS-related dementia must be distinguished from Alzheimer's disease. There are many similarities, however, AIDS-related dementia generally progresses more rapidly and is often associated with peripheral neuropathies and myelopathies.

Planning for the Future

As part of preventive care practice, it is appropriate to counsel patients regarding certain specific issues for the future. One of these is the patient's wishes regarding the medical care she would want to have in the event that terminal debilitating medical illness interfered with her ability to make decisions for herself. Most states have "Living Will" legislation, permitting individuals to write directions concerning the level of support they would want if devastating illness should occur.[382] However, few physicians discuss these issues with patients.[375] This is a subject that must be approached delicately to avoid creating unnecessary anxiety; patients may wonder, for example, whether the physician who raises issues of terminal care may be implying that the patient's health is failing.[378] A reassuring opening statement—for example "It is my practice to discuss these matters with my patients well in advance, at a time when they are healthy"—may make it clear to the patient that no "hidden message" is being communicated.

Patients vary widely in their wishes regarding terminal care, but most prefer the opportunity

Table 9.13 Summary of Recommendations

Patient at average risk

Under age 40
Annual:
  Blood pressure, weight, and pulse measurements
  Updating of medical history
  Review of symptoms and immunization status
  Immunizations as indicated
Additional recommendations:
  PAP testing[*]
Age 40–49
Annual:
  Blood pressure, weight, and pulse measurements
  Updating of medical history
  Review of symptoms and immunization status
  Immunizations as indicated
Additional recommendations:
  PAP testing[*]
  Eye examination every 5 years
Controversial:
  Mammography[1]
Age 50–64
Annual:
  Blood pressure, weight, and pulse measurements
  Updating of medical history
  Review of symptoms and immunization status
  Immunizations as indicated
  Hearing testing as indicated
  Mammography
  Occult blood testing of stool
  Laboratory: TSH and UA; creatinine if taking medications
Additional recommendations
  PAP testing[2]
  Eye examination every 5 years
Controversial:
  Flexible sidmoidoscopy screening[3]
Age 65 and Over
Annual:
  Blood pressure, weight, and pulse measurements
  Updating of medical history
  Review of symptoms and immunization status
  Flu vaccine; other immunizations as indicated
  Hearing testing as indicated
  Mammography
  Occult blood testing of stool
  Laboratory: TSH and UA; creatinine if taking medications
Additional recommendations:
  PAP testing[*]
  Eye examination every 5 years
Controversial:
  Flexible sigmoidoscopy screening

continued on next page

Table 9.13 Summary of Recommendatons *Continued*

Patients at increased risk	
Risk factor	See discussion under
Smoking	*Life-style (Smoking)*
Excessive sun exposure	*Skin Cancer*
Gestational diabetes	*Diabetes Mellitus*
Obesity	*Cardiovascular Disease; Breast Cancer, Life-style (nutrition); Diabetes Mellitus*
Family history of	
Early heart disease	*Cardiovascular Disease*
Cancer	*Breast and Colon Cancer; Family Cancer Syndrome*
Osteoporosis	*Osteoporosis*
Diabetes	*Diabetes Mellitus*

[1] See discussion under *Breast Cancer*.
[2] See Chapter 16.
[3] See discussion under *Colon Cancer*.
TSH, Thyroid-stimulating hormone; UA, urinalysis.

to discuss the matter with their physicians.[375,378] A nondirective discussion, facilitating the patient's efforts to clarify her own wishes, is most helpful. The content of the discussion should be documented in the medical record.

Women are more likely than men to survive a spouse or become caretakers of an ailing spouse. Planning for the future should include a discussion of the need to prepare for such contingencies. Women whose husbands have been diagnosed to have heart disease may benefit from instruction in cardiopulmonary resuscitation (CPR).[374,376] Women should be aided in identifying support groups that will help them to cope with the stresses of their husband's illness.[363] A patient with an ailing spouse should be urged to obtain periodic relief from the role of caretaker.

Summary Guide to Preventive Health Care of Older Women

Recommendations for routine screening in different age groups are summarized in Table 9.13. Forms such as those shown in Figures 9.4 and 9.5 can be helpful in obtaining initial medical history at a patient's first visit and in annual updating. Areas of controversy are noted, with references to discussions in the text of this chapter. Discussions of specific high-risk groups and of counseling for life-style changes are also referenced.

References

Cardiovascular

1. Arnold AM, Mick MJ, Piedmonte MR, Simpfendorfer C: Gender differences for coronary angioplasty. *Am J Cardiol.* 1994; 74(1):18–21.
2. Barrett Connor E, Suarez L, Khaw K, Criqui MH, Wingard DL: Ischemic heart disease risk factors after age 50. *J Chronic Dis.* 1984; 37(12): 903–8.
3. Beard CM, Kottke TE, Annegers JF, Ballard DJ: The Rochester coronary heart disease project. *Mayo Clin Proc* 1989;64:1471–1480.
4. Blair SN, Kohl HW, Paffenbarger RS, Clark DG, Cooper KH, Gibbons LW: Physical fitness and all-cause mortality. *JAMA* 1989;262:2395–2401.

Have <u>YOU</u> had any of the following?

YES	NO		YES	NO	
__	__	Asthma	__	__	Cancer
__	__	Heart murmur	__	__	Liver disease, yellow
__	__	High blood pressure	__	__	jaundice, hepatitis
__	__	Mental breakdown	__	__	Pneumonia
		or emotional problem			
__	__	Rheumatic fever	__	__	Serious injury or accident
__	__	Sugar diabetes	__	__	Thyroid gland trouble
__	__	Tuberculosis (TB)	__	__	Uncontrolled bleeding
__	__	Sexually transmitted	__	__	Exposure to asbestos
		disease (STD)	__	__	Exposure to excessive sun

Obstetric History

Age periods began _____
Age periods stopped _____
Number of pregnancies _____
Number of miscarriages or lost pregnancies _____

Have you had a hysterectomy?   Yes___   No___

Please list any allergies: _____

_____

Have you ever had a bad reaction to a drug?   Yes____   No____

If yes, please list medication and type of reaction:_____

_____

Date of last immunization _____

Check each of the following diseases for which you have received immunization at any time in the past:

Polio __   Tetanus __   Diphtheria ___   Measles ___   Mumps ___   Pneumonia ___   Flu ___

Family Health History   **Hospitalizations**

Family Member	Birth Year	Health (if living)	Cause of death (if deceased)	Date	Location	Reason for hospitalization
				__	_____	_____
				__	_____	_____
Mother	__	_____	_____	__	_____	_____
Father	__	_____	_____	__	_____	_____

Brothers/sisters (Please List)	__	_____	_____
	__	_____	_____
	__	_____	_____

Habits:

Smoking	Now	Ever
Cigarettes	__	__
Other(Cigars etc)	__	__

Number of years smoked _____
Daily amount smoked _____

<u>Alcohol</u> (Please circle)
Beer   Wine   Other Liquors   None

| Children (Please List) | __ | _____ | _____ |
| | __ | _____ | _____ |

Amount per week _____

Figure 9.4 Form for initial health history.

Annual Health Questionnaire

1. Do you have any of the following symptoms?

	Yes	No
Changes in eyesight	—	—
Trouble with hearing	—	—
Cough	—	—
Shortness of breath	—	—
Chest ain	—	—
Frequent Indigestion	—	—
Fequent nausea	—	—
Bowel habit change	—	—
Vaginal bleeding	—	—
Other bleeding	—	—
Skin problem	—	—
Lack of energy	—	—
Memory trouble	—	—

2. Do you have any of the following problems?

	Yes	No
Heart disease	—	—
Diabetes	—	—
High blood pressure	—	—
Cancer	—	—
Asthma or breathing problem	—	—

Other _____

3. Current medications:

_____   _____

_____   _____

4. Have you been hospitalized in the past year? yes____ no____
    If yes, state reason_____

    _____

5. Immunizations:

Date of your last tetanus (DT) shot ____

Have you had a flu shot?   Yes___   No___

        If yes, date ____

Have you had a Pnuemovax shot (immunization against pneumonia)?

        Yes___   No___

        If yes, date ____

Have you had any bad reactions to medications in the past year?

        Yes___   No___

If yes, please give details:_____

_____

Figure 9.5 Form for annual updating of health history.

5. Bourassa MG, Chaitman BR, Davis K, Rogers WJ, Tyras DH, Berger R, Kennedy JW, Fisher L, Judkins MP, Mock MB, Killip T: Angiographic prevalence of high-risk coronary artery disease in patient subsets (CASS). *Circulation.* 1981;64(2):360–7.
6. Chronic disease reports: Mortality trends 1979–1986. *MMWR* 1989;38:189–93.
7. Colditz GA: Cigarette smoking and coronary artery disease. *Adv Exp Med Biol.* 1990;273:311–26.
8. Friedman GP, Loveland DB, Ehrlich SP: Relationship of stroke to other cardiovascular disease. *Circulation* 1968;38:533–541.
9. Gordon T, Sorlie P, Kannel WB: Coronary heart disease, atherothrombotic brain infarction, intermittent claudication—a multivariate analysis of some factors related to their incidence: Framingham study, 16-year follow-up. Section 27, U.S. Government Printing Office, Washington DC, 1971.
10. Herman B, Schmitz PIM, Leyton ACM, Van Luijk JH, Frenken CWGM, Op de Coul AAW, Schulte BPM: Multivariate logistic analysis of risk factors for stroke in Tilburg, the Netherlands. *Am J Epidemiol* 1983;118:514–525.
11. Hermanson B, Omenn GS, Kronmal RA, Gersh BJ: Beneficial six-year outcome of smoking cessation in older men and women with coronary artery disease. Results from the CASS registry [see comments] *N Engl J Med.* 1988;319(21):1365–9.
12. Jajich CL, Ostfeld AM, Freeman DH Jr: Smoking and coronary heart disease mortality in the elderly. *JAMA.* 1984; 252(20):2831–4.
13. Ostfeld AM: A review of stroke epidemiology. *Epidemiol Rev* 1980;2:136–52.
14. Roehmholdt ME, Palumbo PJ, Whisnant JP, Elveback LR: Transient ischemic attack and stroke in a community-based diabetic cohort. *Mayo Clin Proc* 1983;58:56–58.
15. Wenger NK, Speroff L, Packard B: Cardiovascular health and disease in women. *N Engl J Med* 1993;329:247–256.

Cardiovascular: Hypertension

16. Agras WS: Relaxation therapy in hypertension. *Hosp Pract* 1983; May:129–137.
17. Amery A, Birkenhager W, Brixko P, Bulpitt C, Clement D, de Leeuw P, de Plaen JF, Deruyttere M, De Schaepdryver A, Dollery C, et-al: Influence of antihypertensive drug treatment on morbidity and mortality in patients over the age of 60 years. European Working Party on High blood pressure in the Elderly (EWPHE) results: sub-group analysis on entry stratification. *J Hypertens Suppl.* 1986; 4(6): S642–7.
18. Anastos K, Charney P, Charon RA, Cohen E, Jones CY, Marte C, Swiderski DM, Wheat ME, Williams S. Hypertension in women: What is really known? The Women's Caucus, Working Group on Women's Health of the Society of General Internal Medicine. *Ann Intern Med* 1991;115:287–293.
19. Applegate WB: Hypertension in elderly patients. *Ann Intern Med* 1989;110:901–915.
20. Applegate WB, Phillips HL, Schnaper H, Shepherd AM, Schocken D, Luhr JC, Koch GG, Park GD: A randomized controlled trial of the effects of three antihypertensive agents on blood pressure control and quality of life in older women. *Arch Intern Med* 1991;151:1817–1823.
21. Benson H: Systemic hypertension and the relaxation response. *N Engl J Med* 1977;296:1152–1156.
22. Blair SN, Goodyear NN, Gibbons LW, Cooper KH: Physical fitness and incidence of hypertension in healthy normotensive men and women. *JAMA* 1984;252:487–490.
23. Curb JD, Borhani NO, Blaszkowski TP, Zimbaldi N, Fotiu S, Williams W: Long-term surveillance for adverse effects of antihypertensive drugs. *JAMA* 1985;253:3263–3268.
24. Cutler JA, Brittain E: Calcium and blood pressure: An epidemiologic perspective. *Am J Hypertens* 1990;3:137S–146S.
25. Epstein FH: The epidemiology of hypertension, in Robertson JLS (ed.): *Handbook of Hypertension.* Elsevier, New York 1983.
26. Floras JS, Hassan MO, Sever PS, Jones JV, Osikowska B, Sleight P: Cuff and ambulatory blood pressures in subjects with essential hypertension. *Lancet* 1981;2:107–109.
27. Gruchow HW, Sobocinski KA, Barboriak JJ: Alcohol, nutrient intake, and hypertension in US adults. *JAMA* 1985;253:1567–1570.
28. Hamet P, Mongeau E, Lambert J, et al: Interactions among calcium, sodium, and alcohol intake as determinants of blood pressure. *Hypertension* 1991;17:I-150–I-154.
29. Hebert PR, Fiebach NH, Eberlein KA, Taylor JO, Hennekens CH: The community-based randomized trials of pharmacologic treatment of mild-to-moderate hypertension. *Am J Epidemiol* 1988;127:581–590.
30. Hennekens CH: Benefits of treatment of mild to moderate hypertension. *J Gen Intern Med* 1987;2:438–441.
31. Intersalt Cooperative Research Group, Intersalt: An international study of electrolyte excretion and blood pressure: Results for 24 hours urinary sodium and potassium excretion. *Br Med J* 1988;297:319–328.

32. Kaplan NM: Maximally reducing cardiovascular risk in the treatment of hypertension. *Ann Intern Med* 1988;109:36–40.
33. Khaw K-T, Barrett-Connor E: Dietary potassium and stroke-associated mortality. *N Engl J Med* 1987;316:235–240.
34. MacGregor GA, Markanda ND, Sagnella GA, Singer DRJ, Capuccio FP: Double blind study of the sodium intakes and long-term effects of sodium restriction in essential hypertension, *Lancet* 1989;2:1244–1247.
35. Maheswaran R, Gill JS, Davies P, Beevers DG: High blood pressure due to alcohol: A rapidly reversible effect. *JAMA* 1991;262:2395–2401.
36. Mattila K, Haavisto M, Rajala S, Heikinheimo R: Blood pressure and five year survival in the very old. *Br Med J Clin Res Ed.* 1988; 296(6626): 887–9.
37. McClellan WM, Hall WD, Brogan D, Miles C, Wilber JA: Continuity of care in hypertension. *Arch Intern Med* 1988;48:525–528.
38. Perloff D, Sokolow M, Cowan R: The prognostic value of ambulatory blood pressures. *JAMA* 1983;249:1792–1798.
39. Pickering TG, Harshfield GA, Kleinert HD, Blanks, Laragh JH: Blood pressure during normal daily activities, sleep and exercises. *JAMA* 1982;247:992–996.
40. Porter G: Chronology of the sodium hypothesis and hypertension. *Ann Intern Med* 1883;98:720–723.
41. Prevention of stroke by antihypertensive drug treatment in older persons with isolated systolic hypertension. Final results of the Systolic Hypertension in the Elderly Program (SHEP). SHEP Cooperative Research Group. *JAMA,* 1991;265:3255–3264.
42. The 1988 report of the Joint National Committee in Detection, Evaluation, and Treatment of High Blood Pressure. *Arch Intern Med* 1988;148:1023–1038.
43. The effects of nonpharmacologic interventions on blood pressure of persons with high normal levels. Results of the Trials of Hypertension Prevention, Phase. *JAMA* 1992;267:1213–1220.
44. The fifth report of the Joint National Committee on Detection, Evaluation, and Treatment of High Blood Pressure (JNCV). *Arch Intern Med* 1993;153:154–183.
45. The treatment of mild hypertension study. A randomized, placebo-controlled trial of a nutritional-hygienic regimen along with various drug monotherapies. The Treatment of Mild Hypertension Research Group. *Arch Intern Med* 1991;151:1413–1423.
46. Tuck ML, Sowers J, Dornfield L, Kledzik G, Maxwell M: The effect of weight reduction on blood pressure, plasma activity, and plasma aldosterone levels in obese patients. *N Engl J Med* 1981;304:930–933.
47. World Hypertension League: Alcohol and hypertension—Implications for management: A consensus statement by the World Hypertension League. *J Hum Hypertens* 1991;5:1854–1856.

Cardiovascular: Cholesterol

48. Abbott RD, Wilson PWF, Kannel WB, Castelli WP: High density lipoprotein cholesterol, total cholesterol screening and myocardial infarction: The Framingham study. *Arteriosclerosis* 1988;8:207–211.
49. Barrett-Connor-E: Hypercholesterolemia predicts early death from coronary heart disease in elderly men but not women. The Rancho Bernardo Study. *Ann Epidemiol* 1992;2:77–83.
50. Basinski A, Frank JW, Naylor CD, Rachlis MM: Detection and Management of Asymptomatic Hypercholesterolemia. A Policy Document by the Toronto Working Group on Cholesterol Policy. Toronto, Ontario, Canada, Ontario Ministry of Health, 1989.
51. Brett AS: Treating hypercholesterolemia: How should practicing physicians interpret the published data for patients? *N Engl J Med* 1989;321:676–680.
52. Canner PL, Berge KG, Wenger NK, Stamler J, Friedman L, Prineas RJ, Friedwald W: Fifteen year mortality in the coronary drug project: Long term benefits with niacin. *J Am Coll Cardiol* 1986;8:1245–1255.
53. Ettinger WH, Wahl PW, Kuller LH, Bush TL, Tracy RP, Manolio TA, Borhani NO, Wong ND, O'Leary H: Lipoprotein lipids in older people. Results from the Cardiovascular Health Study. The CHS Collaborative Research Group. *Circulation* 1992;86:8585–869.
54. Frick MH, Elo O, Haapa K, Heinonen OP, Heinsalmi P, Helo P, Huttunen JK, Kaitaniemi P, et al: Helsinki heart study: Primary prevention trial with gemfibrizol in middle-aged men with dyslipidemia. *N Engl J Med* 1987;317:1237–1245.
55. Garber AM: Where to draw the line against cholesterol. *Ann Intern Med* 1989;3:625–627.
56. Garber AM, Sox HC, Littenberg B: Screening asymptomatic adults for cardiac risk factors: The serum cholesterol level. *Ann Intern Med* 1989;110:622–639.
57. Periodic health examination, 1993 update: 2. Lowering the blood total cholesterol level to prevent coronary heart disease. *Can Med Assoc J* 1993;148:521–538.
58. Krumholz HM, Seeman TE, Merrill SS, et al: Lack of association between cholesterol and coronary heart disease mortality and morbidity and all-cause mortality in persons older than 70 years. *JAMA* 1994;272:1335–1340.

59. Leaf A. Management of hypercholesterolemia: Are preventive interventions advisable? *N Engl J Med* 1989;321:680–684.

60. Lipid Research Clinics Program. The lipid research clinics coronary primary prevention trials result I. Reduction in the incidence of coronary heart disease. *JAMA* 1984;251:351–364.

61. Manolio TA, Pearson TA, Wenger NK, Barrett-Connor E, Payne GH, Harlan WR: Cholesterol and heart disease in older persons and women. Review of an NHLBI workshop. *Ann Epidemiol* 1992;2:161–176.

62. National Cholesterol Education Program: Second Report of the Expert Panel on Detection, Evaluation, and Treatment of High Blood Cholesterol in Adults (Adult Treatment Panel II). *Circulation* 1994;89:1333–1445.

63. Report of the National Cholesterol Education Expert Panel on Detection, Evaluation, and Treatment of High Blood Cholesterol in Adults. *Arch Intern Med* 1988;148:36–69.

64. Rifkind BM, Segal P: Lipid Research Clinics Program reference values for hyperlipidemia and hypolipidemia. *JAMA* 1983;250:1869–72.

65. Rubin SM, Sidney S, Black DM, Browner WS, Hulley SB, Cummings SR: High blood cholesterol in elderly men and the excess risk for coronary heart disease. *Ann Intern Med.* 1990; 113(12): 916–920.

Cardiovascular: Estrogen Replacement Therapy

66. American College of Physicians: Guidelines for counseling postmenopausal women about preventive hormone therapy. *Ann Intern Med* 1992;117:1038–1041.

67. Barrett-Connor E: Estrogen and estrogen-progestogen replacement: Therapy and cardiovascular diseases. *Am J Med* 1993;95:40S–43S.

68. Belchetz PE: Hormonal treatment of postmenopausal women. *N Engl J Med* 1994;330:1062–1071.

69. Bergkvist L, Adami HO, Persson I, Hoover R, Schairer C: The risk of breast cancer after estrogen and estrogen-progestin replacement. *N Engl J Med* 1989;321:293–297.

70. Bush TL, Cowan LD, Barrett-Connor E, Criqui MH, Karon JM, Wallace RB, Tyroler A, Rifkind BM: Estrogen use and all-cause mortality: Preliminary results from the lipid research clinics program follow-up study. *JAMA* 1983;249:903–906.

71. Ferguson KJ, Hoegh C, Johnson S: Estrogen replacement therapy. A survey of women's knowledge and attitudes. *Arch Intern Med* 1989;149:133–136.

72. Grady D, Rubin SM, Petitti DB, Fox CS, Black D, Ettinger B, Ernster VL, Cummings SR: Hormone therapy to prevent disease and prolong life in postmenopausal women. *Ann Intern Med* 1992;117:1016–1037.

73. Henrich JB: The postmenopausal estrogen/breast cancer controversy. *JAMA* 1992;268:1900–1902.

74. Hivonen E, Malkonen M, Manninen V: Effects of different progestogens on lipoproteins during postmenopausal replacement therapy. *N Engl J Med* 1981;304:560–563.

75. Luciano AA, Turksoy RN, Carleo J: Clinical and metabolic responses of menopausal women to sequential vs. continuous estrogen and progestin therapy. *Obstet Gynecol* 1988;71:39–43.

76. Magos AL, Brincal M, Studd JWW, Wardle P, Schlesinger P, O'Dowd T: Amenorrhea and endometrial atrophy with continuous oral estrogen and progestin therapy in postmenopausal women. *Obstet Gynecol* 1985;65:496–499.

77. Manolio TA, Furberg CD, Shemanski L, Psaty BM, O'Leary DH, Tracy RP, Bush TL: Associations of postmenopausal estrogen use with cardiovascular disease and its risk factors in older women. The CHS Collaborative Research Group. *Circulation* 1993;88:2163–2171.

78. Nabulsi AA, Folsom AR, White A, Patsch W, Heiss G, Wu KK, Szklo M: Association of hormone-replacement therapy with various cardiovascular risk factors in postmenopausal women. The Atherosclerosis Risk in Communities Study Investigators. *N Engl J Med* 1993;328:1069–1075.

79. Nachtigall LE, Nachtigall RH, Nachtigall RD, Beckman EM: Estrogen replacement therapy I: a 10–year prospective study in the relationship to osteoporosis. *Obstet Gynecol.* 1979; 53(3): 277–281.

80. Nachtigall LE, Nachtigall RH, Nachtigall RD, Beckman EM: Estrogen replacement therapy II: a prospective study in the relationship to carcinoma and cardiovascular and metabolic problems. *Obstet Gynecol* 1979;54(1):74–9.

81. Psaty BM, Heckbert SR, Atkins D, Lemaitre R, Koepsell TD, Wahl PW, Siscovick DS, Wagner EH: The risk of myocardial infarction associated with the combined use of estrogens and progestins in ostmenopausal women. *Arch Intern Med* 1994;15:1333–1339.

82. Psaty BM, Heckbert SR, Atkins D, Siscovick DS, Koepsell TD, Wahl PW, Longstreth WT Jr, Weiss NS, Wagner EH, Prentice R, et al: A review of the association of estrogens and progestins with cardiovascular disease in postmenopausal women. *Arch Intern Med* 1993;153:1421–1427.

83. Ross RK, Paganini-Hill A, Mack TM, Arthur M, Henderson BE: Menopausal estrogen therapy and protection from death from ischaemic heart disease. *Lancet* 1981;1:858–860.

84. Stampfer MJ, Colditz GA: Estrogen replacement therapy and coronary heart disease: A quantitative assessment of the epidemiologic evidence. *Prev Med* 1991;20:47–63.

85. Stampfer MJ, Colditz GA, Willett WC, Manson JE, Rosner B, Speizer FE, Hennekens CH: Postmenopausal estrogen therapy and cardiovascular disease. Ten-year follow-up from the nurses' health study. *N Engl J Med* 1991;325:756–762.
86. Sullivan JM, Zwaag RV, Lemp GF, Hughes JP, Maddock V, Kroetz FW, Ramanathan KB, Mirvis DM: Postmenopausal estrogen use and coronary atherosclerosis. *Ann Intern Med* 1988;108:358–363.
87. Weinstein L. Efficacy of a continuous estrogen-progestin regimen in the menopausal patient. *Obstet Gynecol* 1987;69:929–932.

Cardiovascular: Family History

88. Goldstein JL, Brown MS: Familial hypercholesterolemia in Stanbury JB, Wyngaarden JB, Fredrickson DS, Goldsstein JL, Brown MS (eds.): *The Metabolic Basis of Inherited Disease,* New York, McGraw-Hill, 1983.
89. Hopkins PN, Williams RR, Hunt SC: Magnified risks from cigarette smoking for coronary prone families in Utah. *West J Med* 1984;141:196–202.
90. Khaw K-T, Barrett-Connor E: Family history of heart attack: A modifiable risk factor? *Circulation* 1986;74:239–244.
91. Nora JS, Lortscher RH, Spangler RD, Nora AH, Kimberling JH: Genetic-epidemiologic study of early onset schemic heart disease. *Circulation* 61:503.
92. Snowden CB, McNamara PM, Garrison RJ, Feinleib M, Kannell WB, Epstein FH: Predicting coronary heart disease in siblings: A multivariate assessment. *Am J Epidemiol* 1982;115:217–222.
93. Tenkate LP, Boman H, Daiger SP, Motulsky AM: Familial aggregation of coronary heart disease and its relation to known genetic risk factors. *Am J Cardiol* 1982;50:945–953.

Cardiovascular: Obesity and Exercise

94. Barrett-Connor EL: Obesity, atherosclerosis, and coronary artery disease. *Am Intern Med* 1985;103:1010–1019.
95. Barrett-Connor EL, Khaw K-T: Cigarette smoking and increased central obesity. *Ann Intern Med* 1989;111:783–787.
96. Bray GA, Bouchard C: Role of fat distribution during growth and its relationship to health. *Am J Clin Nutr* 1988;47: 551–552.
97. Harris SS, Caspersen CJ, DeFriese GH, Estes EH: Physical activity counseling for healthy adults as a primary preventive intervention in the clinical setting. *JAMA* 1989;261:3590–3598.
98. Hubert HB, Feinleib M, McNamara PM, Castelli WP: Obesity as an independent risk factor for cardiovascular disease: A 26-year follow-up of participants in the Framingham Heart Study. *Circulation* 1983;67:968–977.
99. Lapidus L, Bengtsson C, Larsson B, Pennert K, Rybo E, Sjostrom L: Distribution of adipose tissue and risk of cardiovascular disease and death: A 12 year follow-up of participants in the population study of women in Gothenburg, Sweden. *Br J Med* 1984;289:1257–1261.
100. Peiris AN, Sothmann MS, Hoffmann RG, Hennes MI, Wilson CR, Gustafson AB, Kissebah AH: Adiposity, fat distribution, and cardiovascular risk. *Ann Intern Med* 1989;110:867–872.

Cardiovascular: Aspirin

101. Anti-Platelet Trialists' Collaboration: Secondary prevention of vascular disease by prolonged anti-platelet therapy. *Br Med J* 1988;296:320–331.
102. Boston Collaborative Drug Surveillance Group: Regular aspirin intake and acute myocardial infarction. *Br Med J* 1974;1:1440–1443.
103. Buring JR, Hennekens CH: Prevention of cardiovascular disease: Risks and benefits of aspirin. *J Gen Intern Med* 1990;5:S54–S75.
104. Canadian Task Force on the Periodic Health Examination. Periodic health examination, 1991 update: 6. Acetylsalicylic acid and the primary prevention of cardiovascular disease. *Can Med Assoc J* 1991;145:1091–1095.
105. Hammond EC, Garinkel L: Aspirin and coronary heart disease; Findings of a prospective study. *Br Med J* 1976;2: 269–271.
106. ISIS-2 (Second International Study of Infarct Survival) Collaborative Group: Randomized trial of intravenous streptokinase, oral aspirin, both or neither among 17,187 cases of suspected acute myocardial infarction. *Lancet* 1988;2:349–360.
107. Manson JE, Stampfer MJ, Colditz GA, Willett WC, Rosner B, Speizer FE, Hennekens CH: A prospective study of aspirin use and primary prevention of cardiovascular disease in women. *JAMA* 1991;266:521–527.
108. Paganini-Hill A, Chao A, Ross RK, Henderson BE: Aspirin use and chronic diseases: A cohort of the elderly. *Br Med J* 1989;299:1247–1250.

109. Patrono C: Aspirin as an antiplatelet drug. *N Engl J Med* 1994;330:1287–1294.
110. Peto R, Gray R, Collins, et al: A randomized trial of the effects of prophylactic daily aspirin among male British doctors. *Br Med J* 1988;296:320–332.
111. The Steering Committee of the Physicians' Health Study Research Group: Final report from the aspirin component of the ongoing Physicians' Health Study. *N Engl J Med* 1989;321:129–135.

Cancer: General

112. Boring CC, Squires TS, Tong T: Cancer statistics, 1993. *CA Cancer J Clin* 1990;43:7–26.
113. Eddy DM (ed.): *Common Screening Tests*, Philadelphia, American College of Physicians, 1991.
114. Mettlin C, Dodd GD: The American Cancer Society Guidelines for the cancer-related checkup: An update. *CA Cancer J Clin* 1991;41:279–82.
115. US Preventive Services Task Force: *Guide to Clinical Preventive Services*. Baltimore, MD, Williams & Wilkens, 1989.

Lung Cancer

116. Beckett WS: Epidemiology and etiology of lung cancer. *Clin Chest Med* 1993;14:1–15.
117. Berman BA: Women and smoking: Current trends and issues for the 1990s. *J Subst Abuse* 1991;3:221–238.
118. Eddy DM: Screening for lung cancer. *Ann Intern Med* 1989;111:232–237.
119. Fielding JE: Smoking and women: Tragedy of the majority. *N Engl J Med* 1987;317:1343–1345.
120. Fontana RS, Sanderson DR, Woolner LB, Taylor WF, Miller WE, Muhm JR: Lung cancer screening: The Mayo program. *J Occup Med* 1986;28:746–750.
121. Melamed MR, Flehinger BJ, Zaman MB, Heelan RT, Perchick WA, Nartini N: Survival and mortality from lung cancer in a screened population. The Johns Hopkins study, *Chest* 1984;86:44–53.
122. Surgeon General's 1989 Report on Reducing the Health Consequences of Smoking: 25 Years of Progress; Executive Summary. *MMWR* 1989;38 (suppl S-2):1–32.
123. Tockman MS: Survival and mortality from lung cancer in a screened population. The Johns Hopkins study, *Chest* 1986;89(suppl):3245–3255.

Breast Cancer

124. Brown JT, Hulka BS. Screening mammography in the elderly; A case-control study. *J Gen Intern Med* 1988;3:126–131.
125. Campbell HS, Fletcher SW, Lin S, Pilgrim CA, Morgan TM: Improving physicians' and nurses' clinical breast examination: A randomized controlled trial. *Am J Prev Med* 1991;7:1–8.
126. Claus EB, Risch N, Thompson WD: Autosomal dominant inheritance of early-onset breast cancer: Implications for risk prediction. *Cancer* 1994;73:643–651.
127. Daling JR, Malone K, Voigt L, White E, Weiss NS: Risk of breast cancer among young women: Relationship to induced abortion. *J Nat Cancer Inst* 1994;86:1584–1592.
128. Eddy DM: Screening for breast cancer. *Ann Intern Med* 1989;111:389–399.
129. Eley JW, Hill HA, Chen VW, Austin DF, Wesley MN, Muss HB, Greenberg RS, Coates RJ, Correa P, Redmond K, Hunter CP, Herman AA, Kurman R, Blacklow R, Shapiro S, Edwards BK: Racial differences in survival from breast cancer. *JAMA* 1994;272:947–954.
130. Fletcher SW, Black W, Harris R, Rimer BK, Shapiro S: Report of the International Workshop on Screening for Breast Cancer. *J Nat Cancer Inst* 1993;85:1644–1656.
131. Fletcher SW, Black W, Harris R, Rimer BK, Shapiro S: Screening for breast cancer (letter). *J Natl Cancer Inst* 1994;86:558–559.
132. Foster RS, Lang SP, Costanza MC, Worden JK, Haines CR, Yates JW: Breast self-examination practices and breast cancer stage. *N Engl J Med* 1978;299:265–270.
133. Feuer EJ, Wun LM, Boring CC, Flanders WD, Timmel MJ, Tong T. The lifetime risk of developing breast cancer *J Nat'l Cancer Inst* 1993;85:892–897.
134. Harper AP: Mammography utilization in the poor and medically underserved. *Cancer* 1993;72:1478–1482.
135. Harris JR, Lippman ME, Veronasi U, Willett W: Breast cancer. *N Engl J Med* 1992;327:319–328.
136. Kopans DB: Screening for breast cancer and mortality reduction among women 40–49 years of age. *Cancer* 1994;74:311–312.

137. McGuire LB: Screening for breast cancer. *Ann Intern Med* 1989;111:858–859.

138. Miller AB: Is routine mammography screening appropriate for women 40–49 years of age? *Am J Prev Med* 1992;7:55–62.

139. Miller AB, Baines CJ, To T, Wall C: Canadian National Breast Screening Study 1: Breast cancer detection and death rates among women aged 40 to 49 years. *Can Med Assoc J* 1992;147:1459–1476.

140. Miller BA, Feuer EJ, Hankey BF: Recent incidence trends for breast cancer in women and the relevance of early detection: An update. *CA Cancer J Clin* 1993;43:27–41.

141. Nystrom L, Rutqvist LE, Wall S et al: Breast cancer screening with mammography: Overview of Swedish randomized trials. *Lancet* 1993;341:973–978.

142. Sickles EA, Kopans DB: Screening for breast cancer (letter). *J Natl Cancer Inst* 1994;86:559–560.

143. Steinberg KK, Thacker SB, Smith J et al: A meta-analysis of the effect of estrogen replacement therapy on the risk of breast cancer. *JAMA* 1991;265:1985–1990.

Colon Cancer

144. Allison JE, Feldman R, Tekawa IS: Hemoccult screening in detecting colorectal neoplasm: Sensitivity, specificity, and predictive value. *Ann Intern Med* 1990;112:328–333.

145. Altquist DA, Wienand HS, Moertel CG, et al: Accuracy of fetal occult blood screening for colorectal neoplasia. *JAMA* 1993;269:1262–12

146. Leach FS, Nicolaides NC, Papadopoulos N, Liu B, Jen J, Lahti M et al: Mutations of a MutS homolog in hereditary nonpolyposis colorectal cancer; *Cell* 1993;75:1215–1225.

147. Lipshutz GR, Katon RM, McCool MF, Mayer B, Smith FW, Duff T, Melnyk CS: Flexible sigmoidoscopy as a screening procedure for neoplasia of the colon. *Surg Gynecol Obstet* 1979;148:19–22.

148. Mandel JS, Bond JH, Church TR et al (Minnesota Colon Cancer Study): Reducing mortality from colorectal cancer by screening for fecal occult blood. *N Engl J Med* 1993;328:1365–1371.

149. Nicolaides NC, Papadopoulos N, Liu B, Wei YF, Carter KC, Fraser CM et al: Mutations of two PM2 homologs in hereditary nonpolyposis colon cancer. *Nature* 1994;371:75–80.

150. Ow CL, Lemar HJ, Weaver MJ: Does screening proctosigmoidoscopy result in reduced mortality from colorectal cancer? *J Gen Intern Med* 1989;4:209–215.

151. Selby JV, Friedman GD, Quesenberry CP, Weiss NS: A case-control study of screening sigmoidoscopy and mortality from colorectal cancer. *New Engl J Med* 1992;326:653–657.

152. Simon JB: Occult blood screening for colorectal carcinoma: A critical review. *Gastroenterology* 1985;88:820–827.

153. Winawer SJ, Miller DG, Sherlock P: Risk and screening for colorectal cancer. *Adv Intern Med* 1984;30:471–496.

Ovarian Cancer

154. Andolf E: Ultrasound screening in women at risk for ovarian cancer. *Clin Obst Gyn* 1993;36:423–432.

155. Campbell S, Bhan V, Royston P, Whitehead MJ, Collins WP: Transabdominal ultrasound screening for early ovarian cancer. *Br Med J* 1989;299:1363–1367.

156. Ferucci JT: Screening for ovarian cancer (letter). *JAMA* 1986;255:3169.

157. Ganiats TG: Screening for ovarian cancer (letter). *JAMA* 1986;256:1892.

Cancer-Prone Families

158. Biesecker B, Bochnke M, Calzone K, Markel DS, Garber JE, Collins FS, Weber BL, Genetic counseling for families with an inherited susceptibility to breast cancer *JAMA* 1993;269:1970–4.

159. Gallion HH, Smith SA: Hereditary ovarian carcinoma. *Semin Surg Oncol* 1994;10:249–254.

160. Li FP, Fraumeni JF: Prospective study of a family cancer syndrome. *JAMA* 1982;247:2692–2694.

161. Lynch HT, Follett KL, Lynch PM, Albano WA, Mailliard JL, Pierson RL: Family history in an oncology clinic. *JAMA* 1979;242:1268–1272.

162. Offit K, Brown K. Quantitating familial cancer risk: A resource for clinical oncologists. *J Clin Oncol* 1994;12: 1724–1736.

Skin Cancer

163. Cassileth BR, Temostok L, Frederick BE, Walsh WP, Hurwitz S, Guerry D, Clark WH, DiClemente RJ, Sweet DM, Blois MS, Sagebiel RW: Patient and physician delay in melanoma diagnosis. *J Am Acad Derm* 1988;18:591–598.
164. Elwood JM, Gallagher RP, Hill GP, Spinelli JJ, Pearson JCG, Threlfall N: Pigmentation and skin reaction to sun as risk factors for cutaneous melanoma: Western Canada Melanoma Study. *Br Med J* 1984;288:99–102.
165. Fitzpatrick TB, Sober AJ: Sunlight and skin cancer. *N Engl J Med* 1985;313:818–819.
166. Green A, Siskind V, Bain C, Alexander J: Sunburn and malignant melanoma. *Br J Cancer* 1985;41:393–397.
167. Greene MH, Clark WH, Tucker MA, Kraemer KH, Elder DE, Fraser MC: High risk of melanoma in melanoma-prone families with dysplastic nevi. *Ann Intern Med* 1985;102:458–465.
168. Kopf AW, Rigel DS, Friedman RJ: The rising incidence and mortality rate of malignant melanoma. *J Dermatol Surg Onc* 1982;8:760–761.
169. Lee JAH: The rising incidence of cutaneous malignant melanoma. *Am J Dermatopath* 1985;7(suppl):35–39.
170. Lew RA, Sober AJ, Cook N, Marvell R, Fitzpatrick TB: Sun exposure habits in patients with cutaneous melanoma. *J Dermat Surg Onc* 1983;9:981–986.
171. National Institutes of Health Consensus Development Conference Statement: Precursors to malignant melanoma. *J Am Acad Derm* 1984;10:683–688.

Musculoskeletal
Osteoarthritis

172. Bradley JD, Brandt KD, Katz BP, Kalasinski LA, Ryan SI: Comparison of an antiinflammatory dose of ibuprofen, an analgesic dose of ibuprofen, and acetaminophen in the treatment of patients with osteoarthritis of the knee. *N Engl J Med* 1991;325:87–91.
173. Bradley JD, Brandt KD, Katz BP, Kalasinski LA, Ryan SI: Treatment of knee osteoarthritis: Relationship of clinical features of joint inflammation to the response to a nonsteroidal antiinflammatory drug or pure analgesic. *J Rheumatol* 1992;19:1950–1954.
174. Goldin RH, McAdam L, Louie JS, Gold R, Bluestone R: Clinical and radiological survey of the incidence of osteoarthritis among obese patients. *Ann Rheum Dis* 1976;35:349–353.
175. Leach RE, Baumgard SS, Broom J: Obesity: Its relationship to osteoarthritis of the knee. *Clin Orthop* 1973; 93:271–273.
176. Lowman EW: Osteoarthritis. *JAMA* 1955;157:487–488.
177. Moskowitz RW: Primary osteoarthritis: Epidemiology, clinical aspects, and general management. *Am J Med* 1987;83(suppl 5A):5–10.
178. Roberts J, Burch TA: Prevalence of osteoarthritis in adults by age, sex, race, and geographic area, United States—1960–1962. National Center for Health Statistics: Vital and health statistics: Data from the National Health Survey. US Public Health Service document No. 1000, Series 11, No. 15. Washington, DC, Government Printing Office, 1966.

Osteoporosis

179. Aloia JF, Vaswani AN, Yeh JK, Cohn SH: Premenopausal bone mass is related to physical activity. *Arch Intern Med* 1988;148:121–123.
180. Aloia JF, Vaswani AN, Yeh JK, Ross PL, Flaster E, Dilmanian FA: Calcium supplementation with and without hormone replacement therapy to prevent postmenopausal bone loss. *Ann Intern Med* 1994;120:97–103.
181. Barrett-Connor E, Chang JC, Edelstein SL: Coffee-associated osteoporosis offset by daily milk consumption. The Rancho Bernado Study. *JAMA* 1994;271:280–283.
182. Bickle DD, Genant HK, Cann C, Recker RR, Halloran BP, Strewler GJ: Bone disease in alcohol abuse. *Ann Intern Med* 1985;103:42–48.
183. Bridge, SJ: Osteoporosis and hip fractures. *Clin Ger Med* 1993;9:69–83.
184. Chapuy MC, Arlot ME, Duboeuf F, Brun J, Crouzet B, Arnaud S, Delmas PD, Meunier PJ: Vitamin D3 and calcium to prevent hip fractures in the elderly women. *N Engl J Med.* 1992;327(23):1637–1642.

185. Chesnut CH III: Bone mass and exercise. *Am J Med* 1993;95:34S–36S.

186. Clark AP, Schuttinga JA: Target estrogen/progesterone replacement therapy for osteoporosis: Calculation of health care cost savings. *Osteoporos Int* 1992;2:195–200.

187. Cummings RG, Miller JP, Kelsey JL, Davis P, Arfken CL, Birge SJ, Peck WA: Medications and multiple falls in elderly people: The St. Louis OASIS study. *Age Ageing* 1991;20:455–461.

188. Cummings SR: Are patients with hip fracture more osteoporotic? *Am J Med* 1985;78:487–494.

189. Dalsky GP, Stocke KS, Ehsani AA, Slatopolsky E, Lee WC, Birge SJ: Weight-bearing exercise training and lumbar bone mineral content in postmenopausal women. *Ann Intern Med* 1988;108:824–828.

190. Ettinger B, Genant HK, Cann CE: Long-term estrogen replacement therapy prevents bone loss and fractures. *Ann Intern Med* 1985;102:319–324.

191. Ettinger B, Genant HK, Cann CE: Postmenopausal bone loss is prevented by treatment with low-dosage estrogen with calcium. *Ann Intern Med* 1987;106:40–45.

192. Felson DT, Zhang Y, Hannan MT, Kiel DP, Wilson PW, Anderson JJ: The effect of postmenopausal estrogen therapy on bone density in elderly women. *N Engl J Med* 1993;329:1141–1146.

193. Goldbloom R, Battista RN: The periodic health examination: 1. Introduction. *Can Med Assoc J* 1988;138:617–618.

194. Hall FM, Davis MA, Baran DT: Bone mineral screening for osteoporosis. *N Engl J Med* 1987;316:212–214.

195. Heaney RP: Bone mass, nutrition, and other lifestyle factors. *Am J Med* 1993;95:29S–33S.

196. Hopper JL, Seeman E: The bone density of female twins discordant for tobacco use. *N Engl J Med* 1994;330:387–392.

197. Hussey HH. Editorial: Osteoporosis among women who smoke cigarettes. *JAMA* 1976;235:1367–1368.

198. Kanis JA, Johnell O, Gullberg B, Allander E, Dilsen G, Genari C, Lopes-Vaz AA, Lyritis GP, Mazzuli G, Miravet L, et al: Evidence for efficacy of drugs affecting bone metabolism in preventing hip fracture. *Br Med J* 1992;305:1124–1128.

199. Kiel DP, Baron JA, Anderson JJ, Hannan MT, Felson DT: Smoking eliminates the protective effect of oral estrogens in the risk of hip fractures among women. *Ann Int Med* 1992;116:716–721.

200. Krolne B, Toft B, Nielsen PS, Tondevold E: Physical exercise as prophylaxis against involutional vertebral bone loss: A controlled trial. *Clin Sci* 1983;64:541–546.

201. Lauritzen JB, Petersen MM, Lund B: Effect of external hip protectors on hip fractures. *Lancet* 1993;341:11–13.

202. Mazess RB: On aging bone loss. *Clin Orthop* 1982;165:239–252.

203. Mazess RB: The noninvasive measurement of skeletal mass, in Peck WA (ed.): *Bone and Mineral Research Annual 1*. Amsterdam, Excerpta Medica, 1983, pp 223–279.

204. McBean LD, Forgac R, Finn SC: Osteoporosis: Visions for care and prevention—A conference report. *J Am Dietetic Assoc* 1994;94:668–671.

205. Meunier PJ: Prevention of hip fractures. *Am J Med* 1993;95:75S–78S.

206. Miravet L, et al: Evidence for efficacy of drugs affecting bone metabolism in preventing hip fracture. *Br Med J* 1992;305:1124–1128.

207. Hewcomer AD, Hodgson SF, McGill DB, Thomas PJ: Lactase deficiency: Prevalence in osteoporosis. *Ann Intern Med* 1978;89:218–220.

208. Pritchard KI: Screening for endometrial cancer: is it effective? *Ann Intern Med.* 1989; 110(3): 177–179.

209. Reid IR, Ames RW, Evans MC, Gamble GD, Sharpe SJ: Effect of calcium supplementation on bone loss in postmenopausal women. *N Engl J Med* 1993;329:1281.

210. Richelson LS, Wabner HW, Melton LJIII, Riggs, BL: Relative contributions of aging and estrogen deficiency to postmenopausal bone loss. *N Engl J Med* 1984;311:1273–1275.

211. Riggs BL, Hodgson SE, O'Fallon WM, Chao EYS, Wahner HW, Muhs JM, Cedel SL, Melton LJ. Effect of flouride treatment on the fracture rate in postmenopausal women with osteoporosis. *N Engl J Med* 1990;322:802–809.

212. Riggs BL, Melton LJ III: Involutional osteoporosis. *N Engl J Med* 1986;314:1676–1686.

213. Riggs BL, Melton LJ III: The prevention and treatment of osteoporosis. *N Engl J Med* 1992;327:620–627.

214. Shapiro S, Kelly JP, Rosenberg L, Kaufman DW, Helmrich SP, Rosenshein NB, Lewis JL Jr., Knapp RC, Stolley PD, Schottenfeld D: Risk of localized and widespread endometrial cancer in relation to recent and discontinued use of conjugated estrogens. *N Engl J Med.* 1985; 313(16): 969–972.

215. Simonen O, Laitinen O: Does flouridation of drinking water prevent bone fragility and osteoporosis? *Lancet* 1985;2:432–433.

216. Stall GM, Harris S, Sokoll LJ, Dawson HB: Accelerated bone loss in hypothyroid patients overtreated with L-thyroxine. *Ann Intern Med* 1990;113:265–269.

217. Tinetti ME, Baker DI, McAvay G, Claus EB, Garrett P, Gottschalk M, Koch ML, Trainor K, Horwitz RI: A multifactorial intervention to reduce the risk of falling among elderly people living in the community. *N Engl J Med* 1994;331:821–827.

218. Toft AD: Thyroxine therapy. *N Engl J Med* 1994;331:174–180.

219. Tosteson AN, Rosenthal DI. Melton LJ III, Weinstein MC: Cost effectiveness of screening perimenopausal white women for osteoporosis: Bone densitometry and hormone replacement therapy. *Ann Intern Med* 1990;113:594–603.
220. Williams AR, Weiss NS, Ure CL, Ballard J, Daling JR. Effect of weight, smoking, and estrogen use on the risk of hip and forearm fractures in postmenopausal women. *Obstet Gynecol* 1982;60:695–699.

Vision and Hearing

221. ASHA Committee on Audiometric Evaluation. Guidelines for determining the threshold level for speech. *ASHA* 1979;21:353–356.
222. Bengtsson B: The prevalence of glaucoma. *Br J Ophthalmol* 1981;65:46–49.
223. Comprehensive Adult Eye Evaluation. American Academy of Opthalmology, San Francisco CA, 1995.
224. Dawson DA, Adams PF: National Center for Health Statistics. Current estimates from the Health Interview Surgery, United States, 1986. Vital and Health Statistics Series 10. Number 164, DHHS Publication No. (PHS) 87-1592. Washington, DC, US Department of Health and Human Services, 1987.
225. Five Minute Hearing Test. American Academy of Otolaryngology–Head and Neck Surgery, Inc., Washington, DC, 1989.
226. Gates GA, Caspary DM, Clark W, Pillsbury HC, Brown SC, Dobie RA: Presbycusis. *Otolaryngol Head Neck Surg* 1989;100:266–271.
227. Gennis V, Garry PJ, Haaland KY, Yeo RA, Goodwin JS: Hearing and cognition in the elderly. New findings and a review of the literature. *Arch Intern Med* 1991;151:2259–2264.
228. Hatton ER, Cogan CM, Hatton MN: Common oral conditions in the elderly. *American Family Practice AFP* 1989;40:149–162.
229. Katz M: The human eye as an optical system, in Duane TD (ed.): *Clinical Ophthalmology.* Philadelphia, JB Lippincott, Rev ed, 1988, Vol 1, Chapt 33, pp 1–52.
230. Luntz MH: Clinical types of cataract, in Duane TD (ed.): *Clinical Ophthalmology.* Philadelphia, JB Lippincott, rev ed, 1988, Vol 1, Chapt. 73, pp 1–20.
231. Mashberg A, Barsa P: Screening for oral and oropharyngeal squamous carcinomas. *Cancer* 1984;34:262–268.
232. Nadol JB Jr: Hearing loss. *N Engl J Med* 1993;329:1092–1102.
233. Canadian Task Force on the Periodic Health Examination. Periodic health examination, 1995 update: 3. Screening for visual problems among elderly patients. *Can Med Assoc J.* 1995; 152(8):1211–1222.
234. Olson L: Anatomy and embryology of the lens, in Duane TD (ed.): *Clinical Ophthalmology.* Philadelphia, JB Lippincott, Rev ed, 1988, Vol 1, Chapt 71, pp 1–8.
235. Peterson FT: Accuracy of a 40 dB HL audioscope and audiometer screening for adults. *Ear Hear* 1987;8:180–183.
236. Phelps CD: Examination and functional evaluation of crystalline lens, in Duane TD (ed.): *Clinical Ophthalmology.* Philadelphia, JB Lippincott, Rev ed, 1988, Vol 1, Chapt 72, pp 1–23.
237. Phelps CD: Glaucoma: General concepts, in Duane TD (ed.): *Clinical Ophthalmology.* Philadelphia, JB Lippincott, Rev ed, 1988, Vol 3, Chapt 42, pp 1–8.
238. Snyder JM: Office audiometry. *J Fam Pract* 1984;19:535–548.
239. Uhlmann RF, Rees TS, Psaty BM, Duckert LG: Validity and reliability of auditory screening tests in demented and non-demented older adults. *J Gen Intern Med* 1989;4:90–96.

Depression and Dementia

240. Blazer D: Depression in the elderly. *N Engl J Med* 1989;320:164–166.
241. Blessed G, Tomlinson BE, Roth M: The association between quantitative measures of dementia and of senile change in the cerebral grey matter of elderly subjects. *Br J Psychiatry* 1968;114:796–811.
242. Clarfeld AM: The reversible dementias: Do they reverse? *Ann Intern Med* 1988;109:476–486.
243. *Diagnostic and Statistical Manual of Mental Disorders: DSM-IV.* Washington, DC, American Psychiatric Association, 1994.
244. Folstein MF, Folstein SE, McHugh PR: Mini-mental state: A practical method for grading the cognitive state of patients for the clinician. *J Psychiatr Res* 1975;12:189–198.
245. Knapp MJ, Knopman DS, Solomon PR, Pendlebury WW, Davis CS, Gracon SI: A 30 week randomized controlled trial of high dose tacrine in patients with Alzheimer's disease. *JAMA* 1994;271:985–991.
246. Larson EB, Reifler BV, Featherstone HJ, English DR: Dementia in elderly outpatients: A prospective study. *Ann Intern Med* 1984;100:417–423.

247. Lishman WA: Cerebral disorder in alcoholism: Syndromes of impairment. *Brain* 1981;104:1–20.
248. Mortimer JA: Alzheimer's disease and senile dementia: Prevalence and incidence, in Reisberg B (ed.): *Alzheimer's Disease: The Standard Reference*. New York, Free Press, 1983.
249. Perry K, Curtis M, Dick DJ, Candy JM, Atack JR, Bloxham CA, Blessed G, Fairbaim A, Tomlinson BE, Perry RH: Cholinergic correlates of cognitive impairments in Parkinson's disease: Comparisons with Alzheimer's disease. *J Neurol Neurosurg Psychiatry* 1985;48:413–421.
250. Strachan RW, Henderson JG: Psychiatric syndromes due to avitaminosis B12 with normal blood and bone marrow. *Q J Med* 1965;34:303–309.

Lifestyle: Smoking

251. Daughton DM, Heatley SA, Prendergast JJ, Causey D, Knowles M, Rolf CN, Cheney RA, Hatlelid K, Thompson AB, Rennard SI: Effect of transdermal nicotine delivery as an adjunct to low-intervention smoking cessation therapy. A randomized, placebo-controlled, double-blind study. *Arch Intern Med* 1991;151:749–752.
252. Dept. of Health and Human Services: *The Health Consequences of Smoking: Cancer*. Rockville, MD, 1982.
253. Dept. of Health and Human Services: *The Health Consequences of Smoking: Cardiovascular Disease*. Rockville, MD, 1983.
254. Dept. of Health and Human Services: *The Health Consequences of Smoking: COPD*. Rockville, MD, 1984.
255. Effectiveness of a nicotine patch in helping people stop smoking: results of a randomised trial in general practice. Imperial Cancer Research Fund General Practice Research Group. *Br Med J* 1993;306:1304–1308.
256. Fielding JE: Smoking: Health effects and control. *N Engl J Med* 1985;313:491–498.
257. Fiore MC: The new vital sign. Assessing and documenting smoking status. *JAMA* 1991;266:3183–3184.
258. Fiore MC, Novotny TE, Pierce JP, Giovino GA, Hatziandreu EJ, Newcomb PA, Surawicz, TS, Davis RM. Methods used to quit smoking in the United States. Do cessation programs help? *JAMA* 1990;263:2760–2765.
259. Friedman GD, Petitti DB, Bawol RD, Siegelaub AB: Mortality in cigarette smokers and quitters. *N Engl J Med* 1981;304:1407–1410.
260. Greene HL, Goldberg RJ, Ockene JK: Cigarette smoking: The physician's role in cessation and maintenance. *J Gen Intern Med* 1988;3:75–87.
261. Hollis JF, Lichtenstein E, Vogt TM, Stevens VJ, Biglan A: Nurse-assisted counseling for smokers in primary care. *Ann Intern Med* 1993;118:521–525.
262. Hurt RD, Dale LC, Fredrickson PA, Caldwell CC, Lee GA, Offord KP, Lauger GG, Marusi'c-Z. Neese LW, Lundberg TG: Nicotine patch therapy for smoking cessation combined with physician advice and nurse follow-up. One-year outcome and percentage of nicotine replacement. *JAMA* 1994;271:595–600.
263. Kawachi I, Colditz GA, Stampfer MJ, Willett WC, Manson JE, Rosner B, Speizer FE, Hennekens CH: Smoking cessation and decreased risk of stroke in women. *JAMA* 1993;269:232–236.
264. Kawachi I, Colditz GA, Stampfer MJ, Willett WC, Manson JE, Rosner B, Speizer FE, Hennekens CH: Smoking cessation and time course of decreased risks of coronary heart disease in middle-aged women. *Arch Intern Med* 1994;154:169–175.
265. Kawachi I, Colditz GA, Stampfer MJ, Willett WC, Manson JE, Rosner B, Hunter DJ, Hennekens CH, Speizer FE: Smoking cessation in relation to total mortality rates in women. A prospective cohort study. *Ann Intern Med* 1993;119:992–1000.
266. Kenford SL, Fiore MC, Jorenby DE, Smith SS, Wetter D, Baker TB: Predicting smoking cessation. Who will quit with and without the nicotine patch. *JAMA* 1994;271:P589–594.
267. LaCroix AZ, Lang J, Scherr P, Wallace RB, Cornoni-Huntley J, Berkman L, Curb JD, Evans D, Hennekens CH: Smoking and mortality among older men and women in three communities. *N Engl J Med* 1991;324:1619–1625.
268. Lee EW, D'Alonzo GE: Cigarette smoking, nicotine addiction, and its pharmacologic treatment. *Arch Intern Med* 1993;153:34–48.
269. Li-Wan PoA: Transdermal nicotine in smoking cessation. A meta-analysis. *Eur J Clin Pharmacol*, 1993;45:519–528.
270. Neighbor WE: The physician's role in smoking cessation. *UW Med* 1989;15:22–24.
271. Ockene JK: Smoking intervention: The expanding role of the physician. *Am J Pub Health* 1987;77:782–783.
272. Paulozzi L: The costs of smoking for Washington. *Wash Morb Rep* 1984;1:4.
273. Pederson LL: Compliance with physician advice to quit smoking: A review of the literature. *Prev Med* 1982;11:71–84.
274. Petitti D, Wingerd J: Use of oral contraceptives, cigarette smoking, and risk of subarachnoid hemorrhage. *Lancet* 1978;2:234–235.
275. Pirie PL, McBride CM, Hellerstedt W, Jeffery RW, Hatsukami D, Allen S, Lando H: Smoking cessation in women concerned about weight. *Am J Public Health* 1992;82:1238–1243.

276. Risser NL, Belcher DW: Adding spirometry, carbon monoxide and pulmonary symptom results to smoking cessation counseling: A randomized trial. *J Gen Intern Med* 1989;5:16–22.

277. Rogers RL: Abstention from cigarette smoking improves cerebral perfusion among elderly chronic smokers. *J Am Med Assoc* 1985;253:2970–2974.

278. Rosenberg L, Palmer JR, Shapiro S: Decline in the risk of myocardial infarction among women who stop smoking. *N Engl J Med* 1990;322:213–217.

279. Smoking and cardiovascular disease. *MMWR* 1984;32:677–679.

280. State-specific estimates of smoking attributable mortality and years of potential life lost—United States 1985. *MMWR* 1988;37:689–692.

281. The Surgeon General's 1989 Report on Reducing the Health Consequences of Smoking: 25 Years of Progress. *MMWR Morb Mortal Wkly Rep.* 1989; 38:(Suppl 2) 1–32.

282. Tonnesen P, Norregaard J, Simonsen K, Sawe U: A double-blind trial of a 16-hour transdermal nicotine patch in smoking cessation. *N Engl J Med* 1991;325:311–315.

283. Transdermal nicotine for smoking cessation: Six-month results from two multicenter controlled clinical trials. Transdermal Nicotine Study Group. *JAMA* 1991;266:3133–3138.

284. Willet WC, Green A, Stampfer MJ, Speizer FE, Colditz GA, Rosner B, Monson RR, Stason W, Hennekens CH: Relative and absolute excess risks of coronary heart disease among women who smoke cigarettes. *N Engl J Med* 1987;317:1303–1309.

Lifestyle: Exercise

285. Harris SS, Caspersen CJ, DeFriese GH, Estes EH: Physical activity counseling for healthy adults as a primary preventive intervention in the clinical setting. *JAMA* 261:3590–3598.

286. Koplon JP, Caspersen CJ, Powell KE: Physical activity, physical fitness and health: Time to act. *JAMA* 1989;262:2347.

287. Sorock GS, Bush TL, Golden AL, Fried LP, Breuer B, Hale WE: Physical activity and fracture risk in a free-living elderly chort. *J Gerontol* 1988;43:M134–M139.

288. Surgeon General's Workshop on Health Promotion and Aging: Summary recommendations of the physical fitness and exercise working group. *MMWR* 1989;38:700–707.

289. Taylor PA, Ward A: Women, high-density lipoprotein cholesterol, and exercise. *Arch Intern Med* 1993;153:1178–1184.

290. The President's Council on Physical Fitness and Sports: Progress toward achieving the 1990 national objectives for physical fitness and exercise. *MMWR* 1989;38:449–453.

291. US Preventive Services Task Force: Recommendations for physical exercise in primary prevention. *JAMA* 1989;261:3588–3589.

Nutrition and Obesity

292. Andres R: Mortality and obesity: The rationale for age-specific height-weight tables, in Andres R, Bierman EL, Hazzard WR (eds.): *Principles of Geriatric Medicine.* Mc-Graw-Hill, New York, 1985.

293. Brody JE: Changing nutritional needs put the elderly at risk because of inadequate diets. *NY Times* Feb 8, 1990, p B7.

294. Butrum-R-R. Clifford-C-K. Lanza-E. NCI dietary guidelines: rationale. Am-J-Clin-Nutr. 1988 Sep. 48(3 Suppl). P 888-95.

295. Calcium Supplements. *The Medical Letter* 1989;31:101–103.

296. Committee on Diet and Health: *Diet and Health: Executive Summary.* National Academy Press, Washington DC, 1989.

297. Folsom AR, Kaye SA, Sellers TA, et al: Body fat distribution and 5-year risk of death in older women. *JAMA* 1993;269:483–487.

298. Food and Nutrition Board, National Research Council: *Recommended Dietary Allowances,* 10 ed. Washington DC, National Academy Press, 1989.

299. Gebhardt SE, Mathews RH: Nutritive Value of Foods, Dept. of Agriculture, Washington, DC, US Government Printing Office, 1981.

300. Greenberg ER, Baron JA, Tosteson TD, Freeman DH Jr, Beck GJ, Bond JH, Colacchio TA, Coller JA, Frankl HD, Haile RW, et al: A clinical trial of antioxidant vitamins to prevent colorectal adenoma. Polyp Prevention Study Group. *N Engl J Med* 1994;331:141–147.

301. Gotto AM, Scott LW, Foreyt JP: Diet and health. *West J Med* 1984;141:872–877.

302. Kuczmarski RJ, Flegal KM, Campbell SM, Johnson CL: Increasing prevalence of overweight among US adults. The National Health and Nutrition Examination Surveys, 1960 to 1991. *JAMA* 1994;272:205–211.

303. Morley JE: Nutrition and the older female: A review. *J Am Coll Nutr* 1993;12:337–343.

304. Morris DL, Kritchevsky SB, Davis CE: Serum carotenoids and coronary heart disease. *JAMA* 1994;272:1439–1441.

305. Pennington JAT, Church HN: *Bowes and Church's Food Values of Portions Commonly Used*, 13 ed., New York. 1980.

306. Pi-Sunyer FX: Short-term medical benefits and adverse effects of weight loss. *Ann Intern Med* 1993;119:722–726.

307. Rimm EB, Stampfer MJ, Ascherio A, Giovannucci E, Colditz GA, Willett WC. Vitamin E consumption and the risk of coronary heart disease in men. *N Engl J Med* 1993;328:1450–1456.

308. Stampfer MJ, Hennekens CH, Manson JE, Colditz GA, Rosner B, Willett WC: Vitamin E consumption and the risk of coronary disease in women. *N Engl J Med* 1993;328:1444–1449.

309. Steinberg D: Antioxidant vitamins and coronary heart disease. *N Engl J Med* 1993;328:1487–1489.

310. The effect of vitamin E and beta carotene on the incidence of lung cancer and other cancers in male smokers. The Alpha-Tocopherol, Beta Carotene Cancer Prevention Study Group. *N Engl J Med* 1994;330:1029–1035.

311. US Department of Health and Human Servics, Public Health Service. The Surgeon General's report on nutrition and health. Superintendent of Documents, Washington, DC, US Government Printing Office, 1988.

312. Worthington-Roberts B: Diet and health. *UW Med* 1989;15:13–17.

Bladder and Bowel Function

313. Barrett JA: ABC of colorectal diseases. Colorectal disorders in elderly people. *Br Med J* 1992;305:764–766.

314. Harari D, Gurwitz JH, Minaker KL: Constipation in the elderly. *J Am Geriatr Soc* 1993;41:1130–1140.

315. Houston KA: *Incontinence and the Older Woman*. Clinics in Geriatric Medicine, No 9, 1993, pp 157–71.

316. Merkel IS, Locher J, Burgio K, Towers A, Wald A: Physiologic and psychologic characteristics of an elderly population with chronic constipation. *Am J Gastroenterol* 1993;88:1854–1859.

317. Resnick NM, Yalla SV: Management of urinary incontinence in the elderly. *N Engl J Med* 1985;313:800–803.

318. Towers AL, Burgio KL, Locher JL, Merkel IS, Safaeian M, Wald A: Constipation in the elderly: Influence of dietary, psychological, and physiological factors. *J Am Geriatr Soc* 1994;42:701–706.

Use of Medications

319. Bloom BS: Risk and cost of gastrointestinal side effects associated with nonsteroidal anti-inflammatory drugs. *Arch Intern Med* 1989;149:1019–1022.

320. Sandler DP, Smith JC, Weinberg CR, Buckalew VM, Dennis VW, Blythe WB, Burgess WP: Analgesic use and chronic renal disease, *N Engl J Med* 1989;320:1238–1243.

321. Willcox SM, Himmelstein DU, Woolhandler S: Inappropriate drug prescribing for the community-dwelling elderly. *JAMA* 1994;272:292–296.

Laboratory Screening Test

322. Abrutyn E, Mossey J, Berlin JA, Boscia J, Levison M, Pitsakis P, Kaye D: Does asymptomatic bacteriuria predict mortality and does antimicrobial treatment reduce mortality in elderly ambulatory women? *Ann Intern Med* 1994;120:827–833.

323. Abuelo JG: Proteinuria: Diagnostic principles and procedures. *Ann Intern Med* 1983;98:186–191.

324. Akin BV, Hubbell FA, Frye EB, Rucker L, Friis R: Efficacy of routine admission urinalysis. *Am J Med* 1987;82:719–722.

325. Atkinson RL: Occult thyroid disease in an elderly hospitalized population. *J Gerontol* 1978;33:372–376.

326. Bard RH: The significance of asymptomatic microhematuria in women its economic implications: A ten-year study. *Arch Intern Med* 1988;148:2629–2632.

327. Benbassat J, Froom P, Feldman M, Margoliot S: The importance of leukocyturia in young adults. *Arch Intern Med* 1985;145:79–80.

328. Bennett PH, Knowler WC. Early detection and intervention in diabetes mellitus: Is it effective? *J Chronic Dis* 1984;37:653–666.

329. Bilezikian JP: The medical management of primary hyperparathyroidism. *Ann Intern Med* 1982;96:198–202.

330. Boonstra CE, Jackson CE: Serum calcium; Survey for hyperparathyroidism: Results in 50,000 clinic patients. *Am J Clin Pathol* 1971;55:523–526.

331. Canadian Task Force on the Periodic Health Examination: The periodic health examination. *Can Med Assoc J* 1979;121:1193–1254.

332. Carel RS, Silverberg DS, Kaminsky R, Aviram A: Routine urinalysis (dipstick) findings in mass screening of healthy adults. *Clin Chem* 1987;33:2106–2108.

333. Cebul RD, Beck JR: Biochemical profiles. *Ann Intern Med* 1987;106:403–413.

334. Davidson MB: The effect of aging on carbohydrate metabolism. A review of the English literature and a practical approach to the diagnosis of diabetes mellitus in the elderly. *Progr Endocrinol Metab* 179;28:688–705.

335. Davis PJ, Davis B: Hyperthyroidism in patients over the age of 60 years. *Medicine* 1974;53:161–181.

336. Diagnosis and management of asymptomatic primary hyperparathyroidism. National Institutes of Health Consensus Development Conference. October 29–31, 1990. *Consens Statement* 1990;8:1–18.

337. Elwood PC, Waters WE, Green WJ, Wood MM: Evaluation of a screening survey for anemia in adult non-pregnant women. *Br Med J* 1967;4:714–717.

338. Epstein M, Hollenberg NK: Age as a determinant of renal sodium conservation in normal men. *J Lab Clin Med* 1976;87:411–417.

339. Expert Committee on Diabetes Mellitus, World Health Organization: WHO Technical Report Series 646. Genera: World Health Organization, 1980:1–80.

340. Ferero MS, Klein RF, Nissenson RA, Nelson K, Heath H III, Arnaud CD, Riggs BL: Effect of age on circulation immunoreactive and bioactive parathyroid hormone levels in women. *J Bone Min Res* 1987;2:363–366.

341. Forrest RD, Jackson CA, Yudkin JS: The glycohaemoglobin assay as a screening test for diabetes mellitus: The Tslington Diabetes Survey. *Diabetic Med* 1987;4:254–259.

342. Friedman GD, Goldberg M, Ahuja JN, Siegelaub AB, Bassis ML, Collen MI: Biochemical screening tests: Effect of panel size on medical care. *Arch Intern Med* 1972;129:91–97.

343. Ginsberg JM, Chang BS, Matarese RA, Garella S: Use of single voided urine samples to estimate quantitative proteinuria. *N Engl J Med* 19XX;309:1543–1546.

344. Harris MI, Hadden WC, Knowler WC, Bennett PH: Prevalence of diabetes and impaired glucose tolerance and plasma glucose levels in US population aged 20–24 years. *Diabetes* 1987;36:523–534.

345. Heath H III, Hodgson SF, Kennedy MA: Primary hyperparathyroidism: Incidence, morbidity, and potential economic impact in a community. *N Engl J Med* 1980;302:189–193.

346. Is routine urinalysis worthwhile? *Lancet* 1988; 1:747.

347. Kaplan EB, Sheiner LB, Boeckmann AJ, Roizen MF, Beal SL, Cohen SN, Nicoll CD: The usefulness of preoperative laboratory screening. *JAMA* 1985;253:3576–3581.

348. Kaplan SE, Lippe BM, Brinkman CR, Davidson MB, Geffner ME: Diabetes mellitus. *Ann Intern Med* 1982;96:635–649.

349. Keen H, Jarrett RJ, McCartney P: The ten year follow-up of the Bedford Survey (1962–1972): Glucose tolerance and diabetes. *Diabetologia* 19XX;22:73–78.

350. Kiel DP, Moskowitz MA: The urinalysis: A critical appraisal, in *Office Practice of Laboratory Medicine*. Medical Clinics of North America, Vol 71, 1987, pp 607–624.

351. Klein I, Levey GS: Unusual manifestations of hypothyroidism. *Arch Intern Med* 1984;144:123–128.

352. Medical Practice Committee, American College of Physicians: Periodic health examination: A guide for designing individualized preventive health care in the asymptomatic patient. *Ann Intern Med* 1981;95:729–732.

353. Morris LR, McGee JA, Kitabachi AE: Correlation between plasma and urine glucose in diabetes. *Ann Intern Med* 1981;94:469–471.

354. Morrow LB: How thyroid disease presents in the elderly. *Geriatrics* Apr 1978;33:42–45.

355. Nathan DM, Singer DE, Hurxthal K, Goodson JD: The clinical information value of the glycosylated hemoglobin assay. *N Engl J Med* 1984;310:341–346.

356. National Diabetes Data Group: Classification and diagnosis of diabetes mellitus and other categories of glucose tolerance. *Diabetes* 1979;28:1039–1057.

357. O'Sullivan JB, Mahan CM: Prospective study of 352 young patients with chemical diabetes. *N Engl J Med* 19XX;278:1038–1011.

358. Robuschi G, Safran M, Braverman LE, Gnudi A, Roti E: Hypothyroidism in the elderly. *Endocr Rev* 1987;8:142–153.

359. Rotter SI, Vadheim CM: Diabetes mellitus, in King RA, Rotter JI, Motulsky AG (eds.): *The Genetic Basis of Common Disease,* Oxford University Press, 1990; in press.

360. Rowe JW, Andres R, Tobin JD, Norris AH, Shock NW: Age-adjusted normal standards for creatinine clearance in man. *Ann Intern Med* 1976;84:567–569.

361. Rowe JW, Andres R, Tobin JD, Norris AH, Shock NW: The effect of age on creatinine clearance in man: A cross-sectional and longitudinal study. *J Gerontol* 1976;155–163.

362. Schectman JM, Pawlson G: The cost-effectiveness of three thyroid function testing strategies for suspicion of hypothyroidism in a primary care setting. *J Gen Intern Med* 1990;5:9–15.

363. Shapiro MF, Greenfield S: The complete blood count and leukocyte differential count: An approach to their rational application. *Ann Intern Med* 1987;106:65–74.

364. Shorliffe L. Asymptomatic bacteriuria: Should it be treated? *Urology* 1986;27S:19–25.
365. Singer DE, Coley CM, Samet JH, Nathan DM. Tests of glycemia in diabetes mellitus: Their use in establishing a diagnosis and treatment. *Ann Intern Med* 1989;110:125–137.
366. Singer DE, Samet JH, Coley CM, Nathan DM: Screening for diabetes mellitus. *Ann Intern Med* 1988;109:639–649.
367. Sox HC, Garber AM, Littenberg B: The resting electrocardiogram as a screening test. *Ann Intern Med* 1989;111:489–502.
368. Tape TG, Mushlin AI: The utility of routine chest radiographs. *Ann Intern Med* 1986;104:663–670.
369. Thomas FB, Mazzafern EL, Skillman TG: Apathetic thyrotoxicosis: A distinctive clinical and laboratory entity. *Ann Intern Med* 1970;72:679–687.
370. Von Hoff W, Ballardie FW, Bicknell EJ: Primary hyperparathyroidism: The case for medical management. *Br Med J (Clin Res)* 1983;287:1605–1608.
371. Wesson LG: *Physiology of the Human Kidney*. Grune & Stratton, New York, 1969.
372. Wilson RJ, Rao DS, Ellis B, Kleerekoper M, Parfitt AM: Mild asymptomatic primary hyperparathyroidism is not a risk factor for vertebral fracture. *Ann Intern Med* 1988;109:959–962.
373. Zazove P: Should we screen for hypothyroidism in the elderly? *J Fam Pract* 1994;38:571–573.

General

374. Brody EM: Women in the middle and family help to older people. *Gerontologist* 1981;25:19–29.
375. Dracup K, Heaney DM, Taylor SE, Guzy PM, Breu C: Can family members of high-risk cardiac patients learn cardiopulmonary resuscitation? *Arch Intern Med* 1989;149:61–64.
376. Finucane TE, Shumway JM, Powers, RL, D'Alessandri RM: Planning with elderly outpatients for contingencies of severe illness. *J Gen Intern Med* 1988;3:322–325.
377. Goldberg RJ: Training family members of high-risk cardiac patients in cardiopulmonary resuscitation. *Arch Intern Med* 1989;149:25–26.
378. Hayward RSA, Steinberg EP, Ford DE, Roizen MR, Roach KW: Preventive care guidelines. *Ann Intern Med* 1991;114:758–783.
379. Lo B, McLeod GA, Saika G: Patient attitudes to discussing life sustaining treatment. *Arch Intern Med* 1986;32:930–934.
380. Medical Practice Committee, American College of Physicians: Periodic health examination: A guide for designing individualized preventive health care in the asymptomatic patient. *Ann Intern Med* 1981;95:729–732.
381. Ship JA, Wolff A, Selik RM: Epidemiology of acquired immune deficiency syndrome in persons aged 50 years or older. *J Acquir Immun Defic Syndr* 1991;4:84–88.
382. Sox HC Jr: Preventive health services in adults. *N Engl J Med* 1994;330:1589–1595.
383. Strand J: The living will: The right to death with dignity? *Case Western Reserve Law Rev* 1976;26:485–526.
384. Wallace JI, Paauw DS, Spach DH: HIV infection in older patients: When to suspect the unexpected. *Geriatrics* 1993;48:61–4, 69–70.
385. Zazove P, Mehr DR, Ruffin MT IV, Klinkman MS, Peggs JF, Davies TC: A criterion-based review of preventive health care in the elderly. Part 2. A geriatric health maintenance program. *J Fam Pract* 1992;34:320–347.

Chapter 10

Immunization

Wylie Burke, MD, PhD, Linda Pinsky, MD, and
Wendy H. Raskind MD, PhD

Immunization provides the opportunity for prevention of death and disability from a number of infectious diseases, at low cost and with little risk of serious complications. The development of immunization techniques constitutes one of the most successful advances in the history of preventive health care. Public health strategies, such as mandatory immunization for school entry, have been used in industrialized countries to assure completion of recommended childhood immunizations. However, control of certain diseases requires adult immunization as well. Unfortunately, immunization rates are frequently low, even among adults receiving regular medical care. Clinical practices to address this problem include patient education and routine assessment of the adequacy of childhood immunization and of risk factors that affect immunization schedules.

Taking an Immunization History

A review of the patient's immunization status begins with documentation that routine childhood immunization series have been completed. Recommendations for childhood immunization, as shown in Table 10.1 and reviewed below, are regularly updated, based on available technology and epidemiological risk data.[1,2] For example, recommendations for hepatitis B immunization and a second dose of measles–mumps–rubella (MMR) vaccine were added after 1990, and most adult women will not have had these immunizations. Some childhood immunizations that were missed require correction while others do not.[3–5]

Many adults are unable to provide details of their childhood immunizations. Women who received regular health care as children or who attended public elementary schools in urban or suburban areas of the United States can generally be assumed to have received the recommended series. That is unless immunizations were declined for a specific reason, such as religious beliefs. Older women from rural areas and women who have emigrated to the United States as teenagers or adults may have missed some or all immunizations.[5] When an person's immunization history is in doubt, essential immunizations should be provided, as summarized in Table 10.1.

Routine Adult Immunizations

In the United States, recommendations for immunization are regularly reviewed and updated by the Immunization Practices Advisory Committee (ACIP), under the auspices of the Centers for

Table 10.1 Routine Childhood Immunizations. Recommendations of the Immunization Practices Advisory Committee[1,2]

Currently recommended childhood immunizations	Recommendations for adult women with unknown or incomplete immunization
Diphtheria/tetanus/pertussis (DTP) series	Diphtheria–tetanus series
Oral polio series (OPV)	Inactivated polio series (IPV) **Recommended only for:** Health care workers Those exposed to young children Polio outbreak Travel to area where immunization is required
Measles–mumps–rubella (MMR) (2 doses)	MMR (2 doses if no previous immunization, 1 dose if previous dose received) **Recommended only for:** Individuals born after 1956
Hemophilus influenza	Not needed
Hepatitis B series	Hepatitis B series **Recommended only for:** Health care workers Public safety workers Recipients of blood products Intravenous drug users Household or sexual contact with Hepatitis B carrier

Disease Control.[2,5] Current routine recommendations for adults are summarized in Table 10-2. They include a tetanus–diphtheria (Td) booster every 10 years, an annual influenza vaccination starting at age 65, and a pneumococcal vaccine at or after 65. The recommendation for pneumococcal vaccination remains controversial, as discussed below. Additional recommendations are made for individuals in high-risk groups. These are summarized in Table 10.3 and reviewed in detail in subsequent sections. Contraindications to immunization are summarized in Table 10.4.

Tetanus and Diphtheria

Tetanus and diphtheria are extremely rare diseases. In 1993, 44 cases of tetanus and no cases of diphtheria were reported in the United States; 3 cases of diphtheria were reported in 1992.[6,7] However, these diseases occur almost exclusively in adults who have not been adequately immunized.[6,7] Because immunity wanes over time, risks of infection and mortality increase with age.

Table 10.2 Routine Immunizations. Recommendations of the Immunization Practices Advisory Committee[2,5]

Immunization	Schedule
Tetanus–diphtheria booster (Td)	Every 10 years
Influenza vaccine	Annually, starting at age 65
Pneumococcal vaccine*	One dose, at or after age 65

*Controversial; see discussion in text.

Table 10.3 Immunizations in High-Risk Women

High-Risk group	Immunizations recommended
Health care workers	Hepatitis B Annual flu vaccine
Chronic diseases that increase risk of respiratory infection	Annual flu vaccine Pneumococcal vaccine
Residents of chronic care facilities	Annual flu vaccine
Asplenic Human immunodeficiency virus (HIV) infection Sickle-cell anemia	Pneumococcal vaccine
Intravenous drug users Dialysis recipients Recipients of blood products	Hepatitis B

Diphtheria and tetanus toxoids are at least 95% effective in reducing both the risk and the clinical severity of disease, and the immunization schedule recommended is very inexpensive.

The primary immunizing series of three doses of combined toxoids (the pediatric mixture also contains pertussis toxoid, which is not given to adults) and two booster doses is usually complete at age 5. Adults who did not receive primary immunization or whose immunization status is unknown should be given a full primary series, using a tetanus–diphtheria preparation.[5] All adults should be vaccinated with booster doses every 10 years.

Polio

Routine primary or booster immunizations of adults in this country is not deemed necessary and is recommended only when exposure to polio virus is possible. Adults not adequately immunized

Table 10.4 Contraindications to Immunization

Immunization	Contraindication
All immunizations	Anaphylactic reaction to previous administration Anaphylactic reaction to a vaccine constituent Moderate or severe illness (with or without a fever)
Oral polio vaccine (OPV)	HIV infection Household contact with HIV infection Other immunodeficiency
Inactivated polio vaccine (IPV)	Anaphylactic reaction to neomycin or streptomycin
Measles–mumps–rubella (MMR)	Anaphylactic reaction to egg ingestion or to neomycin Pregnancy Immunodeficiency **Precaution:** Immune gobulin administration within 3 months
Hepatitis B	None identified
Influenza	Anaphylactic reaction to egg ingestion

HIV, Human immunodeficiency virus.

or whose immunity has waned have a small risk of developing paralytic polio from the stool of a child who has recently received the live oral polio vaccine (OPV). Therefore, individuals who have close contact with very young children (parents, grandparents, day-care workers) should be given a booster immunization if previously immunized or a three-dose primary immunization if never vaccinated. Other circumstances leading to potential exposure to polio virus include health care employment and travel to endemic areas.[2,5] Because OPV is a live-virus vaccine it presents a risk to those with human immunodeficiency virus (HIV) infection or other immunodeficiency and should not be used for either these persons or those who have household contact with them.

Vaccine-associated polio, although rare, is more common in adults.[8] Therefore an enhanced-potency (e) inactivated polio virus vaccine (IPV), available since the spring of 1988, is suggested for adults requiring primary immunization. The e-IPV is produced in cultured human diploid cells and may contain trace amounts of streptomycin and neomycin. Adults with a history of anaphylactic reactions to these antibiotics should not receive IPV.[9]

Measles (Rubeola)

Recent measles epidemics among young adults have included some individuals previously vaccinated.[4,5] This observation has led to a modification of the childhood immunization schedule from one to two doses of MMR, the live, attenuated virus vaccine for measles, mumps, and rubella. The second dose is typically administered during grade school. Since measles outbreaks are most likely to occur in settings where young adults congregate, a second dose is recommended for college entrants who have previously received only one dose. Prior to development of the MMR vaccine most persons had clinical or subclinical measles and have developed natural antibodies. Therefore, it is not necessary to vaccinate persons born before 1957. Patients who can reliably document a history of measles also need not be vaccinated. Patients who do not fall into these categories and who have never been immunized against measles should be given a series of two MMR vaccinations. Persons traveling to endemic areas who have had only one MMR should receive a second one, as should health care workers born after 1957. In the event of a measles outbreak, all those exposed should receive a second dose. Measles vaccine is derived from chick embryo cell culture and may contain traces of neomycin. A history of anaphylactic reaction to neomycin or eggs thus is a contraindication to administration of the MMR vaccine. In addition, because it is a live-virus vaccine, it is contraindicated in persons with immunosuppressive disorders.[1,2]

Mumps

As with measles, most persons born before 1957 have developed natural immunity to mumps, even if they did not have clinically apparent disease. Those born after 1957 who are unsure of their mumps disease or vaccination history should receive an MMR vaccination.[2,5] Those who received a killed-virus mumps vaccine, available from 1950 to 1978, may also benefit from receiving the live-virus vaccine. The two-dose MMR schedule recommended to ensure adequate measles immunity may also contribute to increased protection against outbreaks of mumps.

Rubella

The central concern in rubella immunization is the prevention of fetal infection and congenital rubella syndrome.[2,5] Thus, immunity is of particular importance for women of reproductive age and for all individuals who may have contact with pregnant women or young children. Proof of immunity can be established either by a documented rubella vaccination on or after the first birthday or by a positive serologic test. Rubella vaccination (usually given as MMR) is indicated for health care workers, child care workers, and others potentially in contact with susceptible persons.

Influenza

"Flu" results from infection with one of the antigenically and immunologically distinct myxovirus influenza groups. Epidemics are caused mostly by type A viruses whose surface antigen composition undergoes frequent mutational change, the so-called antigenic drift. Since the immune response to these viruses is mounted against the antigen phenotype, past infection or vaccination with one strain may not confer adequate protection against another strain with an altered antigenic profile. For this reason, to prevent or attenuate the severity of disease it is necessary to vaccinate at-risk persons each year with a vaccine that includes the viral strains predicted to be prevalent. The most significant complication of influenza is bacterial pneumonia, which can occur concurrently or as a secondary infection. Between 1977 and 1988, seven epidemics of influenza occurred, each causing more than 10,000 deaths.[9] In the 1988–89 influenza season, 78% of the pneumonia or influenza deaths reported occurred in persons 65 years of age or older.[10] Although influenza vaccination is less effective in elderly populations than in young, healthy adults, 75% reduction in mortality was seen in nursing home residents who had been vaccinated compared with those who had not.[11] The vaccine has also been shown to reduce hospital admissions and deaths related to respiratory infection.[12]

Routine vaccination of persons ages 65 and older has been shown to be cost-effective[13] and should be performed each year in the autumn. Persons with chronic diseases such as cardiovascular, pulmonary, or renal impairment, diabetes, severe anemia, and depressed immunocompetence should be vaccinated as well. It is also recommended that health care personnel and household contacts of high-risk persons be immunized to prevent the spread of influenza to those who are most likely to develop complications. Vaccines should not be given during a febrile illness because an inadequate immune response may occur. A history of egg allergy is a contraindication to vaccination because the vaccine contains traces of egg protein.

To reduce the risk of developing influenza A, high-risk patients who fail to receive influenza immunization may be given amantadine (200 mg/day for persons under 65 years of age and 100 mg/day for the elderly) for the duration of the outbreak. Vaccination remains the best strategy for prevention since postexposure prophylaxis with this drug may not be effective,[14,15] and no drug is yet available for prophylaxis or amelioration of influenza B. The primary usefulness of amantadine is in the reduction of severity and duration of influenza A illness. For this purpose, the recommended dosage of 200 mg/day is begun within 48 hours of onset of symptoms.

Pnuemococcal Pneumonia

Pneumococcus is a common cause of pneumonia, with 150,000 to 570,000 cases per year accounting for 10% to 25% of all pneumonias.[4,15] Even in the era of antibiotics, the overall mortality rate is 5%. Higher mortality risk occurs in persons older than 55, alcoholics, and those with underlying chronic disease or impaired immunity, especially asplenia. Associated bacteremia carries a 15% to 40% mortality rate, and intensive care support has had no impact on this number.[16] Whereas there is general agreement regarding the immunization schedules discussed above, controversy surrounds the topic of pneumococcal vaccine utility. Previous enthusiastic support for routine immunization[17] has been dampened by a raft of negative reports. Efficacy is estimated at 44% to 61% for immunocompetent persons over age 64,[5,18] but this conclusion is based largely on retrospective studies demonstrating protection from bacteremic infection with pneumococcal subtypes included in the vaccine.[19] Randomized prospective trials to assess the effect of the vaccine on mortality or morbidity in the elderly are lacking. One prospective trial of chronically ill persons over age 54 showed no vaccine efficacy,[20] and other studies have demonstrated reduced efficacy in chronically ill and immunosuppressed persons.[19,21] Further, antibody titers wane after 5 years, particularly in the very old, raising concerns that a one-time immunization may offer little benefit.[19,20,21]

However the risk and cost of giving the vaccine are small. The current vaccine formulation, licensed in the United States in 1983, contains polysaccharide components of 23 pneumococcal subtypes, responsible for almost 90% of bacteremic pneumococcal illness.[18] Currently, the ACIP recommends that all persons 65 years or older receive the pneumococcal vaccine, as well as persons at increased risk, as noted in Table 10.3,[5] a recommendation endorsed by many experts.[4,22,23] Given the uncertainties about efficacy, however, the use of this vaccination should be considered a matter of physician discretion and patient preference.

Hepatitis B

Hepatitis B has been recognized as an important cause of long-term mortality and morbidity. The recent development of safe vaccine preparations based on recombinant DNA technology has led to implementation of routine hepatitis B immunization in childhood.[1,2] Immunization is also encouraged in settings of increased risk. For adults, these settings include employment in health or public safety, exposure to blood products, intravenous drug use, and household or sexual contact with persons who are hepatitis B carriers. Over a generation immunity will develop at the population level, reducing the need for adult immunization.

Travel Immunizations

Persons traveling outside the United States may require additional immunizations for diseases that are still frequent in some countries, such as typhus and yellow fever. Other prophylaxis may also be needed; for example, malaria prophylaxis is required when traveling to endemic regions in Central America, Africa, and the Far East. Those contemplating travel to areas other than Canada or Western Europe should be advised to consult a travel clinic, if one is available, for the most up-to-date information on potential exposures and immunization recommendations. If there is no convenient facility providing this information, guidelines can be obtained from the Centers for Disease Control or the US Department of Health and Human Services.[5,24]

References

1. National Vaccine Advisory Committee (NVAC): Standards for pediatric immunization practices. *MMWR* 1993;42 (RR-5):1–13.
2. Immunization Practices Advisory Committee (ACIP): General recommendations on immunization. *MMWR* 1994;43(RR-1):1–38.
3. Williams WW, Hickson MA, Kane MA, Kendal AP, Spika JS, Hinman AR: Immunization policies and vaccine coverage among adults: The risk for missed opportunities. *Ann Intern Med* 1988;108:616–625.
4. Gardner P. Schaffner W: Immunization of adults. *N Engl J Med* 1993;328: 1252–1258.
5. Immunization Practices Advisory Committee (ACIP): Update on adult immunization. *MMWR* 1991;40(RR-12):1–94.
6. National immunization program, CDC: Reported vaccine-preventable diseases—United States, 1993. *MMWR* 1994;43:57–60.

7. Nkowane BM, Wassilak SGF, Orenstein WA, Bart KJ, Schonberger LB, Hinman AR, Kew OM: Vaccine-associated paralytic poliomyelitis—United States: 1973 through 1984. *JAMA* 1987;257:1335–1340.
8. Recommendations of the Immunization Practices Advisory Committee (ACIP): Poliomyelitis prevention: Enhanced-potency inactivated poliomyelitis vaccine—Supplementary statement. *MMWR* 1988;36:795–498.
9. Immunization Practices Advisory Committee (ACIP): Options for the control of influenza. *MMWR* 1994;43(RR-9):1–10.
10. Centers for Disease Control: Pneumonia and influenza mortality—United States, 1988–89 season. *MMWR* 1989;38:97.
11. Patriarca PA, Weber JA, Parker RA, Hall WN, Kendal AP, Bregman DJ, Schonberger LB: Efficacy of influenza vaccine in nursing homes: Reduction in illness and complications during an influenza A(H3N2) epidemic. *JAMA* 1985; 253:1136–1139.
12. Fedson DS, Wajda A, Nicol JP, Hammond GW, Kaiser DL, Roos LL: Clinical effectiveness of influenza vaccination in Manitoba. *JAMA* 1993;270:1956–1961.
13. Riddiough MA, Sisk JE, Bell JC: Influenza vaccination: Cost-effectiveness and public policy. *JAMA* 1983;249:3189–3195.
14. Hayden FG, Belshe RB, Clover RD, Hay AJ, Oakes MG, Soo W: Emergence and apparent transmission of rimantadine-resistant influenza A virus in families. *N Engl J Med* 1989;321:1696–1702.
15. Burman LA, Norrby R, Trollfors B: Invasive pneumococcal infections: Incidence, predisposing factors and prognosis. *Rev Infectious Dis* 1985;7:133–142.
16. Hook EW III, Horton CA, Schaberg DR: Failure of intensive care unit support to influence mortality from pneumococcal bacteremia. *JAMA* 1983;249:1055–1057.
17. LaForce FM, Eickhoff TC: Pneumococcal vaccine: The evidence mounts. *Ann Intern Med* 1986;104:110–112.
18. Recommendations of the Immunization Practices Advisory Committee: Pneumococcal polysaccharide vaccine. *MMWR* 1989;38:64–68, 73–76.
19. Hirschmann JV, Lipsky BA: The pneumococcal vaccine after 15 years of use. *Arch Intern Med* 1994;154:373–377.
20. Simberkoff MS, Cross AP, Al-Ibrahim M, Baltch AL, Geiseler PJ, Nadler J, Richmond AS, Smith RP, Schiffman G, Shepard DS, Van Eeckhout JP: Efficacy of pneumococcal vaccine in high risk patients. *New Engl J Med* 1986;315:1318–1327.
21. Shapiro ED, Berg AT, Austrian R, Schroeder D, Parcells V, Margolis A, Adair RK, Clemens JD: The protective efficacy of polyvalent pneumococcal polysaccharide vaccine. *N Engl J Med* 1991;325:1453–1460.
22. American College of Physicians Task Force of Adult Immunization, Infectious Diseases Society of America: *Guide for Adult Immunization*, ed 2. Philadelphia, American College of Physicians, 1990.
23. LaForce FM: Adult immunizations: Are they worth the trouble? *J Gen Intern Med* 1990;5(suppl);S57–S61.
24. Health Information for International Travel, published annually by Centers for Disease Control National Center for Prevention Services, Division of Quarantine, 1600 Clifton Road NE, Atlanta GA 30333.

Chapter 11

Breast Disease: Detection and Management

Roger E. Moe, MD

Breast cancer is the most frequent cancer incurred by women. One of every three new cancers in women in 1993 was breast cancer (183,000 cases). Consequently, there are no elderly women at low risk for breast cancer in the United States. Indeed, cumulative life time risk for breast cancer is now one out of eight women. Moreover, age-adjusted incidence rates for breast cancer have been increasing.[1,2] Data in the Surveillance, Epidemiology, and End Results (SEER) Program from the National Cancer Institute reveal a 30% increase in incidence from 1975–1979 to 1987–1991 among white females. On the other hand, mortality rates have remained relatively flat in previous reports—up to now. The latest information covering 1989 to 1992 shows an unprecedented fall of 4.7% for all women.[3] This probably reflects better breast cancer awareness, screening and adjuvant therapy. As one current example, 60 to 70% of women in relevant age groups have had recent mammograms in the most populous counties of the State of Washington. Although breast cancer is second only to lung cancer as a cause of deaths from cancer in women over age 50, earliest non-invasive breast cancer is almost 100% curable. So there are great incentives for prevention and earlier detection of breast cancer.

The goals of this chapter are to describe the general clinical context confronting a clinician who manages breast disease, to offer a relatively simple clinical philosophy for evaluating breast disease, to try to cut through confusing ambiguous concepts, and to describe applications as well as limitations of current technology, thus expediting diagnosis of breast cancer.

General Clinical Context

In women over the age of 50, cancer is high on the list of differential diagnoses. Over 70% of breast cancers occur in women over the age of 50. Very elderly women have the highest incidence of breast cancer, but the prevalence or number of cases encountered reflects the smaller number of living women. Benign diseases of younger women, such as fibroadenomas and infectious mastitis, are lower on the list. Fibroadenomas and gross cysts (fluid filled) usually do not develop after the menopause except in some patients who are receiving hormone replacement therapy.

There are other differences in the clinical challenge of evaluating breast disease in older women than in younger women. For example, older women are more apt than younger women to have had breast surgery in the past, which can be a confounding factor in interpreting physical findings and mammographic findings. Women with thickening near a biopsy site are commonly presumed

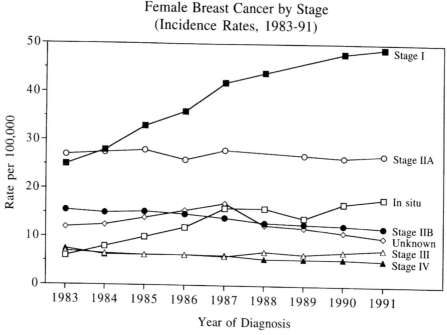

Figure 11.1 SEER Cancer Statistics Review, 1983–1991. Surveillance Program, Division of Cancer Prevention and Control, National Cancer Institute. Courtesy of Dr. David Thomas, Fred Hutchinson Cancer Research Center, Seattle.

to have post surgical scarring; but breast tissue is different from other tissues in the body in that healing in a biopsy area usually occurs with deposition of soft adipose tissue rather than with thick fibrous scar tissue, so it is easy to mistake the density of a cancer as representing a surgical scar.

Comorbidity is also a definite issue.[4] Because of comorbidity, surgical procedures often require modified planning. To reduce surgical morbidity, easy access to needle biopsies for diagnosis can be especially valuable. Again, travel logistics for the elderly warrant attention to avoid unnecessary trips. But in general, the outcome of treatment for breast cancer in elderly patients is as good as it is in younger patients.

How Do Risk Factors Alter Patient Management?

Screening Asymptomatic Patients

Most women who get breast cancer (about 85%) do not have significant risk factors for breast cancer, such as a positive family history. It is important to emphasize this to patients. Many older women who have had no breast problems, and who have a negative family history, think that they don't need mammograms. Age alone in this category of patients warrants monthly self-examinations, annual physical examinations, and annual mammograms. (For patients over the age of 65, Medicare pays for screening mammograms only at 2 year intervals.)

The goal of screening is to find a cancer in lead time before it is large enough to be clinically evident by symptoms or signs. Lead time before a cancer is symptomatic or palpable is longer in elderly women than in women younger than 50 years of age. Lead time in younger patients is about 2 years, and in older patients about 4 years. Accordingly, screening is more apt to be

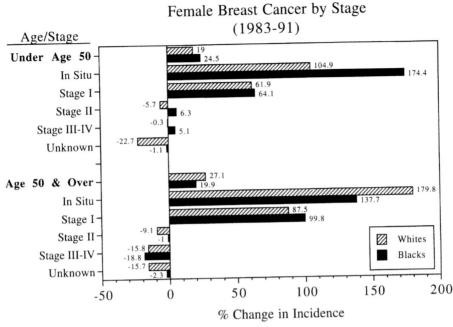

Figure 11.2 SEER Cancer Statistics Review, 1983-1991. Surveillance Program, Division of Cancer Prevention and Control, National Cancer Institute. Courtesy of Dr. David Thomas, Fred Hutchinson Cancer Research Center, Seattle.

productive where lead time is longer. There is general agreement that screening women aged 50 to 65 years reduces the breast cancer mortality rate by nearly 30%.[5] When patients are over 65 years old, evidence for a benefit from screening is less evident, partly because of mortality from comorbid diseases.[6]

Besides longer lead time, screening patients over the age of 50 by mammography is often highly effective in elderly women; internal fibroglandular tissue background density becomes less and less with aging. Most patients in the teens and early twenties have dense fibroglandular tissue. As young patients become older, there is a gradual slope or decrement in this mammographic density. While there is no abrupt fall-off in the density by a certain age, like age 50, which is an approximate age of menopause, normal breast tissue does become less dense with physiologic epithelial involution after the menopause. The proportion of low density adipose tissue to higher density fibroglandular tissue increases until the internal breast tissue is mostly adipose. Such adipose tissue makes a superb low density background against which even very small abnormal breast masses and tissue distortions are readily seen. On the other hand, postmenopausal breast tissue may remain dense in some patients, particularly those who take hormone replacement therapy.

Accordingly, this variation in tissue density underlines a concept of usefulness for surveillance (see figures 11-3 and 11-4). Are mammograms for a given patient useful for revealing a shadow, for example? Or for showing distorted lines of tissue? Or for showing microcalcifications? Or none of these? For individual cases where questions of reliability of surveillance or accurate diagnosis arise, it is very helpful for the clinician to view the mammograms with the radiologist. One doesn't get a good idea of the character of mammograms by only reading a report.

Mammographic equipment and expertise has improved substantially in recent years. For screening, no other technology has supplanted mammography. Ultrasonography is an excellent adjunct

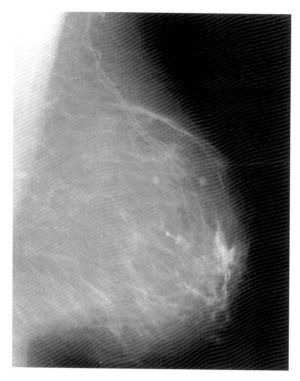

Figure 11.3 Mammogram with low density adipose background. Useful for surveillance.

Figure 11.4 Mammogram with dense fibroglandular background. Cancer can be missed.

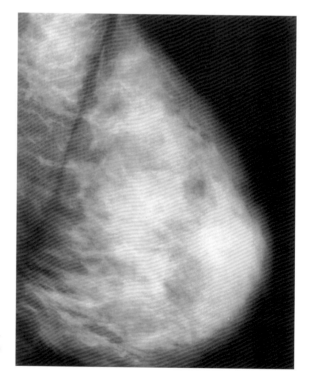

to mammography. MRI is still a research tool; some studies show promising results for detecting breast cancer, but this is expensive technology and is not being used for screening.[7] At this time, the cost of an MRI study of one breast is around $1200.

What Should Be Done With High Risk Patients?

Practical issues arise, such as defining high risk,[8] deciding how often such patients should be followed, and selecting patients who may be candidates for special studies. Which patients should be referred for genetic evaluation? Is prophylactic bilateral mastectomy indicated? Should hormone replacement therapy be withheld?

In general, detailed analyses of risk for breast cancer are carried out in high risk clinics—not in primary care settings.[9] Patients with major risk factors fall into two broad categories, such as family history and biopsy-proved histopathology. From a practical standpoint, family histories are not so easily assessed at this time because family size tends to be smaller than in the past. Women tend to marry later, have fewer children, and have few siblings or none at all. If there only one or two females in a given generation, expression of hereditary breast cancer in that generation might not be evident. To be seen in a high risk clinic, a patient would usually have three relatives with breast cancer, with two or more first degree relatives like a mother and sister with breast cancer, especially premenopausal relatives, particularly if one of the premenopausal relatives like a sister has bilateral breast cancer. Alternatively, an appropriate patient would have three generations of relatives with vertical transmission of breast cancer susceptibility, like a grandmother, mother and sister. Ovarian cancer in the family should be a red flag; breast/ovarian combinations make a hereditary background more likely for breast cancer. If autosomal dominance of breast cancer and autosomal dominance of ovarian cancer exist in the same pedigree, there is potentially a 90% risk that the BRCA-1 gene is carried, with a risk of about 85% for these cancers. It is important to note, that breast cancer susceptibility can be transferred down through the paternal side, even though the father himself does not have breast cancer.

Histopathology, which carries increased risk for future breast cancer, pertains to epithelial proliferative disease.[10] Florid ductal epithelial hyperplasia or severe ductal epithelial atypia are features to look for in pathology reports from biopsies. Severe ductal epithelial atypia usual means that some, but not all, the diagnostic features of non-invasive ductal carcinoma exist. Lobular carcinoma in situ in a biopsy is another feature commonly regarded as a marker for high risk to both breasts. Descriptive terms like "fibrocystic disease" are worthless since there is no precise definition. It should also be noted that fibrosis is common to most breast diseases and is not the tissue at risk for breast cancer—epithelium is the tissue at risk.

The NSABP Breast Cancer Chemoprevention Trial takes in a broader set of risk factors than just family history. Features like the present age of the patient, age of the patient at menarche and at first full term pregnancy, and number of past breast biopsies are taken into account. For example, any patient age 60 or over qualifies on that basis alone, for the study defines high risk as comparable to that of a 60 year-old patient. Candidates for that study are: older ages; family history of breast cancer; early menarche; nulliparity; first full term pregnancy at age past 30; history of benign breast biopsies; lobular carcinoma in situ or ductal carcinoma in situ. Patients are randomized to receive tamoxifen or a placebo. Data on outcomes are not yet available.

Use of prophylactic bilateral mastectomy to prevent breast cancer is a complex issue indeed. Ideally, a multidisciplinary team in a high risk clinic would provide such a consultation. The reasons for this operation should specifically be sorted out for each patient. Cancerophobia with an inaccurate exaggerated idea of the degree of risk is not uncommon. Risk from actual tissue histopathology has also often been vaguely understood. For example, if a patient has had a biopsy showing florid ductal atypia, and the risk for breast cancer is said to be increased by any number—say three times, the question is three times what? Certainly not three times the cumulative lifetime risk of the population. Risk given as a factor like 3X is relative risk compared to a group or cohort which should have been defined; instead, the clinician needs some idea of the actual magnitude of risk. If histopathology is a major factor, then pathology review by a reference pathologist in breast cancer is recommended, because judgment and experience are very important in a pathology decision that may influence prophylactic bilateral mastectomy. At times, features like very dense mammograms or persistent physiologic breast pain or labels like "severe fibrocystic disease" have led to bilateral mastectomy, with no documentation histologically of whether or not any tissue pathology with increased risk existed at all; in these settings, there may in fact be sparse non-proliferative epithelium in a background of fibrosis, lacking the tissue features of increased risk. Moreover, prevention of breast cancer by use of prophylactic bilateral mastectomy is not proved. Presence of familial breast cancer means that genetic susceptibility resides in all the breast cells, some of which may remain after surgery in bits of tissue attached to the skin flaps or attached to subcutaneous tissue.

Hormone replacement therapy is dealt with elsewhere in this book. In general, morbidity of osteoporosis, vaginal dryness, hot flashes, and cardiovascular disease appears to outweigh risk of breast cancer in patients without high risk factors for breast cancer. However, a potential relation of estrogen to breast cancer is not to be casually disregarded. Estrogens are mitogens for human breast cancer, as well as stimulants for biologic growth factor protein production.[11] Likewise, Lupu and Lippman[12] have shown with in vitro studies of human breast cancer cell lines that the erbB2 oncogene signaling pathway can be modulated by estrogen through the estrogen receptor with relevance to emergence, maintenance and control of malignancy. For patients who have been treated for breast cancer, a decision for hormone replacement therapy is a matter of caution. A decision for a patient with a very high probability of cure is a different issue compared to a decision for the patient with multiple positive lymph nodes and high risk of recurrence. For patients who had invasive breast cancer which is estrogen receptor positive with negative lymph nodes, adjuvant therapy with tamoxifen was shown in the NSABP B-14 trial to significantly increase disease free and overall survival. Since estrogen blockade is found to be beneficial,[13] then in patients such as these it seems that estrogen supplementation might incur a potential hazard. At a minimum, the patient's record should show that the patient has been told of the risks and benefits in making such a decision.[14,15]

Clinical Evaluation

Clinical Philosophy

When a patient presents for evaluation in the office, the first goal is direct and simple—discovery of abnormal breast tissue.[16] Once the clinical impression of abnormal breast tissue is reached, the next goal is to diagnose the tissue—to evaluate the tissue in which carcinomas arise, the epithelium. For this, limitations of technology help to define a plan. For example, the epithelium is *not* seen in mammograms or ultrasound images. The epithelium is directly seen only in the microscope. And the epithelium certainly can't be defined by palpation. To "follow" the abnormal tissue does not define it. So a microscopic evaluation is the gold standard. Accordingly, careful records with diagrams and measurements of any abnormalities are set forth with a working diagnosis and time frame for resolution of each problem. Definitive resolution warrants a biopsy unless the problem is gone. These goals and concepts are the clinical philosophy.

How Do Breast Problems Come to Light?

These are the common clinical challenges:

- Mammographic changes
  - New or enlarging shadow or asymmetric density
  - Microcalcifications in a cluster or increasing number
  - Distortion of linear structures (trabeculae)
- Ultrasonic hypoechoic sites
- Local breast thickening or visible change found by the patient
- Breast thickening or visible change found by the doctor
- Symptoms of breast pain and tenderness
- Spontaneous nipple discharge

Initial Diagnostic Steps

History

A symptom of a new lump or thickening or visible change in the breast is a straightforward problem requiring a full diagnostic sequence. A complete history is necessary to assess reproductive physiology, risk factors, family history, abortions, past medication with oral contraceptives, present or recent medication with estrogens and progestins, and past breast problems. That new symptom must be featured and interpreted. Certainly, the time course of the symptom is important, but the fact that the patient's symptom has been noticed for months, or even years, does not rule out a cancer.

Prominent pain and tenderness, even if only in one breast, are most often related to estrogen physiology. A cyclic character with luteal phase correlation can be established in premenopausal women. In postmenopausal women, the first thing one looks for is estrogen intake. In such a patient on estrogen therapy, one doesn't expect the pain and tenderness to remit unless the estrogen dose can be reduced. The mechanism of this pain and tenderness has never been demonstrated; in biopsy tissue, one does not see inflammation or other features which are associated with pain. Indeed, one may see fibrosis and little beyond that. Sometimes ancillary measures like stopping caffeine intake, or trying Vitamin E 400 units per day can mitigate these symptoms. Such pain and tenderness are not characteristic of breast cancer, but 17% of breast cancers present with pain. On rare occasions, pain with breast cancer can be acute, like a low grade infection, but this is exceptional. Inflammatory cancer itself may look a lot worse than it feels to the patient, with low grade pain. The kinds of breast pain or discomfort which are unusual, and which represent a red flag for cancer in some instances, are an internal sensation of pulling or tightening discomfort; internal focal burning; or itching internally or right on the end of the nipple. Itching on the end of the nipple is a sign of Paget's carcinoma, and by itself can warrant a nipple biopsy. Itching on the areola and not on the nipple is rather a sign of eczema, not Paget's carcinoma.

When a patient complains of nipple discharge, the first question to ask is whether or not this is a manually expressed discharge or a spontaneous discharge. A manually expressed discharge is not clinically significant, since it is possible to express fluid from milk ducts in a high proportion of normal women. Mild ducts are hollow tubular structures containing fluid; they aren't dry. So it's no surprise that fluid should be expressible without this being a sign of cancer. The second question to ask is whether or not the discharge comes from one tiny spot on the end of the nipple or from several spots on one or both nipples. If there are multiple sites of discharge, this is more likely not to be a surgical lesion unless one tiny place is a source of bloody discharge. The third question to ask is whether or not the discharge is, or has been, bloody. The fourth question to ask is what medications the patient is taking, because various medicines pertain to nipple discharge, which can be looked up in the PDR. Galatorrhea is a term often applied incorrectly to nipple discharge in a generic fashion. Galactorrhea refers to spontaneous milky discharge from multiple ducts resulting from stimulation by hyperprolactinemia originating from the pituitary gland, and this, of course, warrants a directed endocrine work-up.

Physical Examination

The first part of the physical examination is visual inspection with the patient sitting. When a new patient is evaluated in our Breast Surgery Clinic, she usually automatically lies back into the supine posture at the outset, indicating that she isn't used to be examined in the upright sitting posture. It is true that most breast problems are not reflected in visible breast surface changes, but some are. One looks for indentation of the skin from traction caused by a cancer pulling the skin inward; this indentation can sometimes be accentuated by having the patient contract the pectoral muscles with a maneuver like pressing the hand upon the hips, or raising the arms up over the head and pressing and holding the hands together. The opposite of skin traction is protuberance of the skin; this is a late sign of locally advanced cancer. Another skin change to watch for is surface ulceration. If a surface ulceration or skin edema is caused by breast cancer, this is a sign of locally advanced Stage IIIB (T4) disease.

There are also other skin signs which immediately make one think of cancer. One of these is circumferential 360° skin erythema or a violet color all around the dependent 1/3 of the breast. Sometimes this is a florid red; sometimes it is pale violet. These colors indicate dermal edema, and the main thing to consider is dermal lymphangitic metastatic breast cancer. Skin erythema all the way around the areola is not a sign of infection. On the other hand, erythema from infection only occupies a sector around the areola—not 360°. The reason infectious mastitis present only a sector of erythema based upon the edge of the areola is as follows: infection is typically from oral bacteria which find their way from the mouth into a milk duct through the nipple. Each of the 12 to 16 milk ducts inside the nipple branch out like a tree extending into the breast. But the branches of one central duct do not interconnect inside the breast with the branches of another central duct. So infection does not jump inside the breast from one branching system to another. Inversely, invasive breast cancer cells get outside the ducts and can spread widely through lymphatics and get into skin (dermal) lymphatics; how the actual erythema color arises is not known.

Unlike erythema of the skin around the areola, occasionally one can see erythema of the end of a nipple; this does not refer to erythema of the areola—it refers to erythema of the actual end of the nipple, usually with a thinned out shiny red dermis, somewhat like a second degree burn. All by itself, this is an indication of Paget's carcinoma of the nipple. If the areola is also red (and dry and scaly), it is important to distinguish that the process started on the end of the nipple, that it did not start on the areola as eczema would have. Another nipple feature to watch for is deviation of the nipple away from the natural axis (deviation), or pulling of the nipple inward (retraction). The nipple deviates or is pulled in the direction of the pathology, which is benign or malignant fibrosis. Retraction of the nipple makes a circular declivity; sometimes there is just a circular groove at the base of the nipple, and this is pathologic. Normal inversion of the nipple is a transverse cleft or fish-mouth—not a circular process.

The next part of the physical examination is palpation. With the patient still upright, the lymph nodes in the axillae and supraclavicular areas are palpated. Each nipple is also palpated (not the areola). The nipple should flatten out to 3 or 4 mm; but one is palpating for a thickening like a bee-bee or a piece of thick string (twine), which can indicate a ductal lesion; one is not trying to elicit manual nipple discharge, as already mentioned. Keep in mind that milk ducts, which cause carcinomas, go up the center of the breast to the end of the nipple—not to the areola. Milk ducts do not open onto the areola; glands of Montgomery, not milk ducts, are seen on the areola.

Next, the patient assumes a supine posture, with her arm brought up over her head and resting on a pillow. This flattens the breast out to facilitate more effective palpation. (Upright bimanual palpation is less effective.) The key point is that normal breasts have normal lumps—hundreds of normal lumps. Under the skin is a carpet of normal adipose lumps; these are present in all patients—thin adipose lumps in thin patients, large adipose lumps in corpulent patients. But remember that adipose lumps are not the tissue that causes breast cancer; lumps, yes; cancer, no. Directly beneath the layer of adipose lumps is dense fibroglandular tissue. The surface of this tissue under the adipose layer is not flat and smooth. It has ridges resembling the waves on a lake. These ridges are structural features where the fibroglandular tissue extends connections to the inner surface of the dermis; the fibroglandular tissue doesn't just lie disconnected freely inside the breast—it connects to the skin anteriorly and to the prepectoral fascia posteriorly. The adipose lumps and the fibroglandular ridges are what clinicians typically call "fibrocystic disease", as if these were abnormal or didn't belong in a normal breast. These fibroglandular ridges are camouflaged by adipose lumps in the obese patient; and the fibroglandular ridges are no longer discernible when the fibroglandular tissue involutes with aging and becomes replaced with adipose tissue physiologically. So, the idea is to pick out an abnormal lump from among the numerous normal lumps described above. Palpation with the finger tips yields detailed localized features, augmented by palpation with the broad entire palmar surfaces of the fingers to assess surface uniformity in each quadrant of the breast. There are no set shapes or consistencies of malignancy. In any event, one cannot define epithelium *per se* with palpation; microscopy is required. For that matter, a cancer may be non-palpable; or it may be like a marble, seemingly benign; it may be hard with vague borders; or it may be flat, just a diffuse increase in A-P volume. A flat cancer is easily missed; this can be the case with an infiltrating lobular carcinoma or a poorly differentiated diffusely infiltrating ductal carcinoma. Sometimes bilateral simultaneous mirror image palpation of the breasts tips off the clinician to the asymmetric thickening of a flat cancer in one breast. Anyway, the clinician is not trying to sort things out into "suspicious", or "worrisome", or "not worrisome", or "nothing". The goal is to sort out what is abnormal and go from there.

Acute mastitis from infection is less common in patients 50 years of age and older than it is in young patients. When it does occur, there is not only the erythema described earlier, but palpable induration going under the areola to the central nipple axis from the site of erythema. Typically, this will be so tender that the patient has difficulty tolerating palpation. When there is an abscess, it usually begins in the central nipple axis and works its way up toward the edge of the areola, the pathway of least resistance toward the skin. When there is a patch of erythema some distance away from the areola, separated by white skin, this is not likely to be infectious mastitis. Sometimes one will encounter a chemical mastitis, a periductal inflammatory process relating to benign ductal ectasia in older patients. The inflammatory process is presumably set up by luminal contents which have gotten into the surrounding stroma. This is self-limited and it is not cancer; but it can present just like cancer, and cancer certainly is in the differential, warranting a biopsy.

Imaging

Mammography is essential both for screening and for breast evaluation when breast symptoms or signs are found. There is no other established technology which is as effective as mammography for detecting the earliest evidence of breast cancer. Indeed, microcalcifications are the earliest evidence of breast cancer while the cancer is till non-invasive, preceding formation of a mass. Such microcalcifications are not easily seen with ultrasound, but they are nicely seen in special magnification mammograms (see figures 11.5 and 11.6).

Diagnostic use of mammograms is not merely to find out if a cancer may exist. Mammograms help to define other lesions in the same breast, as well as possible lesions in the opposite breast.

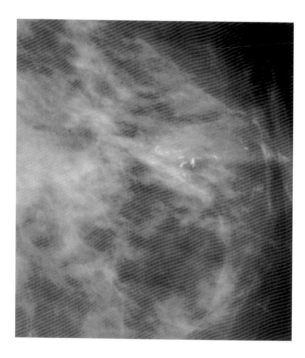

Figure 11.5 Mammogram with malignant microcalcifications.

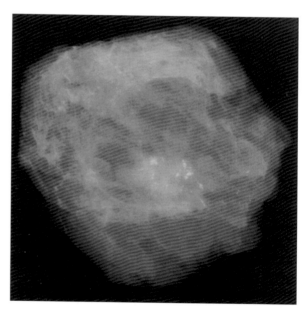

Figure 11.6 Xray of surgical specimen removed with those calcifications in Fig. 11.5.

Moreover, if there is a cancer, mammograms help to define the extent of the changes; particular attention is given to potential spread of a cancer toward the nipple.

Curiously, we still see instances where a palpable abnormality does not show up in a mammogram, so a clinician tells a patient, "It's nothing," or "There's nothing to worry about," and a biopsy isn't done. This is a real trap—an expensive trap, from the medico-legal standpoint. In the first place, if an abnormal lump is palpated, it's there regardless of what the mammograms show. In the second place, it has already been pointed out that mammograms do not specifically define the epithelium, the key cancer tissue. So it's logical that some cancers (10 to 15%) are missed in mammogram readings. In the third place, from mammograms the statement cannot be made that "There is no cancer," or "You do not have cancer." The statement can be made that "No evidence of cancer is seen," certainly not a guarantee. At the same time, most of the missed cancers don't need to be missed. This is where ultrasound imaging comes in.

Ultrasonography is valuable in selected cases, both for detecting a breast cancer and showing the extent of it. While mammography does not sort out details of dense fibroglandular tissue so well, this is the kind of tissue where ultrasound works more effectively. While mammography works beautifully in low density adipose tissue, ultrasound does not work as effectively in this type of tissue. Current 10 megaHerz ultrasound equipment in talented hands can pick up 3 to 4 mm cancers in dense tissue, in some instances. Mammograms often have patches which are asymmetrically more dense than the same areas in the contralateral breast; some of these patches can be thinned out for better detail with localized compression of the tissue in the mammographic machine. On the other hand, ultrasound shows tissue movement and changes in shape during the examination itself, which can tip off the examiner to a firm or stiff or disrupted area; color Doppler blood flow features can sometimes suggest a cancer, too. So ultrasonography will reduce the number of missed cancers. It is well known that ultrasound is commonly used to document fluid-filled cysts, as opposed to solid lumps; so even in this setting of fluid-filled cysts, ultrasound can sort out solid lumps for diagnosis among the fluid-filled lumps (see figures 11-7 to 11.10).

In a study of 79 mammographically detected small breast cancers, visibility on ultrasound was studied retrospectively.[17] Only 1 of 26 cancers detected only by mammographic microcalcifications were demonstrated by ultrasound. However, 47 of 53 cancers (88.7%) detected by other mammographic characteristics were demonstrated with free-hand ultrasound; most of these were not palpable.

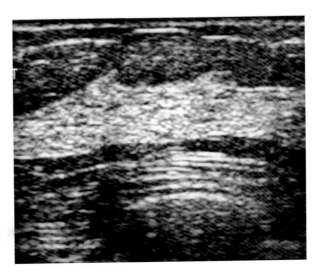

Figure 11.7 Ultrasound image of normal breast tissue—skin at Top, chest wall at bottom. White fibroglandular tissue across middle.

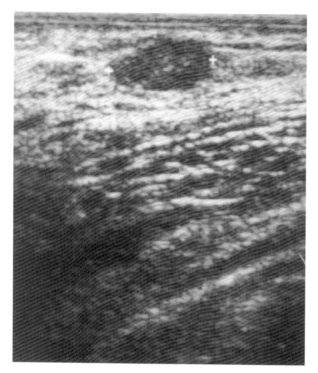

Figure 11.8 Ultrasound image with dark hypoechoic benign lesion at top.

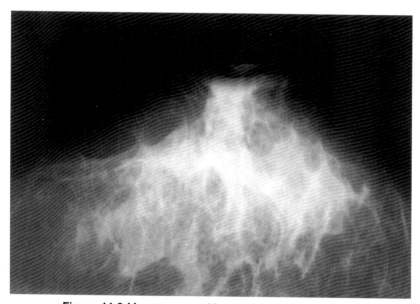

Figure 11.9 Mammogram with cancer which is not seen.

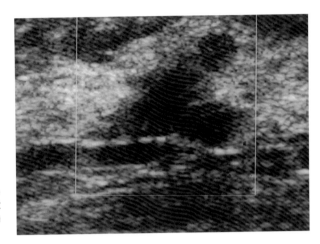

Figure 11.10 Ultrasound image showing dark hypoechoic irregular malignant lesion through middle of photo. Not seen in mammogram.

The clinician should have a low threshold for early use of fine needle aspiration for cytology, or referral for core needle biopsy, which provides histopathology, or open biopsy. Presence or absence of a family history of breast cancer does not change the plan when abnormal tissue is found; a diagnosis is needed. In elderly women, there is no place for labeling an abnormal finding with obfuscating terminology like "fibrocystic disease", or labeling an abnormal lump as a "cyst" and doing nothing. Cysts don't form in elderly women, except for some of those who are receiving estrogens. To the contrary, cysts are one kind of pathology in lobules; lobules normally undergo gradual involution after menopause.

For a patient with a history of spontaneous nipple discharge from one site on the end of the nipple, bloody or not, a ductogram should be done in addition to a cytologic smear of the fluid. This is in addition to other imaging with mammography and ultrasound for a breast mass. High quality ductograms are achieved now, with definition of 2nd and 3rd order ducts. A focal filling defect or intraluminal irregularity indicates the need for a surgical ductectomy (see figures 11.11 and 11.12).

Tailored Breast Imaging

Typically, what happens in breast imaging is that a patient comes in for mammograms, and perhaps a lesion is seen. The referring doctor receives a report; perhaps ultrasound is recommended to the referring physician prompting the patient to come back again for the study. A needle aspiration or biopsy may be recommended, so even a third trip for the patient can ensue once the referring doctor is contacted. The patient may lose a considerable amount of time away from a job and traveling back and forth. In tailored breast imaging, the mammographer makes the decisions as to adding an ultrasound evaluation and a needle aspiration or needle biopsy in one visit by the patient, communicating appropriately with the patient's doctor. Actually, when this sequence is done, including a core needle biopsy and frozen section, a definitive diagnosis can be had in two or three hours. This is efficient management. Moreover, the number of unnecessary surgical biopsies can be reduced, so that positive open biopsies occur about 60 to 65% of the time. If an abnormal focus of tissue is not subjected to microscopic evaluation, a working diagnosis and a plan are needed with specific reevaluation within a time frame, including careful diagrams and actual measurements for any changes.

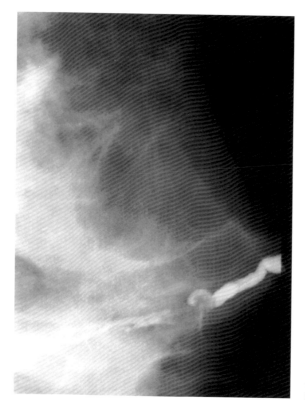

Figure 11.11 Ductogram showing contrast injected through the nipple into a duct with a filling defect.

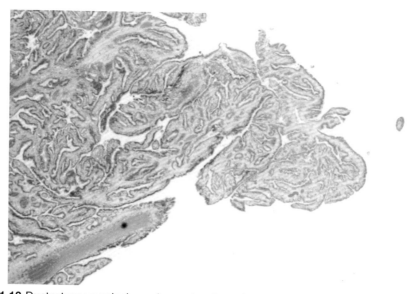

Figure 11.12 Ductectomy surgical specimen showing a benign papilloma removed from the duct.

Biopsies

The gold standard for tissue diagnosis is the microscope. Needle biopsies are being done more frequently, with fewer open surgical biopsies in the current climate of health care reform. For palpable lumps, fine needle aspiration cytology can be easily done in the office when the patient is first seen, particularly if the clinician plans to follow a lump and schedule a reexamination. Fine needle aspiration cytology is not used as often as it could be to expedite early diagnosis of a cancer in patients over 50 years of age. When trained cytologists are available, a cytology report positive for cancer is rarely false; a negative cytology report does not rule out a cancer, however, due to sampling error or technique. In the event of a negative cytology report with an adequate sample of duct epithelial cells read as benign, this is considered in conjunction with mammographic findings and findings on physical examination. Such a triple approach in a clinic with experienced clinicians has been reported.[18] The study group included 234 patients with a breast mass which was evaluated with a physical examination, mammography, and fine needle aspiration cytology. All patients then underwent open surgical biopsy. For the total combined triple tests, the sensitivity was 100% and the specificity was 57%. All patients who had breast cancer had positive findings on at least one of the three tests. Patients who had negative findings on all three of the triple tests had benign lesions, with a negative predictive value of 100%. The authors concluded that such patients with negative findings could be observed.

Stereotactic Needle Biopsy

Breast lesions which are found on mammography and are not palpable can be accessed by x-ray guided needles. This has been done routinely in the past to insert wires into the breast to guide a surgeon to the lesion during open biopsy. More recently, dedicated stereotactic mammography tables have been employed to accurately guide either fine needles for aspiration cytology or 14 guage core cutting needles for paraffin sections. Fine needle cytology can reveal malignant cells, but does not define the presence or absence of invasion. Core needle biopsies show tissue architecture in paraffin sections and can define invasive cancer or non-invasive cancer (see figures 11.13 and 11.14). Typically, 5 or more cores are removed. With an unambiguous diagnosis of invasive cancer, a multidisciplinary team can discuss a treatment plan and options with a patient. Even so, this stereotactic technology has not replaced open surgical biopsy. The indications and limitations of stereotactic needle biopsy as compared to open surgical biopsy are still being sorted out,[19,20] and ultrasound-guided needle biopsies are now part of the picture as well. Stereotactic needle biopsies are probably not needed for radiologically benign lesions which can be followed serially. Stereotactic needle biopsies appear to be useful for lesions with a low probability of malignancy to reduce the number of unnecessary open biopsies. But the role of stereotactic needle biopsy is less clear in highly suspicious mammographic lesions. A diagnosis of non-invasive carcinoma from a core needle biopsy still can leave the possibility of unsampled invasive breast cancer which is contiguous, so that the issue of lymph node dissection is not settled. Again, if breast preservation is to be done, open local surgical resection of the whole cancer with clear surgical margins is still necessary and is not avoided by the stereotactic procedure. On the other hand, if the stereotactic core biopsy is positive for invasive cancer and mastectomy is elected, this can be undertaken directly with axillary lymph node dissection, after appropriate staging; and time is saved in the operating room by not needing a frozen section.

Ultrasound Guided Needle Biopsies

Fine needle aspiration cytologies with ultrasound guidance have been reported from a series of 651 nonpalpable lesions in 586 patients at the University of Texas M.D.Anderson Cancer Center.[21]

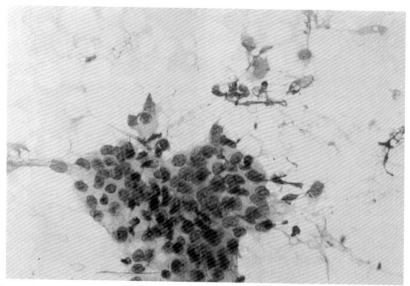

Figure 11.13 Fine needle aspiration breast cytology with a clump of pleomorphic malignant cells. Contiguous single cells show loss of normal cohesiveness.

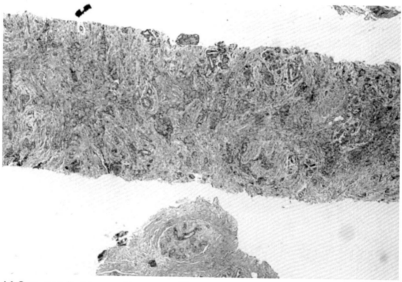

Figure 11.14 Core needle biopsy at low magnification. Malignant cells are seen with structural tissue pattern of invasive cancer.

The sensitivity of ultrasound-guided FNA for diagnosis of malignant lesions was 91%, specificity 77%, and overall accuracy 84%. There was one false positive diagnosis which actually was atypical ductal hyperplasia. Another study was reported from Italy[22] using ultrasound-guided fine needle aspiration cytology for 79 patients with breast lesions less than 1 cm in diameter and non-palpable. The sensitivity was 93% but there were some technical problems with the equipment which led to a specificity of 80%. Ultrasound-guided automated core needle biopsies have also been evaluated[23] but these data pertain to a small number of patients. Ultrasonographically suspicious breast lesions in 181 patients were sampled with a an automated biopsy gun with 14 guage needles guided by a hand-held ultrasound transducer. Only 49 of those lesions were surgically removed; the agreement between the core biopsy and open biopsy was 100%. The remaining 132 cases were followed for 12-36 months with no cancers having emerged. This study is not definitive. But hand-held ultrasound transducer guided FNA or core needle biopsies are relatively easy to do, expeditious, require 20-30 minutes of time, and can produce a diagnosis in two hours. As radiologists become well trained and experienced with this, more widespread use is anticipated with equipment now on the market.

Treatment Counseling

Staging

When a diagnosis of breast cancer is made, staging tests are done to provide precision to treatment planning. For clinical Stage I cancers, up to 2 cm. in diameter with clinically negative lymph nodes, tests include a chest x-ray and liver function blood tests. If a patient has arthritic or skeletal symptoms, a bone scan is done as a baseline; but a positive bone scan is found in only 2 or 3% of asymptomatic patients with cancers under 2 cm. For clinical Stage II patients with positive lymph nodes, tests include a CT of the chest and liver, as well as a bone scan. Similar tests are done for patients with clinical Stage III patients with cancers over 5 cm., skin involvement or inflammatory cancer, and also for recurrent cancer. Pathologic staging follows clinical staging. Pathologic staging is the final description of the clinical presentation, requiring information from complete pathologic evaluation based upon definitive surgery of the cancer and regional lymph nodes. Assessment of the biologic parameters of every cancer is an essential part of the planning process, although there is substantial controversy on just which tests of malignant tissue should be done. All cancers should at least be tested for estrogen receptor proteins and progesterone receptor proteins because the results are prognostic indicators, as well as indicators of potential therapeutic value. Such therapeutic value obviously applies to hormone manipulation; but a choice of chemotherapy agents is also influenced. For example, when ER and PR are both negative, some patients are offered adjuvant therapy with an adriamycin-containing combination. From a practical standpoint, the biologic tests chosen for a cancer reflect the viewpoints of the medical oncologists in a given locality.

Selection of Local Treatment of the Breast

Primary care givers are likely to be asked by the patient for advice and counsel in this area, and subsequently to participate in ongoing care. There are some general guidelines to keep in mind.[24] The overriding treatment plan is ordinarily a plan for cure of the breast cancer. The patient needs to hear that. Also, the treatment plan is aimed for the patient to maintain an active, flourishing, contributing life. She needs to hear that, too. While there is no guarantee for cure, many patients have a high probability of cure. There are many non-cancer diseases like diabetes, rheumatoid arthritis, regional ileitis, coronary artery disease, etc., which are not curable. But breast cancer is a curable disease.

Another guideline is that for invasive breast cancer Stage I and II up to 5 cm., randomized prospective controlled clinical trials with up to ten years and more of follow-up have not shown a survival advantage for mastectomy over breast preservation plus irradiation.[25] Axillary lymph node dissection and relevant adjuvant therapy are used both with breast preservation or mastectomy. Breast preservation is not indicated for multicentric cancer in different parts of the same breast, or for a breast where complete removal of the cancer would grossly deform the breast. Breast preservation also can be done for cancers in the central axis of the breast deep to the nipple, or after removal of the nipple-areolar complex in Paget's disease, provided that the cancer is completely removed with clear margins. There are various reasons why a patient might not choose breast preservation therapy, such as logistics relating to breast irradiation. But, just doing a bigger operation does not yield better survival, provided that standard treatment concepts are followed. Breast surgery in these instances no longer involves removal of pectoral muscles. The patient's muscle power and arm mobility should be normal with either treatment plan. For well informed decision making, each patient should see a multidisciplinary team which includes a radiation oncologist, surgeon, and medical oncologist.

Paradoxically, the most controversy about local treatment of the breast for cancer pertains to non-invasive cancer instead of invasive cancer.[26] The mortality rate of non-invasive breast cancer is very low (see figure 11.15). But unlike data from large well controlled prospective trials of treating invasive breast cancer in Italy, the United States and other countries, data from treatment of non-invasive breast cancer is not conclusive. There aren't nearly as many cases of pure non-invasive breast cancer; the biology is more indolent; and randomized prospective information outside of the NSABP is hard to find. The point is that non-invasive ductal carcinoma is nearly 100% curable by mastectomy alone. This is the gold standard. But why should mastectomy be done for non-invasive breast cancer if it isn't necessary for invasive breast cancer?

For lobular carcinoma in situ, many clinicians do not regard this as a cancer, but rather as a high risk marker for future breast cancer. Regardless, the Cancer Surveillance System of the National Cancer Institute still collects data using this diagnosis which is obtained from pathology reports. For this pathology by itself, neither further breast surgery or breast irradiation are being done. Risk for future breast cancer is regarded as bilateral, approximately 1% per year, often emerging in 15-20 years. So these patients are managed with regular surveillance by annual mammograms and physical examinations and monthly self-examinations. If the breast tissue is dense in mammograms, bilateral ultrasound should be considered as an adjunct. These patients are candidates for the NSABP Chemoprevention Trial.

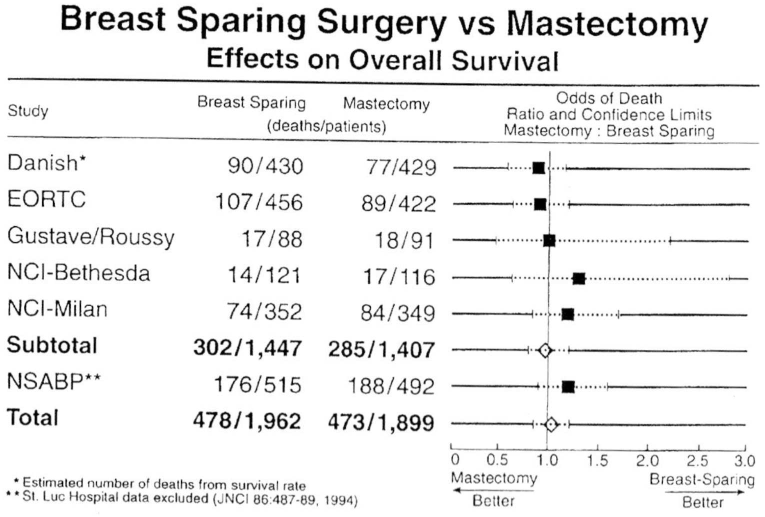

Breast Sparing Surgery vs Mastectomy
Effects on Overall Survival

Study	Breast Sparing	Mastectomy	Odds of Death Ratio and Confidence Limits Mastectomy : Breast Sparing
	(deaths/patients)		
Danish*	90/430	77/429	
EORTC	107/456	89/422	
Gustave/Roussy	17/88	18/91	
NCI-Bethesda	14/121	17/116	
NCI-Milan	74/352	84/349	
Subtotal	302/1,447	285/1,407	
NSABP**	176/515	188/492	
Total	478/1,962	473/1,899	

```
        0   0.5   1.0   1.5   2.0   2.5   3.0
        Mastectomy            Breast-Sparing
          Better                  Better
```

* Estimated number of deaths from survival rate
** St. Luc Hospital data excluded (JNCI 86:487-89, 1994)

Figure 11.15 Graphic comparison of odds ratios of dying from breast cancer treated with breast preservation and irradiation versus mastectomy. Courtesy of *The Journal of The National Cancer Institute*.

Ductal carcinoma in situ is much more common, but it represents heterogeneous pathology and heterogeneous biology. Lagios, at San Francisco, uses selected criteria for observation only.[27] Some of his criteria are cancers which were found because of microcalcifications in mammograms, with all the calcifications removed in follow-up mammograms; disease involving an area of 5 cm. or less; mammograms suitable for surveillance; and all the cancer removed. For ductal carcinoma in situ without using Lagios' criteria, breast preservation with irradiation has been evaluated in NSABP Protocol B-17. Adding irradiation to preservation of the breast for ductal carcinoma in situ was shown to reduce the number of second ipsilateral breast cancers, and to reduce the number of second ipsilateral breast cancers which were invasive.[28] So irradiation was beneficial, reducing the annual number of second ipsilateral breast cancers by 67%. The main patholgy features which predict for recurrence are central necrosis in the cancerous ducts and whether or not the surgical margins of the resected tumor were free of cancer.[29] But more particularly, if mastectomy had been done for those cases with central necrosis or positive margins, this would have been done unnecessarily in 90% of these cases, according to this information. As far as survival is concerned, long term data are sparse. Solin and others report data from a number of institutions using breast preservation and primary irradiation, with a 96% survival at 10 years.[30] This was not a randomized prospective study. Conversely, when a mastectomy is done for ductal carcinoma in situ, immediate reconstruction can be done with excellent cosmetic results. Skin-sparing mastectomy is being done at some centers for added cosmesis (see figures 11.16 to 11.18).

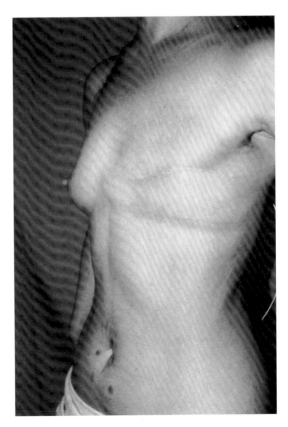

Figure 11.16 Modified radical mastectomy patient prior to reconstructive plastic surgery. Courtesy of Dr. Richard Rand, Chief of Plastic Surgery, University Hospital Medical Center, Seattle.

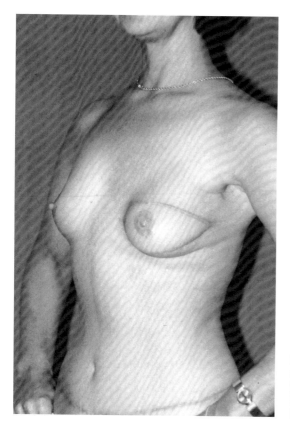

Figure 11.17 Same patient in Fig. 11.16 after reconstructive plastic surgery with a TRAM flap. Courtesy of Dr. Richard Rand, Chief of Plastic Surgery, University Hospital Medical Center, Seattle.

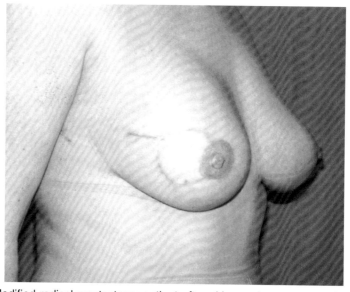

Figure 11.18 Modified radical mastectomy patient after skin-sparing reconstructive plastic surgery with a TRAM flap. Courtesy of Dr. Richard Rand, Chief of Plastic Surgery, University Hospital Medical Center, Seattle.

Special Considerations for the Elderly

Physical limitations and comorbidity need to be taken into account. Mastectomy and axillary dissection are not hazardous procedures. This writer has not had an operative death or has even heard of one in this area. Some of these patients can have a mastectomy under local anesthesia, if necessary, or under a segmental cervical epidural, or be operated in the semi-upright position. Intercostal nerve blocks or wound injection with long acting local anesthetics can aid patient comfort, too. Again, medications often have to be used in lower doses, like narcotics. Mental instability needs to be taken into account as well, but we haven't seen psychotic breaks yet in the several patients we have operated on with mild dementia.

Not all elderly patients with invasive breast cancer require an axillary dissection for staging. If the patient has an estrogen positive cancer, and the patient would be treated with tamoxifen for positive lymph nodes anyway, there are situations where an axillary dissection would add unnecessary morbidity, such as for an infirm patient who is living alone. She could have the breast surgery and then be treated with tamoxifen anyway.

There is no intrinsic reason from age alone why immediate reconstruction can't be done, although there may be selected reasons for not doing this in the individual case. At the same time, physiologic hazards are another issue. Some of these patients have long pendulous breasts, and perhaps with other diseases like diabetes, or a smoking habit; the long skin flaps made in these breasts at surgery can have blood flow compromised by vigorous traction on the skin during the dissection, resulting in skin necrosis and wound complications which delay other therapy.

Elderly patients and their families warrant the same opportunity as younger patients for discussion of treatment options with a multidisciplinary team including the surgeon, radiation oncologist and medical oncologist. Priorities and wishes of each patient should be taken into account. Some patients can say right away that they want no irradiation, for example; others have no preconceived notions. Elderly patients typically have a long enough life expectancy to incur unnecessary morbidity and suffering from recurrent disease if sub-optimal treatment is used. Where chemotherapy is indicated, choice of drugs is on an individual basis. Some patients in age seventies might still receive adriamycin, for example.

In general, the outcome of treatment for breast cancer in elderly patients is as good as it is in younger patients. As mentioned earlier, surveillance with low density adipose tissue mammograms can be excellent. Management of breast cancer in this age group of patients over 50 can be highly rewarding for both the care-giver and the patient.

References

1. JW Berg and RVP Hutter: Breast cancer. *Cancer Supplement* 1995; **75**:257.
2. SS Devesa, WJ Blot, BJ Stone, et al.: Recent cancer trends in the United States. *Journal of the National Cancer Institute* 1995: **87**:175.
3. K Smigel: Breast cancer death rates decline for white women. *Journal of the National Cancer Institute* 1995; **87**:173.
4. WA Satariano: Aging, comorbidity, and breast cancer survival: an epidemiologic view. *Adv. Exp. Med. Biol.* 1993; **330**:1.
5. PC Prorok and RJ Connor: Screening for the early detection of cancer. *Cancer Investigation* 1986; **4**:225.
6. ME Costanza: Issues in breast cancer screening in older women. *Cancer Supplement* 1994; **74**:2009.
7. JC Cross, SE Harms, JH Cheek, et. al.: New Horizons in the diagnosis and treatment of breast cancer using magnetic resonance imaging. *Am. J. Surg.* 1993; 166:749.
8. GA Colditz: Epidemiology of breast cancer. Findings from the nurses' health study. *Cancer* 1993; 71(4 Suppl.):1480.
9. KF Hoskins, JE Stopfer, KA Calzone, et al.: Assessment and counseling for women with a family history of breast cancer. A guide for clinicians. *JAMA* 1995; 273(7):577.

10. DD Page and WD Dupont: Indicators of increased cancer risk in humans. *J. Cell Biochem. Suppl.* 1992; 16G:175.
11. RB Dickson and ME Lippman: Hormonal control of human breast cancer cell lines. *Cancer Surv.* 1986; 5(3):617.
12. R Lupu and ME Lippman: William L. McGuire Memorial Symposium. The role of erbB2 signal transduction pathways in human breast cancer. *Breast Cancer Res. Treat.* 1993; 27:83.
13. IA Jaiyesimi, AU Buzdar, DA Decker and GN Hortobagyi: Use of tamoxifen for breast cancer: twenty-eight years later. *J. Clin. Oncol.* 1995; 13(2):513.
14. Estrogen replacement therapy in women with previously treated breast cancer. ACOG Committee Opinion: Committee on Gynecologic Practice Number 135–April 1994. *Int. J. Gynaecol. Obstet.* 1994; 45(2):184.
15. DJ Marchant: Supplemental Estrogen Replacement. *Cancer* 1994; 74(1Suppl.):512.
16. RE Moe: Clinical Approach to Breast Disease. in *Office Gynecology*, M Stenchever, Ed., (Mosby—Year Book, Inc., St. Louis, 1991), pp. 211–246.
17. AJ Potterton, DJ Peakman and JR Young: Ultrasound demonstration of small breast cancers detected by mammographic screening. *Clin. Radiol.* 1994; 49:808.
18. Z. Kaufman, B Shpitz, M Shapiro, et.al.: Triple approach in the diagnosis of dominant breast masses: combined physical examination, mammography, and fine needle aspiration. *J. Surg. Oncol.* 1994; 56:254.
19. RA Schmidt: Stereotactic needle biopsy. *CA Cancer J. Clin.* 1994; 44:172.
20. SH Parker, F Burbank, RJ Jackman, et. al.: Percutaneous large-core breast biopsy: a multi-institutional study. *Radiology* 1994; 193:359.
21. N Sneige, BD Fornage and G Saleh: Ultrasound-guided fine-needle aspiration of nonpalpable breast lesions. Cytologic and histologic findings. *Am. J. Clin. Pathol.* 1994; 102:98.
22. PR Barbano and G Reali: Ultrasound guided fine needle aspiration of impalpable breast nodules. *Tumori* 1993; 79:418.
23. SH Parker, WE Jobe, MA Dennis, et. al.: US–guided automated large-core breast biopsy. *Radiology* 1993; 187:507.
24. DP Winchester and DC Cox: Standards for Breast—Conservation Treatment. *CA Cancer J. Clin.* 1992; 42:134.
25. J Abrams, T Chen and R Giusti: Survival after breast-sparing surgery versus mastectomy. *Journal of the National Cancer Institute* 1994; 86:1672.
26. B Fowble: Intraductal noninvasive breasr cancer: a comparison of three local treatments. *Oncology* 1989; 3:51.
27. MD Lagios: Duct carcinoma in situ. Pathology and treatment. *Surg. Clin. N. Am.* 1990; 70:853.
28. BF Fisher, J Costantino, C Redmond, et. al.: Lumpectomy compared with lumpectomy and radiation therapy for the treatment of intraductal breast cancer. *N. Eng. J. Med.* 1993; 328:1381.
29. ER Fisher, J Costantino, B Fisher, et. al.: Pathologic findings from the National Surgical Adjuvant Breast Project (NSABP) protocol B-17. Intraductal carcinoma (ductal carcinoma in situ). *Cancer* 1995, 75:1310.
30. LJ Solin, A Recht, A Fourquet, et. al.: Ten-year results of breast-conserving surgery and definiitive irradiation for intraductal carcinoma (ductal carcinoma in situ) of the breast. *Cancer* 1991; 68:2337.

Chapter 12

Cancer in the Older Woman

Joanna M. Cain, MD

Introduction

Cancer is the second leading cause of death (after heart disease) for older women. Since women survive longer than men, the overall number of cancers in older women is greater than in older men. The consequent disability and stress from cancer therapy can precipitate a series of other problems that significantly impact the functional status of older women. However, as a source of disability, cancer alone does not appear to reduce active life expectancy, as only 6.4% of respondents to the National Long-term Care Survey felt cancer contributed to the worsening of their functional status. Of course, this survey was not specifically directed toward women, nor toward the particularly devastating diseases that are unique to older women, such as ovarian and vulvar malignancies. It is of particular concern that advancing age is associated with more advanced disease for most sites examined in women. For those diseases where malignant changes can be detected before they are widespread, early identification through screening affects both the extent of treatment required as well as the likelihood of success. For a number of malignancies in older women, the impact of successful, early treatment on functional status can be significant.[1-5]

The differences noted in both rates of screening and survival from malignant diseases may be representative of social barriers to access as well as attitudes regarding screening in elderly women by both clinician and patient. Of particular import to clinicians is that elderly patients with cancer rated their quality of life higher than did their clinicians. Assumptions that early detection and treatment or even more aggressive treatment are unwarranted for older women as a group need to be replaced with assessments based on present functional status, not age, and present risk for malignant disease, not age.[5,6]

Lung Cancer

The incidence of lung cancer rises progressively to the eighth decade of life. Survival with a diagnosed lung cancer decreases with increasing age for women.[7] Yet, lung cancer is generally thought to be less aggressive in older patients. Screening for lung cancer as a whole, with chest radiographs or with sputum cytology, has not been shown to be effective. However, this has not been specifically assessed in the population of older women. Older women, having a higher frequency of disease per year of age and having a higher incidence of local, rather than distant, disease might well benefit from a screening program. At present, no such screening program is in trial, and no advisory body recommends standard screening for any age group.

Prevention is still focused on prevention of exposure to risk factors such as smoking, whether active or passive.[8] Women have experienced an increase in lung cancers overall while men have had a declining incidence as the incidence of smoking overall falls in men but not in women. The impact of exposure to nicotine may not be fully seen until the present generations of women smokers age, so counseling for smoking cessation is valid at all ages. In addition, cessation of smoking, while not completely protective, does decrease the risk by a significant amount (80%).

Management

The most common symptom of lung cancer is a change or worsening of a cough. Hemoptysis is less common (about 20%) but indicative of central bronchial lesions. Pneumonitis can also be an early symptom. Signs of extrapulmonary extension or spread of the disease are multiple: Pancoast's syndrome (shoulder and arm pain); superior vena cava syndrome, hoarseness, dyspnea, and symptoms of a paraneoplastic syndrome.[9]

Evaluation of a suspected lung cancer starts with a chest radiograph. If a suspicion still exists, then computed tomography (CT) scan should be done to delineate the lesion. This can be followed by a fine-needle aspiration or a flexible fiberoptic bronchoscopy, depending on the site of the lesion. As is always the case, cytology is not as definitive as is direct biopsy, so needle biopsy or brush-sputum cytology that is negative in the face of a visible lesion must be followed by direct biopsy. If there is evidence of metastatic disease, biopsy of this site (for example, lymph nodes) may be possible with less risk than for the primary site.

Further work-up of the lesion after diagnosis includes a careful survey for metastatic disease. Bone scans are important for small-cell lung cancers and for T3 (locally advanced) disease. Further evaluation of the liver (with upper abdomen CT scan) is important when resection is being considered and for small-cell lung cancers. In addition, brain scans for small-cell lung cancers are important.[9]

Therapy of lung cancer depends on its regional spread and cell type. The predominant cell type in women is adenocarcinoma (non–small-cell lung cancer). The most common procedure performed for these and other non–small-cell cancers with negative mediastinal nodes is lobectomy. Localized, but initially inoperable, lung primary tumors may be reduced by chemoradiation to resectable lesions. Management of widespread non–small-cell lung cancers or locally advanced disease is usually by protocol since the differential benefits of the various modalities and combinations are not yet clear. Referral to a cancer center for management is appropriate.

Small-cell lung cancer is an exceptionally aggressive disease, with a high propensity for hematogenous spread. Despite the presence of a small lesion and aggressive chemoradiation, the median survival is only 25% at 5 years. This is a disease in which every small improvement in treatment is a major step forward, and participation in study group protocols can be a major contribution to that step.[10]

Follow-up after successful treatment of lung cancer requires periodic physical examinations including at least chest radiographs or tomography, as indicated by the original disease.

Breast Cancer

One of the most important cancers for surveillance in older women is breast cancer. The risk of cancer increases with increasing age so that by age 65 the risk is 1 in 17, and by age 85 the risk is 1 in 9. In fact, the most significant risk factor for breast cancer is age over 50. Furthermore, the lesions that are identified by screening are more likely to be positive than in younger cohorts of patients. Yet, less than 40% of physicians routinely screen patients over 65 and only 21%

routinely screen women over 75. For breast cancer, the most effective deterrent to advanced disease is education of physicians regarding the efficacy and cost savings of screening in older women.[11,12]

Screening of older women is primarily done by yearly mammography. While breast self-examination is encouraged, it is less effective overall and particularly less effective in the older woman. The American Cancer Society recommends yearly mammography with breast self-examination for women over 50. Every effort should be made to support yearly mammography for older women.[13,14]

Other risk factors for the disease that are especially pertinent to the older woman are the presence of a previous breast cancer, a first-degree relative with breast cancer, early menarche, late first full-term pregnancy, and prior radiation to the chest. Breast cancer remains a disease most prevalent in women born in North America and northern Europe and of upper socioeconomic status.

Management

The presence of a nonpalpable but suspicious finding on a mammogram and any new mass in the breast in an older woman requires evaluation either with fine-needle aspiration or with open biopsy. It is axiomatic that the presence of a negative mammogram does not negate the need for full evaluation of a breast mass. Identification of a nonpalpable, suspicious area may require prebiopsy placement of a guidewire. Further evaluation is dependent on the final pathology diagnosis (including estrogen and progesterone receptors) of the malignancy.[15,16]

The majority of lesions are stage I or II (less than 2 cm), but therapy is generally predicated by the presence or absence of involved axillary nodes. Since the size and palpability of nodes are not reliable, axillary dissection is usually performed as part of staging and treatment planning. In addition, chest radiograph and liver function tests are routinely obtained. Bone scan is of clear benefit in staging node-positive patients but is controversial in staging node-negative, stage I disease.[17]

Therapy is based on the most common presenting stage—I or II. Primary therapy for this group is either modified radical mastectomy or lumpectomy plus radiation. Given the general preference by patients for breast preservation, the latter should be more common. However, there are women who feel that only with removal of the breast will they feel adequately treated. It is important to remember that the treatments are equivalent, even if the general preference is for lumpectomy plus radiation. Following primary therapy, adjuvant therapy to minimize the risk of future recurrence has been shown—even in short-term follow-up—to have a disease-free survival advantage. Many national protocols limit the age for inclusion to less than 71 years, partially because of the toxic effects of drugs included in the regimen. Considering the fact that women at 75 can expect to live more than 7 years, adjuvant therapy is not inappropriate for women with a high performance status. Furthermore, the presence of estrogen receptor positivity is more common in older women, and therapy with tamoxifen can impact the recurrence rate. Avoidance of metastatic breast cancer is clearly in the patient's best interest, since survival after metastases ranges from 18 to 36 months. The best management for breast cancer employs a multidisciplinary approach from the time of initial diagnosis.

Follow-up for women after breast cancer depends on the treatment. However, it is important to note that there may be recurrence in the same breast (with breast-preserving surgery, or the scar area in mastectomies) and the opposite breast, therefore, it is important to screen these areas with examination and mammography.[18,19,20]

Colorectal Carcinoma

Colorectal carcinomas ranked third as a cause of death among women with cancer in 1993. It is predominantly a disease of older women, with the majority of cases occurring in those over 65 years of age. The maximum incidence is at age 80. Women have a slightly higher incidence of colon and lower incidence of rectal carcinomas. Thus, the symptoms and screening for this disease is important for the older woman.[21]

Risk factors for this cancer include a high fat, calorie-dense diet. A history of colonic polyps, previous colon cancer, or inflammatory bowel disease also increases the risk. A family prevalence of the disease should alert physicians to the need for closer screening. Prevention is based on some dietary changes. At present, diets high in calcium, ascorbic acid, and vitamin D are reported to act positively by blocking promoters of neoplastic growth!

The sensitivity of the most easily performed screening test, fecal occult blood test (FOBT), has been fairly low. In patients over 70 years of age, the combination of FOBT with sigmoidoscopy increased detection of cancers and benign adenomas with no increased morbidity from the procedure. Yet, none of the screening trials has shown a decrease in mortality as the consequence of earlier detection. Overall, the recommendations follow the guidelines of the American Cancer Society, which suggests digital rectal examination and FOBT annually for persons over age 50, with sigmoidoscopy every 3 to 5 years beginning at age 50.[22,23,24]

The early symptoms of this disease are subtle, but need attention. First, the presence of rectal bleeding—even if concurrent hemorrhoids are found—is worthy of sigmoidoscopy in the older woman who has not had a recent screening sigmoidoscopy. Second, reports of a change in bowel habits must be taken seriously in older women. Other symptoms suggest more advanced disease, from tenesmus, urgency, pain, and weight loss to outright obstruction and perforation. Taking seriously the subtle changes in bowel and gastrointestinal function of older women is very important for both colorectal cancers and ovarian malignancies. Ascribing these newly reported changes to age is never adequate.[25,26]

There is no reported difference in the aggressiveness of colorectal cancer in older persons. The number of patients with local disease and regional disease (approximately 36% and 40%) at presentation is the same as that for women over 65 years of age. Women have lower survival with increasing age despite this lack of difference in presentation and biological aggressiveness of disease. Again, the reason for this difference is not known, although the clinical status of the patient often dictates the aggressiveness of approach and may be related to the decreased survival.

Management of colorectal cancer is dependent on the staging, which for early or regional cancers is dependent on regional surgical excision of the lesion for all except initially obvious metastatic disease. TNM staging of rectal cancer is directly related to survival. Patients with stage B2 or C disease have a high likelihood of recurrence and are candidates for adjuvant therapy protocols. The National Institutes of Health consensus panel concluded that patients with stage II (Duke's C) colon cancer should be offered a clinical trial. Those who are unable to participate should be offered 5-fluorouracil adjuvant (5-FU) plus levamisole, which is generally a well-tolerated combination in older patients. For rectal carcinoma, the risk for local recurrence is greater and postoperative radiotherapy plus adjuvant chemotherapy for stages II and III are warranted. Adjuvant therapy with chemotherapy (5-FU) plus radiation has significantly reduced distant metastases, local recurrence, and increased overall survival.[27,28,29]

Patients with anal cancer, in particular, have benefited from the effects of combined modality treatments. 5-FU plus mitomycin C have been combined with radiotherapy so successfully that minimal or no resection has been required for a number of patients.

In summary, the most important features of colorectal cancer in older women are the subtlety of the presenting symptoms, requiring vigilance on the part of clinicians not to ascribe these to other changes of aging. Active older patients should be treated aggressively when the disease is diagnosed, as the management of early disease can profoundly influence their survival and quality of life.

Follow-up of patients with colorectal cancers after treatment includes periodic colonoscopy, physical examination, and further testing, depending on the extent of the original disease. If women have received pelvic radiation as part of their treatment, it is important to encourage use of vaginal dilators to prevent strictures of the vaginal canal that impede adequate follow-up and diminish sexual function.

Cancers of the Reproductive Organs

Vulvar Cancer

Invasive vulvar cancer is a disease of older women, being most common in the seventh decade of life. For vulvar cancer, as for other skin malignancies, there is no screening test. However, evaluation of all the skin surfaces and education of patients regarding normal and abnormal skin changes is an important element of preventive care in older women. Of particular concern is the lack of express direction (and permission) for older women to examine the skin of the vulvar area. The fact that this is not an acceptable practice for older (and many younger!) women leads to delays in diagnosis that can be fatal for a disease that, overall, is highly curable.[30]

One of the major correlated conditions is chronic vulvar dystrophy, which is very common in this age group. Approximately 50% of invasive carcinomas will arise within such an area. However, the overall incidence of invasive carcinoma in vulvar dystrophy is actually very low (2% to 4%). In addition, patients who have human papilloma virus (HPV) infections requiring chronic treatment and those who are immunosuppressed have a higher risk for the disease.

Symptoms of the invasive disease process are fairly classic. Local irritation and itching are the most frequent, with a mass or bleeding heralding local extension of the disease. It is valuable to alert older women to these symptoms and to recommend that they report such symptoms promptly.

Management

Initial management of any suspicious skin lesion is outpatient biopsy or removal (dependent on size). This is no different in the vulvar area. However, in the face of concurrent dystrophic changes of the vulva a high index of suspicion must be kept. It is never appropriate to treat lesions of the vulva in older women with topical therapy without adequate clinical evaluation and a low threshold for biopsy. Further metastatic evaluation prior to initial therapy is generally not required. This is because the most common type, squamous cancer, has little propensity for hematogenous transportation and lymphatic transportation is directed toward regional lymph nodes.[30]

This is not true of malignant melanoma of the vulva, however. Consideration of evaluating the areas of hematogenous spread such as chest and liver prior to further local treatment is important, particularly if the lesion is large.[31]

The majority of these cancers are discovered in the early stages where locoregional control is highly successful. The gold standard of therapy is radical vulvectomy with bilateral groin node dissection for invasive squamous lesions of the vulva. The exceptions to this are microinvasive disease (various groups propose less than 1 mm or less than 2 mm below the basement membrane as the diagnostic category for this), where local radical excision with or without uni- or bilateral groin node dissection is equally efficacious. Even the presence of one positive lymph node may not significantly impact the 80%, 5-year, disease-free survival of stages I and II invasive vulvar cancers.[32,33]

Recovery from radical vulvectomy is compromised by early wound disruption in 40% to 50% of cases and later leg lymphedema of variable degree in a significant percentage of patients.

Modification of therapy is necessary for locally advanced disease where primary radiation with concurrent chemotherapy may be more effective. For all vulvar carcinomas, involvement of gynecologic oncologists in treatment planning is essential to achieve the excellent outcome that can be obtained for the majority of patients.

Follow-up of vulvar cancers is concentrated on local inspection of the vulva and the groin, with biopsy of any suspicious area. In addition, because the oncogenic stimulus is widespread, these patients need evaluation of vaginal and cervical mucosa with cytology screening and visual inspection. Generally, the pattern for follow-up is more frequent in the first 2 years (every 3 to 4 months) and then extends to every 6 months until 5 years have elapsed. These patients must continue to have yearly, careful evaluations after 5 years because the possibility of recurrence or new primary still exists.

Cervical Cancer

One of the more controversial areas in the care of older women is the issue of the frequency of cytologic screening that is best for prevention of cervical cancer. Cervical cancer remains a disease of the older woman, with 41% of the annual deaths from cervical cancer occurring in women over age 65. Older women present with late disease and have the largest potential benefit from an improved screening protocol. It is estimated that women over 65 would benefit most from the use of opportunistic screening and a regular recall schedule, with a 63% improvement in 5-year mortality. In addition, the tumor-cell kinetics of cervical cancer found in older women are skewed toward more aneuploid, rapidly growing tumors—another reason to screen for earlier detection. Whether the present increases in precancerous, dysplastic lesions of the cervix in younger women portends increases in invasive cervical cancer as this cohort ages is unknown. However, potential further increases in invasive cervical cancer in this population argues even more strongly for better attention to screening and to eliminating the barriers to screening in older women.[34,35]

Older women at risk for development of invasive cervical malignancies are those who have a previous history of dysplasia or radiation for cervical malignancy. Those who have a history of treatment for or infection with HPV infections and women with acquired immunodeficiency syndrome (AIDS) have higher incidences of invasive disease. Women who smoke have a higher incidence of high grade dysplasias and cervical cancer. The disease development is multifactorial and dependent on individual genetic factors that are poorly understood at present. Of considerable importance is the fact that older women can be exposed to the more closely correlated subtypes of HPV at any age and thus increase the likelihood of disease. Assumptions of decreased risk from sexual exposure is not warranted on the basis of age alone.

The classic symptoms of cervical cancer do not vary in the older woman. The presence of a watery or mucoid discharge, postmenopausal bleeding, postcoital bleeding, and new onset sacral or lower back pain can all be symptoms of a cervical cancer. Late symptoms of unilateral leg edema and neuropathy generally herald a poor prognosis.

Management

There are several areas of special concern for cervical cytology in older postmenopausal women, particularly those not receiving estrogen replacement therapy. First, the presence of endometrial cells in cytologic findings can be indicative of endometrial carcinoma. Therefore, the appropriate follow-up for this is an endometrial biopsy rather than colposcopy and cervical biopsy. Second, the severe atrophy that accompanies estrogen deprivation can lead to cytologic interpretations of intraepithelial neoplasia. This can be diagnosed with colposcopy and treated with estrogen therapy in women for whom this is appropriate. Finally, the ascent of the squamo-columnar junction with atrophic changes in older women leads to a higher frequency of cytologies that lack endocervical cells. While this is somewhat assisted by the use of the cytobrush or small Calgi swabs to access the area, in some patients this may still not result in adequate sampling of the endocervix. Whether or not the presence of endocervical cells in the older age population reflects the adequacy of sampling for cervical cancer is controversial. However, careful repeat screening may be considered particularly if there are high risk factors present.[36]

All cytologic findings of intraepithelial neoplasia (vaginal or cervical) should be followed by colposcopy with vaginal, cervical, or endometrial biopsies as indicated. If there is a question of invasion, then further evaluation with a cervical conization is required to establish the depth. If frank invasion is present on biopsy, then proceeding to therapy is appropriate.

Work-up of an invasive cervical cancer depends on the histologic type and the stage of the lesions. Neuroendocrine, small-cell, and glassy-cell tumors are among the most aggressive histologic types and are the most likely to metastasize early. For these subtypes, consideration of distant disease with chest radiograph, liver function tests, and even bone scans and abdominal–pelvic CT scans for the small-cell tumors are appropriate. With extensive pelvic disease (stage IIA and above), abdominopelvic CT is useful in planning radiation therapy and will indicate whether radiographically enlarged nodes are present.[37,38-43]

Early invasive cancer diagnosed on adequate cervical conization (less than 3 mm from the basement membrane with no confluence or lymphatic or vascular invasion) can be treated conservatively with a simple vaginal or abdominal hysterectomy. Removal of the ovaries at the same time is appropriate for the older woman, but they are exceptionally rare sites for primary metastases from cervical cancer.

The most common cancer cell type is squamous cell, and the second most common tye is adenocarcinoma. For these types, therapy for the most common stage—stage I cervical cancer— is generally a choice between radical hysterectomy with pelvic and para-aortic node dissection and primary radiation therapy. The general pattern of spread for squamous-cell carcinoma is lymphatic through pelvic and then para-aortic echelons of lymph nodes. For this reason, both primary therapies must encompass the entire area at risk. The outcome of each approach is essentially equivalent while the immediate and long-term risks differ. For sexually active older women, the preservation of normal vaginal function is more successful with radical surgery than with radiation therapy. However, the acute stress of surgery and the immediate complications may contraindicate it as an option for older women with significant concurrent medical problems.[44-49]

The remainder of patients with more extensive cervical cancer are best treated primarily with radiation therapy. The more common acute complaints are mild nausea and mild diarrhea. Long-term complications include rectal or vesicovaginal fistulas at rates that average around 1%. Rectal stricture, small bowel obstruction, and ureteral stricture are also potential long-term complications.

The most important features of cervical cancer in older women are attention to an opportunistic and planned screening program and modification of therapy for the most common stage I tumors based on general health and activity.

Follow-up after successful treatment is centered around potential recurrence in the cervical area (with cervical preservation with radiation) or in the vaginal/pelvic areas. These patients are also at risk for vaginal and vulvar dysplasia and carcinomas; thus, careful inspection of these areas on follow-up is mandatory. Patients receiving radiation need to use vaginal dilators in order to prevent strictures of the vagina that would impede follow-up and diminish sexual function. The general follow-up pattern depends on the disease type but every 3 to 4 months for the first year with physical examination and cytology, then every 6 months until 5 years have elapsed, then yearly thereafter.

Endometrial Cancer

The most common form of uterine cancer is endometrial, which is the most common gynecologic malignancy in the United States. The peak incidence is between ages 50 and 69, with the majority diagnosed after menopause. The classic risk factors of obesity, nulliparity, late menopause, and prolonged high dose, unopposed estrogen all point to faulty estrogen processing in an estrogen-rich environment as the key to the etiology of this disease. The threshold for this interaction is unknown, but it is of interest that more recent reviews have found no increased risk of endometrial cancer in women who exclusively used conjugated equine estrogen preparations of 0.625 mg/day or less. This relationship is further supported by the high rate of cancers of the endometrium in women whose only risk factor was hormone-secreting tumors. Both birth control pill use greater than 12 months and cigarette smoking (although this benefit is vastly overweighted by the detrimental effects of smoking) decrease the incidence of this cancer.[50]

There is no classic screening for endometrial cancer, although recommendations for endometrial biopsies in high-risk women at menopause have been made. Of particular interest in the older patient is the group of patients receiving tamoxifen for postmenopausal breast cancer. Overall, patients on tamoxifen had thicker endometriums and larger uterine volumes by transvaginal sonography. The primary pathology found in asymptomatic sampling is polyps. However, the National Surgical Adjuvant Breast Project (NSABP) study of prevention of breast cancer with tamoxifen has reported initially increased numbers (3%) of endometrial cancers in that patient population. The proper interval for screening women with increased risk factors and particularly on prolonged tamoxifen is not defined. Until a clear protocol can be defined for asymptomatic women on tamoxifen, our present policy is to sample 6 months after initiation of therapy and then yearly after that until the risk pattern is more clear.

All women with postmenopausal bleeding from the uterus need to have an explanation for this symptom, which is the most common presentation of endometrial cancer. The finding on a PAP smear of endometrial cancer or endometrial cells in a postmenopausal patient not on estrogen replacement can be a grave prognostic sign and also requires evaluation.[51]

Postmenopausal women have a progression of the squamo-columnar junction higher into the cervical canal and often develop relative strictures of the endocervix. It can be quite difficult in patients with a low endometrial or a high endocervical lesion to differentiate between the two sites of adenocarcinoma. For this population, fractional curettage and clinical examination are the best assistants to making a diagnosis of site. However, even with the most accurate information it may be quite impossible to differentiate between the two diagnoses.[52,53]

Initial evaluation of a patient with endometrial cancer should include a chest radiograph and liver function tests because this malignancy has a higher tendency to metastasize to the lung and the liver. Further evaluation with CT scans or bone scans should be individualized, depending on risk of distant disease by stage, histology, or symptomatology.

Management

Endometrioid adenocarcinoma is the major histologic type of endometrial cancer whose clinical behavior depends on the differentiation. There are subtypes that have significantly different prognoses and management. Of particular importance in the management of endometrial cancers is identification of serious papillary adenocarcinomas of the endometrium, which are more common in older women. These tend to show deep myometrial invasion and involvement of the peritoneal surface. Consequently, the overall survival is decreased in this group.[54]

Staging of this disease is reflective of the primary initial modality of therapy: Surgery. Most women have stage I disease that surgical removal of the uterus and ovaries alone will cure.

However, among patients with stage I disease are those who have deep myometrial invasion, high histologic grade, or unusual and prognostically grave cell types that warrant more aggressive staging and management, including lymph node sampling. The majority of patients with positive lymph nodes results do not have clinically apparent nodal disease. However, their long-term survival is significantly decreased because of this finding, even in the presence of adjuvant pelvic radiation (50% long-term survival).[55]

The involvement of the cervix (stage II) with endometrial cancer presents a particular management challenge, as the pattern of drainage through lymphatics in the parametrium and pelvis is slightly different. Approaches to this problem have included varying combinations or pre- and/or postoperative radiation, with hysterectomy to radical hysterectomy. These are also appropriate approaches for the puzzling presentation of adenocarcinoma in a patient with endocervical or stage II endometrial adenocarcinoma.

Management of metastatic disease, whether peritoneal, pulmonary, or hepatic, rarely results in a long-term response. Of particular importance, however, is identifying patients with well-differentiated to moderate-differentiated tumors or with estrogen/progesterone-positive tumors that are likely to respond to hormonal manipulation. Progesterone has been the major hormonal therapy for this disease, and in this setting it can be highly successful in stabilizing disease for prolonged periods, even years. Tamoxifen, also, has had some success in this setting.

Follow-up of endometrial cancer should include periodic physical examinations and cytology screening because a likely site of recurrence is the vaginal apex. The use of chest radiographs on a routine basis has not been shown to be cost-effective. However, a high index of clinical suspicion must be kept and chest radiographs obtained if pulmonary symptoms warrant it. Again, evaluations every 3 to 6 months for the first 5 years are appropriate.

Ovarian Cancer

Among the gynecologic malignancies, epithelial ovarian cancer is the leading cause of death, and it reaches its highest risk of development in women around 80 years of age. There is a striking difference in length of survival for women over 65 with this disease. One study by Markman and coworkers[56] showed a median survival of 24 months for elderly patients and a median survival for younger patients that exceeded 4 years. Another study by Hightower and coworkers[57] showed a survival advantage of 18 months for younger patients with stages III and IV disease. Of particular importance in this study was the fact that older patients underwent fewer operations, had lower tumor debulking rates, and were more likely to have their surgery done by general surgeons versus gynecologists or gynecologic oncologists. Given the fact that older patients tolerate radical surgery and cytotoxic treatment generally as well as their younger counterparts, these data raise concerns that the older woman is not being offered the most successful and more aggressive treatment modalities and is not being referred to or does not have access to gynecologic oncologists. As noted previously in this chapter, older patients rate their own quality of life significantly higher than do their physicians. Given a general medical sense about the overall failure of therapy for ovarian epithelial malignancies and a mistaken view of older women's perceptions of quality of life, women with this diagnosis may not be adequately treated or referred to appropriate treatment facilities or specialists. In fact, up to 40% of women 85 years of age and older were not offered a definitive cancer treatment. In the treatment of this disease it is important to recognize that for the active older woman the treatment can and should be as aggressive as it is in the younger woman. Otherwise, we are shortening lives on the basis of bias, rather than factual evidence.[56,57]

Risk factors for the development of epithelial ovarian malignancies include those physiological events that increase the number of ovulations over a lifetime. For example, nulliparity, early menarche, and late menopause all increase the risk for this disease, while multiparity and prolonged use of birth control pills decrease the risk. There is a small (5%) genetic risk for development, often combined with a risk for breast cancer or colon cancer. There is a wide geographical and ethnic variation in rates with the highest for white women in industrialized countries, thought to be related to average family size.[58]

Prevention of ovarian cancer in older postmenopausal patients cannot center on prevention through the use of oral contraceptives or patterns of reproduction. There is no effective mass screening available, including the use of serum Ca-125 or transvaginal ultrasonography. Therefore, the best prevention is removal of the ovaries. Given the relatively low incidence of this disease, this is appropriate only when other surgical procedures are anticipated.[59]

Symptoms of ovarian cancer are subtle and usually are indicative of advanced disease. Early symptoms are usually dependent on torsion of the ovary or direct pressure on surrounding structures. Symptoms of new urinary urgency or pressure, changes in bowel function, and vague symptoms of gastrointestinal distress should all raise the question of ovarian cancer. Classic late symptoms include early satiety, regurgitation of gastric contents, and stretching abdominal pain from ascites. Patients may complain of difficulty with deep breathing because of the intra-abdominal tension on the diaphragm. In addition, pleural effusions or involvement can elicit local or back pain and dyspnea. Because the early symptoms are subtle, it is very important to keep this diagnosis in mind.

Management

Diagnosis of a pelvic mass usually requires only a pelvic examination. Unless there is a significant clinical reason to suspect another diagnosis, the use of ultrasonography and computed tomography does not add to the preoperative evaluation. There are, however, two other cancers that should be considered with pelvic masses in older women. Both breast and ovary can present as a pelvic metastases as the initial finding. Initial history and physical then must be directed to rule out the likelihood of these cancers.

There are no sensitive and specific means to rule out malignancy in ovarian-pelvic masses. Some guidance can be obtained from ultrasound characteristics of the mass in that clear cysts less than 5 cm are rarely malignant. However, transabdominal and transvaginal aspiration of ovarian cysts in this age group are strongly discouraged because of the risk of spread with a potentially confined ovarian malignancy. Given the fact that virtually all ovarian masses in older women will require a surgical diagnosis and therapy, there is little reason to take such a risk in this age group.[60-63]

Surgical therapy is the initial modality for this malignancy. Debulking, or removal of maximal tumor burden, is a major factor in length of survival. The ability to rapidly perform all the indicated procedures has diminished the risks in older women for aggressive tumor debulking. However, in the face of extensive unresectable disease, an alternative approach with interval debulking may be safer and potentially as efficacious. Early ovarian cancer confined to the ovaries may require only adequate surgical and careful staging as the full extent of therapy. Management of patients suspected to have ovarian cancer should be done by individuals trained in the overall treatment of these malignancies, such as gynecologic oncologists.

The other modalities of therapy for ovarian cancer are radiation therapy and chemotherapy. The majority of treatment in the United States is with peripherally administered chemotherapy. The two most active families of chemotherapeutic drugs are the taxenes, from which paclitaxel is derived, and the platinum agents, usually cisplatin or carboplatinum. These are given in varying doses and schedules, depending on the disease process and response.[64-66]

Ca-125 is a monoclonal antibody test that identifies an antigen present on many, but not all, ovarian cancers. The fact that this antigen is variably expressed, and expressed by tissues not associated with ovarian malignancy has made it too nonspecific for screening. It has, however, been a useful tool in evaluating response to therapy with chemotherapy.[67]

Evaluating response to therapy when the Ca-125 has returned to normal and there is no palpable disease is desirable but difficult to accomplish at present. Computed tomography scans are reasonable for evaluating the presence of large disease or retroperitoneal disease, but they fail to detect the small disease of concern.[68] Second-look laparotomies also fail to completely evaluate all disease, as for stage III lesions that are found to be negative, more than half recur. The use of additional surgeries in patients with ovarian cancer, regardless of age, should then be confined to those circumstances where evidence of disease presence will alter management, will provide information regarding a protocol in which the patient has chosen to participate, or where there is a lesion that is felt to be resectable after chemotherapy has been completed.[69]

There is little data regarding the quality of life experienced by women undergoing treatment for ovarian cancer. Therefore, the options for treatment and the side effects of drugs must be discussed with patients on an individual basis. As noted previously, assumptions about patients' perceptions of quality of life and about their potential tolerance of therapy can be quite erroneous. Ovarian cancer is a disease where constant, honest communication is a major factor in determining therapy. The therapy of this malignancy is best guided by clinicians with special training in this area.

References

1. Kain CD, Reilly N, Schultz E: The older adult: A comparative assessment. *Nurs Clin North Am* 1990;25:833–848.
2. Manton K: The linkage of health status changes and disability. *Compr Gerontol* 1987;1:16–21.
3. Kant AK, Glover C, Horm J, Schatzkin A, Harris TB: Does cancer survival differ for older patients? *Cancer* 1992;7:2734 to 2740.
4. Oddone EZ, Feussner JR, Cohen HJ: Can screening older patients for cancer save lives? *Clin Geriatr Med* 1992;8:51–67.
5. Pearlman RA, Uhlman RF: Quality of life in chronic disease: Perceptions of elderly patients. *J Gerontol* 1988;43:25–30.
6. Frame P: A critical review of adult health maintenance: Part 8: Prevention of cancer. *J Family Practice* 1986;22:511–520.
7. Filderman AE, Shaw C, Matthay RA: Lung cancer in the elderly. *Clin Geriatr Med* 1986;2:363–383.
8. Stockwell HG, Goldman AL, Lyman GH, et al: Environmental tobacco smoke and lung cancer risk in non-smoking women. *J Natl Cancer Inst* 1992;84:1417–1422
9. Livingston RB: Lunch cancer. *Prim Care Update Ob/Gyns* 1994;1:97–100.
10. McCracken JD, Janaki LM, Crowley JJ, et al: Concurrent chemotherapy/radiotherapy for limited small-cell lung carcinoma: A Southwest Oncology Group Study. *J Clin Oncol* 1990;8:892–896.
11. Feuer EJ, Wun LM, Boring CC, Flanders WD, Timmel M, Tong T: The lifetime risk of developing breast cancer. *J Natl Cancer Inst* 1993:85;892–7
12. Black JS, Sefcik T, Sapoor W: Health promotion and disease prevention in the elderly. *Arch Intern Med* 1990;150:389–391.
13. American Cancer Society: 1989 survey of physicians' attitudes and practices in early cancer detection. *CA Cancer J Clin* 1990;40:77.
14. O'Malley MS, Fletcher SW: Screening for breast cancer with breast self-examination. *JAMA* 1987;257:2196–2199.
15. Ellis G: Breast cancer. *Prim Care Update Ob/Gyns* 1994;1:17–25.
16. Donegan WL: Evaluation of a palpable breast mass: Current concepts. *N Engl J Med* 1992;327:937–942.
17. Cutler SJ: Classification of extent of disease in breast cancer. *Semin Oncol* 1974;1:91.
18. Mansour EG, Gray R, Shatila, AH, et al: Efficacy of adjuvant chemotherapy in high-risk node-negative breast cancer: An intergroup study. *N Engl J Med* 1989;320:485–490.
19. Fisher B, Constantino J, Redmond C, aet al: A randomized clinical trial evaluating tamoxifen in the treatment of patients with node-negative breast cancer who have estrogen-receptor-positive tumors. *N Engl J Med* 1989;320:479–484.
20. Elwood JM, Godolphin W: Oestrogen receptors in breast tumors: Associations with age, menopausal status and epidemiological and clinical features in 735 patients. *Br J Cancer* 1980;42:635–644.
21. Smith DH: Colorectal cancer. *Prim Care Update Ob/Gyns* 1994;1:64–67.
22. Wagner JL, Duffy B, Sandeep W, et al: Costs and effectiveness of colorectal cancer screening in the elderly. Preventive Health Services under Medicare Paper 5, Office of Technology Assessment, Washington DC, US Government Printing Office, 1990.

23. Shelly JV, Friedman GD: Sigmoidoscopy in the periodic health examination of asymptomatic adults. *JAMA* 1989;261:595–598.

24. Mettlin C, Dodd GD: The American Cancer Society guidelines for the cancer-related checkup: An update. *CA Cancer J Clin* 1992;41:279–282.

25. Joseph RR: Aggressive management of cancer in the elderly. *Clin Geriatr Med* 1988;2:363–383.

26. Wetle T: Age as a risk factor for inadequate treatment. *JAMA* 1987;258:516.

27. Moertel CG, Fleming TR, MacDonald JS, Haller DG, Laurie JA, Goodman PJ: Levamisole and fluorouracil for adjuvant therapy of resected colon carcinoma. *N Engl J Med* 1990;833:352–358.

28. Krook JE, Moertel CG, Gunderson LL, et al: Effective surgical adjuvant therapy for high-risk rectal carcinoma. *N Engl J Med* 1991;324:709–715.

29. Smith DE, Muff NS, Shetabi H: Combined preoperative neoadjuvant radiotherapy and chemotherapy for anal and rectal cancer. *Am J Surg* 1986;151:577–580.

30. Morley GW: in Knapp R, Berkowitz RS (eds.): *Gynecologic Oncology.* New York, McGraw-Hill, 1993, pp 292–293.

31. Friedman RJ, Rigel DS, Kopf AW: Early detection of malignant melanoma: The role of physician examination and self-examination of the skin. *Cancer* 1985;35:130–134.

32. Figge DC, Gaudenz R: Invasive carcinoma of the vulva. *Am J Obstet Gynecol* 1974;119:382–395.

33. Hopkins MP, Reid GC, Vettrano I, Morley GW: Squamous cell carcinoma of the vulva: Prognostic factors influencing survival. *Gynecol Oncol* 1991;43:113–117.

34. Mandelblatt J, Gopaul I, Wistreich M: Gynecological care of elderly women. Another look at Papanicolaou testing. *JAMA* 1986;256:367–371.

35. Fahs M, Mandelblatt J, Schechter CB, Muller C: Cost-effectiveness of cervical cancer screening for the elderly. *Ann Intern Med* 1992;117:520–527.

36. Mandelblatt J, Schechter C, Fahs M, Muller C: Clinical implications of screening for cervical cancer under Medicare: The natural history of cervical cancer in the elderly. What do we know? What do we need to know? *Am J Obstet Gynecol* 1991;164:644–651.

37. Goodwin JS, Samet JM, Key CR, Humble C, Kurtvirt D, Hunt C: Stage of diagnosis of cancer varies with the age of the patient. *J Am Geriatr Soc* 1986;34:20–26.

38. Fletcher A: Screening for cancer of the cervix in elderly women. *Lancet* 1990;335:97–99.

39. Minagawa Y, Kigawa J, Kanamori Y, Itamochi H, Terakawa N: Tumor cell kinetics in elderly patients with cervical cancer. *Obstet Gynecol* 1993;82:610–614.

40. Bowling A: Implications of preventive health behavior for cervical and breast cancer screening programmes; A review. *Family Pract* 1989;6:224–231.

41. Richart FM, Barron BA: A follow-up study of patients with cervical dysplasia. *Am J Obstet Gynecol* 1969;105:386–389.

42. Slattery ML, Overall JC, Abbott TM French TK, Robison LM, Gardner J: Sexual activity, contraception, genital infections, and cervical cancer: Support for a sexually transmitted disease hypothesis. *Am J Epidemiol* 1989;130:248–250.

43. Layde PM, Broste SK: Carcinoma of the cervix and smoking. *Biomed Pharmacother* 1989;43:161–164.

44. Tamimi HK, Ek M, Hesla J, Cain JM, Figge DC, Greer BE: Glassy cell carcinoma of the cervix-redefined. *Obstet Gynecol* 1988;71:837.

45. Van Nagell JR, Powell D, Gallion HH, et al: Small cell carcinoma of the uterine cervix. *Cancer* 1988;62:1586.

46. Sevin BU, Nadji M, Averette HE, Hilsenbeck S, Smith D, Lampe B: Microinvasive carcinoma of the cervix. *Cancer* 1992;70:2121–2128.

47. Kenter GG, Ansink AC, Heintz AP, Aartsen EJ, Delemarre JF, Hart AA: Carcinoma of the uterine cervix stage I and IIA: Results of surgical treatment: Complications, recurrence and survival. *Eur J Surg Oncol* 1989;15:55–60.

48. Montana G, Fowler WC, Varia MA, Walton LA, Mack Y: Analysis of results of radiation therapy for stage IB carcinoma of the cervix. *Cancer* 1987;60:2195.

49. Perez CA, Breaux S, Bedwinek JM, et al: Radiation therapy alone in the treatment of carcinoma of the uterine cervix: Analysis of complications. *Cancer* 1989;54:235.

50. Rubin GL, Peterson HB, Lee NC, Maes EF, Wingo PA, Becker S: Estrogen replacement therapy and the risk of endometrial cancer: Remaining controversies. *Am J Obstet Gynecol* 1990;162:148–154.

51. Gusberg SB, Kardon P: Proliferative endometrial response to theca-granulosa cell tumors. *Am J Obstet Gynecol* 1971;111:633–643.

52. Pritchard KI: Screening for endometrial cancer: Is it effective? *Ann Intern Med* 1989;110:117.

53. Lahti E, Blanco G, Kauppila A, Apaja-Sarkkinen M, Taskinen PJ, Laatikainen T: Endometrial changes in postmenopausal breast cancer patient receiving tamoxifen. *Obstet Gynecol* 1993;81:660–664.

54. Chen JL, Tros DC, Wilkinson EJ: Endometrial papillary carcinoma: Two clinical pathological types. *Int J Gynecol Pathol* 1985;4:279.

55. Creasman WT, Morrow CP, Bundy L, Homesley HD, Graham JE, Heller PB: Surgical pathological spread patterns of endometrial cancer. *Cancer* 1987;60:2035–2041.

56. Markman M, Lewis JL Jr, Saigo P, et al: Impact of age on survival of patients with ovarian cancer. *Gynecol Oncol* 1993;49:236–239.
57. Hightower RD, Nguyen HN, Averette HE, Hoskins W, Harrison T, Steren A: National survey of ovarian carcinoma IV: Patterns of care and related survival for older patients. *Cancer* 1994;73:377–383.
58. Greene M, Clark J, Blayney D: The epidemiology of ovarian cancer. *Semin Oncol* 1984;11:209.
59. Schaprio MM, Matchar DB, Young MJ: The effectiveness of ovarian cancer screening: A decision analysis model. *Ann Intern Med* 1993;118:838–843.
60. Ries LA: Ovarian cancer: Survival and treatment differences by age. *Cancer* 1993;71:524–529.
61. Goldstein SR, Subramanyam B, Snyder JR, Raghavendra BN, Beller U, Beckman EM: The postmenopausal cystic adnexal mass: The potential role of ultrasound conservative management. *Obstet Gynecol* 1989;73:8–10.
62. Edmonson JH, Su J, Krook JE: Treatment of ovarian cancer in elderly women. *Cancer* 1993;71:615–617.
63. Trimbos JB, Hacker NF: The case against aspirating ovarian cysts. *Cancer* 1993;72:828–831.
64. Bicher A, Sarosy G, Hohn E, et al: Age does not influence taxol dose intensity in recurrent carcinoma of the ovary. *Cancer* 1993;71:594–600.
65. Piver MS, Baker V: The potential for optimal cytoreductive surgery at a tertiary medical center: A prospective study. *Gynecol Oncol* 1986;24:1.
66. Griffiths CT, Parker LM, Fuller AF: Role of cytoreductive surgical treatment in the management of advanced ovarian cancer. *Cancer Treat Rep* 1979;63:255.
67. Lavin, PT, Knapp RC, Malkasian G, Whitney CW, Berek JC, Bast RC Jr: Ca 125 for monitoring of ovarian carcinoma during primary therapy. *Obstet Gynecol* 1987;69:223–227
68. Clarke-Pearson DI, Bandy LC, Dudzinski M, Heaston D, Creasman WT: Computed tomography in evaluation of patient with ovarian carcinoma in complete clinical remission. *JAMA* 1986;255:627–630.
69. Young RC: A second look at the Second look laparotomy. *J Clin Oncol* 1987;9:1311.

Chapter 13

Benign Gynecologic Tumors in the Older Woman

Marvin C. Rulin, MD

When we first see or feel a pelvic tumor, the main thrust of the initial management is to determine whether the mass is benign or malignant. We must therefore focus attention on characteristics of some malignancies as well as benign tumors to distinguish them from each other. In this chapter we describe the gross appearance, etiology, pathogenesis, diagnosis, and treatment of benign pelvic tumors most likely to be found in older women. Histologic descriptions are omitted unless a lesion has special microscopic characteristics.

Vulva

Benign tumors of the vulva can be classified in several ways, but we will follow the approach of Kaufman, Friedrich, and Gardner[1] and divide tumors into two categories, cystic and solid. Our rationale is based on clinical practicality because the physical nature of the lesion often dictates management.

Cysts

Epidermal Inclusion Cysts

These cysts, often erroneously called sebaceous cysts, are the most common benign tumors of the vulva. Although the etiology is uncertain most dermatologists believe they are caused by obstruction of pilosebaceous ducts. These cysts develop in the labia major, are often multiple, less than 1 cm in diameter, round, and yellowish-white. Surgical excision can be accomplished easily under local anesthesia, but intervention is seldom necessary because the cysts are invariably benign and usually asymptomatic. Infection is unlikely, but when it occurs, incision and drainage may be necessary.

Hidradenomas

Hidradenomas arise from apocrine sweat glands, but Woodworth and coworkers[2] make a strong case that some originate in the eccrine sweat glands. Hidradenomas usually occur singly as a well-circumscribed, raised nodule, located on the inner aspect of the labia majora or the labia minora. They are freely movable and may be firm or soft in consistency. Contents of the cyst may erode through the surface as red, granular appearing tissue. Though benign, their histologic appearance may look alarming to the untrained eye because of marked glandular proliferation. Treatment consists of simple local excision.

Cysts of the Canal of Nuck

The canal of Nuck is a rudimentary peritoneal sac that extends along the round ligament through the inguinal canal. The sac should become obliterated during embryonic development, but if it remains open the patient is at risk for hernia formation, cyst formation, or both. When cysts develop, they are analogous to hydrocele in the male scrotum. One would expect canal of Nuck cysts to present early in the reproductive age group, but they may be small and slow-growing, not becoming symptomatic until later in life.

It is important to recognize this potential entity to avoid attempts at local resection. When symptomatic, with or without a demonstrable hernia, the mass should be treated like a hernia with exploration and excision of the sac.

Bartholin Gland Cysts

Though very common and virtually always benign in women under 40 years of age, Bartholin gland cysts become progressively less common with advancing age. When older women present with a swelling in the area of the Bartholin gland, posterolateral to the vaginal fourchette, one must be concerned about a benign or malignant tumor. Biopsy of the lesion is critical in older women to rule out adenocarcinoma.

Solid Tumors

Acrochordons

Acrochordons are polypoid fibroepithelial tumors of unknown etiology, often referred to as skin tags. They are soft, pedunculated, flesh-colored lesions that have a wrinkled appearance. They develop on the vulva, inner aspect of the thigh, or the perianal area as small lesions seldom exceeding 1 cm in diameter. Because these tumors have no malignant potential and seldom become very large, treatment is often unnecessary. When an acrochordon becomes annoying, it can be treated under local anesthesia by excision or by suture ligating the pedicle and allowing the lesion to slough off.

Seborrheic Keratosis

Seborrheic keratosis occasionally involves the vulva, appearing as a sharply defined, slightly raised verrucous lesion. Lesions may be single or occur in clusters. They may be flesh-colored or much darker with a somewhat oily appearance. Treatment is not necessary as long as the diagnosis is certain. Local excision or curettage of very small lesions is effective.

Nevis

Pigmented nevi usually appear during the reproductive years, but dyplastic nevi can present later in life. Nevi may be flat, somewhat raised, or pedunculated, and vary in color from light tan to dark brown. They are usually asymptomatic but may become irritated. The importance of nevi lies in their relationship to malignant melanomas. About one half of malignant melanomas arise in pre-existing pigmented nevi. Those that are flat or multiple have greater malignant potential than single raised nevi. Because of their malignant potential, flat nevi should be excised with 1-cm free borders around and deep to the lesions. Raised or hairy nevi are usually benign.

Basal Cell Carcinomas

Carcinomas are beyond the scope of this chapter, but basal cell carcinomas behave more like benign tumors than malignant ones. They are slow-growing and locally invasive but very rarely metastasize to lymph nodes or other organs. Perrone and coworkers[3] tried to distinguish the characteristics of one case of basal cell carcinoma of the vulva that had spread to the regional lymph nodes from those lesions that remained localized. The metastasizing tumor had an advanced clinical stage, invading the subcutaneous fat, urethra, and vagina, suggesting long-standing disease with deep invasion before metastasis occurred.

Basal cell carcinomas of the vulva are not common but occur principally in postmenopausal women. Siegler and Green[4] reported a median age of 63, and Palladino and coworkers[5] found an average age of 65.8 years. The tumors appear most frequently in the labia majora as slightly raised nodules with central ulceration and pearly rolled edges. They may or may not be pigmented. They may be asymptomatic or cause itching, burning, ulceration, bleeding, or discharge. Because basal cell carcinomas can invade deeply and in rare circumstances can spread to lymph nodes. They are best treated by wide and deep local excision with free margins to ensure total removal.

Mesodermal Tumors

Fibromas, lipomas, lymphangiomas, and hemangiomas occur in the vulva as they do in many other tissues containing mesodermal elements. They usually do not require attention that is different from similar tumors elsewhere in the body. Cherry hemangiomas are dilated capillaries that occur chiefly in older women. They present as bright-red to dark-blue soft papules, which are often multiple and usually only a few millimeters in diameter. They are seldom symptomatic but may bleed if traumatized. If bleeding is a recurring problem, the lesions can be excised or treated by cryosurgery or electrocoagulation under local anesthesia.

A rare but interesting lesion is the granular cell tumor. These tumors are ubiquitous, occasionally appearing on the vulva. Majmudar and coworkers[6] identified eight cases from Grady Memorial Hospital, Atlanta, Georgia, in a 5-year period. Half the cases were in women more than 45 years of age. Granular cell tumors have a characteristic histologic appearance with a tendency to induce a hyperplastic epithelial response. They appear in the labia majora as a firm, slow-growing nodule, less than 4 cm in diameter. They tend to be asymptomatic unless the overlying skin breaks down. Although almost always benign, there are malignant variants that metastasize to other organs. Simple local excision is indicated for diagnosis and treatment.

Vagina

Urethral Caruncles

Although, strictly speaking, urethral caruncles do not arise from the vagina, they are most often found by gynecologists during pelvic examination. Urethral caruncles develop after menopause, probably as a result of vaginal atrophy and subsequent ectropion of the posterior urethra. They appear at the urethral meatus as a smooth but occasionally friable red lesion. They are usually single, sessile, and less than 1 cm in diameter. Most are asymptomatic, but they can occasionally cause pain, dysuria, or bleeding.

Because urethral caruncles are benign and usually asymptomatic, treatment is often not necessary, but care should be taken to distinguish these lesions from carcinoma of the urethra. Marshall and coworkers[7] reported on 394 urethral lesions, 356 of which were caruncles. Of the 38 lesions that were not, 20 were mistakenly diagnosed clinically as caruncles. Six were carcinomas of the urethra. These findings suggest that when the diagnosis is obvious and the patient is asymptomatic, invasive treatment is not necessary. If any doubt exists as to the diagnosis, biopsy can be performed under local anesthesia. Troublesome bleeding can be controlled by direct pressure with sterile gauze pads, but electrofulguration or sutures may be necessary. Benign symptomatic lesions can be treated with topical or systemic estrogen, with surgical excision reserved for resistant cases.

Prolapsed Urethral Mucosa

Prolapse of the urethral mucosa appears in premenarchal girls and postmenopausal women, suggesting lack of estrogen as an etiological factor. It appears as a ring of red edematous tissue surrounding the opening of the urethra. It is usually painless but may bleed or cause difficulty in voiding. The diagnosis is apparent if the physician takes care to identify the urethral opening completely surrounded by mucosa. Friedrich[8] has reported excellent results in treating postmenopausal women with cryosurgery. He recommends the freeze, thaw, freeze technique, with repeat treatment in 6 to 8 weeks, if necessary. Topical or systemic estrogen should be advised as follow-up therapy.

Vaginal Fibroepithelial Polyps

These lesions are rare but occur most commonly in older women, appearing as polypoid folds in the vaginal epithelium. They may appear worrisome histologically but are benign and should not be mistaken for malignancy. They are treated by simple local excision.

Cervix

Cervical Polyps

Very few benign tumors arise in the cervix, but polyps of the cervix or endocervix are common. Their etiology is uncertain but thought to be caused by inflammatory or atrophic changes. Polyps may be smooth or friable, red or grayish, pedunculated or sessile, single or multiple. They vary in size from a few millimeters to 3 cm across their most dependent surface. When pedunculated, the stalk may be thick and vascular or thin and avascular, and it may arise anywhere along the endocervical canal.

Postcoital bleeding and leukorrhea are the symptoms classically associated with cervical polyps, but most polyps are asymptomatic and found incidentally during a pelvic examination. Unless the pedicle appears thick, polyps can be easily managed in the office. The pedicle is grasped with a hemostat and with a gentle twisting motion avulsed from its base. Bleeding is not usually a problem but when present can be controlled with silver nitrate sticks or Monsell's solution. Though virtually always benign, the removed polyp should be fixed in formalin and submitted for histologic examination.

Two caveats are important. (1) If the pedicle is thick and does not twist readily, the procedure should be abandoned and scheduled in a surgical suite where ligation and excision can be carried out. (2) If the patient seeks care because of postmenopausal bleeding and a cervical polyp is found, do not assume the polyp is the case of the bleeding. Endometrial carcinoma must be ruled out! (See endometrial lesions.)

Endometrium

Ultrasonographic Findings

The development of transvaginal ultrasonography has afforded us a noninvasive look at the endometrial lining heretofore available only by hysteroscopy. Although screening of asymptomatic postmenopausal women has not yet been proven to be cost-effective, wider use of ultrasonography has revealed new findings about the endometrium in pre- and postmenopausal women. Figure 13.1 shows a sonogram with a thin endometrial stripe representing the double layer of apposed endometrial linings from the anterior and posterior walls of the uterus. This double thickness results from a normally empty endometrial cavity.

Fleischer and coworkers[9] suggested that a single layer of thickness of 2 to 3 mm was normal in postmenopausal women. Nasri and Coast[10] reported on 63 women with postmenopausal bleeding. Among the 37 women with a double-layer thickness of 5 mm or less, the endometrium was either inactive or no tissue was obtained by dilation and curettage (D&C). The other 26 women with an endometrial lining of more than 5 mm all had endometrial pathology including polyps, hyperplasia, pyometra, or carcinoma. Smith and colleagues[11] found no pathology in 22 women with postmenopausal bleeding when the endometrial lining was 8 mm or less double thickness. Nine women with thicker linings as depicted in Figure 13.2 all had endometrial pathology, including four cancers. It now appears clear that an endometrial stripe of 5 mm or less is very reassuring even when associated with postmenopausal bleeding, but a thicker lining may represent polyps, hyperplasia, or carcinoma.

Endometrial Biopsy

Although ultrasonography provides valuable information about the endometrial lining, histologic analysis remains the foundation for definitive diagnosis and treatment. The classic indication for endometrial biopsy is postmenopausal bleeding, but any abnormal bleeding after age 40 requires endometrial biopsy. Suspicious ultrasonographic findings as described above are a newer but nonetheless important indication as well. In the past, D&C was the standard method to obtain

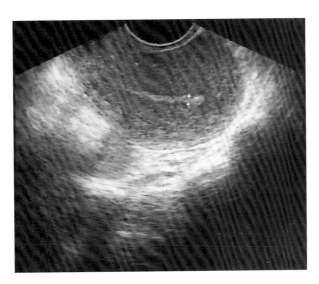

Figure 13.1 Ultrasound view of an atrophic endometrial lining less than 0.5 cm thick.

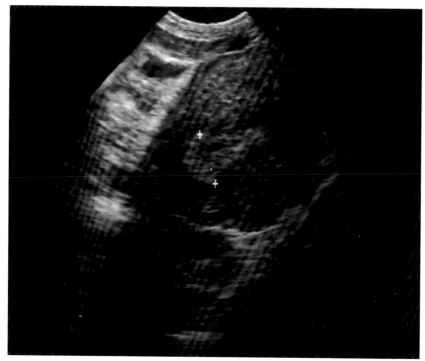

Figure 13.2 Ultrasound view of an endometrial lining 1.2 cm thick.

endometrial tissue, but newer office biopsy techniques have taken over. Traditional D&Cs often required hospitalization and anesthesia, with substantial cost and some risk. Furthermore, Stock and Kanbour[12] showed that D&C was incomplete in 60% of cases undergoing immediate postcurettage hysterectomy. In 1982, Grimes[13] reviewed the literature comparing D&C to Vabra aspiration, a suction biopsy procedure performed in the office usually without anesthesia. He found that Vabra aspiration was safer, less expensive, and obtained more adequate specimens. A meaningful comparison of accuracy in diagnosing endometrial cancer could not be made, but Vabra aspiration had an accuracy rate of 96% while that of D&C was thought to be 90% or lower.

Kaunitz and coworkers[14] subsequently found that a thin, plastic, endometrial suction curette, the Endometrial Pipelle, caused less pain than Vabra aspiration and obtained at least as much tissue, a finding confirmed by others. But the ultimate question is how accurate is the Pipelle in detecting endometrial cancer? Stovall and colleagues[15] performed Pipelle biopsies in the office on 40 women who were to undergo hysterectomy in less than 4 weeks for known endometrial cancer. Of these, 39 revealed endometrial cancer and 1 showed atypical hyperplasia. Histologic grade of the tumor correlated with hysterectomy findings in 83% of cases.

Guido and coworkers[16] performed Pipelle biopsies at the time of hysterectomy for previously diagnosed endometrial cancer. They detected 54 of 65 (83%) cancers. Of the 11 missed cases, 5 were confined to polyps and 4 others were localized to less than 5% of the endometrial surface. The other 2 showed atypical hyperplasia. The difference in sensitivity of these two studies may be related to the extent of the tumor in differing patient populations.

Based on the data above, endometrial suction biopsy performed in the office is the initial procedure of choice to diagnose abnormal endometrial histology, including carcinoma. Thin, flexible, plastic devices are better-tolerated by patients than rigid devices, without sacrificing accuracy. If the initial biopsy shows complex or atypical hyperplasia a full D&C, complemented by either pelvic ultrasonography or hysteroscopy, should be done to rule out a small focus of carcinoma.

Polyps

Endometrial polyps are localized concentrations of endometrial tissue attached by a pedicle. They are covered by endometrial lining on all surfaces. Polyps may be very small, a few millimeters in size, or much larger, filling the endometrial cavity or even protruding through the endocervical canal. A moderate-sized polyp, detected by ultrasonography, is shown in Figure 13.3. Polyps may reflect the same histology as the remainder of the endometrium; they may be hyperplastic or neoplastic, but most commonly in the older woman, they simply reflect an atrophic change in the endometrium. Not surprisingly endometrial polyps are common in older women, being found at autopsy in as many as 10% of women with intact uteri.

Before the advent of ultrasonography, endometrial polyps usually went undiscovered unless a woman had postmenopausal bleeding. They were then identified grossly or microscopically by endometrial sampling or D&C. Because polyps are common and usually asymptomatic, if they are found in a woman with postmenopausal bleeding, we should not assume they are the cause of the bleeding. Benign polyps have been found in approximately 20% of uteri removed for endometrial cancer.

Do polyps undergo malignant change? Pettersson and coworkers[17] estimate that the risk of subsequent carcinoma is twice that of the general population, but it is important to look at the histology of the polyp to assess risk. Those polyps that are atrophic are of very little concern, however, those that show atypical hyperplasia are of major concern and may already exist in a field of cancer.

How should endometrial polyps be managed? When they are discovered by ultrasonography in

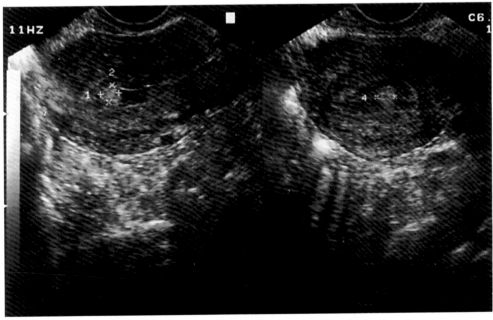

Figure 13.3 Ultrasound view of a 1-cm endometrial polyp.

asymptomatic women, endometrial sampling should be performed in the office. When the histology of the polyp reveals atrophy, no further intervention is necessary. If the polyp is hyperplastic, hysteroscopy and D&C should be performed to rule out carcinoma. If the polyp is associated with postmenopausal bleeding, thorough sampling of the remainder of the endometrium is critical.

Hematometra and Pyometra

Fluid collections that may represent blood or pus may be found on ultrasonography. These findings have been viewed with alarm in the past but in 1994 Goldstein[18] called attention to the lining of the collection rather than the fluid. In his study, 27 postmenopausal women had endometrial fluid collections with a single-layer lining of 3 mm or less. Nine women underwent D&C and had scant tissue reported as inactive endometrium. Eighteen women were followed conservatively, six cases resolved and 12 remained unchanged. Of the three women with thickened endometria one had a polyp and two had hyperplasia.

Hematometra is present when the endometrial cavity contains blood that cannot escape. In the older woman the obstruction to the outflow of blood usually results from atrophic changes in the cervical canal, especially if the cervix has previously been coned, cauterized, radiated, or ablated by laser. Hematometra are often asymptomatic but may cause cramping pain as the uterus tries to expel the blood. The major concern is the possibility of an occult endometrial cancer.

How should we manage older women with hematometra? As stated above, if the patient is asymptomatic and the fluid collection is found on ultrasonography, attention should be focused on the endometrial lining. If the lining is 3 mm or less, observation alone constitutes satisfactory management. If the patient is symptomatic or the endometrial lining exceeds 3 mm, the endometrium must be thoroughly sampled. Dilation of a severely stenotic postmenopausal cervix is seldom successful without anesthesia. Intravenous sedation and paracervical block are usually needed. Care must be taken in probing the endocervical canal to avoid creation of a false passage. Ultrasound guidance may be helpful.

Pyometra is similar to hematometra except that the retained fluid in the endometrial cavity is pus rather than blood. The pus is usually sterile and patients are rarely septic. Principles of treatment are similar to those described for hematometra. Older literature cautioned against curettage in the presence of pyometra, but modern suction techniques appear to be safe. Coverage with intravenous broad-spectrum antibiotics to avert septicemia is probably a good idea, but no controlled studies have been done to support that contention. Antibiotics are clearly indicated—before and after D&C—in the rare patient who is symptomatic with or without fever.

Hyperplasia

Endometrial hyperplasia was first described as a precursor to carcinoma by Cullen in 1900.[19] This concept was reintroduced in the 1930s by Taylor[20] and reinforced in the 1950s by Gusberg and coworkers.[21] It was generally accepted in the literature until the 1980s, when the theory of a progressive continuum of hyperplasia to carcinoma was challenged. Some of the controversy developed because of varying definitions and interpretations of the pathology of hyperplasia.

A standard classification of hyperplasia proposed by the International Society of Gynecological Pathologists should help clarify the pathology and, consequently, the clinical management of this condition. Hyperplasia is either simple or complex, based on its *architecture*. The glands in simple hyperplasia (Figure 13.4) have round to slightly irregular shapes, are increased in proportion to stroma, but there is no crowding. In complex hyperplasia (Figure 13.5) the glands exhibit budding and papillary foldings. They are crowded together with little intervening stroma. Nuclei show

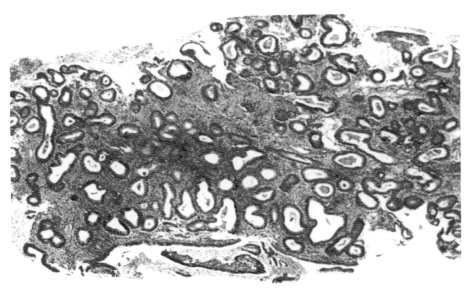

Figure 13.4 Microscopic appearance of simple hyperplasia.

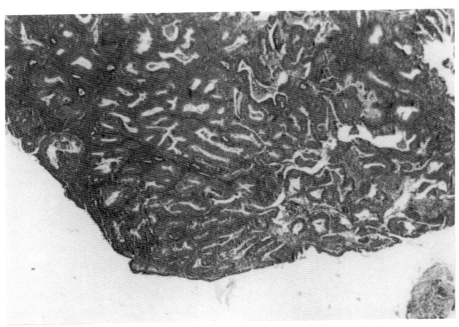

Figure 13.5 Microscopic appearance of complex hyperplasia.

increased stratification but maintain polarity. Atypical hyperplasia refers to cellular changes described as *cytologic* atypia. These changes (Figure 13.6) are characterized by large nuclei of varying size and shape that have lost polarity. Nucleoli are prominent and mitoses present, but there is still some intervening stroma between glands. Atypical hyperplasia may be simple or complex, based on its architecture. The present of cytologic atypia is the critical factor affecting progression to carcinoma.

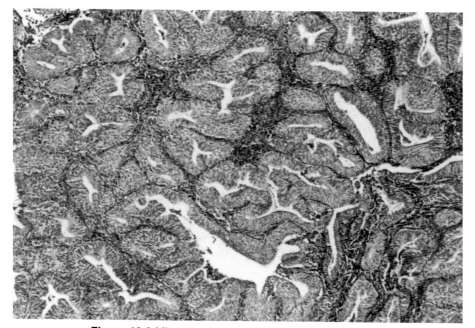

Figure 13.6 Microscopic appearance of cytologic atypia.

Kurman and coworkers[22] reported on 170 untreated patients followed for a mean of 13.4 years after D&Cs that showed varying degrees of hyperplasia. Progression to cancer occurred in 1% of women with simple hyperplasia, 3% with complex hyperplasia, 8% with simple atypical hyperplasia, and 20% with complex atypical hyperplasia. Furthermore, 25% of patients who were diagnosed with complex atypical hyperplasia by D&C had an associated well-differentiated carcinoma found at the time of hysterectomy. Janicek and Rosenshein[23] report an association of endometrial cancer in 43% of women diagnosed with atypical hyperplasia by a variety of sampling techniques.

Management

Given the long-standing confusion of terminology, there is no unanimity of opinion regarding treatment, but certain trends have emerged based on the classification described above. Ferency and Gelfand[24] treated 85 peri- and postmenopausal women with progestins and followed them for 2 to 12 years. Of those, 65 had simple or complex hyperplasia without atypia, and 20 had cytologic atypia. All were diagnosed by D&C under anesthesia. Those without atypia were treated with medroxyprogesterone acetate (MPA) 10 mg/day for 14 days per month. Eighty percent of the lesions regressed completely, 20% persisted. Most of the persistence occurred in women with complex hyperplasia. None developed cancer. Similar results have been reported by Kurman and coworkers[22] and by Gal and colleagues.[25]

Women who had cytologic atypia were treated with 20 mg/day of MPA continuously for six months. Only 5 (25%) lesions regressed, 10 (50%) persisted, and 5 (25%) progressed to endometrial cancer. Studies by Gal[25] and by Wentz[26] showed remission in 92% and 100% of lesions with cytologic atypia using megesteral acetate. Gal used 40 mg/day for 9 to 104 months; Wentz used 80 mg/day in 4 divided doses for 6 weeks. Logical interpretation of these data would suggest the following plan of management.

Simple Hyperplasia Without Atypia

Treat with MPA, 10 mg/day for 10 to 14 days per month for 3 months. Repeat a 10-day course of treatment every 3 months until withdrawal bleeding ceases, then convert to hormone replacement therapy. Subsequent biopsy is unnecessary unless abnormal, unpredictable bleeding occurs. For refractory cases, pelvic ultrasonography should also be obtained to determine endometrial thickness and to rule out an ovarian tumor.

Complex Hyperplasia Without Atypia

Treat with MPA, 20 mg/day, or megesterol acetate, 40 mg/day for 6 to 12 weeks. Following withdrawal, give MPA 10 mg/day for 14 days each month until withdrawal bleeding ceases. Principles governing subsequent biopsy and ultrasonography are similar to those listed above. If patients have progestin-related side effects, such as vaginal dryness, supplementary estrogen can be given.

Hyperplasia With Cytologic Atypia

Hysterectomy with bilateral salpingo-oophorectomy is the treatment of choice for women who are good operative risks. If patients are to be treated nonsurgically either because they are poor operative risks or because they prefer to avoid surgery, pelvic ultrasonography and thorough D&C should be performed to rule out an existing endometrial cancer or ovarian neoplasm. If neither is found, treat with megesterol acetate, 40 to 80 mg/day for 6 months. Repeat an endometrial biopsy, and if regression is demonstrated use MPA, 10 mg/day for 14 days each month until withdrawal bleeding ceases. Follow-up sampling every 6 to 12 months is indicated.

Atrophy

Fully one third of endometrial biopsies performed on women with postmenopausal bleeding will reflect atrophic changes. This may be manifested by too little tissue for analysis or by a small amount of tissue that is diagnosed by the pathologist as atrophic or inactive endometrium. Although such a finding is physiological in the postmenopausal woman, it creates concern for many physicians because the cause of bleeding has not been demonstrated. A careful examination before biopsy to rule out cervical, vaginal, or vulvar lesions will help allay some concern. If the bleeding does not recur, further testing is unnecessary; however, if bleeding persists or recurs, further investigation must be carried out to be certain that a small endometrial lesion or a rare tubal neoplasm has not been missed. Pelvic ultrasonography can detect both of these conditions and, at the same time, can offer reassurance if the endometrial stripe is 5 mm thick or less. If the endometrium shows a localized lesion hysteroscopy and D&C should be performed.

Uterine Leiomyomas

Myomas of the uterus develop from smooth muscle cells in the uterine wall. Their etiology is uncertain, but clinically they seem to be estrogen-dependent. They never appear in premenarchal girls, nor do they arise in postmenopausal women. Nevertheless, they can present problems in the older woman. The usual life-cycle of uterine myomas is growth during the reproductive years and degeneration in the peri- and postmenopausal years as the blood supply to the uterus diminishes. Most commonly the process is gradual, with asymptomatic hyaline degeneration of the myoma.

Myxomatous and calcific degeneration also occur. These bear little clinical significance, but when calcifications in the uterus appear on X-ray examination or with other imaging techniques it is important to recognize their benign nature.

Most myomas in postmenopausal women are asymptomatic. However, occasionally degeneration may occur somewhat rapidly, producing necrosis of parts of the myoma. Pain and/or rapid enlargement of the myoma can result. Pain can usually be controlled with analgesics and, if the process is not extensive, the pain will resolve. Myomas very rarely—if ever—undergo malignant degeneration, but when a tumor of the uterus enlarges rapidly in a postmenopausal woman, a sarcoma must be ruled out because it can arise de novo. When faced with an enlarging uterine mass in a postmenopausal woman, hysterectomy is indicated so that the tumor can be thoroughly analyzed histologically.

The diagnosis of uterine myomas can often be made by pelvic examination, but frequently in older women they are first detected incidentally by ultrasound (US) scan, computed tomography (CT), or magnetic resonance imaging (MRI) as patients are being tested for a variety of other conditions. The appearance of myomas by any of these techniques is usually characteristic and seldom is biopsy or other invasive testing necessary.

The most significant concern about myomas in the postmenopausal woman may be their influence on the decision to initiate hormone replacement therapy (HRT). Because myomas seem to be responsive to estrogen, they are often listed as a contraindication to HRT. Lamminen and coworkers[27] showed by automatic image analysis that leiomyoma cells had no proliferative activity after the climacteric, but when combined with estrogen and progesterone in vitro the quantitative proliferative index increased considerably. Despite this laboratory finding, review of the literature fails to reveal any studies describing an adverse clinical outcome. Maheux and coworkers[28] reported on 10 premenopausal women with myomas who were treated with a gonadotropin-releasing hormone (GnRH) agonist for 1 year, producing a pseudomenopause. Their myomas decreased in volume by 49% within 3 months. Adding back low doses of conjugated estrogens and medroxyprogesterone acetate did not result in an increase in mean myoma volume. This study closely simulates what probably happens clinically in the natural or surgical menopause. The proven benefits of HRT, therefore, seem to far outweigh the theoretical risk of enlarging uterine myomas.

Tamoxifen-Induced Uterine Enlargement

Tamoxifen is a nonsteroidal drug used widely as adjunctive therapy for women with breast cancer. It is also being studied in a large, multicenter trial for its protective effect against breast cancer. Tamoxifen binds to estrogen receptors resulting in contrasting effects, an antiestrogenic action on breast tissue, but an estrogenic effect on the uterus. Concern has been reported regarding a possible link between tamoxifen and the development of endometrial cancer.[29]

The majority of patients taking tamoxifen will show no demonstrable effect on their uteri but Goldstein[30] has described a new, benign finding observed by ultrasonography. The endometrium of five asymptomatic women, 57 to 82 years old, seemed to reveal bizarre, sonolucent areas suggestive of endometrial polyps. Using intrauterine fluid instillation, the lesions were shown to be located subendometrially, deep in the myometrium. Endometrial biopsy in all five cases showed inactive endometrium.

We call attention to this report, even though it is as yet unconfirmed by others, because of the widespread use of tamoxifen in older women. Given the speculation about tamoxifen's association with endometrial cancer, the findings described above should not give rise to an overly aggressive plan of management.

Adnexal Masses

Evaluation of adnexal masses is a very important part of the gynecological care of older women. Ovarian cancer is a devastating disease that is the most frequent cause of death among all gynecological cancers. Early diagnosis has escaped us in the majority of cases, leaving physicians with a strong temptation to intervene surgically for all adnexal masses in older women. Benign tumors, however, are not uncommon in postmenopausal women. Rulin and Preston,[31] in a review of 150 adnexal masses in postmenopausal women, proven by laparotomy, found 103 benign conditions and 47 malignancies. The proportion of benign to malignant lesions decreased with advancing age but did not become even until after the age of 70. The types of benign adnexal masses, subdivided into cystic and solid categories, are listed in Table 13.1 The more common tumors are described briefly, then an overall approach to the diagnosis and management of adnexal masses in postmenopausal women is presented.

Cystic Masses

The most common cystic neoplasms arise from the surface epithelium of the ovary and develop by invagination into the underlying stroma. As the surface of the invagination closes, an epithelial-lined cyst forms. For reasons not understood, the epithelium undergoes metaplasia and may take on mucosal characteristics of the fallopian tube, endocervix endometrium, or even the urinary bladder. Epithelial inclusion cysts are most prevalent in the fifth and sixth decades of life.

Table 13.1 Benign Adnexal Masses

Cystic	*N*
Serous cystadenoma	22
Mucinous cystadenoma	17
Simple cyst	11
Mature teratoma	7
Paratubal cyst	4
Hydrosalpinx	4
Endometrioma	3
Functional cyst	3
Solid	
Fibroma/Thecoma*	10
Uterine myoma	10
Brenner's tumor	6
Nongenital tract	4
Residual ovary	2

*Includes two adenofibromas.

Simple Cysts

The term *simple cyst* is not universally recognized but is used at some institutions to describe cysts that have clear fluid and smooth walls in which no epithelium can be recognized. The absence of epithelium is probably secondary to pressure atrophy and fibrosis, leaving no route of escape for the fluid. These cysts tend not to exceed 3 cm in diameter and are asymptomatic.

Serous Cystadenomas

Serous cystadenomas are lined by epithelium resembling tubal mucosa. The lining can vary from an indifferent cuboidal epithelium to tall columnar cells. The cyst wall is usually smooth, but papillary excrescences may project into the cyst cavity or outward from the surface of the ovary. Serous cystadenomas contain clear fluid, are usually but not always unilocular, and may vary in diameter from less than 5 cm to more than 10 cm. Cysts as large as 30 cm have been reported. Approximately 10% are bilateral, but that percentage increases in older women. Benign serous and mucinous cystadenomas have malignant and borderline counterparts that are beyond the scope of this chapter.

Mucinous Cystadenomas

Mucinous cystadenomas are lined by mucin-containing cells resembling those of the endocervix or intestine. The capsule is usually thick, smooth, and opaque. The interior of the mass is typically multilocated and contains tenacious mucinous material. Only 5% to 10% are bilateral, but mucinous cystadenomas can grow to enormous size.

Mature Cystic Teratomas

Mature teratomas are by far the most common tumors arising from germ cells. They are found predominately in young women but are discovered in postmenopausal women as well. In our series, they constituted 11% of the ovarian cysts found. It is doubtful that teratomas arise in this age group, but they can be present and go unrecognized for many years. When palpable, they may feel cystic or softly solid in consistency. They often have characteristic ultrasonographic findings and may reveal calcification or a toothlike structure on roentgenogram.

Teratomas in the older age groups are almost always mature and benign. When small, they are usually asymptomatic and require no treatment. Larger teratomas, 5 cm or more, may cause symptoms of pelvic pressure or complete torsion, causing acute abdominal pain. In young women ovarian cystectomy is the treatment of choice, but in postmenopausal women oophorectomy is preferred with strong consideration given to removal of the contralateral ovary as well. The decision to use laparoscopy or laparotomy depends on the skill and experience of the surgeon.

Other Cystic Masses

Hydrosalpinx usually results from infection that causes a purulent exudate while closing the fimbriated end of the tube. The exudate is resorbed, but a clear transudate persists. In the majority of cases among postmenopausal women the process is inactive and asymptomatic. A mass may be palpated on pelvic examination or detected by imaging. Size varies but ultrasonographic appearances may be characteristic, showing a fluid-filled, oblong structure overlying a normal-appearing ovary. If the hydrosalpinx is small and the findings characteristic, surgical intervention is not necessary.

Paratubal or parovarian cysts may also be discovered by pelvic examination or ultrasonography. They have virtually no malignant potential, and when small and asymptomatic require no treatment.

Functional cysts and endometriomas are not expected in postmenopausal women but can occasionally be present, especially in the first few years after the last menstrual period. Endometriomas may represent an old inactive process, however, endometroid carcinoma must be ruled out.

Solid Masses

Fibroma and Thecomas

Fibromas and thecomas are described together because, although each can occur in pure form, elements of both tissues are usually present. The tumors arise from the matrix of the ovarian cortical stroma and are composed of connective tissue (fibroma) and gonadal mesenchyme (thecoma). When thecal cells predominate, estrogen activity may result. More commonly, there is a preponderance of fibrous tissue, and the tumor is hormonally inactive. Occasionally glandular elements are present—an adenofibroma. For the sake of expedience all these variations will be referred to as fibromas.

Fibromas are diagnosed most commonly in the 40 to 60 year-old age group. They may be small, very large, unilateral, or bilateral. The cut surface is usually white and trabeculated but may be yellowish, depending on the concentration of thecal elements. Small fibromas are usually asymptomatic and are found incidentally, but large ones may cause pelvic pressure or complete torsion, producing acute abdominal pain. When the pedicle is chronically compressed, partial obstruction of venous return can occur with resultant transudation of fluid into the peritoneal cavity. Ascites, therefore, is sometimes associated with large ovarian fibromas. Meigs' syndrome consists of fibroma, ascites, and hydrothorax, the latter probably resulting from permeation of ascitic fluid through diaphragmatic lymphatics. Excision of the fibroma stops the process and ascitic fluid is resorbed. Small asymptomatic fibromas require no treatment.

Brenner's Tumors

Brenner's tumors are composed of well-circumscribed nests of characteristic epithelial cells embedded in fibrous stroma. The epithelial cells are round or polygonal, have clear margins, and contain clear cytoplasm. Traditionally Brenner's tumors were thought to stem from Walthard cell rests or granulosa cells, but recent studies support the concept of differentiation of ovarian surface epithelium into Wolffian duct epithelium found in the urinary tract.

Brenner's tumors are not rare, especially in older women. About 50% are discovered in women over the age of 50. In our series, they comprised one third of solid, benign ovarian tumors, and 4% of all adnexal masses. They are almost benign and rarely exceed 10 cm in diameter. The diagnosis is rarely made clinically. When a solid mass presumed to be a fibroma is detected and excised, histologic examination reveals the true diagnosis. Treatment in the postmenopausal woman is bilateral oophorectomy.

Other Solid Adnexal Masses

Other benign solid masses may be discovered on pelvic examination, US, CT, or MRI. These may arise from the ovary or fallopian tube, but more often than not they are lesions of adjacent structures. The most common extraovarian mass situated in the adnexa is a leiomyoma arising from the uterus but extending laterally into the adnexal area. This is especially true of myomas that are contained between the leaves of the broad ligament. Ultrasonographers can often make this distinction, but when the ovary is obscured by the mass, a solid tumor of the ovary cannot be ruled out. Laparoscopy is the procedure of choice to make the diagnosis. If a uterine myoma is found and the patient is asymptomatic, further surgery is unnecessary. Virtually all other nonovarian masses need to be excised or at least biopsied for histologic examination. Care must be exercised to exclude lesions of the colon and avoid injury to them.

Ovarian remnant syndrome is the presence of ovarian tissue in the pelvis after hysterectomy with intended bilateral salpingo-oophorectomy. Patients may present with a small mass that may or may not be painful. Retention of ovarian tissue is more common when the initial surgery was performed for adhesive conditions such as endometriosis or pelvic inflammatory disease. Price and coworkers[32] believe that the syndrome is more prevalent than is generally recognized. The ovarian remnant is usually embedded in retroperitoneal adhesions and may cause ureteral compression. Meticulous dissection is required to remove the ovary and avoid injury to adjacent structures.

Management of an Adrenal Mass

We have just described specific benign adnexal masses, but most often we do not know in advance their precise histology; nor do we know for certain whether a mass is benign or malignant. How should we manage the patient in whom an adnexal mass is detected? Since most adnexal masses are asymptomatic until they reach very large sizes, we must use criteria other than symptoms to determine when to operate. In 1971, Barber and Garber[33] described three cases of ovarian cancer in postmenopausal women who were found to have ovaries that were palpable on pelvic examination but not enlarged by premenopausal standards. They coined the term Postmenopausal Palpable Ovary (PMPO) syndrome and advocated abdominal hysterectomy and bilateral salpingo-oophorectomy for all such cases. That became the standard of care in the 1970s and 1980s. Emergence of sophisticated imaging techniques, especially high-resolution vaginal ultrasonography has enabled us to accurately determine the size and internal characteristics of masses. Testing for tumor markers reveals additional information, and the development of operative laparoscopy has afforded new opportunities for diagnosis and treatment. How can we best utilize these technologies to individualize the management of an adnexal mass?

By far the most important question that must be answered is whether the mass is benign or malignant. Granberg and coworkers[34] classified ovarian tumors in women of all ages by their gross appearance and related those findings to whether the mass was benign or malignant. Only one among 296 (0.3%) unilocular cysts was malignant, and it had macroscopically visible vegetation on the inner cyst wall. Four of 203 (2%) solid tumors were malignant. Rates of malignancy increased when lesions were multilocular or had vegetations inside the cyst lining. Because ultrasonography can detect these characteristics, it is logical to analyze its accuracy in predicting whether a mass is benign or malignant.

Herrman and coworkers[35] prospectively assessed by ultrasonography 312 women who subsequently underwent laparotomy for an adnexal mass. Benign tumors were predicted correctly in 177 of 185 cases (95.6%). Among 48 purely cystic tumors under 10 cm in diameter there were no malignancies. Andolf and Jörgensen[36] reviewed cystic lesions diagnosed by ultrasonography in women more than 50 years of age. Among 58 anechoic lesions less than 5 cm in diameter, none were malignant. There were 3 malignancies among 33 anechoic lesions greater than 5 cm in diameter, and 8 malignancies in 18 cysts, which contained several septa. Goldstein and coworkers[37] reported on 42 postmenopausal women with unilocular cysts without septation. Twenty-six were operated on, and the cysts were found to be benign. The other 16 were followed conservatively, and only one required surgery for increasing size. It, too, was benign.

There are isolated case reports in the literature of malignancy in a purely cystic, less than 5 cm in diameter cyst. Maiman, Seltzer, and Boyce[38] surveyed 156 members of the society of gynecologic oncologists concerning ovarian neoplasms found to be malignant after laparoscopic surgery. Twenty-nine responders reported a total of 42 cases. In 13 cases the masses were 8 cm or less, cystic, and unilocular. The denominator from which these 13 cases is taken is impossible to know, but in a 1988 survey of the American Association of Gynecologic Laparoscopists, 24% of the members reported performing almost 37,000 operative laparoscopies; ovarian cysts were the third most common indication.

Because studies use different age groups and classify lesions by different sizes, it becomes impossible to simply add numerators and denominators to arrive at an accurate determination of prevalence. However, it is clear that purely cystic unilocular lesions 5 cm or less in diameter with no internal echoes have an extremely low rate of malignancy, probably below 1%. As size and presence of internal echoes increases, the risk of malignancy rises.

Doppler color flow ultrasonography is a relatively new imaging technique used transvaginally that is potentially capable of differentiating benign from malignant masses. Fast-growing tumors such as ovarian cancer contain newly formed blood vessels that have little smooth muscle in their walls. Vascular resistance is therefore decreased and pulsatility increased. When compared with standards, indices can be calculated for any tumor. In a study of 115 pelvic masses, Timor-Tritsch and coworkers[39] prospectively compared Doppler color flow-directed measurements with Sassone and coworkers'[40] scoring system based on traditional ultrasonographic findings. Sensitivity for diagnosing malignancies was 94% for each technique. By adding color flow resistance and pulsatility indices to traditional ultrasonographic criteria, specificity was improved from 87% to 99% and positive predictive value increased from 60% to 94%. At the time of this writing, Doppler color flow-directed ultrasound machines are very expensive and their usefulness and cost-effectiveness in the diagnosis of pelvic masses have not be established, but the technology holds promise for the future.

Tumor Markers

There are currently at least 20 tumor markers for ovarian cancer but all are nonspecific and relatively insensitive in detecting early disease. CA-125 is the only one approved by the FDA for monitoring ovarian cancer and has become the most widely used marker in assessing ovarian cysts preoperatively. Malkasian and coworkers'[41] multicenter center study contained 58 postmenopausal women with ovarian cancers of varying stages and 34 with benign ovarian neoplasms. Using 35 U/ml as the cut-off, sensitivity was 81% and specificity 91%. CA-125 was not elevated in most borderline tumors or mucinous carcinomas. The ability of CA-125 to detect stage I ovarian cancer has been reported to be as low as 23% and no higher than 81%. At this time the clinical value of tumor makers has not been established in differentiating benign from malignant tumors, however, when the CA-125 level is more than 35 U/ml in a postmenopausal woman, cancer must be ruled out. Normal values (35 U/ml or less) associated with ovarian cysts may be somewhat reassuring if benign characteristics are found by transvaginal ultrasonography.

Laparoscopy or Laparotomy?

The development of operative laparoscopy has opened a whole new approach and much controversy to the management of adnexal masses. Although improvement in operative mortality, serious morbidity, and total hospital costs have not been demonstrated, less postoperative pain, faster return to normal activities, and decreased hospital stays make operative laparoscopy an attractive choice over traditional laparotomy for the surgical management of benign ovarian tumors. The most prevalent controversy centers on the consequences of laparoscopic surgery performed for unsuspected ovarian cancers, but there are others.

What is the role of laparoscopic puncture in the diagnosis and treatment of pelvic masses? Aspiration of ovarian cysts for cytologic analysis has been associated with a 60% false-negative rate. Even in vitro irrigation of cysts failed to improve on the accuracy of cytologic analysis, indicating that the poor yield does not result from deficiencies in technique but rather the pathophysiology of the tumor. Aspiration as a method of treatment is no better. Recurrence rates are as high as 40%. Those cysts that do not recur probably have inactive linings that require no surgical intervention in the first place.

One should not be tempted to use laparoscopy for cases in which laparotomy would not be considered just because laparoscopy is thought to be a less traumatic procedure. A mass should be assessed as to whether or not it requires surgery and then, based on the characteristics of the mass, the condition of the patient, and the skill and experience of the surgeon, a decision should be made about operative approach. The amount of tissue to be removed should not be compromised by this decision. Once surgery has been decided on, how safe and effective is operative laparoscopy in the postmenopausal woman? Parker and Berek[42] initially reported a pilot study of 25—subsequently expanded to 48—carefully screened adnexal masses, treated by laparoscopy. All masses were predicted to be benign based on ultrasonography findings of a purely cystic mass less than 10 cm in diameter with distinct borders, no irregular solid parts, thick septa, ascites, or matted bowel. Serum CA-125 levels were less than 35 U/ml. All masses were proven to be benign. Of the 48 masses, 45 were successfully removed by laparoscopy, 3 required laparotomy: 1 for a bowel injury, 1 because of an inconclusive frozen section, and 1 to remove metastic breast cancer found independently along with a benign cyst. All patients recovered. Average operating time was 63 minutes, average postoperative hospital stay was 12 hours, and return to normal activity averaged 5 days.

In skilled, experienced hands laparoscopy has a definite role in the management of adnexal masses in older women, but screening criteria must be followed to minimize the risk of encountering a malignant tumor. As operative laparoscopy gains wider usage, an unsuspected ovarian cancer will occasionally be found even after careful screening. Two possibilities create concern, delay in treatment and spillage of cancer cells. In the Society of Gynecologic Oncologists' survey, definitive treatment was delayed by a mean of 4.8 weeks when ovarian cancer was found unexpectedly. This should not happen if careful inspection and frozen section of the cyst lining are carried out at the time of operation and the surgeon and patient are always prepared for a possible laparotomy. Laparoscopic technique requires aspiration of the cyst to remove it through a small puncture wound. In the process, tumor cells can be spilled into the peritoneal cavity. Retention of tumor cells is possible despite through lavage. Recent studies, however, indicate that rupture of malignant ovarian cysts does not alter the prognosis, once the influence of advanced tumor grade and the presence of adhesions and/or ascites have been discounted.

Summary

Constructing an algorithm based on the information given above is tempting, but too many variables still exist to develop a definitive plan. Some principles need to be reinforced. At present, ultrasonography is the most accurate and cost-effective method of predicting whether a mass is benign or malignant. When CA-125 levels are normal it is somewhat reassuring but when elevated further investigation is required to rule out cancer. Purely cystic ovarian enlargements less than 5 cm in diameter are rarely malignant and if asymptomatic can be followed by repeat ultrasonography in 3 months and again 6 months later. If no growth occurs, further follow-up need not be done more than yearly. Purely cystic tumors between 5 and 10 cm in diameter are in the gray zone. They are expected to be benign, however, in women who are good surgical risks they should be removed because the incidence of malignancy begins to increase and cysts of that size probably have active linings. The choice of laparoscopy versus laparotomy depends on the skill and experience of the surgeon. Cystic masses greater than 10 cm and smaller ones containing internal echoes should have an exploratory laparotomy in which the surgeon and patient are prepared for definitive cancer staging and treatment.

References

1. Kaufman RH, Friedrich EG Jr, Gardner HL: *Benign Diseases of the Vulva and Vagina*, ed 3. Chicago, Year Book Publishers, 1989.
2. Woodworth H, Dockerty MB, Wilson RB, Pratt JH: Papillary hidradenoma of the vulva. A clinical pathologic study of 69 cases. *Am J Obstet Gynecol* 1971;110:501–508.
3. Perrone T, Twiggs LV, Adcock LL, et al: Vulval basal cell carcinoma: An infrequently metastasizing neoplasm. *Int J Gynecol Pathol* 1987;6:512–516.
4. Siegler AM, Green HJ: Basal cell carcinoma of the. *Am J Obstet Gynecol* 1951;62:1219.
5. Palladino US, Duffy JL, Guves GJ: Basal cell carcinoma of the vulva. *Cancer* 1969;24:460–470.
6. Majmudar B, Castellano PZ, Wilson RW, Siegel RJ: Granula cell tumors of the vulva. *J Reprod Med* 1990;35:1008–1014.
7. Marshall FC, Uson AC, Melicow MD: Neoplasm and urethral caruncles of the female urethra. *Surg Gynecol Obstet* 1960;110:723.
8. Friedrich EG Jr: Cryosurgery for urethral prolapse. *Obstet Gynecol* 1977;50:359–361.
9. Fleischer AC, Kalemeris GC, Machin JE, Entman SS, James RE: Sonographic depiction of normal and abnormal endometrium with histopathologic correlation. *J Ultrasound Med* 1986;5:445–452.
10. Nasri MN, Coast GJ: Correlation of ultrasound findings and endometrial histopathology in postmenopausal women. *Br J Obstet Gynecol* 1989;96:1333–1338.
11. Smith P, Bakos O, Heimer G, Ulmsten U: Transvaginal ultrasound for identifying endometrial abnormality. *Acta Obstet Gynecol Scand* 1991;70:591–594.
12. Stock RS, Kanbour A: Prehysterectomy curettage. *Obstet Gynecol* 1975;45:537–541.
13. Grimes DA: Diagnostic dilation and curettage: A reappraisal. *Am J Obstet Gynecol* 1982;142:1–6.
14. Kaunitz AM, Masciello A, Ostrowski M, Rovina EZ: Comparison of endometrial biopsy with the Endometrial Pipelle and Vabra Aspirator. *J Reprod Med* 1988;33:427–431.
15. Stovall TG, Photopulos GJ, Poston WM, Ling FW, Sandles LG: Pipelle endometrial sampling in patients with known endometrial cancer. *Obstet Gynecol* 1991;77:954–956.
16. Guido RS, Kanbour-Shakir A, Rulin MC, Christopherson WA: Pipelle endometrial sampling: Sensitivity in the detection of endometrial cancer *J Reprod Med* in press.
17. Peterson B, Adami HO, Lindgren A, et al: Endometrial polyps and hyperplasia at risk factors for endometrial carcinoma. *Acta Obstet Gynecol Scand* 1985;64:653.
18. Goldstein S. Postmenopausal fluid collections revisited: Look at the doughnut rather than the hole. *Obstet Gynecol* 1994;83:738–740.
19. Cullen TS: *Cancer of the Uterus*. Appleton, New York, 1900.
20. Taylor HC Jr: Endometrial hyperplasia and carcinoma of the body of the uterus. *Am J Obstet Gynecol* 1932;23:309.
21. Gusberg SB, Moore DB, Martin F: Precursors of corpus cancer II. A clinical and pathological study of adenomatous hyperplasia. *Am J Obstet Gynecol* 1954;68:1472.
22. Kurman RJ, Kaminski PF, Norris HS: The behavior of endometrial hyperplasia: A long term study of "untreated" hyperplasia in 170 patients. *Cancer* 1985;56:403–412.
23. Janicek MF, Rosenshein, NB: Invasive endometrial cancer in uteri resected for atypical endometrial hyperplasia. *Gynecol Oncol* 1994;52:373–378.
24. Ferency A, Gelfand M: The biologic significance of cytologic atypia in progestogen-treated endometrial hyperplasia. *Am J Obstet Gynecol* 1989;160:126–131.
25. Gal D, Edman CD, Vellios F, Forney PJ: Long-term effect of megesterol acetate in the treatment of endometrial hyperplasia. *Am J Obstet Gynecol* 1983;146:316–322.

26. Wentz WB: Progestin therapy in endometrial hyperplasia. *Gynecol Oncol* 1974;2:362–367.
27. Lamminen S, Rantala I, Helin H, Rorarius M, Tuimala R: Proliferative activity of uterine leiomyoma cells as measured by automatic image analysis. *Gynecol Invest* 1992;34(2):111–114.
28. Maheux R, Lemay A, Blanchet P, Friede J, Pratt X: Maintained reduction of uterine leiomyoma following addition of hormonal replacement therapy to a monthly luteinizing hormone-releasing hormone agonist implant: A pilot study. *Hum Reprod* 1991;6:500–505.
29. Gal D, Kopel S, Bashevkin M, et al: Oncogenic potential of tamoxifen on endometria of postmenopausal with breast cancer—a preliminary report. *Gynecol Oncol* 1991;42:120–123.
30. Goldstein SR: Unusual ultrasonographic appearance of the uterus in patients receiving tamoxifen. *Am J Obstet Gynecol* 1994;170:447–451.
31. Rulin MC, Preston AL: Adnexal masses in postmenopausal women. *Obstet Gynecol* 1987;70:578.
32. Price FV, Edwards R, Buchsbaum HJ: Ovarian remnant syndrome: difficulties in diagnosis and management. *Obstet Gynecol Surv* 1990;45:151–156.
33. Barber RK, Garber EA: The postmenopausal palpable ovary syndrome. *Obstet Gynecol* 1971;38:921.
34. Granberg S, Wikland M, Jansson I: Macroscopic characterization of ovarian tumors and the relation to the histologic diagnosis: Criteria to be used for ultrasound evaluation. *Gynecol Oncol* 1989;35:139–144.
35. Herrman UJ Jr, Locher GW, Goldhirsch A: Sonographic patterns of ovarian tumors: Prediction of malignancy. *Obstet Gynecol* 1987;69:777–781.
36. Andolf E, Jörgensen C: Cystic lesions in elderly women, diagnosed by ultrasound. *Br J Obstet Gynecol* 1989;96:1076–1079.
37. Goldstein SR, Subramanyam B, Snyder JR, Beller U, Raghavendra BN, Beckman EM: The postmenopausal cystic adnexal mass: The potential role of ultrasound in conservative management. *Obstet Gynecol* 1989;73:8–10.
38. Maiman M, Seltzer V, Boyce J: Laparoscopic excision of ovarian neoplasms subsequently found to be malignant.
39. Timor-Tritsch IE, Lerner JP, Monteagudo A, Santos R: Transvaginal ultrasonographic characterization of ovarian masses by means of color flow-directed doppler measurements and a morphologic scanning system. *Am J Obstet Gynecol* 1993;168:909–913.
40. Sassone AM, Timor-Tritch IE, Artner A, Westhoff C, Warren W: Transvaginal sonographic characterization of ovarian disease. *Obstet Gynecol* 1991;78:70–76.
41. Malkasian GD Jr., Knapp RC, Lavin PT, Zurawski VR Jr, Podratz KC, Stanhope CR, Mortel R, Berek JS, Bast RC Jr, Ritts RE: Preoperative evaluation of serum CA 125 levels in premenopausal and postmenopausal patients with pelvic masses: Discrimination of benign from malignant disease. *Am J Obstet Gynecol* 1988;159:341–346.
42. Parker WH, Berek JS. Management of the adnexal mass by operative laparoscopy. *Clin Obstet Gynecol* 1993;36:413–422.

Chapter 14

Hypertension and Arthrosclerosis

George N. Aagaard, MD

Hypertension is a major risk factor for stroke, coronary heart disease, congestive heart failure, and kidney failure. For several years an intensive educational campaign has been waged to make physicians and the public more aware of hypertension and its possible consequences. One good result of these efforts has been that many people have become aware of their elevated blood pressure. A questionable outcome is that many patients with mild hypertension may have received drug therapy when other methods of treatment may have been more appropriate. This is an important problem since 70% of newly discovered hypertension is in the "mild" range (diastolic 90 to 100 mm Hg). This discussion of hypertension suggests ways in which physicians can help older women with high blood pressure.

The determination of blood pressure is an important part of the examination of an older woman. It is important to give the patient an opportunity to relax for 5 minutes in the sitting or supine position. My usual practice is to take a series of readings first in the supine position, continuing until the pressure is stable. Next, the pressure is checked in the standing position. Going from supine to standing in that order gives the best opportunity to detect a postural drop in pressure, a not uncommon problem in older patients. Finally, the blood pressure is taken in the sitting position, with a series of readings until it is stabile.

Blood pressure may vary considerably between visits and will usually be higher on the first visit. Therefore, if blood pressure is elevated on the initial visit it should be rechecked at two subsequent visits.

In dealing with populations, blood pressures differ slightly with age and between genders. The National Health and Nutrition Survey of 1971 to 1974 showed that the average systolic pressure increased from age 7 years to age 74, while diastolic pressure tended to peak at 50 years. Hamilton reported mean blood pressures of 159.1/92.4 mm Hg in females aged 60 to 64 years, and 175.3/93.1 mm Hg for ages 70 to 74.[1] The systolic pressures probably reflect changes in the large arteries caused by aging. The mean systolic pressure of women is slightly lower than that of men until age 50 years. The diastolic pressure of women averages slightly lower than men until the seventh decade.

In evaluating older women it is important to recognize that falsely high diastolic pressure is not uncommon. Spence and coworkers have pointed out that pseudohypertension should be considered if the diastolic pressure is 110 mm Hg or greater and there are no clinical signs of secondary hypertension change (funduscopic changes, abnormal electrocardiogram, cardiomegaly on chest radiograph, or impaired kidney function).[2] Spence studied 24 subjects who were over 60 years of age. In 12, diastolic pressure measured by the indirect method with a regular size adult cuff was 30 mm Hg or more higher than the direct arterial reading.

Messerili and coworkers have suggested a clinical test for pseudohypertension, which he has called the Osler maneuver.[3] The examiner identifies the pulsating radial or brachial artery. The pressure in the cuff is then pumped up until it exceeds the systolic pressure, obliterating the pulse. If the artery, no longer pulsating, is definitely palpated the test is positive. The assumption is that the thickened and stiff arterial wall resists the external pressure of the cuff, resulting in a falsely high reading.

Prevalence of Hypertension

The prevalence of hypertension in the 1976 to 1980 National Health Survey was 44% in whites 65 to 74 years of age, and 60% in blacks. Hypertension was diagnosed when three readings taken on a single visit averaged 160/95 mm Hg or greater. The World Health Organization has also recognized 160/95 mm Hg as the beginning level of hypertension. With time, the level at which hypertension has been diagnosed has been moved significantly lower. The Fifth Report of the Joint National Committee sets less than 130 and less than 85 mm Hg as the normal range of systolic and diastolic blood pressures, respectively. Readings of 130–139/85–89 mm Hg are classified as high-normal. Mild hypertension begins at 140 mm Hg systolic and 90 mm Hg diastolic.

Isolated systolic hypertension (an elevated systolic pressure with a normal diastolic pressure) is more common in elders. It is probably a manifestation of the increased stiffness of the arteries that occurs with age. The Fifth Report suggests that isolated systolic hypertension should be diagnosed when the systolic pressure is over 140 mm Hg and the diastolic pressure is under 90 mm Hg.

Health Risks of Hypertension

It is important to consider the risks associated with hypertension because physicians must evaluate the hazards of an illness in making a decision regarding therapy. Life insurance data show that mortality increases with both systolic and diastolic pressure independently. The increased mortality begins at 128 to 137 mm Hg systolic and 78 to 82 mm Hg diastolic. In such studies the mortality of a group with blood pressure in a given range is compared with the mortality of the general population of the same age. The latest report of the National Committee states that mortality is lowest for adults at an average systolic pressure less than 120 mm Hg and an average diastolic less than 80 mm Hg.[4]

It is difficult to separate the effect of age and elevated blood pressure on mortality and the incidence of cardiovascular disease. Both mortality and cardiovascular disease incidence increase sharply with each decade after 55 years. The effect of age is much more powerful, but hypertension has an unfavorable effect on both mortality and cardiovascular disease incidence.

The Framingham study reported increased annual mortality and increased incidence of cardiovascular disease (coronary heart disease, congestive heart failure, cerebrovascular disease, and intermittent claudication) with increased blood pressure in women.[5] The unfavorable influence of an elevated diastolic pressure appeared to be less marked in women aged 65 to 74 than in those aged 55 to 64.

Other studies also suggest that hypertension has relatively less impact on older than middle-aged women. Fry observed 704 hypertensives in a London suburban practice over a twenty year period.[6] He found that in hypertensives the ratio of observed to expected deaths was 6.21 in women age 30 to 39 years and 0.80 in women 70 years and older. This suggests that the older hypertensives had a more favorable outlook than the normotensive women of their own age.

Mattila and coworkers followed 561 very old people—all were 85 years of age or older—for 5 years.[7] The greatest mortality was observed in those with the lowest systolic and diastolic pressures. Mortality was lowest in subjects with systolic pressure of 160 mm Hg or greater and with diastolic pressure of 90 mm Hg or greater. Those with lower blood pressure were leaner and had lower levels of blood glucose, serum cholesterol, and hematocrit. This suggests that the subjects with the lowest blood pressure were in a poorer state of health and that this may have contributed to their poor survival rate. However, it is important to note that the very old subjects with blood pressure greater than 160 mm Hg systolic and 90 mm Hg diastolic had the best five-year survival record.

Anderson and Cowan examined 423 men and women of age 70 to 89 years.[8] Mean systolic and diastolic blood pressures were 167.1 and 87.3 mm Hg, respectively. They found no relationship between systolic or diastolic pressure and survival.

It is difficult to interpret these studies, which suggests that hypertension has less impact on older women. In cross-sectional studies it is possible that the most vulnerable subjects have been eliminated, leaving a more resistant population. This could falsely make the incidence of complications and the death rate appear to be low. However, this criticism does not apply to the prospective survival–type study.

Another factor that may confound the studies on the influence of hypertension on health in the elderly is the possibility of pseudohypertension. It is possible that some of the subjects who apparently had higher readings were really normotensive. Efforts to identify pseudohypertension were made in only a few studies. It is likely that pseudohypertension is more frequent with increasing age.

The presence of left ventricular hypertrophy (LVH) definitely increases the chances of complications of hypertension, especially coronary heart disease manifestations. This is true whether LVH is diagnosed by electrocardiogram or echocardiography. Evidence of LVH is often present on echocardiography when the electrocardiogram is normal. LVH by echocardiography may be present when BP is normal. Normotensive children with a hypertensive parent may show LVH by echocardiogram when the blood pressure is still normal. Obese normotensive adults may show increased left ventricular mass.[9,10]

Hyperinsulinemia, evidence of insulin resistance, increased blood glucose, and central obesity have been observed in a significant number of hypertensive patients. In fact, young people with normal blood pressure but with a hypertensive parent are more likely to have hyperinsulinemia along with evidence of dyslipidemia than are controls.[11]

Efficacy of Drug Treatment

Great controversy exists over the blood pressure level at which drug therapy of hypertension is indicated. There is no doubt that hypertension is a risk factor for stroke, coronary heart disease, and congestive heart failure. The difficult questions are: Does drug treatment of hypertension reduce morbidity and mortality? At what level of blood pressure does this favorable effect occur? These questions are not easily answered because factors other than blood pressure must be considered.

In general, it is true that the higher the pretreatment diastolic pressure, the greater the favorable effect of drug treatment. The VA study of moderate-to-severe hypertension (diastolic pressure 115 mm Hg and 129 mm) showed a profound effect of drug treatment on deaths and complications in treated subjects as compared with controls.[12] However, in the mild-to-moderate hypertensive patients, drug therapy did not have a significant effect on those with entering diastolic pressures of 90 to 104 mm Hg but did cause a decrease in morbidity and mortality in those in the 105 to 114 mm Hg stratum.[13]

Many clinical trials have been reported since the VA study. They vary considerably in design and results. The US Public Health Service study of mild-to-moderate hypertension showed no significant effect of drug treatment in a group of subjects, 80% of whom had baseline diastolic pressures of 90 to 104 mm Hg and 20% of 105 to 114 mm Hg.[14] The Australian study of mild hypertension had subjects with entry diastolic pressures of 95 to 109 mm Hg.[15] A small but significant benefit was found in complication rate. It is interesting to note that in 50% of the placebo-treated subjects diastolic pressure fell below 95 mm Hg and remained so for the three-year study period.

The British Medical Research Council study had subjects with entry diastolic pressures of 90 to 109 mm Hg.[16] The investigators found a small but significant reduction in strokes in the subjects who received the active drugs. However, the report states that one would have to treat 850 patients for one year to prevent one stroke.

Several studies have combined large clinical trials in an effort to determine if larger numbers might reveal significant results of treatment. MacMahon, Cutler and coworkers studied data from nine prospective trials involving 30,000 to 40,000 subjects. The authors found 37% fewer strokes and 23% fewer cardiac deaths and nonfatal myocardial infarctions in drug-treated patients versus placebo-treated controls.[17] Collins, Peto, and coworkers reviewed 14 reports of randomized trials and found a 42% reduction in strokes and a 14% reduction in manifestations of coronary heart disease.[18] These studies illustrate the point that drug treatment is more effective in preventing strokes and deaths from stroke than in preventing coronary heart disease manifestations.

Does Drug Treatment of Hypertension Increase the Risk of Myocardial Infarction or Sudden Cardiac Death?

A disappointing finding of most clinical trials of hypertension treatment has been the failure to show that drug treatment reduces the frequency of manifestations of coronary heart disease. In fact, there is evidence that drug treatment may have an adverse effect.

Steward followed 169 patients with severe hypertension.[19] He found that those under treatment whose diastolic pressure was below 90 mm Hg had a greater risk of having a myocardial infarction than those with pressures of 100 to 109 mm Hg.

The Multiple Risk Factor Intervention Trial Research Group also showed that intensively treated subjects had an increased death rate from coronary heart disease.[20] The report suggests that this may have been due to cardiac arrhythmias secondary to diuretic therapy. However, the data in the report also suggest that low blood pressure during treatment may have been a factor.

Cruickshank and coworkers found that mortality from myocardial infarction followed a J-shaped curve in hypertensives receiving drug therapy.[21] Below a diastolic pressure of 85 mm Hg mortality increased. This was true for subjects who had some evidence of ischemic heart disease on entry into the study. In a 12-year study of hypertensive men Samuelsson and coworkers found that cardiovascular morbidity was lowest at a treatment diastolic pressure of 86 to 89 mm Hg and increased when diastolic pressure was below 86 mm Hg.[22] This was true for all of the subjects in the study and was not limited to those who had evidence of ischemic heart disease on entry into the study.

Farnett and coworkers reviewed 13 studies that stratified cardiovascular outcomes by level of achieved blood pressure.[23] Their studies showed a consistent J-shaped relationship for cardiac events and diastolic blood pressure. The beneficial threshold point was 85 mm Hg. Below that level there was an increased risk of cardiac events.

Langer and coworkers reported a study of men 75 years and older. Those who took antihypertensive drugs and had a decrease of 5 mm Hg or greater had higher all-cause mortality and cardiovascular mortality rates.[24]

Floras treated 34 symptom-free hypertensive patients without clinical evidence of coronary heart disease.[25] Average clinical blood pressure was 176/108 mm Hg before treatment and 151/95 mm Hg after 5 months of treatment with a beta blocker. Intra-arterial blood pressure was measured for 24 hours before treatment and after 5 months of treatment. During sleep, mean hourly diastolic pressures of 50 mm Hg or less were recorded in 11 patients.[25] Only two had had pressures in this range before treatment. After treatment, some patients had diastolic pressures during sleep of 30 mm Hg or less. Such low diastolic pressures are a matter of concern because myocardial perfusion occurs during diastole and is dependent on diastolic pressure. Patients with myocardial ischemia or left ventricular hypertrophy might have poor perfusion at such low diastolic pressures. Also, patients with silent coronary artery stenosis might be at risk for coronary thrombosis if coronary blood flow were reduced.

It is possible that patients with coronary heart disease may be more likely to suffer a myocardial infarction if blood pressure is lowered excessively with drug therapy. Because older women are more likely to have coronary artery narrowing than younger women, it seems wise to be cautious in our use of drug therapy. This is especially true in those with mild hypertension, because in such patients drug therapy may more readily reduce diastolic pressure to levels at which risk of myocardial infarction may be increased.

Hygienic Methods of Treatment

Hygienic methods of treatment of hypertension include weight reduction in patients who are over ideal body weight, restriction of dietary salt, moderation of alcohol intake, avoidance of tobacco, recreational exercise, and psychological and behavioral methods. In general, these measures promote health and make patients feel and function better. Properly applied, they do not have troublesome adverse effects. Some, such as restricting diet, may require a measure of self-discipline. Recreational exercise, on the other hand, may give pleasure and entertainment and add to the enjoyment of life.

Hygienic methods will bring the blood pressure of most women with mild hypertension to a satisfactory level without the need for drugs. In patients with moderate or severe hypertension, these methods may make it possible to control blood pressure with fewer drugs and with smaller doses of drugs. Hygienic methods should, therefore, be the foundation of every treatment program for hypertension.

Reduction of Body Weight

In populations, there is a correlation between body weight and blood pressure. It is also true that in populations an upward change in body weight correlates with an increase in blood pressure. Conversely, reduction of body weight is a powerful method of lowering blood pressure. Stamler and coworkers followed a group of overweight men for 5 years.[26] Their average weight loss was 12 pounds. The average blood pressure decrease was 13/10 mm Hg. Reisin and coworkers reported a significant decrease in blood pressure in hypertensive patients who had a average weight loss of 10 kg over a 6-month period.[27] In general, it can be said that a reduction of 10 to 15 pounds in weight will reduce blood pressure to the same degree as the administration of full doses of an antihypertensive drug.

It is possible that weight loss causes a decrease in sympathetic nervous system activity or catecholamine metabolism. Young and Landsberg measured norepinephrine turnover rate in cardiac muscle.[28] They found an increase with forced feeding and a decrease with fasting. Jung and coworkers followed obese women on a low carbohydrate diet.[29] The authors found a decrease of urine 4-hydroxy-3-methoxy-mandelate and in plasma norepinephrine concentration.

Another mechanism that may contribute to the blood pressure lowering effect of weight loss may be its effect on glucose metabolism and insulin sensitivity. In recent years it has been noted that hypertension may be preceded by higher blood glucose levels with an oral glucose challenge, higher plasma insulin levels, insulin resistance, and obesity.[11] Weight reduction will shift glucose and insulin blood levels toward normal and reduce blood pressure. Thus, a reduced risk of diabetes, coronary heart disease, and hypertension may result.

It is encouraging to note that weight reduction will reduce blood pressure in subjects with high-normal readings. Thus, it appears that hypertension can be prevented by caloric restriction and exercise.[30]

Many physicians take a pessimistic view of the prospects of helping patients to reduce body weight. Perhaps, they are influenced by results reported in the management of morbid obesity. Fortunately, in hypertension we are dealing with patients who are, on the average, only 25% over ideal body weight. They have a powerful motivation for weight reduction in their elevated blood pressure. An additional inducement is the fact that a reduction in weight is likely to have a favorable effect on blood lipids.

It is important for physicians to take an active and continuing role in helping hypertensive patients to reduce weight and to monitor weight carefully so that the benefits of a lowered blood pressure may continue. I recommend that patients check their weight each morning under standard conditions. If weight increases more than 2 pounds above the maximum that the patient and physician have agreed on, the diet should be restricted until the weight returns to within the desired range.

Restriction of Dietary Salt

Population studies show a correlation of salt intake and blood pressure. Page and coworkers have published an excellent review of this subject.[31] Oliver and coworkers observed people of the Yanomamo tribe who live in the area that borders Venezuela and Brazil.[32] Salt had never been introduced into their culture. Blood pressure did not increase on the average after the second decade of life. Averages for females over 50 years of age were 106 mm Hg systolic and 64 mm Hg diastolic.

An increase in salt intake in individuals may cause an increase in blood pressure. Mark and coworkers gave young men with borderline hypertension an oral salt load.[33] Blood pressure and vascular resistance was increased and blood flow was decreased. These responses were not observed in normotensive controls.

Dietary salt restriction was reported by Allen to be effective in lowering blood pressure in hypertensives.[34] Some of the patients had extremely high diastolic pressures. Kempner described dramatic reductions in blood pressures following the use of the rice and fruit diet.[35] Allen's diet and Kempner's diet were very low in sodium. (The rice and fruit diet was also extremely monotonous!) This approach to the treatment of hypertension has been judged impractical by some because of the extremely low sodium content of the above-mentioned diets.

However, Morgan and coworkers obtained an average decrease of 7.3 mm Hg diastolic pressure in persons who followed a diet with 70 to 100 mEq of sodium.[36] Hunt and Margie had good results in persons who reduced salt intake so that sodium excretion was consistently 75 mEq/day or less.[37] Of subjects with entry diastolic pressure of 90 to 104 mm Hg, 85% became normotensive over the 4-study. A satisfactory result was obtained in 50% of those subjects who had diastolic blood pressures of 115 mm Hg or higher on entering the study. It should be noted that these subjects also lost weight during the study: an average of 12 pounds during the first 3 months.

My practice has been to suggest a diet with approximately 45 mEq (1,000 mg) of sodium. This is attainable if the patient can avoid processed foods with a high sodium content, such as cold-cuts, ham, and canned soup and vegetables. Foods must be prepared without using salt. It is possible to prepare tasty meals without salt if creative use is made of spices, wine, tomatoes, onions, and other sources of flavoring. Table 14.1 shows the sodium content of some foods that are basic to the American diet, and illustrates that an attractive diet is possible. Today, chefs working in many restaurants and for airlines will make low-sodium foods available to their patrons.

Differences exist between hypertensive patients in their sensitivity to salt. In general, older patients tend to show a greater response than younger ones. This may be related to the increased blood volume and decreased renin level that are common in older hypertensives.

Moderation of Alcohol Intake

Patients should be advised to limit intake of alcoholic beverages to 1 ounce of ethanol per day (2 ounces of 100 proof whiskey, 8 ounces of wine, or 24 ounces of beer). Patients withdrawing from heavy alcohol consumption may have increased blood pressure that usually decreases after a few days.

Avoidance of Tobacco

Although tobacco is not a cause of hypertension, it is a major risk factor for coronary heart disease. Therefore it is important to help hypertensive women who are smokers to break their ties with nicotine. If necessary, every available source of help should be enlisted to accomplish this purpose.

Exercise

In general an exercise program of 30 minutes followed 3 to 7 days per week will be associated with a decrease in blood pressure. Boyer and Kasch observed middle-aged men over a span of 6 months in an exercise program. Blood pressure was reduced by 13.5/11.8 mm Hg.[38]

Hagberg and colleagues worked with hypertensive adolescents who followed an endurance exercise training program for 8 months. Diastolic pressure decreased an average of 7 mm Hg. Subjects with increased cardiac output or peripheral resistance on entry to the study also showed a decrease in these measures.[39]

Korner and coworkers used a bicycle ergometer in an exercise program for mild hypertensive

Table 14.1 Sodium Content of Some Basic Foods

Milk, 2 glasses	260 mg
Bread, 2 slices	250 mg
Butter, 2 pats	100 mg
Meat, 6 oz.	150 mg
Egg, 1	60 mg

patients.[40] Subjects did 30 minutes of exercise at a workload of 60% to 70% of their calculated capacity. The exercise was preceded and followed by 5-minute warm-up and cool-down periods. Patients participated 3 or 7 days per week and showed an average diastolic decrease of 11/9 mm or 16/11 mm Hg respectively. They also observed a decrease in peripheral resistance and plasma norepinephrine, and an increase in cardiac output.

Exercise has other benefits that may be significant to the older hypertensive woman. It may help to reduce body weight. This is important because many older women can maintain weight on a very modest energy intake. Exercise will help them to burn additional calories. It has been estimated that adding a 1-mile walk to daily activity while keeping food intake constant will cause a weight reduction of 1 pound per month, or 12 pounds per year.

Exercise may also have beneficial psychological effects. Patients may feel more relaxed. A walking program may offer a chance to expand the horizons of daily life. Many older women are sedentary because no one has ever suggested a program of exercise. In one instance, an 80-year-old woman did not like to walk in the rainy winter weather. A program of dancing in her living room to the music of a record player was suggested and followed. She found that she loved to dance the hula and was soon dancing for 45 minutes daily.

An exercise program should be started with minimal intensity and duration and slowly increased as tolerated. Walking is the best exercise because most patients have the necessary skill and no special equipment or facility is required. Ten minutes of walking is a good beginning for a sedentary woman. The duration can be increased by one minute each day, if tolerated, until the patient is walking 20 or 30 minutes daily. The pace should always be comfortable, never at a level that causes shortness of breath or pain. A good guide is to walk at a pace at which one can carry on a conversation with a companion.

Patients who cannot walk because of disabilities may be able to use a stationary bicycle. Exercise can be done in front of the television set, so the patient can be informed or entertained while fulfilling an exercise program. Swimming is an excellent exercise for some of those who cannot walk, however, pools are not always readily available. Many women who cannot walk may exercise their shoulders and arms by sitting on a small chair or stool and swinging small weights. The number of repetitions and the amount of the weight load can be gradually increased as tolerated. If possible, an exercise program should be comfortable, convenient, enjoyable, and readily available. Sports, such as tennis or golf, are excellent supplements to an exercise program because of the companionship and the competition they provide, however, they do not serve well for a basic exercise program.

Psychological and Behavioral Methods

Blood pressure is markedly influenced by emotions, going up with anger and fear and going down in relaxed states and during sleep. Any form of stress may raise blood pressure. In even mild and moderate hypertensive persons the blood pressure increase caused by stress is likely to be greater and to last longer than in normotensives.

Older hypertensive women may be under considerable stress. Theirs may not be the stereotypical placid, rocking-chair existence. Older women may be lonely because of loss of spouse, family, and friends. There may be insecurity and isolation because of fear of going outside the home. Intergenerational relationships may deteriorate because of differences in tastes or in standards of behavior. The need for understanding and support may be great, and the physician should provide this and also assist his patient in finding additional resources if needed.

Suggestions can be made that will help the patient to avoid stressful situations. It may be possible to help the patient to cope more effectively with the situation or to perceive it in a less disturbing light. It is important to try to help the patient to avoid anger, anxiety, and a sense of hurry or time pressure, and to recognize these feelings even when they occur to a mild degree.

Meditation, relaxation, and biofeedback techniques have been studied in hypertension. Studies differ widely in design, in adequacy of baseline readings, in duration of treatment and follow-up, and in well-matched control subjects. Shapiro and coworkers reviews these techniques in detail.[41]

In my experience these techniques have not had a significant blood-pressure lowering effect. However, I believe that they may be useful in some patients who achieve a sense of quietness when practicing relaxation or meditation. These patients may become more sensitive to their own feelings of anger, anxiety, or time pressure, and as a result may be more successful in avoiding the situations that cause these feelings.

The support of an interested physician is an important element in the treatment of the hypertensive older woman. Two noteworthy studies suggest that psychosocial support may have a significant beneficial effect in preventing the development of coronary heart disease manifestations. Medalie and Goldcourt followed a large group of men at high risk for coronary heart disease.[42] Men who had a loving and supportive wife had a lower incidence of angina. Frasure-Smith and Prince followed a large group of patients who had been hospitalized for acute myocardial infarction.[43] Patients in the experimental group were called by telephone once a month to administer a short questionnaire designed to detect stress. Those subjects who showed an increase in stress since the previous monthly score were visited at home by a nurse who explored the cause of stress and continued monthly visits for the remainder of the 1-year follow-up period. The experimental group had a decrease in cardiac deaths of 47% as compared with the control group. I believe that these studies illustrate how important family, community, and physician support can be in the prevention of the cardiovascular complications of hypertension.

Drug Treatment of Hypertension

The decision to initiate drug therapy in a woman with hypertension should be based on the total health picture of the patient and on the published results of efficacy and safety of drug therapy. Drugs should not be prescribed unless blood pressure is consistently at least 145/95 mm Hg in a patient who has one or more risk factors for a complication and has made a sincere effort to follow the hygienic measures.

Start slowly with drug therapy. Use small initial dosages and increase slowly with small increments and at long intervals. Ambulatory hypertension is not an emergency. The chance of obtaining the patient's compliance with the drug treatment program is increased if disturbing adverse effects can be avoided in the beginning. Fatigue, lassitude, disturbed sleeping patterns, impaired sexual desire and function, and postural hypotension are common, unless skill is used in beginning drug therapy. In general, older patients are more vulnerable to the adverse effects of antihypertensive drugs. They are also more likely to have silent coronary heart disease. One should avoid lowering blood pressure too quickly or by too much.

The pattern of drug treatment has changed in recent years because the majority of hypertensive persons have mild-to-moderate blood pressure levels when first diagnosed. These patients are more likely to respond satisfactorily to a single drug. One can, therefore, prescribe a single drug with the expectation that it will be effective in reducing blood pressure to a satisfactory level. If the response is not adequate or if adverse effects are significant, a second drug may be added, or the second drug may be substituted for the first. Several years ago diuretics and beta blockers were the drugs of first and second choice because they have been shown in large clinical trials to reduce morbidity and mortality. Other groups of drugs are effective in lowering blood pressure but have not been studied in large clinical trials in which an effect on morbidity and mortality has been demonstrated. Drugs that are useful in the management of hypertension will be discussed below. Table 14.2 summarizes information regarding the different groups of drugs. An effort will be made to suggest situations in which drugs may be of special value.

Diuretics

1. The mild diuretics have diuretic, natriuretic, and chloruretic effects. However, they may vary in promptness of onset and in duration of action. These drugs reduce extracellular volume and plasma volume. They may also act by reducing the sodium content of vascular smooth muscle. With chronic use, peripheral resistance may be reduced. Diuretics, in addition to their own blood pressure lowering effects, may increase the blood pressure reduction of other drugs such as some of the adrenergic inhibitors and the vasodilators. They will usually prevent salt and water retention, which may occur if other types of antihypertensive drugs are given alone. The effects of these drugs is quite limited in patients with impaired renal function, and increasing the dose usually will not increase the response.

   In general, these drugs are well tolerated, especially if given in small doses; however, hypokalemia is a significant risk, particularly in older women. The cause for the vulnerability of this group is not known. In some cases it may be because of an inadequate diet with low potassium stores. It is important to check serum potassium before prescribing the mild diuretics. This is especially true in women who are receiving digitalis. Siscovick and coworkers have emphasized that the risk of sudden cardiac death is increased in hypertensive persons who are receiving a thiazide without a potassium-sparing diuretic. The increased risk also occurred in patients who were receiving moderate doses of thiazide (50 mg/day) as compared with low doses (25 mg/day or less).[44]

   Other adverse effects are hyperuricemia, hyperglycemia, skin rashes, gastrointestinal distress, and vasculitis. These drugs may also cause an increase in total cholesterol and triglycerides.

2. Loop diuretics usually cause a prompt and copious diuresis. This may be a disadvantage in some women, especially those who have questionable urinary sphincter control. They may be immobilized until the surge of diuresis is spent. These drugs can cause fluid and electrolyte depletion. With increased dosage they are usually effective even in patients with impaired renal function. In women with normal renal function, these drugs have no advantages over the mild diuretics and may cause significant problems.

3. Potassium-sparing diuretics include triamterene and amiloride. They are usually weak diuretics and natriuretics and are usually given with a diuretic such as thiazide, so that satisfactory diuresis is obtained and excess potassium loss is prevented. These diuretics should not be given with angiotensin converting enzyme inhibitors.

   Adverse effects include nausea and leg cramps. Renal failure has been attributed to these drugs. This hazard may be increased by concommitant use of nonsteroidal anti-inflammatory drugs (NSAIDs).

   Spironolactone is an aldosterone antagonist. It causes sodium excretion and potassium retention. It, too, is often used with a thiazide diuretic. It should not be used in patients with impaired renal function, in patients who are receiving an angiotensin converting enzyme inhibitor, nor together with potassium supplementation because of the possibility of hyperkalemia. Breast tenderness may be a problem.

Table 14.2 Antihypertensive Drugs

Drug	Adult daily dose	Remarks
Diuretics		
Bendroflumethazide	2.5–5	AE: Hypokalemia, especially in women. Lethargy, depression.
Chlorthalidone	12.5–50	Hyperuricemia. Limited response with impaired kidney function.
Hydrochlorothiazide	12.5–50	
Indapamide	2.5–5	
Metolazone	0.5–5	
Loop Diuretics		
Bumetanide (Bumex)	0.5–5	Powerful agents. Dehydration is a hazard. Best reserved for
Ethacrynic acid	25–100	impaired kidney function. Copious response may limit mobility.
Furosemide	20–320	
Potassium-Sparing Diuretics		
Amiloride	5–10	AE: Hyperkalemia: Do not use with potassium supplements.
Spironolactone	25–100	Menstrual irregularities reported with spironolactone.
Triamterene	50–150	
Adrenergic-Inhibiting Drugs		
1. Beta-adrenergic blockers[*]		
Propranolol	40–240	
Acebutolol	200–1200	Has intrinsic sympathomimetic (ISA) effect. Some cardioselectivity.
Atenolol	25–100	Cardioselective.
Carteolol	2.5–10	Cardioselective.
Metoprolol	25–100	Cardioselective.
Nadolol	20–160	
Penbutolol	10–40	ISA
Pindolol	5–60	ISA
Timolol	5–40	
2. Alpha-Beta Blocker		
Labetalol	200–1200	Has alpha blockade. Same AE as beta blockers.
3. Alpha-1-Receptor Blockers		
Doxazosin	1.0–16	All may cause postural hypotension. Titrate dose using standing
Prazosin	1.0–20	blood pressure.
Terazosin	1.0–20	
4. Central Acting Alpha$_2$ Agonists		
Clonidine	0.1–1.2	Available as a patch. Avoid rapid withdrawal. May lead to blood
Guanabenz	4–64	pressure overshoot. Dry mouth and sedation significant AE.
Guanfacine	1–3	
Methyldopa	250–2000	
5. Peripheral-Acting Adrenergic Antagonists		
Guanadrel	10–75	May cause exercised-induced and postural hypotension.
Guanethidine	10–100	
Rauwolfia Alkaloid		
Reserpine	0.05–0.25	AE: Depression, lethargy.
Direct Vasodilators		
Hydralazine	50–200	AE: Headache, tachycardia, angina. Need diuretic and beta blocker
Minoxidil	2.5–80	or other adrenergic inhibitor.
Calcium Antagonists		
Diltiazem	90–360	Caution with conduction defects and reduced ejection fraction.
Verapamil	80–480	
Dihydropyridine Calcium Antagonists		
Amlodipine	2.5–10	The drugs in this group are more potent vasodilators. May cause
Felodipine	5–20	headache, flushing, peripheral edema, and tachycardia.
Isradipine	2.5–10	
Nicardipine	60–120	
Ni fedipine	30–120	
Angeotensin-Converting Enzyme (ACE) Inhibitors		
Captopril	12.5–150	Should reduce dose or discontinue diuretic when starting these
Enalapril	2.5–40	drugs. Also if serum creatinine is 2.5 mg or more, hyperkalemia a
Lisinopril	5.0–40	risk with renal impairment or in patients receiving potassium-
Ramipril	1.25–20	sparing diuretics.

[AE], Adverse effects.

[*]*Comment.* All beta blockers may cause fatigue, depression, and increase symptoms of peripheral vascular disease (coldness of extremities, and so forth). None should be used in patients with a history of asthma. Drugs with ISA do not reduce heart rate and may cause fewer metabolic adverse effects (unfavorable lipid effects).

Adrenergic-Inhibiting Drugs

The sympathetic nervous system is obviously important in the regulation of blood pressure. Drugs may reduce sympathetic nervous system activity in various ways, many of them involving some aspect of the synthesis or release of norepinephrine. Drugs may also block adrenergic receptors or in other ways prevent sympathetic stimulation of end-organs.

1. *Beta-adrenergic blockers.* see Table 14.2 for a list of drugs. These drugs reduce the rate and force of cardiac contraction. This may be the mechanism through which they lower blood pressure. They also reduce renin release. Some beta blockers are cardioselective, blocking beta-1 receptors but not beta-2. These drugs should cause less bronchoconstriction. However, freedom from bronchoconstriction is only relative. Even cardioselective beta blockers may cause broncho-constriction in asthmatic patients. Intrinsic sympathomimetic activity is present in some beta blockers. This may permit blood pressure reduction without significant reduction of heart rate. Beta blockers have been shown to reduce recurrence rates of myocardial infarction, and they are commonly used in the treatment of angina and cardiac arrhythmias. However, they have not been shown to reduce the frequency of coronary heart disease complications in hypertension.

    Adverse effects of beta blockers include bronchoconstriction. They should not be used in asthmatics, in patients with chronic obstructive pulmonary disease, and in patients with a slow resting heart rate or heart block. Patients who experience an upper respiratory infection with bronchitis while taking a beta blocker may have a persistent cough that may not stop until the drug is discontinued.

    Other adverse effects include disturbances of sleep, cognitive function, and memory, and lassitude. Gastrointestinal complaints, especially flatulence, are common. Many patients will tolerate the lassitude and other complaints if the drug is started in low doses. These drugs may cause an increase in triglyceride concentration, a decrease in high-density lipoproteins, and a reduction in the ratio of total cholesterol to high-density lipoproteins.[44]

    In diabetics, beta blockers may accentuate the degree of hypoglycemia with insulin overdosage and mask the symptoms and signs (tachycardia and anxiety). Cardioselective beta blockers have a theoretical advantage in diabetics.

2. *Labetalol (Normodyne).* This drug acts both as a noncardioselective beta blocker and as an alpha-1 blocker. Flamenbaum and coworkers reported that labetalol was equally effective as monotherapy in blacks and whites.[46] A multicentered study showed that it was effective when used with small dosages (25 mg twice a day) of hydrochlorothiazide. Standing blood pressure is reduced more than supine, which means that postural hypotension may be a problem. In a long-term study Lund-Johanson reported that peripheral resistance was reduced and that cardiac output, which had been reduced early in the study, was increased at the end of the study.[47]

    Adverse effects include dizziness, which is probably related to its alpha-1 blocking effect. The adverse effects ascribed to the beta blockers may also be a problem. These include fatigue, sleep disturbances, and gastrointestinal distress. McGonigle and coworkers[48] have reported a reduction in total cholesterol without any change in high-density lipoproteins, while Frishman and coworkers[49] have reported no change.

3. *Clonidine.* This drug acts centrally on alpha-2 receptors and causes a reduction in sympathetic outflow; a reduction in norepinephrine release and plasma level; a decrease in peripheral resistance; a small decrease in cardiac output; and a decrease in renin release. This drug does not have as great a blood pressure lowering effect as monotherapy, but it may be quite effective when used with a mild diuretic.

    Adverse effects of clonidine include dry mouth and drowsiness, which may be a difficult problem for those who work at desks or who must drive. Taking 75% of the daily dose before bedtime may be useful in reducing daytime drowsiness. However, sleep disturbance may also be a problem with this drug.

Withdrawal hypertensin may be a problem with clonidine. If the drug is abruptly discontinued after a significant blood pressure reduction has been achieved with clonidine, the result may be a sharp increase in blood pressure and heart rate. Because of the possibility of a withdrawal reaction, clonidine is not recommended for older women who might forget to take daily drug doses.

Transdermal clonidine is now available. Patches may be applied once weekly. More consistent plasma levels of the drug may be an advantage. However, a significant number of patients may have local skin reactions. This method of administration may be useful with forgetful patients.

4. *Methydopa.* The exact mechanism of action is still uncertain, but this drug probably acts through central depression of sympathetic activity via alpha-2 receptors. For many years it was widely used as a step two drug, following a diuretic. Sedation, fatigue, and loss of libido must be avoided by careful dosing. Postural hypotension may be a problem in some patients.

5. *Guanabenz and Guanfacine.* These are other centrally acting drugs. They are similar to Clonidine in actions and in adverse effects.

6. *Guanethidine.* This drug probably acts at the peripheral sympathetic neuroeffector junction by inhibiting norepinephrine release. It was once widely used as a step four drug when the first three drugs did not lower blood pressure satisfactorily. Postural and exertional hypotension are significant problems. Diarrhea may be severe. The drug may aggravate bronchial asthma. Guanadrel is similar to guanethidine in action and may cause postural hypotension.

7. *Prazosin (Minipress).* This drug acts as a selective antagonist to peripheral postsynaptic alpha-1 receptors. This selective action leaves the presynaptic alpha-2 receptors able to inhibit release of norepinephrine, thus decreasing the tachycardia that often occurs with alpha-1 blockade. Another explanation may be that prazosin acts on both resistance and capacitance vessels and thus reduces venous return to the heart. Prazosin has been reported to cause a reduction in total cholesterol and triglycerides and an increase in high-density liproteins.

Adverse effects of prazosin include a marked hypotensive response after taking the first dose (probably 5% of patients). To minimize the danger of this response the first dose can be given in the evening, when the patient is ready to get into bed. Other adverse effects that have been reported are headache, drowsiness, nervousness, and lassitude.

Vasodilators

Hydralazine. This direct vascular smooth muscle vasodilator effects mainly the arterial side of the circulation, and has little effect on the capacitance vessels. Hence, return venous flow is increased with increased heart rate and cardiac output. Therefore angina may occur in patients with coronary heart disease. This drug has been widely used as a third step drug and still may be useful when blood pressure is difficult to control. It should usually be given along with a diuretic and an adrenergic inhibitor.

Adverse effects are tachycardia, angina, headache, and sodium and water retention. Headaches can usually be avoided if the drug is started in small doses. Some patients acetylate hydralazine at a slow rate and show a therapeutic response and/or adverse effects at low doses.

Minoxidil. This very potent vasodilator is useful in severe hypertension. It is usually given with a beta blocker and a diuretic, as noted above with hydralazine. Abnormal hair growth may be a distressing adverse effect, especially in women.

Calcium Channel Blockers

Calcium ions play an important role in the function of cardiac and vascular tissues and the specialized cardiac conduction system. Reduction of calcium concentration within the cell will reduce activity. Thus vasodilitation, reduced force of cardiac contraction, or slowed sinus node firing or auricular-ventricular (AV) conduction may be caused by this group of drugs. They differ in the extent to which they effect various functions.[50]

Verapamil, nifedipine, and diltiazem have been available for the longest time. All have vasodilator effects, with nifedipine being the most potent. Verapamil and diltiazem both cause negative chronotropism and inotropism. Thus they are less likely to cause a reflex increase in heart rate. In hypertensive patients with impaired left ventricular function they could theoretically cause further impairment. However, the reduced left ventricular afterload and the improved coronary circulation might compensate for such effects. Verapamil and diltiazem should be used with caution in such patients.

These drugs will probably have an important place in the treatment of hypertensive patients with cardiovascular complications or associated diseases. Hypertensive patients with angina may benefit from the coronary vasodilatation that is a part of the main action of these drugs. Calcium antagonists have great advantages over the beta blockers in hypertensive persons with asthma or diabetes. Thus far they do not appear to have any adverse effects on plasma lipids, which may give them an advantage over diuretics and beta blockers. These drugs appear to have a special place in the treatment of older hypertensive patients.[51]

Adverse effects of the calcium antagonists vary considerably. In general they are well tolerated. Constipation has been a common complaint reported with verapamil use. Tachycardia, headaches, and palpitation are more common adverse effects with use of nifedipine and the dihydropyridines. Flushing, dizziness, and skin rashes are not uncommon. Swelling of the feet may require stopping the drug. It is probably related to vasodilatation and not to sodium retention. In fact, in some patients these drugs cause a natriuresis. Some patients complain of fatigue and reduced tolerance for exercise, especially with verapamil.

Verapamil and diltiazem should be used only with great caution if at all with beta blockers. Increased AV block may occur. These drugs may reduce the renal clearance of digoxin and cause an increase in plasma digoxin levels. Therefore the dose of digoxin should be reduced or the plasma level carefully monitored.

Angiotensin-Converting Enzyme Inhibitors (ACEI)

These drugs reduce the production of angiotensin 2, a potent vasoconstrictor that also causes the increased release of aldosterone and stimulation of the sympathetic nervous system. Angiotensin 2 also causes the degradation of bradykinin, an endogenous vasodilator. Thus inhibitors of angiotensin-converting enzyme may lower blood pressure through at least two mechanisms: reducing angiotensin 2 and increasing bradykinin. These drugs are effective in reducing peripheral resistance. They may also dilate the large arteries.

One would expect that the ACEIs would be most effective in high-renin hypertension, and therefore less effective in elders and blacks in whom low renin is common. Nonetheless, these drugs are often effective in and well tolerated by elders.

Initially, captopril, the first of these drugs to become available, was used almost exclusively in severe hypertension and almost always with a diuretic and an adrenergic inhibitor. It is clear now that these drugs can be effective as monotherapy in older patients.[52,53]

ACEIs cause a blood pressure decrease similar to a beta blocker. The VA study of captopril showed a good response at a daily dose of 37.5 mg. The addition of hydrochlorothiazide increased the diastolic blood pressure response by 4 to 6 mm Hg.

Adverse effects of the ACEIs appear to be about half as frequent as with beta blockers. Early reports of skin rash and loss of taste sensation with captopril have declined with the use of smaller doses. Neutropenia and proteinuria are uncommon but are more likely to occur in patients with decreased renal function and collagen diseases, that is, lupus or scleroderma. These adverse effects may be related to the SH (sulfur-hydrogen) group in captopril. They are less common with enalapril, which has no SH group. Neutropenia when it has occurred, has usually resolved quickly when the drug was stopped.

The most common adverse effects of ACEIs appear to be dizziness, headache, fatigue, diarrhea, and upper respiratory symptoms. Cough is fairly common and is dose-related. The drug has been discontinued in approximately 6% of patients because of adverse effects.

These drugs may cause acute renal failure if they are given to patients with severe bilateral renal artery stenosis.

Conclusion

Hypertension is a common finding in older women. It deserves careful and thoughtful consideration. Initial efforts at treatment should focus on hygienic measures because they are frequently effective in lowering blood pressure and have a beneficial effect on quality of life, mental status, and plasma lipids.

The decision to start drug therapy should be based on the total health picture of the patient.

All-cause mortality and risk of and mortality from cardiovascular disease increase with age. Age is more important than blood pressure in older women.

Drug treatment of hypertension in older women should be initiated with a low dosage and increased in small increments and at long intervals.

Drug dosage should be slowly and carefully reduced if diastolic pressure falls below 85 mm.

References

1. Hamilton M, Pickering GW, Fraser Roberts JA: Etiology of essential hypertension: Arterial pressure in the general population. *Clin Sci.* 1954;13:11–35.
2. Spence JO, Sibbald WJ, Cape RD: Pseudohypertension in the elderly. *Clin Sci Molecular Med.* 1978;55:399s–s.
3. Messerli, Franz H, Ventura HO, Amodeo C: Osler's maneuver and pseudohypertension. *N Engl J Med* 1985;1548–1551.
4. Fifth Report of the Joint National Committee on Detection, Evaluation, and Treatment of High Blood Pressure: Publ. No. 93-1088. Washington, DC, National Institutes of Health, 19XX. *Arch Int Med* 1993: 153: 154–183.
5. *Framingham Study: An Epidemiological Investigation of Cardiovascular Disease*, Kannel RB, Gordon T (eds.): Shurtleff, D. Sec. 30 NIH 74-599 Washington DC, National Institutes of Health, 1974.
6. Fry J: Natural history of hypertension: A case for selective non-treatment. *Lancet* 1974;2:431–433.
7. Mattila K, Haavisto M, Rajala S: Blood pressure and five year survival in the very old. *Br Med J* 1988;296:887–889.
8. Anderson F, Cowan NR: Survival of healthy older people. *Br J Prev Soc Med* 1976;30:231–232.
9. Devereux RB, Koren MJ, de Simone G: Methods for detection of left ventricular hypertrophy: Application to hypertensive heart disease. *Eur Heart J* 1993;14:8–15.
10. Devereux RB, de Simone G, Koren MJ: Left ventricular mass as a predictor of hypertension. *Am J Hypertens* 1991;4:603s–607s.
11. Reaven GM: Insulin resistance, hyperinsulinemia, and hypertriglyceridemia in the etiology and clinical course of hypertension. *Am J Med* 1991;90(2A):7s–12s
12. VA Cooperative Study Group on Antihypertensive Agents: Effects of treatment on morbidity in hypertension, results in patients with diastolic blood pressures averaging 115 through 129 mm Hg. *JAMA* 1967;202(II):1028–1034.

13. VA Cooperative Study Group on Antihypertensive Agents: Effects of treatment on morbidity in hypertension, II. Results in patients with diastolic blood pressure averaging 90 through 114 mm Hg. *JAMA* 1967;213(7):1143–1152.

14. US Public Health Service Hospitals Cooperative Study Group: Treatment of mild hypertension: Results of a ten-year intervention trial. *Circ Res* 1977;40(suppl I):1–98.

15. Australian therapeutic trial in mild hypertension. *Lancet* 1980;1:1261–7.

16. Medical Research Council Working Party: MRC trial of treatment of mild hypertension: Principal results. *Br Med J* 1985;291:97–104.

17. MacMahon S, Cutler JA, Stamler J: Antihypertensive drug treatment. Potential, expected, and observed effects on stroke and on coronary heart disease. *Hypertension* 1989;13(5 Suppl):145s–150s.

18. Collins R, Peto R, MacMahon S: Blood pressure, stroke, and coronary heart disease. Part 2. Short-term reductions in blood pressure: Overview of randomised drug trials in their epidemiological context. *Lancet* 1990;Vol 1:827–838.

19. Stewart I, McD G: Relation of reduction in pressure to first myocardial infarction in patients receiving treatment for severe hypertension. *Lancet* 1979;IX:861–865.

20. Multiple Risk Factor Intervention Trial Research Group, 1982: Multiple risk factor intervention trial: Risk factor changes and mortality results. *JAMA* 1982;248:1465–1477.

21. Cruickshank JM, Thorp JM, Zacharias FJ: Benefits and potential harm of lowering high blood pressure. *Lancet* 1987;1:581–584.

22. Samuelsson, Wilhelmsen L, Andersson OK: Cardiovascular morbidity in relation to change in blood pressure and serum cholesterol levels in treated hypertension. *JAMA* 1987;258:1768–1776.

23. Farnett L, Mulrow CD, Linn WD: The J-curve phenomenon and the treatment of hypertension. Is there a point beyond which pressure reduction is dangerous? *JAMA* 1991;265:489–495.

24. Langer RD, Criqui MH, Barrett-Connor EL: Blood pressure change and survival after age 75. *Hypertension* 1993; 22;551–559.

25. Floras JS: Antihypertensive treatment, myocardial infarction, and nocturnal myocardial ischaemia. *Lancet* 1988; 2:994–996.

26. Stamler J, Farinaro E, Mojonnier LM: Prevention and control of hypertension by nutritional-hygienic means. *JAMA* 1980;243:1819–1823.

27. Reisin E, Abel R, Modan M: Effect of weight loss without salt restriction on the reduction of blood pressure in overweight hypertensive patients. *N Engl J Med* 1978;298:1–6.

28. Young JB, Landsberg L: Suppression of sympathetic nervous system during fasting. *Science* 1977;196:1473–1475.

29. Jung RI, Shetty PS, Barrand M: Role of catecholamines in hypotensive response to dieting. *Brit Med J* 1979;1:12–13.

30. Stamler, R, Stamler J, Gosch FC: Primary prevention of hypertension by nutritional hygienic means. Final report of a randomized, controlled trial. *JAMA* 1989;262:1801–1807.

31. Page LB, Damon A, Moellering RC Jr.: Antecedents of cardiovascular disease in six Solomon Islands societies. *Circ* 1974;49:1132–1146.

32. Oliver W, Cohen EL, Neel JV: Blood pressure, sodium intake and sodium related hormones in the Yanomamo Indians, a no-salt culture. *Circulation* 1975;52:146–151.

33. Mark AL, Lawton WQ, Abboud FM: Effects of high and low sodium intake on arterial pressure and forearm vascular resistance in borderline hypertension. *Cir Res* 1975;36 & 37 (suppl I): 194–198.

34. Allen FM: Arterial hypertension. *JAMA* 1920;74:652– .

35. Kempner W: Treatment of hypertensive vascular disease with rice diet. *Am J Med* 1948;X:Vol 4:545–577.

36. Morgan T, Adam W, Gillies A: Hypertension treated by salt restriction. *Lancet* 1978;1:227–230.

37. Hunt JC, Margie JO: Influence of diet on hypertension management, in Hunt JC (ed.): *Hypertension Update: Dialogues in Hypertension.* Health Learning Systems Inc., Bloomfield, NJ.

38. Boyer JL, Kasch FW: Exercise therapy in hypertensive men. *JAMA* 1970;211:1668–1671.

39. Hagberg JM, Ehsani AA, Goldring D: Effect of weight training on blood pressure and hemodynamics in hypertensive adolescents, *J Pediatr* 1984;104X:147–151.

40. Korner PI, et al: Long-term antihypertensive action of regular exercise. Its role in a new Treatment strategy, in Yamori, Lenfant (eds.): *Prevention of Cardiovascular Diseases: An Approach to Active Long Life.* Elsevier Science Publishers, 1987; p 213.

41. Shapiro AP, Schwartz GE, Ferguson DCE: Behavioral methods in the treatment of hypertension—A review of their clinical status. *Ann Int Med* 1977;86:626–636.

42. Medalie JH, Goldbourt, U: Angina pectoris among 10,000 men, II. Psychosocial and other risk factors as evidenced by a multivariate analysis of a five year incidence study. *Am J Med* 1976;60:910–921.

43. Frasure-Smith N, Prince R: The ischemic heart disease life stress monitoring program: Impact on mortality. *Psychosomatic Med* 1985;47:431–445.

44. Siscovick DS, Raghunathan TE, Psaty BM: Diuretic therapy for hypertension and the risk of primary cardiac arrest. *N Engl J Med* 1994;330:1852–1857.

45. Weinberger MH: Antihypertensive therapy and lipids. Evidence, mechanisms and implications. *Arch Int Med* 1985;145:1102–1105.
46. Flamenbaum W, Weber, MA, McMahon FG: Monotherapy with labetalol compared with propranolol. *J Clin Hypertens* 1985;1:56–69.
47. Lund-Johansen P: Short and long-term (six-year) hemodynamic effects of labetalol in essential hypertension. *Am J Med* 1983;75:24–31.
48. McGonigle RJS, Williams L, Murphy MJ: Labetalol and lipids. *Lancet* 1981;1:163– .
49. Frishman WH, Michelson EL, Johnson BF: Multiclinic comparison of labetalol to metoprolol in treatment of mild to moderate systemic hypertension. *Am J Med* 1983;75:54–67.
50. Van Zweiten PA, van Meel JC, Timmermans PB: Pharmacology of calcium entry blockers: Interaction with vascular alpha adrenoreceptors. *Hypertension* 1983;(suppl 5)8–17.
51. Kaplan NM: Calcium entry blockers in the treatment of hypertension. Current status and future prospects. *JAMA* 1989;262:817–823.
52. VA Cooperative Study Group on Antihypertensive Agents: Low-dose captopril for the treatment of mild to moderate Hypertension. I. Results of a 14 week trial. *Arch Intern Med* 1984;144:1947–1953.
53. VA Cooperative Study Group on Antihypertensive Agents: Captopril: Evaluation of low doses, twice-daily doses and the addition of diuretic for the treatment of mild to moderate hypertension. *Clin Sci* 1982;63:443s.

Chapter 15

Depression, Dementia, and Delirium

Edward A. Walker, MD

Although gynecologists will continue to play a vital role as secondary and tertiary care specialists in the treatment of diseases of women, it is becoming increasingly clear that they will also be primary care "gatekeepers" in the new health care system. It is likely that many otherwise healthy women will continue to obtain regular pelvic examinations, contraception, and obstetrical care from gynecologists, allowing these providers to account for a significant percentage of the total de facto primary care for women.

Research on the process of primary care has shown that approximately 50% to 60% of visits have a significant behavioral component that influences outcome. For example, the prevalence of current psychiatric disorders in primary care clinics has been repeatedly shown to be about 25%.[1] Yet only 15% of the mental health care in the United States occurs in the traditional specialty mental health sector (psychiatrists, psychologists, and other therapists), and 60% of this mental health care is provided by primary care physicians.[7]

Because women share a disproportionate burden of these affective and anxiety symptoms, having two to three times the risk for depression compared with men,[8] it is likely that gynecologists will increasingly assume the duties of mental health providers. This will become even more apparent as the "baby boomer" cohort advances in age and the natural longevity of women slowly increases the relative proportion of this gender and age group in primary care. Thus, the recognition of psychiatric disorders in these older women will become increasingly important.

This chapter focuses on the recognition and treatment of three of the most common psychiatric diagnoses in older women: depression, delirium, and dementia. A biopsychosocial model of care will be presented including the collaborative role of the consultation-liaison psychiatrist who can be of great assistance in the management of these disorders.

Psychological Responses to Aging

The aging process is as variable and unique as the women who undergo it. For some women the later years are a rich and fulfilling continuation of their previous well-integrated life, however, for others it can represent a disquieting, uncertain shift from well-defined roles such as motherhood. In many ways the response to aging is the sum of the previous adaptations to the physical, psychological, and social factors that have been active throughout the woman's whole life. The biopsychosocial model provides a useful paradigm to understand the impact of these factors in the psychological adjustment of the elderly woman.[2]

Biologically, the aging process slowly diminishes physical ability and shifts the endocrine milieu from reproduction to the menopause. Despite the fact that most women now live a third of their lives in the postmenopausal period, very little is actually known about the long-term effects of the physiological changes that occur in this period. The aging process causes decreases in muscle mass, cardiopulmonary reserve, microsomal enzyme activity (slowing of the principal drug metabolism pathway), and sensory acuity, while increasing the rate of bone demineralization. Most women adapt gracefully to these physiological changes, but others can find their changing physical appearance and ability to be stressful.[9]

Studies of psychological function have documented both static and dynamic properties of the aging brain. Knowledge acquired over the course of the socialization process (eg, facts about the past) tends to remain stable during the aging process, while there is a gradual decline in acquisition and retrieval of new information and a decrease in the fluidity of thought as reflected in the solution of novel problems (eg, decreased creativity and increased reliance on routine). Additionally, the sociocultural stereotypes that emphasize the desirability of physical beauty and youthful sexuality can sometimes present adjustment challenges for some women as they attempt to redefine their self-image during aging.[6]

Social forces are among the most potent factors shaping the adjustment to later life. Aging can bring a change in the defining roles of wife and mother, and social isolation can gradually increase as children leave the home, friends move away during retirement, and spouses die. Due to differences in longevity, there are over five times as many widows as widowers in the United States, and half the women over age 65 are widows. Financial difficulties and failing health can further worsen this isolation, leading to more serious problems with depression.

Major Depression

It is important to distinguish between the symptom of depressed mood and the diagnosis of Major Depressive Disorder. Depression as a symptom is common across all age groups. Transient depression is a normal response to disappointment, bereavement, and other forms of loss and stress. However, when depression becomes more severe, lasting, and disabling it is important to consider the diagnosis of major depression.

The prevalence of current major depression in a primary care clinic is about 5%, (similar to hypertension), and a woman has about a 1 in 5 chance of having a major depression at some time in her life. The criteria for a major depressive episode are shown in Table 15.1.

Patients with severe major depression can often be identified as you walk into the consulting room. A depressed woman may appear fatigued, sad, and disinterested. She may speak slowly or have difficulty concentrating, often taking several seconds to respond to your questions. Sometimes, however, patients are significantly more depressed than they look, and a routine screening process may be helpful in identifying patients with the disorder. The need for screening is supported by studies of recognition rates of major depression in primary care settings, which show that the diagnosis is missed from 50% to 90% of the time.

Probably the easiest screening technique is to simply ask about the quality of sleep. Most patients with middle of the night or early morning awakening have a moderately severe major depression. Difficulty falling asleep may also be a clue to a more agitated form of depression mixed with anxiety. A positive response to the sleep question can be further explored by a review of the DSM-III-R criteria listed in Table 15.1 or by use of a formal screening questionnaire, such as the Beck Depression Inventory. Scores of 10 to 20 on the Beck Inventory are associated with mild-to-moderate depression, and scores of 20 or greater indicate moderate-to-severe depression

Table 15.1 Criteria for Major Depression

A. Five (or more) of the following symptoms have been present during the same 2-week period and represent a change from previous functioning; at least one of the symptoms is either (1) depressed mood or (2) loss of interest or pleasure.
Note: Do not include symptoms that are clearly due to a general medical condition, or mood-incongruent delusions of hallucinations.
1. Depressed mood most of the day, nearly every day, as indicated by either subjective report (eg, feels sad or empty) or observation made by others (eg, appears tearful). **Note:** In children and adolescents, can be irritable mood.
2. Markedly diminished interest or pleasure in all, or almost all, activities most of the day, nearly every day (as indicated by either subjective account or observation made by others).
3. Significant weight loss when not dieting or weight gain (eg, a change of more than 5% of body weight in a month), or decrease or increase in appetite nearly every day. **Note:** In children, consider failure to make expected weight gains.
4. Insomnia or hypersomnia nearly every day.
5. Psychomotor agitation or retardation nearly every day (observable by others, not merely subjective feelings of restlessness or being slowed down).
6. Fatigue or loss of energy nearly every day.
7. Feelings of worthlessness or excessive or inappropriate guilt (which may be delusional) nearly eery day (not merely self-reproach or guilt about being sick).
8. Diminished ability to think or concentrate, or indecisiveness, nearly every day (either by subjective account or as observed by others).
9. Recurrent thoughts of death (not just fear of dying), recurrent suicidal ideation without a specific plan, or a suicide attempt, or a specific plan for committing suicide.
B. The symptoms do not meet criteria for a Mixed Episode.
C. The symptoms cause clinically significant distress or impairment in social, occupational, or other important areas of functioning.
D. The symptoms are not due to the direct physiological effects of a substance (eg, a drug of abuse, a medication) or a general medical condition (eg, hypothyroidism).
E. The symptoms are not better accounted for by Bereavement, that is, after the loss of a loved one, the symptoms persist for longer than 2 months or are characterized by marked functional impairment, morbid preoccupation with worthlessness, suicidal ideation, psychotic symptoms, or psychomotor retardation.

American Psychiatric Association: Diagnostic and Statistical Manual of Mental Disorders, Fourth ed. Washington DC: APA 1994

and suggest further evaluation or referral. This questionnaire screening can easily be accomplished by the clinic nurse or even the receptionist.

While most physicians can recognize major depression in a suicidal, psychologically minded patient who presents complaining of severely depressed mood, the more typical primary care presentation is the patient who has one or more medically unexplained physical symptoms masking the depression. Complaints of headache, abdominal pain, premenstrual distress, chronic fatigue, backache, and gastrointestinal distress commonly lead to no medical etiology, and are frequently found to be somatoform presentations of major depression.

Major depression can coexist with other medical conditions. Two large population studies have shown that approximately 50% of people subsequently diagnosed as having a major depression first presented to a primary care provider with physical complaints. Another frequent presenting situation is the perimenopausal woman whose adjustment to menopause is complicated by a coexisting major depression. Contrary to popular belief menopausal women are no more likely to have a major depression than age-matched premenopausal women; however, the adjustment to menopause is frequently a catalyst for the development of major depression in vulnerable individuals. Women who appear to have problems adapting to hormone replacement therapy may be experiencing comorbid major depression.

A serious misdiagnosis can occur if the physician mistakes the cognitive slowing and memory problems of major depression for the more lasting cognitive impairments of dementia. Failure to recognize this depressive *pseudodementia* can result in inadequate treatment of reversible major depression symptoms and the possible incorrect labeling of the patient as having an untreatable, irreversible dementia. Simple screening for major depression symptoms at the time of presentation can prevent this tragic error, and all patients who have both mood and cognitive symptoms should be treated with antidepressants as part of the evaluation of dementia (see below).

The management of the patient with major depression is facilitated by an understanding of the biopsychosocial model. Social environment, early family experiences, and biology all contribute to the establishment and maintenance of the depression cycle. It is useful to think of this model as actually *three* models, each with a *diagnosis* and *treatment* component.

The Biological Model of Depression

Diagnosis

Major depression results in a destabilization of the balance of neurotransmitters in the brain with concomitant dysregulation of sleep, appetite, and sexual drives. Thinking and concentration are impaired as are normal interest and energy.

Treatment

Antidepressant medications are powerful regulators of these systems. Although all antidepressants are effective, the side-effect profiles suggest that some are less appropriate for the older woman. Medications such as amitriptyline (Elavil), doxepin (Sinequan or Adepin), and imipramine (Tofranil) may be too anticholinergic for an older patient and may cause a reversible delirium or dementia. Trazodone (Desyrel) causes significant hypotension and could lead to a nocturnal hip fracture. Thus, care needs to be take to use the most gentle agents available.

The emergence of a new class of antidepressants, the selective serotonin reuptake inhibitors (SSRIs) promises to be an important factor in future geriatric psychopharmacology. These agents, fluoxetine (Prozac), sertraline (Zoloft), and paroxetine (Paxil) have remarkably benign side-effect profiles while retaining full antidepressant action. They should be started in smaller doses than recommended for younger adults, however, as some women will do better on lower dosages. Recommended doses for *younger adults* are fluoxetine 20 mg, sertraline 50 mg, and paroxetine 20 mg.

For older patients quarter or half doses are frequently used to start. This can be done by cutting the pills or, in the case of fluoxetine, opening the capsule into a liquid such as juice or water, drinking a quarter or half and refrigerating the remainder. Because these agents are mildly activating they should be taken in the morning. To avoid gastric upset they are best taken after breakfast.

A small number of patients may experience an increase in nervousness or initial insomnia as a result of the medication. This an often be managed by using a very small amount of a sedating antidepressant such as nortriptyline (10 mg qhs) or trazodone (50 mg qhs). In patients who cannot tolerate SSRIs at all due to significant agitation, it is best to use one of the least anticholinergic tricyclic antidepressants. Desipramine (25 to 50 mg q AM), and nortriptyline (10 mg qhs) have gentle side-effect profiles that are usually well tolerated in older patients. Initial doses should be kept low and increased slowly. Although elderly patients will generally respond to lower doses, be sure to provide an adequate clinical trial of at least 6 weeks at final dose level. This final level can vary widely but should be at least 50 to 100 mg for desipramine, and 25 to 50 mg for nortriptyline. Watch for the development of mental status changes, particularly cognitive problems such as orientation and memory difficulties that may be signs of developing delirium (see below).

If you feel you are not getting a good antidepressant response there may be other factors present such as marital problems, a comorbid personality disorder, or chronic psychosocial stressors that are preventing the full antidepressant response, and a referral to a consultation-liaison psychiatrist may be helpful.

Although smaller doses and longer titration periods are generally used in older women, patients in this age group are not necessarily more fragile, but have more variability. Thus, some elderly women will require and tolerate full antidepressant dosages. It is important to use an adequate dose for a sufficient length of time before concluding that an antidepressant is not working properly. This usually means at least a 6-week trial on each agent at the maximal tolerated dose. One of the most frequent psychopharmacologic errors to be avoided is low-dosing combined with weekly switching of antidepressant medications.

An important additional concern is women with a history of bipolar affective (manic-depressive) disorder. Although these patients may appear to meet criteria for a current major depression, closer questioning may reveal a history of prior manic episodes as well. In contrast to women with unipolar depression who will respond appropriately to antidepressants, women with bipolar disorder may be at risk for the precipitation of a manic episode when treated with even small doses of antidepressant medication. This can be avoided by asking about prior psychoactive medication treatment and hospitalizations. Onset of bipolar disorder is usually before age 30, and geriatric onset is extremely rare. It is therefore likely that a good history will elicit prior treatment clues (eg, lithium, carbamazepine, and haldol) or a manic episode severe enough to warrant hospitalization. It is important not to be confused by reports of "mood swings" that are frequent, lower amplitude reactions to environmental stressors commonly associated with the maladaptive coping strategies used by women with personality disorders.

In summary, it is useful to have familiarity with and confidence in using antidepressants. You may be pleasantly surprised at the relatively rapid and complete response in most of your patients. However, after an antidepressant has been used without significant improvement in an adequate dose and for a sufficient time, or if signs or symptoms of confusion or memory problems develop, consultation with a psychiatrist may be helpful in planning further treatment. As we shall see next, sometimes the apparent "failure" of antidepressant therapy is due to the presence of severe psychosocial distress.

The Social Model of Depression

Diagnosis

Clinicians frequently observe that adequate doses of antidepressants have blunted responses. Social factors can interact with pharmacological approaches and render medications less effective. Distress such as domestic violence, financial difficulties, and bereavement, or other forms of social isolation such as prolonged medical illness can all overpower medications. The older woman is statistically more likely to outlive her mate and may be unable to maintain a standard of living based on the partner's earnings. Decreasing physical function may further impair socialization.

Treatment

Understanding more about the patient's current living situation is essential. Frequently a scheduled interview time that allows for a greater depth of understanding will assist the clinician with this task. A social work assessment can also clarify the dimensions of the problem as well as point to community resources available to the patient. Patients frequently are isolated and lonely, and involvement in social events such as senior groups and church-sponsored activities will often be helpful. The victim of domestic violence or elder abuse is unlikely to respond to any treatment intervention until the assaultive behavior stops. The patient may also be entitled to financial assistance of which she is unaware. Changing the resources of the current environment, when possible, can be a powerful intervention in the management of depression and may significantly potentiate pharmacological approaches.

The Psychological Model of Depression

Diagnosis

In addition to current environment, prior social history contains clues for enhancing treatment response. Every woman grows up in a family where she learns the skills of interpersonal relationships, trust, coping, and problem-solving. In some families parents are unable to provide a protected, loving environment for the child. Sometimes this is due to parental psychiatric disorders, alcohol abuse, personality disorders, and exposure of the child to episodes of emotional, physical, and sexual abuse. This can later lead to dysfunctional adult coping behaviors and depression.

Women who grow up in homes where they are not taken care of properly can learn "automatic thoughts" or negative beliefs about themselves that leap into action in times of ambiguity. "I **ALWAYS** do things wrong." "Nobody wants to spend time with a loser." One negative outcome can be focused on to the exclusion of hundreds of successful outcomes. Many patients see themselves as chronically worthless, ineffective, and depressed. These cognitive mechanisms can be crucial in maintaining a chronic depression originally initiated in childhood and adolescence and can account for an apparent "nonresponse" to antidepressant medication.

Treatment

The treatment of patients with these adverse life experiences can be complicated, especially when the experiences have been severe, such as in cases of repeated incest. Formal psychotherapy is frequently helpful for these patients but often is not available due to lack of adequate insurance coverage. Self-help books such as *Feeling Good* by David Burns and *Control Your Depression* by Peter Lewinsohn are often useful in giving the patient "homework" exercises to review at your next appointment.

Briefer forms of psychotherapy can actually be done in 10-minute office visits using supportive listening and affirmation. Because medical training emphasizes the development of problem-solving and action-oriented skills, clinicians frequently underestimate the power of supportive listening (to paraphrase an old cliche, "don't just do something, stand there"). Basic communication skills learned in the first year of medical school such as *reflection* ("that must be difficult for you") and *legitimation* ("anyone with that much pain/stress/disease would understandably feel depressed") become important therapeutic interventions despite their apparent simplicity.

Frequently, however, patients with more severe stressors will need consultation with a behavioral specialist for more formal psychotherapy. This can range from a few sessions to many months of therapy in patients with severe childhood stressors such as emotional or sexual abuse. A consultation-liaison psychiatrist can help you estimate the severity of the personality components of the depression as well as the appropriateness of the patient for psychotherapy. Whether or not the patient begins formal psychotherapy, your 15-minute office visit is likely to be an important part of her overall improvement.

The biopsychosocial model assists the physician in obtaining a comprehensive history so that the relative contribution of each factor can be assessed and treated. The consultation-liaison psychiatrist can be particularly helpful to the gynecologist in understanding the interrelationships of these factors and should be consulted in more complicated patients who present with severe suicidality, psychosis, prior manic-depressive illness, personality disorders, substance abuse, and chronic pain.

Somatization as a Form of Depression

In psychologically minded women the awareness of psychosocial distress will usually lead to a complaint of anxiety or depression during a clinic visit. However, in non-Western cultures, and in individuals who have not learned the cultural cues associated with psychological mindedness (the awareness of feelings and their impact on emotional and physical health), the process of reporting distress may take the form of a physical symptom. The transduction of psychological or social distress into physical symptoms is known as somatization.

Somatization has been conservatively estimated to influence up to one half of all primary care visits. In a study of 1,000 patients followed over 3 years Kroenke and coworkers[4] studied the new appearance of the 14 most common presenting physical symptoms (eg, chest pain, abdominal pain, headache). They showed that, on average, only 10% of the time could an organic cause be found for these symptoms.

Why does somatization occur? Women may present medically unexplained physical symptoms for a number of reasons. First, depression and anxiety can present as dramatic physical processes. Patients with panic disorder frequently assume they are having life-threatening cardiac disease, and depressed patients experience either a psychomotor retardation and fatigue or a distressing agitation that they may associate with prior severe illness.

Second, in managed care environments distressing physical symptoms may get more immediate attention compared with "less critical" emotional complaints, thus encouraging the report of physical symptoms. "Chest pain" may get you a prompt evaluation, whereas "depression" might be handled as time permits. This is often justified by pointing out the consequences of failure to rule out a myocardial infarction. Interestingly, the Kroenke study found that nearly 90% of the time chest pain was not organic in origin, while other studies of depression have shown a 10% to 20% suicide rate. This illustrates the common double-standard that is frequently applied to complaints that are psychosocial in nature.

Finally, reimbursement incentives connected with disability can reward the production and maintenance of physical symptoms. Depression is frequently viewed as a moral failure by patients and their families, and patients can become trapped economically as they lose employment and become dependent on disability payments for their life needs.

Some patients will have large numbers of medically unexplained physical symptoms across several organ systems. Recent research has shown that the number of these symptoms is highly correlated with number of lifetime psychiatric disorders, severity of personality pathology, and high health care utilization. Regardless of severity, however, there are several useful strategies that can be employed to manage patients who have multiple medically unexplained symptoms (Table 15.2). Psychiatric consultation may also be beneficial to help constitute a long-term treatment plan that decreases utilization and increases the quality of the interaction for both the patient and the gynecologist.

INSTRUCTIONS FOR ADMINISTRATION OF
MINI-MENTAL STATE EXAMINATION

Orientation

1) Ask for the date. Then ask specifically for parts omitted, for example, "Can you also tell me what season it is?" One point for each correct.

(2) Ask in turn "Can you tell me the name of this hospital?" (town, county, etc.). One point for each correct.

Registration

Ask the patient if you may test his memory. Then say the names of 3 unrelated objects, clearly and slowly, about one second for each. After you have said all 3, ask him to repeat them. This first repetition determines his score (0–3) but keep saying them until he can repeat all 3, up to 6 trials. If he does not eventually learn all 3, recall cannot be meaningfully tested.

Attention and Calculation

Ask the patient to begin with 100 and count backward by 7. Stop after 5 subtractions (93, 86, 79, 72, 65). Score the total number of correct answers.

If the patient cannot or will not perform this task, ask him to spell the word "world" backwards. The score is the number of letters in correct order (eg, dlrow = 5, dlorw = 3).

Language

Naming: Show the patient a wrist watch and ask him what it is. Repeat for pencil. Score 0–2.

Repetition: Ask the patient to repeat the sentence after you. Allow only one trial. Score 0 or 1.

3-Stage Command: Give the patient a piece of plain blank paper and repeat the command. Score 1 point for each part correctly executed.

Reading: On a blank piece of paper print the sentence, "Close your eyes," in letters large enough for the patient to see clearly. Ask him to read it and do what it says. Score 1 point only if he actually closes his eyes.

Writing: Give the patient a blank piece of paper and aks him to write a sentence for you. Do not dictate a sentence, it is to be written spontaneously. It must contain a subject and verb and be sensible. Correct grammar and punctuation are not necessary.

Copying: On a clean piece of paper, draw intersecting pentagons, each side about 1 in, and ask him to copy it exactly as it is. All 10 angles must be present and 2 must intersect to score 1 point. Tremor and rotation are ignored.

Estimate the patient's level of sensorium along a continuum, from alert on the left to coma on the right.

Patient _____
Examiner _____
Date _____

"MINI-MENTAL STATE"*

Maximum Score	Score	

Orientation

5   (   )   What is the (year) (season) (date) (day) (month)?

5   (   )   Where are we: (state) (county) (town) (hospital) (floor).

Registration

3   (   )   Name 3 objects: 1 second to say each. Then ask the patient all 3 after you have said them. Give 1 point for each correct answer. Then repeat them until he learns all 3. Count trials and record.

Trials _____

Attention and Calculation

5   (   )   Serial 7's. 1 point for each correct. Stop after 5 answers. Alternatively spell "world" backwards.

Recall

3   (   )   Ask for the 3 objects repeated above. Give 1 point for each correct.

Language

9   (   )   Name a pencil, and watch (2 points)

Repeat the following "No ifs, ands or buts." (1 point)

Follow a 3-state command:
   "Take a paper in your right hand, fold it in half, and put it on the floor" (3 points)

Read and obey the following:
   Close your eyes (1 point)
   Write a sentence (1 point)
   Copy design (1 point)

TOTAL SCORE _____

ASSESS level of consciousness along a continuum

Alert	Drowsy	Stupor	Coma

Figure 15.1 Folstein Mini-Mental State Examination. (From Folstein MD, Folstein SE, McHugh PR: "Mini-mental state," a practical method for grading the cognitive state of patients for the clinician. *J. Psychiatr Res* 12;1975:189–198. © 1975, Pergamon Press, Lt.)

Table 15.2 Suggestions for Managing Patients with Multiple Medically Unexplained Symptoms

1. Schedule regular visits that focus on the impact of stress and life events.
2. Use conservative medical interventions (eg, exercise, diet and life-style changes).
3. Avoid narcotic medications and surgery whenever possible.
4. Do not challenge the physical basis of the symptom.
5. Reassure that no serious disease exists.
6. Treat existing depression and anxiety disorders.

Dementia and Delirium

Cognitive impairment is a common finding in elderly women. Although some very mild decreases in memory and abstraction ability are normal signs of aging, some women develop more serious deficits such as dementia and delirium. In the general population, 5% of those over age 65 have severe dementia and an additional 10% have mild dementia. By age 80, nearly 20% of the population has severe dementia. Organic mental disorders in the elderly are even higher in medical inpatient settings where the rates of delirium and dementia are found to be 30% to 50%. Both delirium and dementia reflect organic changes in brain function and can have superficially similar presentations of cognitive processing dysfunction, yet the pathophysiology of each is unique.[5]

Dementia and delirium are serious psychiatric disorders, and a prompt psychiatric consultation can make a significant difference in quality of life for both the patient and her family. A useful tool in diagnosing dementia and delirium is the Folstein Mini-Mental State Examination (Figure 15.1).[3] A score below 25/30 on this instrument is highly suggestive of an ultimate diagnosis of dementia and/or delirium and should result in a timely psychiatric referral.

Dementia

Dementia is marked by significant impairment of short- and long-term memory, which may be accompanied by impaired abstract thinking or judgment, aphasia, apraxia, agnosia, constructional difficulty, or personality change (Table 15.3).

The term *dementia* is used for several conditions that can result from potentially reversible metabolic, endocrine, or infectious etiologies, although most frequently it represents an *anatomical* insult to the brain accompanied by an irreversible loss of neuronal mass due to cell death. This is frequently seen on neuroimaging studies as widened sulci representative of decreased brain size.

Dementia should not be confused with the cognitive slowing and memory problems found in major depression. Frequently, elderly individuals are labeled with dementia before depression is thoroughly ruled out. The detection of a depressive *pseudodementia* allows the clinician to focus on vigorous antidepressant treatment. As the depressive component resolves there may be a concomitant resolution or decrease in the dementia symptoms as well. Even in cases of a well-established dementia, a decrease in severity of symptoms will be a welcome relief to caregivers.

Dementia is associated with Alzheimer's disease, multi-infarct disease, advanced acquired immunodeficiency syndrome (AIDS), and alcoholism as well as with several less common neurode-generative disorders such as Creutzfeld-Jakob disease. Onset is usually insidious, and the diagnosis is frequently made retrospectively by family members. While there is a normal, age-related decrease in memory known as benign senescent forgetfulness, dementia progresses into patterns of gradually worsening memory problems. In early phases keys are misplaced, word finding is occasionally difficult, and details of appointments are often forgotten. Later, the patient may leave burners on after cooking, the checkbook may be hopelessly unbalanced, and the patient may get lost in a

Table 15.3 DSM-IV Diagnostic Criteria for Dementia

A. The development of multiple cognitive deficits manifested by both
  1. Memory impairment (impaired ability to learn new information or to recall previously learned information).
  2. One (or more) of the following cognitive disturbances:
    (a) Aphasia (language disturbance).
    (b) Apraxia (impaired ability to carry out motor activities despite intact motor function).
    (c) Agnosia (failure to recognize or identify objects despite intact sensory function).
    (d) Disturbance in executive functioning (eg, planning, organizing, sequencing, and abstracting).
B. The cognitive deficits in Criteria A1 and A2 each cause significant impairment in social or occupational functioning and represent a significant decline from a previous level of functioning.
C. The course is characterized by gradual onset and continuing cognitive decline.
D. The cognitive deficits in Criteria A1 and A2 are not due to any of the following:
  1. Other central nervous system conditions that cause progressive deficits in memory and cognition (eg, cerebrovascular disease, Parkinson's disease, Huntington's disease, subdural hematoma, normal-pressure hydrocephalus, and brain tumor).
  2. Systemic conditions that are known to cause dementia (eg, hypothyroidism, vitamin B_{12} or folic acid deficiency, niacin deficiency, hypercalcemia, neurosyphilis, and HIV infection).
  3. substance-induced conditions
E. The deficits do not occur exclusively during the course of a delirium.
F. The disturbance is not better accounted for by another Axis I disorder (e.g., Major Depressive Disorder, Schizophrenia).

HIV, Human immunodeficiency virus.
American Psychiatric Association: Diagnostic and Statistical Manual of Mental Disorders, Fourth ed. Washington DC: APA, 1994

familiar neighborhood. In still later stages the patient may gradually lose orientation and even be unable to recognize her own children.

Early detection can help either in preventing progression (control by hypertension in multi-infarct dementia) or allowing the family to prepare for the increasing disability that lies ahead. Newer nootropic pharmacological agents such as Tacrine (Cognex) may be helpful in slowing the progression of Alzheimer's disease. If a patient is suspected of having an early dementia, a psychiatric consultation may be helpful in clarifying the diagnosis and suggesting a treatment plan that is helpful to both the patient and her family. Even in cases of rapidly progressive dementia the gynecologist can be an important supportive resource for the patient's caregivers as they try to cope with the difficulties of providing 24-hour-a-day care or making the decision to place the patient in an assisted-living or nursing-home situation.

Delirium

Delirium, by contrast, is a disorder of brain *physiology*. In delirium the brain experiences a global disruption of its metabolic equilibrium. This can be caused by hypoxia, electrolyte imbalances, hypoglycemia, internal toxins (metabolic byproducts not cleared in liver and kidney disease), external toxins (drugs of abuse as well as side effects of medications), and central nervous system infections. Although it frequently occurs in the presence of dementia, delirium also happens to patients without other brain pathology (Table 15.4).

Delirium presents with the sudden onset of mental status changes marked by disorientation and confusion, inability to remember new information, and either obtunded or hypervigilant conscious-ness. Delirium symptoms will wax and wane over hours from near-normal mental status to insignifi-

Table 15.4 DSM-IV Diagnostic Criteria for Delirium

A. Disturbance of consciousness (ie, reduced clarity of awareness of the environment) with reduced ability to focus, sustain, or shift attention.

B. A change in cognition (such as memory deficit, disorientation, language disturbance) or the development of a perceptual disturbance that is not better accounted for by a pre-existing, established, or evolving dementia.

C. The disturbance develops over a short period of time (usually hours to days) and tends to fluctuate during the course of the day.

D. There is evidence from the history, physical examination, or laboratory findings that the disturbance is caused by the direct physiological consequences of a general medical condition.

cant impairment of orientation. The patient with delirium may be difficult to interview because of apparent "sleepiness" or may even be thought to have "schizophrenia" due to disorganized thinking.

It is important to recognize that delirium is a medical emergency until proven otherwise. Delirium is often caused by life-threatening metabolic diseases, and proper treatment of the underlying medical disease will usually resolve the mental status changes. The treatment of delirium involves attention to both specific and general factors. Specifically, it is important to correct the underlying metabolic abnormality (eg, infection, blood pH, oxygen saturation) while providing general support-ive care, such as frequent orientation of the confused patient and removal of ambiguous environmen-tal cues that may be interpreted as threats. Haldol 0.5 mg qhs or twice a day is frequently very helpful in managing the patient. Benzodiazepines, although initially sedating for an agitated, delirious patient may actually worsen the delirium over time and should be avoided.

In an office setting, however, delirium may be less obvious. Older women placed on multiple medications by several physicians may experience more subtle forms of delirium. In cases where there is suspicion of mental status change, the clinician can do a simple memory test—such as ask the patient to repeat the names of three objects immediately and then in 5 minutes, or to say the months of the year backwards. In outpatient settings, polypharmacy is frequently the cause and simplifying medication plans can be helpful. Watch particularly for anticholinergic medications, such as tricyclic antidepressants and benadryl, and other psychotropic medications, such as benzodi-azepines and analgesics. These are sometimes combined with over-the-counter medications by the patient without the knowledge of the physician.

Summary

Changes in the health care system are increasingly calling upon the gynecologist to be a mental health provider for the aging woman. The biopsychosocial model suggests a thorough and efficient approach to the diagnosis of major depression and organic brain disorders such as delirium and dementia. Knowledge of the biomedical, social, and psychological dimensions of the patient assists in the formulation of better integrated treatment plans for these psychiatric disorders. Psychiatric consultation can be additionally helpful, particularly in patients with complex combinations of medical, social, and developmental stressors, and may assist the gynecologist in providing effective and comprehensive treatment.

Case One

A 68-year-old woman presents with a 6-month history of chronic lower abdominal pain, a weight loss of 30 pounds, fatigue, and diarrhea, and states that she is sure she has colon cancer. Multiple physical examinations and diagnostic tests including laparoscopic surgery, lower gastrointestinal, stool occult blood, and STD (sexually transmitted disease) cultures have yielded no explanation. On further questioning she reports early morning awakening, loss of appetite, poor concentration, anhedonia (diminished pleasure), and feelings of worthlessness and guilt. The physician suspects a Major Depressive Disorder (biological diagnosis) and starts the woman on 25 mg of desipramine each morning (biological treatment). She is told to return in 2 weeks and to increase the desipramine to 50 mg after 1 week. Two weeks later, she has minimal improvement and is told to increase the dose to 75 mg and return in 1 week. Upon return no improvement is noted.

The physician then learns that the woman is in an abusive relationship with her alcoholic husband who beats her several times a week (social diagnosis). The physician recommends that she leave her home for a women's shelter (social treatment) and return to the office in 1 week. At follow-up the patient "never felt so good" and feels the medicine is "miraculous." Another follow-up is scheduled for 2 weeks.

The patient returns stating that "she feels worse depression than before" and blames the doctor and the medication. The physician, surprised at the woman's return to her abusive home environment, inquires about her family history. Her father was also an abusive alcoholic who regularly struck the patient's mother. The patient, who was the oldest of three girls, frequently took over the mother's role in the family and was also a victim of her father's abuse.

The physician recommends leaving the abusive home again and arranges a psychiatric consultation. After 10 sessions with a therapist the patient improves markedly.

Case Two

Am 81-year-old woman is brought in by her daughter with the complaint of "confusion." The daughter states that the patient has been slowly "failing," but has had a recent sharp decline in her ability to care for herself. She cannot remember appointments, thinks it is 1927, and sees vivid patterns on her blank walls at bedtime. On mental status testing she is oriented to name only and cannot even repeat three objects immediately. Her Folstein Mini-Mental State Examination score is 14/30. The physician recognizes a delirium and searches for a medical cause. Examination of the patient's medications reveals prescriptions from several doctors including valium and amitriptyline for sleep, and Percocet for joint pain. The physician recommends a tapered discontinuation of these medications, asks the daughter to make arrangements for someone to live with the patient for a few days, and requests a follow-up visit in 1 week.

A week later the patient is markedly better. She is now oriented times 3, and has no more visual hallucinations. On further evaluation, however, it appears that the memory problems are more subtle. She still has residual short-term memory impairment and word-finding problems. Her ability to abstract is somewhat impoverished. Her Mini-Mental State score is now 24/30, consistent with moderate dementia. The daughter recalls that this has been a slow, almost unnoticed process, which the family has decided was "just aging." A consultation visit with a psychiatrist is obtained and further medical work-up shows an abnormal computed tomographic finding of decreased cortical mass consistent, with a diagnosis of Alzheimer's disease. The family, the gynecologist, and the psychiatrist then begin to plan for the future special needs of this patient.

References

1. Barrett JE, Barrett JA, Oxman TE, et al: The prevalence of psychiatric disorders in a primary care practice. *Arch Gen Psychiatry* 1988;45:1100–1106.
2. Engel GL: The clinical application of the biopsychosocial model. *Am J Psychiatry* 1980;137:535–544.
3. Folstein MF, Folstein SE, McHugh PR: Mini-mental state: A practical method for grading the cognitive state of patients for the clinician. *J Psychiatr Res* 1975;12:189–198.
4. Kroenke K, Mangelsdorff AD: Common Symptoms in ambulatory care: incidence, evaluation, therapy and outcome *Am J Med* 1989;86:262–6.
5. Perry SW, Markowitz J: Organic mental disorders, Talbott JA, Hales RE, Yudofsky SC (eds.): in *American Psychiatric Press Textbook of Psychiatry*. Washington, DC, American Psychiatric Press, 1988, pp 281–282.
6. Poon LW, Siegler IC: Psychological aspects of normal aging, In Sadavoy J, Lazarus LW, Jarvik LF (eds.): *Comprehensive Review of Geriatric Psychiatry*. American Association of Geriatric Psychiatry, Washington DC, American Psychiatric Press, 1991, pp 117–145.

7. Regier DA, Goldberg ID, Taube CA: The de facto US mental health care system. *Arch Gen Psychiatry* 1978;35:685–693.
8. Regier DA, Myers JK, Kramer M, et al: The NIMH epidemiologic catchment area program. *Arch Gen Psychiatry* 1984;41:934–941.
9. Warheit GJ, Longino CF, Bradsher JE: Sociocultural aspects, in Sadavoy J, Lazarus LW, Jarvik LF (eds.): *Comprehensive Review of Geriatric Psychiatry*. American Association of Geriatric Psychiatry, Washington DC, American Psychiatric Press, 1991, p 105.

Chapter 16

Lower Urinary Tract Disorders in Older Women

Gretchen Lentz, MD and Morton A. Stenchever, MD

By the early part of the next century, 20% of Americans will be over the age of 65. The inevitable aging process leads to many physiological changes in the lower urinary tract, making lower urinary tract dysfunction common in the older female. Furthermore, the multisystem alterations that occur with aging also interact with the function of the genitourinary system. These changes may include neurological deficits, mental status changes, hormonal deficiency, medication effects, and mobilization problems, which can all interact and upset the balance involving the bladder functions of storing and emptying. The result of the interplay of many of these factors may be urinary incontinence. Yarnell and St. Leger[1] found that approximately 5% to 15% of community-dwelling elderly have incontinence. Diokno and coworkers[2] found the prevalence to be 37.7% in elderly Michigan residents. This rises to 40% in hospitalized patients aged 70 or older in Warshaw's and coworkers[3] survey and over 50% in institutionalized patients according to Ouslander and coworkers.[4,5] Urinary incontinence is responsible for 40% to 60% of all nursing-home admissions. Norton and coworkers[6] found that incontinence has considerable social consequences in addition to the medical aspects.

This chapter reviews the physiology of micturition, with consideration of age-related changes, anatomical relationships of the female genitourinary tract, the pertinent history, diagnostic issues, and therapy for many common conditions affecting the lower urinary tract. The International Continence Society (ICS) has standardized the terminology of lower urinary tract function.[7] The terminology in this chapter adheres to the ICS nomenclature.

Anatomy and Physiology of Micturition

Continence is a function of the urethra's ability to prevent the flow of urine and the bladder's ability to store urine. Micturition is dependent on the ability of the urethra to relax and the detrusor muscle of the bladder to contract. Both the urethra and the bladder are under neurological control via the autonomic nervous system. Simply stated, the sympathetic portion of the autonomic nervous system maintains continence because stimulation of alpha-adrenergic receptors (which occur primarily in the urethra and rarely in the bladder) causes contraction of the urethral musculature, and stimulation of beta-adrenergic receptors (which occur primarily in the bladder and rarely in the urethra) causes relaxation. The neurotransmitter for the sympathetic system is norepinephrine. On the other hand, the parasympathetic nervous system stimulates contraction of the detrusor muscle and relaxation of the urethral musculature. The neurotransmitter involved here is acetylcholine (Figure 16.1).

The factors that affect urethral closure involve urethral tone, which is affected by the elasticity of the urethral wall, the presence of smooth and striated muscles in the urethra, and the vascular component supplying the urethra and bladder neck. In addition, urethral pressure is supported by the vaginal levator muscle attachments, which DeLancey[8] has shown is primarily supportive of the mid-60% of the urethral length. The fascial and connective tissue supports that suspend the urethra to the posterior region of the pubic symphysis are important because they maintain the proximal urethra and the bladder neck in an intra-abdominal position.

The act of voiding involves four basic autonomic and somatic nervous system feedback loops. The first (loop I) connects the cerebral cortex to the brain stem and inhibits micturition by modifying sensory stimuli that emanate from the second loop. The second loop (loop II) originates in the sacral micturition center (S2 to S4) and the detrusor muscle wall itself. Sensory fibers of this loop run to the brain stem, where a modulation by loop I takes place. If cerebral inhibition is not imposed via loop I, the stimuli returns to the sacral micturition center and allows activation of loop III. Loop III involves the sensory nerve flow from the pressure receptors of the bladder wall to the sacral micturition center with return motor fibers to the urethral sphincter striated muscle. This allows the voluntary relaxation of the urethral sphincter as the detrusor contracts. Loop IV is initiated in the frontal lobe of the cerebral cortex and extends to the sacral micturition center and on to the urethral striated muscle allowing urethral voluntary muscles to relax, thus initiating the voiding mechanism (Figure 16.2). A variety of conditions, such as demyelinating diseases,

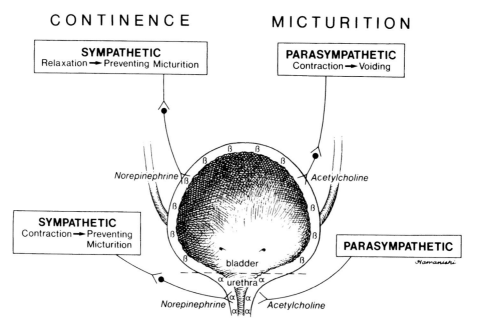

Figure 16.1 The innovation of the bladder and urethra. Parasympathetic fibers arising in S2–S4 have long preganglionic fibers and pelvic ganglia close to the bladder and urethra. These parasympathetic fibers excrete acetylcholine. Sympathetic fibers that have long postganglionic fibers discharge norepinephrine to beta-receptors, primarily in the bladder, and alpha-receptors, primarily in the urethra. (Redrawn and modified from Raz S: *Urol Clin North Am* 1978;5:323–.)

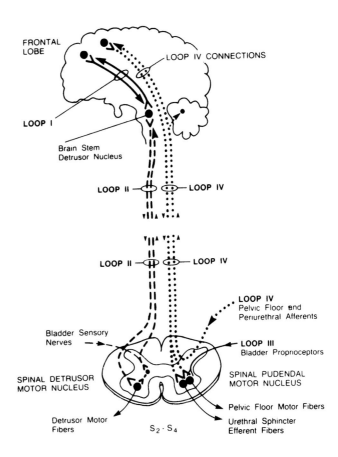

Figure 16.2 Central nervous system feedback loops. (From Williams ME, Fitzhugh CP: Urinary incontinence in the elderly. *Ann Intern Med* 1982;97:895–; with permission.)

Parkinson's disease, cerebral vascular conditions, disease of the lower urinary tract, and central nervous system (CNS) tumors, may interfere with any or all of these loops and cause malfunction of the system. Table 16.1 summarizes the importance of each loop and the way in which pathological conditions may effect the loops. Furthermore, medications that affect the autonomic nervous system by stimulating or blocking either the action of acetylcholine or norepinephrine, thereby affecting CNS transmission, may effect micturition and continence. Table 16.2 lists common medications often used by aging patients and the specific effects these medications may have on the micturition process.

Sympathetic receptors are influenced by estrogen and progesterone with estrogen-stimulating alpha-receptors and progesterone-influencing beta-receptors. Hormone withdrawal during the aging process affects these, and hormone replacement therapy (HRT) may reverse the effects that are observed.

Asmussen and Ulmsten[9] consider the bladder and urethra a functional unit, with the bladder's subfunction being to store urine and the urethra's to allow it to pass. For urine to exit the urethra, the maximal urethral pressure must be lower than the intravesical pressure. Intravesical pressure depends on the volume of urine in the bladder, the part of the intra-abdominal pressure that is transmitted to the bladder, and the tension in the bladder wall that is related to muscular and nervous system activity. Normal resting pressure within the bladder is 20 to 30 cm of water.

Table 16.1 Neurological Control of Micturition: Clinical Considerations on Central Nervous System Reflex Loops

Loop	Origin	Termination	Function	Association conditions
I	Frontal lobe	Brain stem	Coordinates volitional control of micturition	Parkinson's disease, brain tumors, trauma, cerebrovascular disease, multiple sclerosis, lower urinary tract disease
II	a. Brain stem b. Bladder wall	Sacral micturition center Brainstem	Detrusor muscle contraction to empty bladder	Spinal cord trauma, multiple sclerosis, spinal cord tumors
III	Sensory afferents of detrusor muscle	Striated muscle of urethral sphincter via pudendal motor nervous and micturition center	Allows relaxation of urethral sphincter in synchrony with detrusor contraction	Multiple sclerosis, spinal cord trauma or tumors, diabetic neuropathy, local urinary tract disease
IV	Frontal lobe	Pudendal nucleus	Volitional control of striated external urethral sphincter	Cerebral or spinal trauma or tumor, multiple sclerosis, cerebrovascular disease, lower urinary tract disease

From Ostergard DR: The neurologic control of micturition and integral voiding reflexes. *Obstet Gynecol Surv* 1979;34:417–; with permission.

The intra-urethral pressure depends on striated and smooth muscle fibers within the urethral wall, the vasculature of the urethral submucosal cavernous plexus, the elasticity of the urethral wall, and the part of the intra-abdominal pressure that is transmitted to the urethra. The urethral closure pressure is defined as the maximal urethral pressure minus the bladder pressure. For continence to be present, the urethral closure pressure (UCP) must be greater than the intravesicle pressure. Asmussen and Ulmsten[9] have demonstrated that the highest pressure zone in the urethra is just proximal to the mid-point of the total length of the urethra and just above the urogenital diaphragm (Figure 16.3). Enhorning and coworkers[10] and Asmussen and Ulmsten[9] have noted that the submucosal cavernous plexus of vessels, the bulk of smooth and striated musculature, and the majority of autonomic nervous system fibers are the most prominent in this area. In addition, pressure recording within this area oscillates in synchrony with the heartbeat, making it likely that the submucosal cavernous plexus is important in helping to maintain continence. The structure is also under the influence of estrogen. The oscillations that correlate with the heartbeat in young women can be as great as 25 cm of water. In postmenopausal women not on estrogen replacement therapy (ERT), it may be as little as 5 cm of water. In addition, this cavernous plexus is more thick-walled and less elastic in older women. Estrogen is therefore important to the urethral closure mechanism because of its effect on the alpha-adrenergic receptors, the elasticity and maintenance of the subcavernous plexus, and also because of its positive effect on the epithelium of the urethra itself. When the urethra is properly supported and most of the functional urethra is in its normal position above the urogenital diaphragm, it will receive an increase in intra-abdominal pressure simultaneously with the effect of the increase on the bladder. Thus, a sudden increase in intra-abdominal pressure should not, under normal circumstances, cause incontinence. If the functional

Table 16.2. Drugs with Possible Effects on the Lower Urinary Tract

Class	Possible side effects	Drug and usual indication	Action
Antihypertensives	Incontinence	Reserpine— hypertension Methyldopa— hypertension	Pharmacological sympathectomy by depleting catecholamines
Dopaminergic agents	Bladder neck obstruction	Bromocriptine— galactorrhea Levodopa— Parkinson's disease	Increased urethral resistance and decreased detrusor contractions
Cholinergic agonists	Decreased bladder capacity and increased intravesical pressure	Digitalis—cardiotropic	Increased bladder wall tension
Neuroleptics	Incontinence	Major tranquilizers: prochlorperazine, promethazine, trifluoperazine, chlorpromazine, haloperidol	Dopamine receptor blockade, with internal sphincter relaxation
β-adrenergic agents	Urinary retention	Isoxsuprine— vasodilator Terbutaline— bronchodilator	Inhibited bladder muscle contractility
Xanthines	Incontinence	Caffeine	Decrea sed urethral closure pressure

From Corlett RC: Gynecologic urology: I. Urinary incontinence. *Female Patient* 1985;10:20–; with permission.

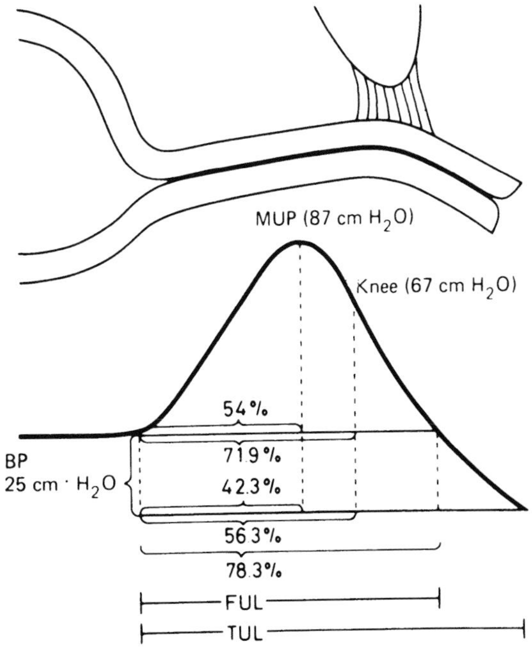

Figure 16.3 The location of maximal urethral pressure in relation to the urogenital diaphragm (average value of 25 normal women). *Knee* indicates the location of the urogenital diaphragm seen on X-ray film and transformed to the pressure curve. (From Asmussen M, Ulmsten U: On the physiology of continence and pathophysiology of stress incontinence in the female. *Contrib Gynecol Obstet* 1983;10:32–35.)

urethra is displaced from its usual anatomical relationships, it would be below the urogenital diaphragm. Then an increase in intra-abdominal pressure to the bladder will not equally affect the urethra but, rather, will be additive to the intravesicular pressure. In such instances, stress incontinence is a common finding. These issues are discussed later in this chapter when incontinence is considered.

Age-Related Changes in Anatomy and Physiology

There are many age-related anatomical and physiological changes in the lower urinary tract (Table 16.3). Histologic bladder changes in women from age 74 to 102 from studies of cadavers show marked trabeculation and diverticula formation. In studies of cadavers, Levy and Wight[11] have shown increased collagen content with age.

With age, the ability to inhibit a detrusor contraction (delay voiding), bladder capacity, urethral closure pressure, bladder compliance, and urinary flow rates all decrease. Detrusor contractility may also decrease. Residual urine increases to 50 to 100 ml (but probably no more than 25 cc). Uninhibited detrusor contractions probably increase with age such that 15% to 20% of normal women aged 60 to 70 demonstrate this finding, and this increases with advancing age. The significance of this finding on cystometry must be placed in context of the clinical picture. The elderly also excrete a larger proportion of their daily fluid intake at night compared with younger people. This can lead to nocturia up to two times per night in the majority of normal elderly women.

It has been commonly stated that urinary incontinence prevalence increases with age, but few studies have addressed this issue.[12] These normal physiological changes in the lower urinary tract do not necessarily cause incontinence, but they probably predispose the aging woman to incontinence when additional pathological insults occur.[13]

Lower Urinary Tract Evaluation

A great number of tests and procedures are available to the physician for the evaluation of urinary tract symptoms and incontinence. These range from very simple tests that can be performed in the doctor's office to more sophisticated tests that require specialized equipment and expertise. Several of these are discussed.

History and Physical Examination

Despite the present era of sophisticated laboratory testing, a detailed medical, urological, and neurological history is essential in the initial evaluation of a patient who complains of lower urinary tract problems. Although the bladder has been called an "unreliable witness," the history and physical examination certainly help direct the investigation. Resnick[14] points out the importance of transient causes of incontinence in the elderly using the mnemonic DIAPPERS (delirium, infection, atrophic vaginitis/urethritis, pharmaceuticals, physiological, endocrine, restricted mobility, stool impaction). Many of these causes can be identified by careful history-taking. Specific information regarding urology includes establishing duration and frequency of symptoms, the extent to which the symptoms affect the patient, daytime and nighttime voiding frequency, irritative symptoms (urgency, frequency, dysuria), voiding difficulty, hematuria, postvoid dribbling and urinary leakage; in short, questions must be asked which seek to distinguish stress from urge incontinence. Stress incontinence involves the loss of urine secondary to activities that suddenly increase intra-abdominal pressure—straining, coughing, sneezing, lifting, running. Urge incontinence is leakage of urine associated with a strong desire to void. Asking about the use of pads to

Table 16.3 Age-Related and Age-Associated Factors Affecting Micturition

Factors	Potential effects on micturition*
Age-Related	
Decreased estrogen	Thinner and more friable vaginal and urethral mucosa, predisposing to atrophic vaginitis and associated symptoms; diminished supporting tissue surrounding bladder outlet and urethra, predisposing to stress incontinence; increased likelihood of vaginal vault prolapse, urinary symptoms, and infection
Lower urethral pressure (women)	Increased likelihood of incontinence
Prostatic hyperplasia	Increased likelihood of urinary symptoms and urinary retention

Altered bladder function:
  Decreased capacity
  Increased residual urine
  Involuntary contractions (detrusor motor instability)
	Increased likelihood of urinary symptoms, incontinence, and infection

Increased nocturnal urine production	Nocturia, incontinence at night
Altered immune function	Increased susceptibility to infection
Altered central and peripheral neurotransmission; changes in neurotransmitters, receptors, nerve conduction	Increased likelihood of bladder and urethral dysfunction
Age Associated	

Disorders that impair mobility:
  Degenerative joint disease
  Hip fracture
  Peripheral vascular disease
  Stroke
  Parkinson's disease
	More difficulty getting to a toilet or toilet substitute, predisposing to functional incontinence

Central nervous system diseases affecting cognition and bladder function:
  Dementia
  Stroke
  Parkinson's disease
	Decreased ability to manage toileting independently, predisposing to functional incontinence
	Increased incidence of detrusor hyperreflexia and urge incontinence

Other general medical conditions: Diabetes mellitus	Polyuria; increased risk of a contractile bladder, urinary retention, and overflow incontinence

Congestive heart failure
  Venous insufficiency
  Chronic lung disease
	Nocturia
	
	Precipitation or exacerbation of stress incontinence

Medications: Autonomic agents	Predispose to incontinence and/or urinary retention by effects on bladder and urethral function
Diuretics	Precipitate or exacerbate urge incontinence
Psychotropics	Autonomic effects (some); affect mental status and/or mobility and may contribute to incontinence
Lower urinary tract disorders: Asymptomatic bacteriuria	May increase likelihood of symptomatic infections and exacerbate urinary symptoms and incontinence
Benign prostatic hyperplasia Cancer of the prostate	Urinary symptoms and urinary retention
Bladder tumors and stones	Urinary symptoms

*Although all of the effects listed may occur, the precise role of many of the factors listed in producing disorders of micturition in the elderly remains unclear.

From Ouslander JG, Bruskewitz R: Disorders of micturition in the aging patient. *Adv Intern Med* 1989;34:165–190; with permission.

manage incontinence is helpful in gauging the severity of the leakage and how problematic it is for the patient. Other relevant questions include those regarding the history of previous pelvic surgery, enuresis, pregnancy, bowel dysfunction, gynecological symptoms—especially pelvic relaxation—and prescription drugs. A history of neurological disease or trauma may be pertinent to the problem.

On physical examination a neurological examination is frequently indicated. Neurological evaluation of the lower urinary tract includes assessment of T10–S4 sensation, motor strength, tone, and reflexes. Pudendal nerve motor function is evaluated by eliciting the bulbocavernous reflex and anal wink and assessing rectal sphincter tone. Certainly a complete neurologic examination is necessary if the history indicates other problems.

In addition to the usual pelvic examination, inspection for estrogen effect and vaginal wall support with a Sims' speculation or posterior blade of a bivalve speculum are important. A stress test can be performed to directly observe urinary leakage by having the patient stand and cough repetitively with a moderately full bladder.

Urolog

A 3-day voiding diary as shown in Figure 16.4 may be helpful in delineating the severity of the patient's frequency-urgency symptoms or incontinent episodes. The patient records the amount of fluid intake, time and amount of each void, and number and activity related to the incontinence episodes. The voiding diary may also identify the patient with excessive fluid intake, explaining her complaints of urgency and frequency. Lenz and Stanton[15] showed that a 3-day urinary diary is as accurate as a longer diary for assessing urinary habits in women complaining of frequency and urgency (Abstract AUGS, 1992, Cambridge, Mass).

Urinalysis and Culture

Urine may be collected for analysis and culture either by catheterizing the patient or by collecting a clean voided sample. Such a sample can be collected by first preparing the periurethral area of the vulva with an antiseptic solution and catching a mid-stream urine specimen. This is sent for urinalysis, culture, and sensitivity testing. The presence of red blood cells can signal cystitis or upper urinary tract damage caused by infection, renal cell carcinoma, or other kidney disease. The

DAY 1

Time	Fluid intake (oz.)	Amount voided (cc)	Activity or symptoms	Leakage volume

DAY 2

Time	Fluid intake (oz.)	Amount voided (cc)	Activity or symptoms	Leakage volume

Figure 16.4 Urinary diary

presence of red blood cells, white blood cells, or bacteria may suggest cystitis, asymptomatic bacteria, urethritis, infected urethral diverticulum or an upper urinary tract infection, such as pyelonephritis. Lower urinary tract infection is often accompanied by urgency, frequency, dysuria, and at times incontinence. Treating the infection with specific antibiotic therapy may alleviate the symptoms completely.

Test for Residual Urine

This test can be very helpful in evaluating a patient with a cystocele, one who may have overflow incontinence or voiding dysfunction. The patient is asked to urinate and the spontaneously voided amount of urine is measured. She is then catheterized and the residual urine left in the bladder is measured and may be sent for culture and analysis. If the patient has voided at least 100 to 150 ml, the residual urine should be less than 50 ml. Larger residual volumes are suggestive of inadequate bladder emptying and large amounts may indicate overflow incontinence. Overflow incontinence may be seen in patients with a neurological impairment, as a result of medications affecting micturition such as anticholinergic drugs, after stress incontinence surgery, or rarely with acute infection. In the case of neurogenic bladder, the patient may have a demyelinating disease, diabetic neuropathy, Parkinson's disease, or a tumor, trauma, or vascular accident involving the brain or spinal cord. Inadequate bladder emptying may be seen with anatomical abnormalities, such as large cystocele or vaginal prolapse, or in the elderly with impaired detrusor contraction. The residual volume can also be accurately measured by ultrasonography although this does not allow for sterile specimen for culture.

Office Cystometrics

A good deal of information can easily be gained about bladder capacity and function in an office setting. After the patient is catheterized to obtain a residual urine, the catheter is left in place and attached to a graduated asepto-syringe without bulb. Warm sterile saline is then infused through the syringe, carefully measuring the amount introduced. When the patient first has the urge to void, the amount is noted. In a normal patient, this urge generally occurs with 150 to 200 ml of saline in the bladder. Following this, saline infusion continues until the patient has a strong urge to void. This usually occurs when 400 to 500 ml has been infused. Women with detrusor instability or bladder hypersensitivity frequently have their first urge to void at levels far below 150 ml and have bladder capacities considerably less than 400 to 500 ml. Patients with poorly contractile neurogenic bladders will often be able to tolerate much larger volumes. Normal women can maintain bladder capacities of greater than 500 ml but generally with great conscious effort.

A cough stress test can be done by leaving 300 to 500 cc of saline in the bladder. The catheter is removed and the patient is asked to cough. If fluid spurts instantaneously from the urethral meatus, stress incontinence may be present. If a delayed loss of fluid or prolonged leakage is noted, detrusor instability may be present with a cough-induced uninhibited detrusor contraction.

Q-Tip Test

Q-tip testing is performed to assess the degree of urethral mobility. Greater mobility tends to be observed with stress incontinence. A moistened or lubricated (2% Xylocaine jelly) Q-tip is gently inserted through the urethra into the bladder. It is gently drawn back to the internal urethral meatus. The patient is asked to cough or perform a Valsalva maneuver, and the deflection of the Q-tip is noted in degrees from the horizontal. The resting angle from horizontal is measured with a goniometer or is estimated. A Q-tip angle of greater than 30 degrees during straining suggests mobility (relaxation of anatomic support of the urethrovesical junction) and roughly correlates with stress incontinence. Most authors define a positive test as greater than 30°. The role of the Q-tip test is controversial because it is not a good diagnostic test for stress incontinence. Montz and Stanton[16] re-evaluated the Q-tip test and discovered that 32% of patients with a positive Q-tip test had either pure detrusor instability or pure sensory urgency after complete urological work-up. Of the patients who had a negative Q-tip test, 29% were diagnosed as pure, genuine stress incontinence. Other studies have also found the Q-tip test to be unreliable in differentiating genuine stress incontinence (GSI) from other lower urinary tract disorders. In 1993 Caputo and Benson[17] reported the inaccuracy of the Q-tip test in measuring urethrovesical junction mobility compared with perineal ultrasonography. The Q-tip test had a sensitivity of 25%, specificity of 78%, positive predictive value of 67%, and negative predictive value of 37%. These results suggest that the Q-tip is not accurate for assessing hypermobility either.

Marshall or Bonney Test

To perform this test, 250 ml of saline is left in the bladder and the catheter is removed. The patient is asked to cough while in the recumbent position. If urine spurts from the urethral meatus, stress incontinence may be present. Gentle elevation of the bladder neck using the index finger and the middle finger on either side of the urethra may then be performed. Care should be taken not to obstruct the urethra, only to replace it behind the pubic symphysis. The patient is then asked to cough and is observed for loss of urine. If the urine is not lost the Bonney test is said to positive. This test can be repeated with the patient in the standing position because it frequently requires this to demonstrate stress incontinence.

There is a good deal of controversy as to whether or not the Bonney test is of value. This is because it is difficult to compare the results of a Bonney test with more sophisticated cystometric studies. Elevation of the urethrovesical junction using an Allis clamp or the examiner's fingers to predict the outcome of incontinence surgery has now been shown to be inaccurate and unreliable. The test probably obstructs the urethrovesical junction and proximal urethra and is almost always positive. Nevertheless, some clinicians find they gain useful information in directing the patient's evaluation.

Uroflowmetry

The urinary flow rate is the initial measurement in the evaluation of many voiding dysfunctions. Although urethral obstruction is more common in the male, uroflowmetry is a simple screening test for detecting severe voiding disorders in the female. If uroflowmetry equipment is not available, the patient can be asked to urinate while she times her void with a stopwatch. The amount voided should be recorded. It is important to remember that urinary flow rate varies significantly with the voided volume. Furthermore, it can vary in an individual from one voiding episode to another, so several urinary flow rate studies should be done.

Endoscopy

The lower urinary tract is easily accessible for evaluation via endoscopy. Endoscopy is frequently used as part of the evaluation for urinary tract dysfunction. Not all physicians believe it is necessary for an incontinence work-up, but others believe useful information is gained in visualizing the urethra and bladder neck. Local anesthetic, such as 2% Xylocaine, frequently works well alone for analgesia, but some patients may also require parenteral analgesics.

Urethroscopy allows visualization of the urethra for evaluation of urethral diverticulum, periurethral gland inflammation, atrophic urethritis, fibrosis with loss of urethral mucosal coaptation known as a "drain-pipe" urethra, bladder neck incompetence with increased intra-abdominal pressure, or other urethral pathology. Xylocaine local anesthetic can cause reddening of the urethral mucosa, which may alter urethral assessment. At cystoscopy, findings might include fistula, trabeculation (thought to be secondary to high intravesical pressure), mucosal abnormality, carcinoma in situ of the bladder, bladder diverticulum, bladder polyps, calculi, abnormal ureteral implantation, uretero-cele with reflux. Cystoscopy is routinely used for advanced gynecological malignancy investigation to exclude tumor extension into the lower urinary tract.

Originally, carbon dioxide gas was used for urethroscopy. Currently available equipment allows for the performing of pressure readings within the urethra and the bladder, but caution must be exercised to avoid rapid instillation of carbon dioxide into the lower urinary tract. This may in itself stimulate detrusor contraction and lead to a reflex opening of the vesicle neck, thus giving the operator a false impression of function and pathology. Today a water system is more commonly used (either saline or sterile water). A water system is probably better for diagnosing detrusor hyperactivity because it is less irritating to the detrusor muscle. With either system the bladder may be visualized and pathology noted. Equipment is relatively simple to operate, quite inexpensive, and can be easily used in the office setting. Few serious complications occur with urethroscopy and cystoscopy. However, urinary tract infections can commonly (3–5%) occur therefore many physicians give prophylactic antibiotics. Patients can have irritative symptoms, burning sensation with urination, bleeding, or lower abdominal discomfort for a few days after the procedure.

Endoscopy is also routinely used in surgical procedures for stress incontinence to confirm correct suture placement at the bladder neck, to evaluate tension when tying the supporting sutures, to be sure that no suture has been placed in the bladder, and to ensure efflux of urine from the ureters once the sutures have been tied.

Cystometry

Cystometry is used to assess detrusor activity, sensation, capacity, and compliance. It can measure changes in bladder pressure in response to filling and voiding and involves the use of a pressure transducer.[18] Cystometry can be performed in a number of ways. Single-channel cystometry can be performed without sophisticated equipment, but it is limited because increases in abdominal pressure can be mistaken for detrusor contractions. Sand and coworkers[19] found simple standing cystometry to be an accurate, reproducible, fairly sensitive test for detecting detrusor instability, although the test was repeated on two occasions. Subtracted cystometry (2 or 3 channels) involves the simultaneous recording of pressure within the bladder and abdominal cavity. A subtracted pressure (intravesical minus intra-abdominal) allows for estimation of the true detrusor pressure. Multichannel urodynamic studies can add urethral pressure measurement and electromyography. Video cystourethrography can add another dimension to testing. Dynamic evaluation of bladder filling (with radiopaque fluid) and voiding with fluoroscopy can add visualization of structural abnormalities. Because some women are incontinent due to both a stress urinary incontinence component and a detrusor instability component, it is important to define the causes of incontinence for the individual patient before undertaking therapy. This is discussed more thoroughly later when the specific types of incontinence are considered.

At least simple cystometry should be done in patients with stress incontinence if over age 50 or for mixed symptoms of urgency, frequency, or urge incontinence. Specialized testing may be recommended when (1) the diagnosis is uncertain after basic evaluation; (2) a conservative treatment trial fails; (3) hematuria without infection is present (indicates need for cystoscopy and intravenous pyelogram); (4) voiding dysfunction is suspected; (5) examination detects severe pelvic prolapse;

(6) high postvoid residual urine is found; or (7) neurological impairment is evident. Other indications to consider include age over 60 (because of the higher incidence of detrusor instability), failed prior incontinence surgery, symptoms of urgency, frequency, and urge incontinence are present and simple cystometry is negative, prior gynecological cancer treated with radial pelvic surgery or radiation, and continuous urinary incontinence or leakage without warning.

Ambulatory urodynamics, or continuous urodynamic monitoring, has been developed analogous to Holter monitoring. Pressure transducers are placed in the bladder and either the vagina or rectum. The patient can be observed during several cycles of natural bladder filling (with urine, not retrograde filling with saline or sterile water), storing, and emptying. Events such as urgency, cough, and incontinence can be marked by the patient and evaluated later in relation to the pressure changes. Van Waalwijk and van Doorn[20] studied healthy female volunteers to compare standard urodynamics with ambulatory monitoring. On standard testing 18% had uninhibited contractions, and on ambulatory testing, 69%. Studies on ambulatory patients with symptoms of urge incontinence have shown similar increases in detection of detrusor contractions.[21] The appropriate indications for using this technique are not clearly defined, but it may be useful for evaluating the patient with urgency and urge incontinence symptoms who has a negative traditional multichannel study.

Ultrasonography has often been used to measure residual urine, but there is interest in finding a wider role for ultrasonography in urodynamic studies. Ultrasonography may prove to be a noninvasive way to evaluate urinary tract function and structure, and to avoid using a urethral catheter, which may greatly affect the function of the bladder, bladder neck, and urethra. As ultrasound resolution continues to improve and advances are made in the ability to study blood and urine flow, new information regarding the dynamics of lower urinary tract function may emerge.

Urodynamic evaluation of the lower urinary tract represents an important diagnostic aid for assessment of urinary function. But it should be viewed in the context of the patient's complaints and serve to complement clinical impressions.[22] Reliance on one urodynamic study to determine the diagnosis would be a mistake. Most urodynamic studies are conducted in a laboratory setting, and this leads to a number of potential problems. These studies are a brief picture of physiological events performed in an artificial setting. Although the results are reproducible, they do not always accurately reflect the patient's problem in day-to-day life.

Lower Urinary Tract Infections

Urinary tract infections (UTI) are more common among women than men of all ages, except infancy. The incidence of UTI in women increases greatly at the onset of sexual activity, but the prevalence is highest in the older population. Komaroff[23] estimates as many as 25% of women in the United States experience an episode of acute dysuria annually.

UTI symptoms can include frequency, urgency, dysuria, hematuria, and pyuria; back, pelvic, and flank pain; and fever and chills. Occasionally, incontinence is associated with acute or chronic infection. Two bacterial pathogens, *Escherichia coli* and *Staphylococcus saprophyticus* cause 90% of episodes of acute uncomplicated cystitis (AUC). A variety of organisms can also be found with much lower frequency, including *Klebsiella, Pseudomonas, Proteus, Streptococcus faecalis,* and *Chlamydia.* The microbiology of bacteriuria changes in elderly women. Although *E. coli* remains the predominant causative organism, *Proteus, Klebsiella, Providencia, Pseudomonas,* and *Citrobacter* play larger roles. In addition, Nicolle and coworkers[24] found that in elderly women infections are more likely to be localized to the upper renal tract instead of the bladder and may require prolonged treatment. Bacteriuria also increases after menopause.

The pathogenesis of AUC involves many factors. The narrow spectrum of pathogens responsible for AUC suggests that these microorganisms have specific virulence factors that enable them to colonize and infect the urinary tract.[25] The *E. coli* that cause AUC originate in fecal flora, colonize the vaginal introitus and periurethral area, and ascend into the bladder via the short female urethra. According to Buckley and coworkers[26], this ascent is facilitated by urethral manipulation, most often with coitus. Other properties promoting infection include bacterial virulence factors such as adhesions (P. fimbriae), toxins, and bacterial invasiveness. Stamm[27] has shown host characteristics to be important in the pathogenesis of AUC including women who do not secrete blood group antigens into their bodily fluids. Certain glycolipids on nonsecretor epithelial cells may provide binding sites for bacteria. Immune and hormonal factors may also play a role. Since colonization of the introitus is a critical step, the host vaginal microbial ecology influences susceptibility to infection. Behavioral factors may likewise contribute to the pathogenesis. Hooton and Stamm[28] also showed that the use of a diaphragm plus spermicide appears to alter normal vaginal microflora in such a manner as to predispose to *E. coli* colonization and an increased risk for urinary tract infections. It is likely that antibiotic use and lack of estrogen do the same thing.

It is not clear why older women may actually be more vulnerable to UTIs. The reasons advanced include a shortened urethra in the female often made apparently shorter by hormone withdrawal; the close proximity of the vulva, vagina, and rectum to the urethra (areas where multiple bacterial flora are present); poor hygiene brought about because of physical or mental incapacitation; the habit some women have of wiping their anus toward the urethra; chronic mild trauma from sexual intercourse; and the loss of estrogen's effect on the reproductive and urinary tracts in postmenopausal women. In some women, urinary tract obstruction that may occur because of pelvic relaxation problems or impaired detrusor contractility may also play a role in UTI. Certain medical conditions such as diabetes contribute as well.

The absence of estrogen mentioned above deserves further comment. Raz and Stamm[29] found that lack of estrogen in postmenopausal women is associated with markedly reduced *Lactobacillus* colonization, increased vaginal pH, increased colonization, and a tenfold increased risk for AUC. These changes can be reversed with topical estrogen preparations.

Asymptomatic UTI

In 1987, Nicolle and coworkers[24] reported that more than 10% of women over the age of 70 who are otherwise healthy have positive urine culture. Boscia and coworkers[30] state that symptomatic bacteriuria increases from about 20% at age 70 to 80% at age 80. Most elderly women with bacteriuria do not have symptoms of UTI. Patients with acute UTI and asymptomatic bacteriuria have been compared and the microorganisms were found to be similar. *E. coli* is present 70% to 80% of the time. Organisms isolated from women with asymptomatic infection are characterized by a lower prevalence of virulence factors. Despite the lack of symptoms, 50% to 90% of women with asymptomatic bacteriuria will have host response to infection, as evidenced by inflammation within the urinary tract (pyuria).

Asymptomatic bacteriuria has been shown to be associated with significant morbidity only in pregnant women. Increased mortality for women with asymptomatic bacteriuria has been reported in some studies,[31] but these studies failed to identify potential confounding factors. There is currently no compelling evidence to support screening of nonpregnant populations for bacteriuria or for treatment of asymptomatic bacteriuria when identified. In 1987 Boscia and coworkers[30] compared treated and untreated geriatric groups with asymptomatic UTI. No long-term morbidity was found, including no increase in hypertension, renal scarring, or renal failure.

Diagnosis

The previous definition of UTI was based on the culture showing concentrations of 10^5 or more CFU (colony-forming units) per milliliter of coliform bacterium. More recently, Stamm[32] reported that a significant percentage of women with acute dysuria from coliform infection in fact have lower growth cultures, of 10^2 to 10^4 CFU/ml. White blood cells (pyuria) are found in UTI and red blood cells may be present as well in either microscopic or macroscopic numbers, especially when the infection is acute. The leukocyte esterase dipstick has a 75% to 96% sensitivity in detecting pyuria associated with infection and is a simple screening method for AUC. A culture should be performed in atypical or complicated cases. Because impaired bladder emptying can predispose to recurrent infections in the elderly, a postvoid residual volume should be measured.

Treatment

In the acute situation, leukocyte esterase dipstick test or microscopy may be performed. If pyuria is present, the patient can be started on a general antibiotic regimen known to be effective against most urinary pathogens, such as a sulfa preparation or fluoroquinolone. If a culture was sent for a complicated case, when the laboratory report on the sensitivities of the organism is received, a narrower spectrum antibiotic may be substituted. The current trend in therapy of AUC is use of short course, especially 3-day antimicrobial regimens. Three days appears to more effective than a single dose. Single-dose therapy has been advocated by some for uncomplicated UTIs because of compliance concerns, reduced cost, fewer side effects, and less alterations in microbial flora in the gastrointestinal tract and vagina. A Mayo Clinic study compared single-dose (3 trimethoprim-sulfamethoxazole tablets) to a 10-day course with significantly lower relapse rate in the group treated for 10 days (3% versus 15%). If single-dose therapy is to be used, the best results have been found using trimethoprim-sulfamethoxazole or a fluoroquinolone.[27] This is also true of the 3-day regimens. Cephalexin, amoxicillin, and nitrofurantoin have had poorer treatment results with 3-day courses.

Approximately 20% of women with AUC develop recurrences. Recurrent UTIs are usually reinfection. Many individuals will stop taking drug therapy as soon as the symptoms disappear, and if the same organism is found, it likely represents reinfection. Retreat with a short course of antibiotics and address behavioral modification techniques such as estrogen replacement therapy, voiding after intercourse, improved perineal hygiene, and fluid intake habits. However, if different organisms are found, a recurrent infection may have been what has occurred. For such individuals, long-term use of lower dose antibiotics may be appropriate.

Some recommend that elderly women should be treated with a 2-week course of antimicrobial therapy because of the higher likelihood of upper tract infection. An equally reasonable approach is to treat elderly women with typical UTI symptoms with 3 days of trimethoprim-sulfamethoxazole, trimethoprim alone, or norfloxacin. Relapses when the therapy is stopped may suggest an upper urinary tract infection, and at this point symptomatic patients can be retreated with 14 days of antimicrobial therapy.

A preliminary study by Privette and coworkers[33] suggested estrogen may be helpful in preventing recurrent UTI in elderly women. More recently, Raz and Stamm[29] reported that the intravaginal administration of estriol prevented recurrent UTI in postmenopausal women.

Avorn and coworkers[34] recently reported, in a randomized, double-blind, placebo-controlled trial, that regular intake of 300 ml of cranberry juice beverage per day in women with a mean age of 78 years decreased the odds of bacteruria with pyuria to 40% of that of the control group. However, women with irritative bladder symptoms without infection may find that cranberry juice aggravates their symptoms.

Frequent catheterization and manipulation of the lower urinary tract may lead to urinary tract infections. In general, indwelling catheters left in place for 24 hours will lead to bacteriuria in as many as 50% of the patients. When left in place for more than 30 days, they will cause bacteriuria in almost everyone. There is no good evidence that prophylactic antibiotic use for chronically catheterized patients prevents symptomatic infection. Furthermore, treating asymptomatic bacteriuria does not reduce complications in patients with prolonged catheter drainage. The patients with catheters should be monitored for the presence of symptomatic infection. Postoperative (particularly gynecological, urological, and transplant patients) and debilitated patients seem to be at greatest risk. When indwelling catheters are necessary, they should be at least a 16 French. Smaller catheters plug easily with normal urine debris and increase the risk of infection. The best prevention strategy is high fluid intake and output to keep the system open.

Urethral Diverticulum

Urethral diverticula is a relatively uncommon disorder in women and may present with a confusing array of symptoms and physical findings. Although prevalence rates of 1.9% to 4.7% have been recorded, the true incidence of urethral diverticula in the general female population remains unknown. Urethral diverticula have been reported in women of all ages. Davis and Telinde[35] observed that only 2 of 121 cases of urethral diverticula presented symptoms prior to age 15, with the majority presenting at ages 20 to 40. Lee[36] found most patients at the Mayo Clinic to be between ages 30 and 50, although the age range was 19 to 76 years. Nonetheless, elderly women can develop diverticula. The disease occurs more frequently in blacks than whites, with a ratio as high as 6 to 1 in Anderson's study.[37]

Proposed etiologies for urethral diverticula include congenital, acute, and chronic inflammatory conditions, and trauma.[38] While a variety of etiological conditions may be responsible, an infectious etiology is probably the most common, perhaps stemming from infection and obstruction of the periurethral glands. Resultant retention cyst formation and rupture into the lumen of the urethra could give rise to the diverticulum.[39] Although *N. gonococcus* has been implicated as the cause of this condition by some authors, *Chlamydia, E. coli,* and most bacteria associated with cystitis have been found in diverticula.

The presenting symptoms vary considerably and include dysuria, postvoid dribbling, dyspareunia, urinary frequency and urgency, recurrent urinary tract infection, urinary incontinence, hematuria, and anterior vaginal wall pain and swelling (particularly after voiding). Some urethral diverticula are asymptomatic (10% to 20% of women with urethral diverticulum may be asymptomatic) and are found incidentally on routine pelvic examination. A high index of suspicion is essential in making the diagnosis. Pelvic examination is essential to detect periurethral mass, tenderness, possibly purulent discharge from urethra or demonstration of urine leakage with palpation, urethral hypermobility, and associated pelvic pathology. All periurethral masses do not represent urethral diverticula, so the differential diagnosis of an anterior vaginal wall mass must be considered. Possibilities include an infected Skene duct cyst, a vaginal or suburethral cyst, an ectopic ureterocele, a urethral or vaginal tumor, or a simple urethrocele. Induration or firmness of the diverticulum should raise suspicion of cancer or stones within the diverticulum.

Diagnosis

A voiding cystourethrogram (VCUG) is the most useful radiographic test to confirm the presence and extent of a urethral diverticulum. Cystourethroscopy is essential to identify the diverticular communication site in the urethra and to see if multiple diverticula are present. Intravenous urogram (IVU) and ultrasonography may be helpful. The technique of double catheter balloon insufflation (or retrograde positive-pressure urethrography) is somewhat difficult to perform and uncomfortable for the patient, but it is useful mainly in ambiguous cases. Bhatia and coworkers[40] found that women with urethral diverticula have biphasic curves on urethral pressure profilometry, but Summitt and Stovall[41] found a pressure depression in women without diverticulum as well. Urodynamic evaluation is indicated if the patient has urinary incontinence. Urine culture was positive 33% (3 of 9 patients) of the time in Summit and Stovall's study.

Treatment

While some advocate conservative treatment for small and asymptomatic diverticula, most agree it is beneficial to treat the diverticulum, especially if it is associated with lower urinary tract symptoms or if it is more than 1 cm in size. Operative excision and repair of the diverticulum can be accomplished by a transvaginal route with a vaginal flap technique. It is important to investigate for the possibility of multiple diverticula. Lee[36] noted 18 such instances in 85 patients investigated at the Mayo Clinic.

Major complications following the repair of a urethral diverticulum include urethrovaginal fistula, which has been reported in about 5% of repairs, and urethral stricture which occurs occasionally. Recurrence rates have been estimated to be 5% to 10%. If a diverticulum recurs immediately after an operation, it probably represents a second diverticulum that was overlooked or an inappropriate repair. If there is a recurrence after 1 year, it is probably a new lesion. Stress incontinence secondary to the dissection of the bladder neck may occur. Occasionally, irritative symptoms such as frequency, urgency, and dysuria develop.

Genuine Stress Incontinence

The International Continence Society definition of genuine stress incontinence (GSI) is the involuntary loss of urine occurring when, in the absence of a detrusor contraction, the intravesical pressure exceeds the maximal urethral pressure. In the continent women in the resting state, the urethra closure pressure is greater than the intravesical pressure and the sudden increase in intra-abdominal pressure generated by either a cough or the strain of lifting is generally transmitted equally to both the bladder and the bladder neck and urethra. This is true because the bladder neck and proximal urethra are above the urogenital diaphragm and are essentially intra-abdominal organs. This phenomenon was demonstrated by Enhorning and coworkers[10] using simultaneous intra-urethral and intravesical pressure measurements. In the women with GSI, the proximal urethra and bladder neck are frequently displaced below the urogenital diaphragm and are no longer intra-abdominal organs. With an increase in intra-abdominal pressure, the force generated is additive to the intravesical pressure and is usually enough to overcome urethral closure pressure. These anatomical changes may come about because of relaxation of pelvic support structures including the urogenital diaphragm musculature or because of damage to the supports of the urethra and upper vagina to the pubic symphysis. Stress urinary incontinence is thought to be secondary to neuromuscular weakness of the pelvic support structures resulting in hypermobility. Child-bearing, trauma, loss of hormonal support to these tissues, connective tissue disorders, and general stress and strain over the years may cause or accentuate this process.

In the past, a number of other reasons have been given for the cause of stress incontinence.

One of these was felt to be the shortening of the urethra that occurs with time. Lapides and coworkers[42] measured urethral length before and after operations for correction of stress incontinence using calibrated intra-urethral catheters and found that, in incontinent cases, the urethra did appear to be shorter. However, during the procedure downward traction was exerted in order to give the most accurate measurement. Since the bladder neck of many women will funnel, the accuracy of these authors' measurements has been suspect. In studies using bead chain cystourethrography by multiple investigators, no difference in urethra length has been noted before or after surgical repair. Thus, urethral length does not seem to be a major factor in the cause of stress incontinence.

Jeffcoate and Roberts[43] introduced the concept of the importance of the posterior urethral vesicle angle for the maintenance of stress incontinence. They believed that a normal posterior urethrovesical (PUV) angle of less than 120° was an important aspect for the maintenance of continence because this angle was usually greater than 120° in patients suffering from stress incontinence. They had noted that the relationship to the bladder neck and the urethra to the pubic symphysis was not the major anatomical feature in the etiology of stress incontinence because many patients with bladder descent but with normal PUV angles were continent, whereas some incontinent women had bladders and urethras reasonably well positioned to the pubic symphysis but had lost their PUV. Normal continent women will demonstrate a bladder base nearly parallel to the horizontal in the standing position and will have a PUV angle of 90° to 100°. Such bladders, when visualized on cystourethrocystography will be noted to have this angle maintained with cough, and funneling of the bladder neck does not occur. With stress incontinence, there is almost a complete loss of the PUV angle and funneling and posterior descent of the vesicle neck does occur. Attempt to measure the PUV using chain cystourethrocystography and the Q-tip test has demonstrated that the change in the PUV angle is not a predictive finding in patients with genuine stress incontinence. Fantl and coworkers[44] demonstrated that 83 cystourethrograms done by the chain cystourethrogram technique and interpreted by three radiologists utilizing five specific radiologic landmarks failed to identify any agreement in interpretation with a variation in interpretation being from 19.3% to 54.2%. Fantl's group could find no statistically significant difference in the distribution of radiographic characteristics between patients with stress incontinence and detrusor instability using this test. Therefore, it must be concluded that tests which measure PUV are not sensitive enough to determine whether the patient has stress incontinence, and a complete urologic urodynamic workup is indicated in most instances. It is fairly well accepted that PUV angle is not as critical as the position of the bladder neck within the abdominal cavity.

Many women with pelvic relaxation have large cystoceles. A cystocele is a herniation of the bladder into the vagina and can be seen as a bulge in the anterior vaginal wall when the patient is in the lithotomy position or is standing. If these patients have well-supported bladder necks, they will usually be continent. If the urethra and bladder are involved in the anatomical defect forming a cystourethrocele, the patient will often be incontinent. Alternatively, genital prolapse by itself is not diagnostic of genuine stress incontinence due to the significant number of patients who remain continent despite pelvic relaxation. Incontinence in a patient with a cystocele is rare, whereas it is quite common in patients with cystourethroceles.

Several of the different theories reviewed above have attempted to explain stress urinary incontinence based on angles, pressures, or various structures. More recently, partial denervation of the pelvic floor has been investigated in the etiology of prolapse and incontinence.[45] Overall, poor urethral support appears to be an important factor in the loss of urine associated with increases in intra-abdominal pressure. Our understanding of stress urinary incontinence is far from complete.

One specific subtype of GSI deserves mention: intrinsic sphincter deficiency (ISD). This is a much less frequent cause of GSI, which tends to occur after prior incontinence surgery, trauma, or radiation. The bladder neck is usually well supported and there is no evidence of hypermobility. Patients will easily leak urine, often with gravity alone as the urethra no longer functions as a sphincter, hence the term "drain-pipe urethra."

Nonsurgical Treatment for Genuine Stress Incontinence

Therapy for stress incontinence can be divided into nonoperative and operative approaches. Nonsurgical management of stress urinary incontinence includes simple strategies such as fluid management, prompted voiding, and behavior modification techniques aimed at strengthening pelvic floor muscles.[46] These techniques have virtually no side effects but do require patient motivation and instructor time. Drug therapy is also often appropriate.

Education about pelvic floor musculature is key in the nonsurgical management of stress urinary incontinence. "Progressive resistance exercise in the functional restoration of the perineal muscles" is the title of Arnold Kegel's[47] 1948 paper. In 1856 Kegel[48] suggested that patients contract their pubococcygeal muscles 5 times on awakening, 5 times on arising, and 5 times every half-hour throughout the day. These muscles can be demonstrated to the patient by asking her to contract the muscles that it takes to stop the urinary stream during urination. Once she knows which muscles to contract, Kegel exercises may be performed. Since most patients will not follow a rigorous schedule as laid down by Kegel, it will probably suffice to ask them to exercise these muscles by contracting them 10 times to the count of 10 several times per day. Bump and coworkers[49] concluded that brief verbal directions were not adequate instruction for patients before undertaking a Kegel exercise program. Some other form of education is also necessary such as vaginal and abdominal muscle palpation with verbal feedback while the patient attempts levator ani muscle contraction.[50] Wells'[51] 1990 review of pelvic floor muscle exercises for stress urinary incontinence show varied success rates. Cures ranged from 30% to 70% in patients who continued to use the techniques.

Controversy exists regarding who is the ideal patient to benefit from pelvic floor muscle exercise. Wilson and coworkers[52] found better success in younger women who had a milder degree of incontinence and no prior surgery. In 1988 Henalla and coworkers[53] reported the opposite: severity of incontinence, prior surgery, and older age did not matter. Although studies show conflicting results, it makes sense to encourage patients to try nonsurgical management because there is no risk involved.

Several other techniques for increasing strength and awareness of pelvic floor musculature are available. These include electrical stimulation, interferential therapy, vaginal weighted cones, and perineometers. Unfortunately, the best method of training, the optimal exercise schedule, treatment duration, and long-term effectiveness with any modality are not known.

In addition to exercises, medications are a useful adjunct in the nonsurgical therapy program. Iosif and coworkers[54] demonstrated the presence of estrogen receptors in the lower urinary tract. In the older woman, atrophy of the urethral mucosa and the underlying blood vessels occurs, which leads to a decrease in urethral closure pressure. Fantl and coworkers[55] however found no direct estrogen effect on urethral function in incontinent women. Rud[56] hypothesized that estrogen may affect the function of the pelvic floor musculature and paraurethral connective tissue, rather than affecting the urethra directly. Currently, there is no study confirming the efficacy of estrogen in treating stress incontinence, but most believe it to contribute positively to intrinsic urethral pressure.

Other drugs and combinations of drugs have been studied to determine whether they are of aid in preventing stress incontinence. Alpha-adrenergic stimulation from the sympathetic nervous system helps maintain the smooth muscle tone of the intrinsic urethral sphincter. Medical therapy with alpha-agonist drugs can therefore be beneficial in treating this condition. Alpha-agonists include phenylpropanolamine (available in Ornade Spansules), ephedrine, and pseudoephedrine (marketed over-the-counter in Dexatrim, Sudafed, and Rondec), and imipramine (which also has anticholinergic side effects and benefits patients with mixed incontinence).

Kiesswetter and coworkers[57] studied 30 stress incontinent women with clinical and urodynamic assessment. These authors compared a continence profile before and after treatment with an alpha-adrenergic stimulant, midodrine; a cholinesterase inhibitor, distigmine bromide; a tricyclic antidepressant, imipramine; and an estriol, triodurin. In each case, the patients were treated for 4 weeks and re-evaluated. Finally, a suspensory sling operation was performed. The continence profile as described by the authors improved 45% with the sling procedure as compared with an improvement of 9% for midodrine, 8.9% for imipramine and 7.9% for a combination of estriol and distigmine bromide. Urethral pressures increased by a mean value of 8.1% after operation, 8.3% after midodrine, 7.9% after imipramine, and 3.5% after the estrogen and distigmine bromide combination. The combination of estriol plus midodrine and estriol plus imipramine were favored by patients over single-drug therapy, however, little difference was noted in urodynamic assessment. Table 16.4 from the Agency for Health Care Policy and Research (AHCPR) guide summarizes the outcome of stress incontinence treatment.

Surgical Treatment of Genuine Stress Incontinence

Before 1950, the operative procedure of choice for treating stress incontinence was primarily a vaginal procedure that included plication of the bladder neck (Kelly procedure) with an anterior colporrhaphy to reduce a cystocele, if it existed. The advantages of this approach are the low operative morbidity and the convenience of vaginally repairing other pelvic floor relaxation defects (uterine prolapse, enterocele and/or rectocele). However, concern exists because of the widely ranging success rates reported in the literature—from 31% to 88%.

With Green's[58] attempt to grade degrees of posterior urethrovesical (PUV) angle loss, Bailey[59] and others stated that success rates for curing stress incontinence using the vaginal approach varied according to the etiology of the stress incontinence. Patients showing a complete loss of PUV

Table 16.4 Outcome of Stress Incontinence Treatments*

| | Treatment options | | | | |
| | Behavioral technique | | | Surgical technique | |
Outcome	Pelvic muscle exercise %	Bladder training %	Pharmacologic: Alpha-agonist %	Retropubic suspension %	Needle suspension %
Cured	12	16	0–14	78	84
Improved	75	54	19–60	5	4
Total	87	70	19–74	83	88
Side effects	None		Minimal to 20	–	
Complications	None		5–33	20	

*The numbers used represent the average reported outcome within a given management option (eg, behavioral, pharmacological, or surgical) based on the literature review. The numbers do not apply equally across specific treatments within a given management option (eg, pelvic muscle exercise versus oxybutynin versus retropubic suspension) because the studies lack uniformity in many critical issues, including outcome criteria, types of subjects, treatment protocol, follow-up period, analytical method. The reader is referred to the guideline text for details. From Urinary Incontinence Guideline Panel: Urinary incontinence in adults: Clinical practice guideline. AHCPR Publication No. 92-0038. Rockville, MD, Agency for Health Care Policy and Research, Public Health Service, US Department of Health and Human Services, March 1992.

angle had a 90% success rate when followed for 5 to 10 years after bladder neck plication and anterior colporrhaphy, but only 50% of patients with lesser PUV angle loss remained continent over that time period. With the introduction of the suprapubic urethrovesical suspension operations, the 5-year cure rate for patients like those in the latter group has passed 90% in most series. Beck and coworkers[60] have reported the best surgical outcome following a modified anterior colporrhaphy with a vaginal retropubic urethropexy. Sutures are placed in the retropubic space to incorporate the pubourethral ligament and the periosteum of the posterior pubic symphysis. In 1979 Stanton and Cardozo[61] published the first prospective study comparing anterior colporrhaphy with an abdominal retropubic urethropexy. Patients who underwent anterior colporrhaphy had a 36% objective cure rate compared with an 85% cure rate for the Burch colposuspension. The only prospective, randomized, surgical trial for genuine stress incontinence was published by Bergman and coworkers[62] in 1989. Cure rates at 1-year follow-up were 65% for anterior colporrhaphy compared with 91% for the abdominal approach. Elia and Bergman's[63] 1994 five 5-year follow-up of this study showed objective success rates of 37% for anterior colporrhaphy and 82% for retropubic urethropexy. In comparing results, it is likely that patient selection, surgical techniques, and skills differ. But, the long-term success rate of anterior colporrhaphy and Kelly plication for treatment of genuine stress incontinence may be considerably lower than that of retropubic urethropexy.

Pereyra[64] originally described the vaginal and suprapubic bladder neck needle suspension operation in 1959. Pereyra designed a special needle to guide sutures from the vaginal incision through the space of Retzius and through the rectus fascia on both sides. There have been many surgical variations and evolution of the needle suspension urethropexy procedure, including changing suture material. Pereyra himself modified his procedure several times. Stamey added cystoscopy and modified the Pereyra procedure utilizing a small tube of dacron material to buttress the suture thereby keeping it from pulling through. Stamey[65] reported that about 3% of the patients in his series required removal of this suprapubic suture because of pain or infection. Raz[66] next modified the procedure by using wide dissection to free the endopelvic fascia from the back of the pubic symphysis and by inserting helical sutures into the deep endopelvic fascia, including part of the vaginal wall. The sutures are then tied above the anterior rectus fascia via a small suprapubic incision.

In 1987 Gittes[67] described a "no-incisions" procedure similar to Pereyra's original report. He avoided a vaginal incision and sutured the full thickness of the vaginal wall. The sutures were elevated using a blind needle technique and tied to the rectus fascia. Six of the 40 patients (15%) noted recurrence within 1 year, although no objective urodynamic studies were reported. No long-term follow-up is available.

Peattie and Stanton[68] published a series of the Stamey procedures in elderly women and showed a subjective cure rate of 68% and an objective cure rate of only 39%. In Bergman's[69] 1989 prospective, randomized trial, the objective cure rate at 1-year follow-up was 70% for the Pereyra operation and 87% for the Burch. Recent 5-year objective success rates were 43% and 82%, respectively. The author found a lower incidence of positive Q-tip test in women after the Burch procedure and hypothesized that the retropubic suspension may give better anatomical support of the bladder neck.

Needle suspension procedures have an advantage of short operative time, relatively low intraoperative morbidity, and there are now reports of outpatient procedures. The main disadvantage appears to be the lower success rate over time compared with retropubic urethropexy. This may be related to the support of the urethrovesical junction relying on the paraurethral sutures.

Retropubic urethropexy operations are thought to alleviate genuine stress incontinence by elevating and stabilizing the proximal urethra into a higher retropubic position. Two retropubic urethropexy procedures are in common use. The Marshall–Marchetti–Krantz (MMK) suprapubic urethrovesical suspension operation was first reported in 1949. Paravaginal tissue at the level of the urethrovesical junction and another pair more distally are sutured bilaterally to the pubic symphysis utilizing interrupted sutures.[70] Today, polyglycol suture is ideal for this procedure, but permanent sutures such as silk or nylon may also be used. Because of the acute elevation of the urethra against the symphysis pubis, one complication can be prolonged voiding difficulty. The problem of osteitis pubis occurs infrequently after an MMK procedure, but when it does occur, it can be disabling (0.5% to 5%).[71]

The second procedure in common use, the retropubic colposuspension, was first described by Burch[72] in 1961. In this case, the upper vaginal wall is sutured to Cooper's ligaments on either side also using a polyglycol suture.[73] Few modifications have occurred since then, but Stanton[74] more specifically described placement of the elevating sutures. Many authors advocate using permanent suture. These operations have a success rate in excess of 90% when performed properly. Gillon and Stanton[75] looked specifically at elderly woman treated with colposuspension for GSI. Three- to 5-year objective cure rate was reported as 89%. Complications are similar to those in the MMK procedure and can include prolonged voiding dysfunction, infection, and postoperative detrusor instability. Wiskind and Stanton[76] recently reported that 26.7% of the patients required corrective prolapse surgery after colposuspension. Of these, 22% required rectocele repair and 11% enterocele repair.

In a study of 29 women investigated urodynamically before and after a MMK procedure, Beisland and coworkers[77] found that no major changes in urethral pressure profile could be demonstrated. These authors did demonstrate a good correlation between the clinical results and the changes in transmission of increased abdominal pressure to the urethra. The procedure did not increase urethral pressure. Those patients with low maximal urethral pressure preoperatively continued to have insufficient urethral sphincter function after the operation. These authors concluded that patients with a low urethral closure pressure but with good transmission of pressure to the urethra are not suitable candidates for urethropexy. Insufficiency of the urethral sphincter in postmenopausal women is most often associated with atrophy of the urethra and vaginal epithelium as well as decreased blood supply to the periurethral tissue. Beisland and coworkers therefore suggested that such patients should be treated with a combination of alpha-receptor-stimulating drugs and estrogen and not by operation. Further studies have demonstrated that MMK and Burch procedures most likely work by partially mechanically obstructing the bladder neck in addition to replacing the bladder neck behind the pubic symphysis.

The surgical approach of choice may prove to be an abdominal retropubic urethropexy, but with only one randomized trial published there is clearly controversy over this issue. Both the MMK procedure and the Burch retropubic colposuspension have been associated with the best long-term success rates.

The paravaginal repair was originally described by White in 1909 and is now advocated by Richardson, Baden, Walker, Shull, and Lyons as an abdominal approach for correction of a cystocele. Proponents have also suggested its use for the treatment of GSI.[78,79] This procedure is appropriate when the cystocele is secondary to a lateral vaginal wall detachment from the arcus tendineus fasciae pelvis. The advantages cited include low complication rate, almost immediate return of normal voiding, and success rates of 95%. Its routine use for genuine stress incontinence treatment is still under investigation.

In situations where these procedures fail to alleviate the stress incontinence, the operations may be re-performed if hypermobility is still present, or a urethral sling procedure using a variety of materials may be fashioned. More recent evidence suggests that sling procedures may also be advantageous in women at increased risk of failing primary standard incontinence procedures, such as women with low urethral pressure.[80] Currently, the most popular of these is the use of a strip

Table 16.5 Surgical Outcome for Female Intrinsic Sphincter Deficiency*

| | Treatment options | | | |
| | Bulking technique | | | Artificial |
Outcome	Teflon %	Collagen %	Sling operation %	urinary sphincter %
Cured	59	69	89	92
Improved	16	25	6	4
Cured/improved	75	94	95	96
Complications	6	–	31	32

*The numbers used represent the average reported outcome within a given management option (eg, bulking, sling, or artificial sphincter) based on the literature review. The numbers do not apply equally across specific treatments within a given management option (eg, Teflon versus sling versus sphincter) because the studies lack uniformity concerning many critical issues, including outcome criteria, types of subjects, treatment protocol, follow-up period, analytical method. The reader is referred to the guideline text for details. From Urinary Incontinence Guideline Panel: Urinary incontinence in adults: Clinical practice guideline. AHCPR Publication No. 92-0038. Rockville, MD, Agency for Health Care Policy and Research, Public Health Service, US Department of Health and Human Services, March 1992.

of anterior rectus fascia. Other choice of materials include autologous graft with fascia lata or inorganic materials (Mersilene mesh, Marlex, GoreTex). Although the sling procedure has been reported to have uniformly good results (objective surgical cure rate is 70% to 95% by Beck and coworkers[81]), it is technically a more difficult operation than the MMK and Burch procedures because of the necessity of dissecting the bladder neck free by both a vaginal and an abdominal approach. There is also a higher frequency of morbidity. Complications include urinary retention (15% to 25%), voiding difficulty, erosion of the sling, and infection, particularly if foreign material is used for the sling. In most instances, it is reserved as a back-up procedure.

Periurethral injection therapy for stress urinary incontinence works most effectively in women who have intrinsic sphincter deficiency (ISD). These women constitute a small proportion of women with incontinence. They have a poorly functioning intrinsic urethral sphincter, an immobile urethrovesical junction, and typically have had prior surgery for incontinence, trauma, or radiation. Injection substances have been used as far back as 1923 when Murless tried injecting a sclerosing agent into the anterior vaginal wall. Polytetrafluoroethylene paste has been used by several authors including Poliatano, but is difficult to inject and has been associated with granuloma formation and distant migration of the particles. Periurethral collagen injection therapy has recently been FDA-approved and can be injected in the doctor's office. This substance is biodegradable and easy to use. Appell and coworkers[82] report success rates of 80% to 90% in carefully selected patients.

The success rates for treating ISD with bulking agents versus surgery is given in Table 16.5.

Detrusor Instability

Detrusor instability is defined as involuntary uninhibited contraction of the bladder during the storage phase of urination. The term *detrusor dyssynergia* is no longer accepted by the International Continence Society (ICS), thus avoiding confusion with detrusor-sphincter dyssynergia, which is a voiding abnormality. Urgency and urge incontinence are often associated with detrusor instability. Urge incontinence is the involuntary loss of urine associated with a strong desire to void. This may be divided into motor urge incontinence, which is associated with uninhibited detrusor contractions, and sensory urge incontinence, which is not caused by uninhibited detrusor contractions. Subtracted cystometry is necessary to make the proper diagnosis of detrusor instability and to help differentiate the two types.

The prevalence of detrusor instability is unknown. Approximately 35% (10% to 63%) of incontinent women seeking treatment have detrusor instability according to Webster and coworkers.[83] Elderly patients demonstrated a 17% prevalence of detrusor instability in Diokno and coworkers'[84] study of community-dwelling patients.

The loss of urine is painless and consists of a large volume. Leakage may occur in any position and often with a change of position or running water. Stress incontinence disappears at night, but urge incontinence continues with nocturia and sometimes enuresis. Cantor and Bates[85] identified three key symptoms clinically associated with the presence of detrusor instability on cystometric evaluation. These are nocturia, urge incontinence, and nocturnal enuresis. Although urgency, frequency, and the mentioned symptoms seem to correlate with the diagnosis of detrusor instability, this can be misleading and patients with what appears to be simple stress incontinence can also have detrusor instability.

The diagnosis is made using provocative subtracted dual-channel cystometry, which detects spontaneous involuntary detrusor pressure changes within the bladder as the bladder is filled. This technique will also allow for the detection of a detrusor instability component in patients with genuine stress incontinence so that both issues may be addressed. A gradual increase in detrusor pressure without phasic contractions is more appropriately regarded as poor bladder compliance.

Detrusor instability during cystometry is uninhibited detrusor contractions of more than 15 cm water pressure that occur spontaneously or after provocation while the patient is attempting to inhibit micturition. The significance of uninhibited contractions without urgency-related symptoms is unclear and are not infrequently seen when studying elderly women. Alternatively, during cystometry some patients with urgency may exhibit "subthreshold" detrusor contractions of less than 15 cm water as described by Coolsaet and coworkers.[86] This finding may be important, although it does not meet the ICS definition precisely.

The cause of detrusor instability is unknown and called "idiopathic." Historically, Frewen writes "urge incontinence is a psychosomatic disorder in which emotional factors play a predominant role." This has not been confirmed.[87] When the overactive detrusor response during filling is known to be secondary to a neurological condition, it is termed *detrusor hyperreflexia*. The detrusor area of the motor cortex may easily be injured by vascular insufficiency so that small ischemic events to large cerebrovascular accidents may result in incontinence. In addition, spinal cord compression, demyelinating diseases, multiple sclerosis, and distal neuropathies are all neurological diseases that may cause detrusor hyperreflexia. The prevalence of neurologically induced detrusor dysfunction is not known. Current estimates are that approximately 5% to 10% of all detrusor overactivity may be secondary to neurological dysfunction.

Treatment of detrusor instability is generally not surgical, except in intractable cases. Although patients with both stress incontinence and detrusor instability may require an operation after medical therapy has been tried, it is not infrequent, however, to find that when the detrusor instability component is treated, the operative procedure is not necessary. In like manner, individuals with both components who are subjected to surgery first may find they are still incontinent after the procedure because of the detrusor instability component. In some instances when the anatomical defect is repaired, the urge incontinence component gradually disappears. This may be the case in some patients with severe cystocele and elevated postvoid residual urine.

Nonsurgical management of idiopathic detrusor instability includes behavioral therapy, drug therapy, and electrical stimulation, although the latter is still under investigation. Bladder re-training is one behavioral therapy. This is a program of progressively lengthening the period between voiding with or without the addition of medications or biofeedback techniques. The patient must resist the urge to void, postpone voiding, and urinate according to a rigid time schedule. The goal is to reach a voiding interval of 2 to 3 hours. Bladder re-training is thought to work because it re-establishes bladder control mechanisms that are under cortical (voluntary) control. This requires patient education and motivation as well as positive reinforcement. Millard and Oldenburg[88] demonstrated improvement in 74% of women with detrusor instability using such techniques. Cystometric studies before and after therapy revealed a reversion to stable bladder function. Interestingly, this behavioral therapy appears to control stress incontinence, as shown by multiple authors including Burgio and coworkers.[89]

Although bladder re-training is the behavioral intervention most commonly used, there are other infrequently used techniques such as hypnosis, biofeedback, and psychotherapy.

Estrogen is a major part of the therapy of detrusor instability in the elderly, since not only will it improve the vasculature of the bladder neck and urethra and the condition of the epithelium of the urethra and trigone, it may also stimulate the development of alpha-adrenergic receptors. Fantl's[55] study of postmenopausal women with urinary incontinence found the estrogen-supplemented group with detrusor instability to have less urine loss than the non–estrogen-supplemented group, although this was of borderline statistical significance (P = .06).

Anticholinergic drugs will help relax the detrusor muscle and may be useful in the therapy of detrusor instability. Unfortunately, the anticholinergic effects extend to other organs, thereby often limiting their use. Dry mouth, constipation, palpitations, and blurred vision are the most frequent side effects. Propantheline (Pro-Banthine) at doses of 15 to 30 mg 4 times a day may be tried in conjunction with bladder training. Anticholinergic drugs are contraindicated in women with narrow angle glaucoma, and caution is advised in woman with cardiac arrhythmias. These possibilities should be addressed in prescribing for an older woman.

Antispasmodic agents have a direct relaxant effect on smooth muscle. These agents also have anticholinergic effects and similar side effects to the anticholinergic drugs. Flavoxate (Urispas) can be used at doses of 200 mg every 6 hr. Meyhoff and coworkers[90] randomized, double-blind, cross-over study failed to show flavoxate was better than placebo, however. Oxybutynin chloride (Ditropan), 5 mg every 8 to 12 hr, was effective in treating detrusor instability as shown by Holmes and coworkers.[91]

Tricyclic antidepressants also seem to be beneficial in treating detrusor instability, although studies are limited. The mechanism of action is incompletely understood, but these drugs have anticholinergic, antispasmodic, and local anesthetic properties that affect the bladder. Imipramine can be given in much lower doses than when used for treating depression (10 to 50 mg 2 times a day). The elderly must be cautioned regarding orthostatic hypotension and usual anticholinergic side effects.

Certain calcium channel blockers have been shown to have an effect on bladder contractibility and anticholinergic properties. Unfortunately, no bladder-specific calcium channel blocker is available in the United States. Terodiline, a more bladder-specific calcium channel blocker has been shown in multiple trials to reduce incontinence. Unfortunately, serious ventricular arrhythmias have occurred in patients in Europe and trials in the United States have been halted.

Most elderly women with detrusor instability will respond very well to a combination of estrogen replacement therapy, an anticholinergic drug, and behavioral therapy. Most drug trials have been of short duration but do seem to help patients. Drugs may improve bladder capacity without improving the warning time between urgency and urinary leakage. Medications should be used only in conjunction with a bladder retraining program. No pharmacological agent has proved better than another.

Electrical stimulation is the application of electric current to stimulate or inhibit the pelvic viscera or their nerve supply in order to directly induce a therapeutic response. Vaginal or anal plug electrodes are used for electrical stimulation to induce reflex inhibition of the detrusor muscle (probably activates inhibitory sympathetic nerve fibers). Ericksen and coworkers[92] reported a 45% reversion to normal on cystometry in patients with detrusor instability. Clinical trials have shown good success, but standardization of methods is needed before this technique becomes standard treatment for detrusor instability.

True Incontinence

True incontinence is the loss of urine without abnormal bladder function. It is usually seen in the case of fistulas or other damage to the urinary tract. Such damage may be congenital or secondary to trauma, such as that occurring secondary to injury, operative procedures, and irradiation.

The diagnosis of a fistula should be aimed at determining the site of the fistula, that is, vesicovaginal, urethrovaginal, or ureterovaginal. Each will need to be corrected surgically in a different fashion. Urethrovaginal fistulas are generally seen following the repair of a urethral diverticulum or postoperatively following surgery to correct incontinence. These injuries are rare and must be repaired operatively.

Vesicovaginal fistulas are the most common genitourinary fistula. Diagnosis is aided by instilling methylene blue dye into the bladder and noting that it passes directly into the vagina. Cystoscopy and intravenous pyelogram should be carried out to determine that the ureters are not involved and to identify the site of the fistula. If the fistula is free of the ureteral orifices, it may lend itself to vaginal repair. If the fistula is near the ureteral openings, it is probably best to repair it via a transvesical approach. This approach is often most suited to repeat attempts at repair. Ureterovaginal fistulae most often require a mobilization of the ureter and reimplantation into the bladder.

In all cases of fistula, the operator must ensure that the blood supply to the area is adequate. For fistulae that follow trauma or operative injury, generally this is not a serious problem. However, for fistulae secondary to irradiation injury, the blood supply is generally compromised. Procedures to cover a vesicovaginal fistula with a myelocutaneous flap is probably the best solution for correcting the problem. For ureterovaginal fistulae following irradiation therapy, reimplantation of the ureter into the bladder is appropriate.

Overflow Incontinence

The International Continence Society's definition of overflow incontinence is the involuntary loss of urine associated with overdistension. This condition occurs when a bladder is overfilled because of its inability to empty. The problem is most often neurological and is seen in conditions that interfere with normal bladder reflexes, decreased bladder sensation, decreased detrusor muscle activity, or outflow obstruction of the urethra. Some of these conditions are multiple sclerosis, diabetic neuropathy, trauma, and tumors of the central nervous system. The patient generally complains of voiding small amounts of urine and still having the feeling that there is urine in the bladder. The patient may frequently lose small amounts of urine. Complete general medical and neurological evaluations are necessary to identify the cause of the problem. Therapy is generally directed at the primary cause. The patient may need to be trained in techniques of intermittent self-catheterization. Pharmacological therapy has not been rewarding in treating this condition.

References

1. Yarnell JWG, St. Leger AS: The prevalence, severity and factors associated with urinary incontinence in a random sample of elderly. *Age Ageing* 1979;8:81–85.
2. Diokno AC, Brock BM, Brown MB, Herzog AR: Prevalence of urinary incontinence and other urological symptoms in the noninstitutionalized elderly. *J Urol* 1986;136:1022–1025.
3. Warshaw GA, Moore JT, Friedman SW, et al: Functional disability in the hospitalized elderly. *JAMA* 1982;248:847–850.
4. Ouslander JG, Kane RL, Abrass IB: Urinary incontinence in elderly nursing home patients. *JAMA* 1982;248:1194–1198.
5. Williams ME, Pannill, FC: Urinary incontinence in the elderly: physiology, pathophysiology, diagnosis, and treatment. 1982;97:895–907.
6. Norton P, MacDonald L, Stanton S: Distress associated with female urinary complaints and delay in seeking treatment. *Neurourol Urodyn* 1987;6:170–.
7. Abrams P, Blaivas JG, Stanton SL, et al: Standardization of terminology of lower urinary tract function. *Neurourol Urodyn* 1988;7:403–427.
8. DeLancey JO: Correlative studies of periurethral anatomy. *Obstet Gynecol* 1986;68:91–97.
9. Asmussen M, Ulmsten U: On the physiology of continence and pathophysiology of stress incontinence in the female. *Contrib Gynecol Obstet* 1983;10:32–50.
10. Enhorning G, et al: Simultaneous recording of intravesical and intraurethral pressure. *Acta Chir Scand* 1971;276 (suppl):1–68.
11. Levy BJ, Wight TN: Structural changes in the aging submucosa: New morphologic criteria for the evaluation of the unstable human bladder. *J Urol* 1990;144:1044–1055.
12. Jewett MA, Fernie GR, Holliday PJ, Pim ME: Urinary dysfunction in a geriatric long-term care population: Prevalence and patterns. *J Am Geriatr Soc* 1981;29:211–214.
13. Resnick NM, Yalla SV: Management of urinary incontinence in the elderly. *N Engl J Med* 1985;313:800–805.
14. Resnick NM, Yalla SV, Laurima E: The pathophysiology of urinary incontinence among institutionalized elderly persons. *N Engl J Med* 1989;320:1–.
15. Lentz GL, Wiskind A, Stanton SL: Periurethral contigen *Bard* collagen injection for stress urinary incontinence: Preliminary results. *Neurourol Urodynam* 1991;10:451.
16. Montz FJ, Stanton SL: Q-tip test in female urinary incontinence. *Obstet Gynecol* 1986;67:258–260.
17. Caputo RM, Benson JT: The Q-tip test and urethrovesical junction mobility. *Obstet Gynecol* 1993;82:892–896.
18. Hodgkinson CP, Cobert N: Direct urethrocystometry. *Am J Obstet Gynecol* 1960;79:648–663.
19. Sand PK, Brubaker LT, Novak T: Simple standing incremental cystometry as a screening method for detrusor instability. *Obstet Gynecol* 1991;77:453–457.
20. Van Waalwij K, van Doorn ES, Remmers A, Janknegt RA: Conventional and extramural ambulatory urodynamic testing of the lower urinary tract in female volunteers. *J Urol* 1992;147:1319–1325.
21. Porru D, Usal E: Standard and extramural ambulatory urodynamic monitoring for the diagnosis of detrusor instability and primary nocturnal enuresis. *Neurourol Urodyn* 1993;12:323–.
22. Katz GP, Blaivis JG: A diagnostic dilemma: When urodynamic findings differ from the clinical impression. *J Urol* 1983;129:1170–1174.
23. Komaroff AL: Acute dysuria in women. *N Engl J Med* 1984;310:368–375.
24. Nicolle LE, Muyr P, Harding GKM, Norris M: Localization of site of urinary infection in elderly institutionalized women with asymptomatic bacteriuria. *J Infect Dis* 1988;157:65–70.
25. Fowler JE Jr, Stamey TA: Studies of introital colonization in women with recurrent urinary infections. VII. The role of bacterial adherence. *J Urol* 1977;117:472–476.
26. Buckley RM, McGuckin M, MacGregor RR: Urine bacterial counts after sexual intercourse. *N Engl J Med* 1978;298:321–324.
27. Stamm WE: Controversies in single dose therapy of acute uncomplicated urinary tract infections in women. *Infection* 1992;20:S272–275.
28. Hooton TM, Hillier S, Johnson C, Roberts PL, Stamm WE: *Escherichia coli* bacteriuria and contraceptive method. *JAMA* 1991;265:64–69.
29. Raz R, Stamm WE: A controlled trial of intravaginal estriol in postmenopausal women with recurrent UTIs. *N Engl J Med* 1993;329:753–756.
30. Boscia JA, Abrutyn E, Kaye D: Asymptomatic bacteriuria in elderly person: Treat or do not treat? *Ann Int Med* 1987;106:764–766.
31. Baldassarre JS, Kaye D: Special problem of urinary tract infection in the elderly. *Med Clin North Am* 1991;75: 375–390.

32. Stamm WE, Counts GW, Running KR, et al: Diagnosis of coliform infection in acutely dysuric women. *N Engl J Med* 1982;137:213–.

33. Privette M, Cade R, Peterson J, Mars D: Prevention of recurrent UTIs in postmenopausal women. *Nephron* 1988;50:24–27.

34. Avorn J, Monane M, Gurwitz JH, Glynn RJ, Choodnovskiy I, Lipsitz LA: Reduction of bacteruria and pyuria after ingestion of cranberry juice. *JAMA* 1994;271:751–754.

35. Davis HJ, Telinde RW: Urethral diverticula: An assay of 121 cases. *J Urol* 1958;80:34–39.

36. Lee RA: Diverticulum of the female urethra: Postoperative complications and results. *Obstet Gynecol* 1983;61:52–58.

37. Andersen MJ: The incidence of diverticular in the female urethra. *J. Urology* 1967;98:96–98.

38. Lee RA: Diverticulum of the urethra: Clinical presentation, diagnosis and management. *Clin Obstet Gynecol* 1984;27:490–498.

39. Davis BL, Robinson DG: Diverticula of the female urethra: Assay of 120 cases. *J Urol* 1970;104:850–853.

40. Bhatia NN, McCarthy TA, Ostergard DR: Urethral pressure profiles of women with urethral diverticula. *Obstet Gynecol* 1981;58:357–8.

41. Summitt RL, Stovall TG: Urethral diverticula: Evaluation by urethral pressure, profilometry, cystourethroscopy and the voiding cystourethrogram. *Obstet Gynecol* 1992;80:695–699.

42. Lapides J, Ajemian EP, Stewart BH, et al: Physiopathology of stress incontinence. *Surg Gynecol Obstet* 1960;11:224–231.

43. Jeffcoate TNA, Roberts H: Observations of stress incontinence of urine. *Am J Obstet Gynecol* 1952;64:721–738.

44. Fantl JA, Beachley MC, Bosch HA, et al: B-chain cysto-urethrogram: An evaluation. *Obstet Gynecol* 1981;58:237–240.

45. Smith ARB, Hosker GL, Warrell DW: The role of partial denervation of the pelvic floor and the etiology of genitourinary prolapse and stress incontinence of urine: A neurophysiological study. *Br J Obstet Gynaecol* 1989;96:24–28.

46. Herzog R, Fultz N, Normolle D, et al: Methods used to manage urinary incontinence by older adults in the community. *J Am Geriatr Soc* 1989;37:339–347.

47. Kegel AH: Progressive resistance exercise in the functional restoration of the perineal muscles. *Am J Obstet Gynecol* 1948;56:238–248.

48. Kegel AH: Stress incontinence of urine in women: Physiologic treatment. *J Int Coll Surg* 1956;25:487–499.

49. Bump RC, Hurt WG, Fantl JA, Wyman JF: Assessment of Kegel pelvic muscle exercise performance after brief verbal instruction. *Am J Obstet Gynecol* 1991;165:322–327.

50. Bo K, Larsen S, Oserd S, et al: Knowledge about and ability to correct pelvic floor muscle exercises in women with urinary stress incontinence. *Neurourol Urodyn* 1988;7:261–261.

51. Wells T: Pelvic (floor) muscle exercise. *J Am Geriatr Soc* 1990;38:333–337.

52. Wilson PD, Al Samarri T, Deakin M, Kolbe E, Brown ADG: An objective assessment of physiotherapy for female genuine stress incontinence. *Br J Obstet Gynaecol* 1987;94:575–582.

53. Henalla SM, Kirwan P, Castleden CM, Hutchins CJ, Breeson AJ: The effect of pelvic floor exercises in the treatment of genuine urinary stress incontinence in women at two hospitals. *Br J Obstet Gynaecol* 1988;95:602–606.

54. Iosif CS, Batra S, Ek A, Astedt B: Estrogen receptors in the human female lower urinary tract. *Am J Obstet Gynecol* 1981;141:817–820.

55. Fantl JA, Wyman JF, Anderson RL, Matt DW, Bump RC: Postmenopausal urinary incontinence: Comparison between non-estrogen-supplemented and estrogen-supplemented women. *Obstet Gynecol* 1988;71:823–828.

56. Rud T: Urethral pressure profile in continent women from childhood to old age. *Acta Obstet Gynecol Scand* 1980;59:331–335.

57. Kiesswetter H, Hennrich F, Englisch M: Clinical and urodynamic assessment of pharmacologic therapy of stress incontinence. *Urol Int* 1983;38:58–63.

58. Green TH Jr: Development of a plan for diagnosis and treatment of urinary stress incontinence. *Am J Obstet Gynecol* 1962;83:632–648.

59. Bailey KV: The clinical investigation into uterine prolapse with stress incontinence. Treatment of modified Manchester colporrhaphy. *J Obstet Gynecol Br Commonwealth* Part I 1954;61:291–; Part II 1956;63:663–; Part III 1963;70:947–958.

60. Beck RP, McCormick S, Nordstrom L: A 25-year experience with 519 anterior colporrhaphy procedures. *Obstet Gynecol* 1991;78:1011–1018.

61. Stanton SL, Cardozo LD: Results of the colposuspension operation for incontinence and prolapse. *Br J Obstet Gynaecol* 1979;86:693–697.

62. Bergman A, Ballard CA, Koonings P: Comparison of three surgical procedures for genuine SUI: Prospective randomized study. *Am J Obstet Gynecol* 1989;160:1102–1106.

63. Elia G, Bergman A: Prospective randomized comparison of three surgical procedures for stress urinary incontinence: Five year follow-up. *Neurourol Urodyn* 1994;13:498.

64. Pereyra AJ: A simplified surgical procedure for the correction of stress incontinence in women. *Western J Surg* 1959;67:223–226.

65. Stamey TA: Cystoscopic suspension of the vesicle neck for urinary incontinence. *Surg Gynecol Obstet* 1973;136:547–54.

66. Raz S: Modified bladder neck suspension for female stress incontinence. *Urology* 1981;18:82–85.

67. Gittes RF: No-incision pubovaginal suspension for stress incontinence. *J Urol* 1987;138:568–570.

68. Peattie A. Stanton SL: The Stamey operation for correction of genuine stress incontinence in elderly women. *Br J Obstet Gynaecol* 1989;96:983–986.

69. Bergman A, Koonings P, Ballard C: Primary stress urinary incontinence and pelvic relaxation: Prospective randomized comparison of three different operations. *Am J Obstet Gynecol* 1989;161:97–101.

70. Marchetti AA, Marshall VF, Shultis LD: Simple vesicle urethral suspension for stress incontinence of urine. *Am J Obstet Gynecol* 1957;74:57–63.

71. Lee RA, Symmonds RE, Goldstein RA: Surgical complications and results of modified Marshall-Marchetti-Krantz procedure for urinary incontinence. *Obstet Gynecol* 1979;53:447–450.

72. Burch J: Urethrovaginal fixation to Cooper's ligament for correction of stress incontinence, cystocele and prolapse. *Am J Obstet Gynecol* 1961;81:281–289.

73. Burch JC: Cooper's ligament urethrovesical suspension for stress incontinence. *Am J Obstet Gynecol* 1968;100:764–774.

74. Stanton SL: Colposuspension, Stanton SL, Tanagho E (eds.): *Surgery of Female Incontinence,* ed. 2. Heidelberg, Springer-Verlag, 1986, p. 95.

75. Gillon G, Stanton SL: Long-term follow-up of surgery for urinary incontinence in elderly women. *Br J Urol* 1984;56:478–481.

76. Wiskind AK, Creighton SM, Stanton SL: The incidence of genital prolapse after the Burch colposuspension. *Am J Obstet Gynecol* 1992;167:399–404.

77. Beisland HO, Fossberg E, Sander S: Urodynamic studies before and after retropubic urethropexy for stress incontinence in female. *Surg Gynecol Obstet* 1982;155:333–336.

78. Richardson AC, Edmonds PB, Williams NL: Treatment of urinary incontinence due to paravaginal fascial defect. *Obstet Gynecol* 1981;57:357–362.

79. Shull BL, Baden WF: A six year experience with paravaginal defect repair for stress urinary incontinence. *Am J Obstet Gynecol* 1989;160:1432–1439.

80. Horbach NS, Blanco JS, Ostergard DR, Bent AE, Cornella JL: A suburethral sling procedure with polytetrafluoroethylene for the treatment of genuine stress incontinence in patients with low urethral closure pressure. *Obstet Gynecol* 1988;71:648–652.

81. Beck RP, McCormick S, Nordstrom L: The fascia lata sling procedure for treating recurrent genuine stress incontinence of urine. *Obstet Gynecol* 1988;72:699–703.

82. Appell RA, Macaluso JN, Deutsch JS, Goodman JR, Prats LJ, Wahl P: Endourologic control of incontinence with GAX collagen: The LSU experience. *J Endourol* 1992;6:275.

83. Webster GD, Sihelnik SA, Stone AR: Female urinary incontinence: The incidence, identification, and characteristics of detrusor instability. *Neurourol Urodyn* 1984;3:235.

84. Diokno AC, Brown MB, Brock BM, Herzog AR, Normolle DP: Clinical and cystometric characteristics of continent and incontinent noninstitutionalized elderly. *J Urol* 1988;140:567–571.

85. Cantor TJ, Bates CP: A comparative study of symptoms and objective urodynamic findings in 214 incontinent women. Br J Obstet Gynaecol 1980;87:889–92.

86. Coolsaet BLRA, Bloc C, van Venrooij GEPM, Tan B: Subthreshold detrusor instability. *Neurourol Urodyn* 1985;4:309–.

87. Frewen WK: Urgency incontinence. *J Obstet Gynecol Br Commonwealth* 1972;79:77–79.

88. Millard RJ, Oldenberg BF: The symptomatic urodynamic and cyclodynamic results of bladder re-education programs. *J Urol* 1983;130:715–719.

89. Burgio KL, Whitehead WE, Engel BT: Urinary incontinence in the elderly: Bladder-sphincter biofeedback and toileting skills training. *Ann Intern Med* 1985;103:507–515.

90. Meyhoff HH, Gerstenberg TC, Nordling J: Placebo: The drug of choice in female motor urge incontinence? *Br J Urol* 1983;55:34–37.

91. Holmes DM, Montz FJ, Stanton SL: Oxybutynin versus propantheline in the management of detrusor instability. *Br J Obstet Gynaecol* 1989;96:607–612.

92. Ericksen BC, Bergman S, Mjolnerod OK: Effects of anal electrostimulation with the "Incontan" device in women with urinary incontinence. *Br J Obstet Gynaecol* 1987;94:147–156.

93. US Senate Special Committee on Aging. Aging America: Trends and Projects. USDHHS, No. PF3377 (1085); 1985–1986. Washington, DC, US Department of Health and Human Services, 19XX.

Chapter 17

Pelvic Support Problems

Morton A. Stenchever, MD

Pelvic support structures frequently weaken as women age. Such stresses as congenital anatomical weakness, childbirth, physical injury, and damage sustained by chronic straining or by surgical intervention, all contribute to this phenomenon. In addition, the withdrawal of estrogen stimulation to pelvic support tissue and its blood supply further aids this weakening. This chapter addresses the specific conditions that are a result of the weakening of the pelvic support structures and discusses their diagnosis and treatment.

Anatomical Considerations

Pelvic Diaphragm

The pelvic diaphragm is the major muscle group that, with its fascia, supports the pelvic organs. It consists of two muscles: the coccygeus and levator ani muscles. These muscles have evolved from the tailwagging musculature of quadripeds. They are strong muscles with interwoven bundles and they completely close off the pelvis, except for openings for the urethra, vagina, and rectum, which they encircle. The levator ani muscle is the largest and has three components named for their origin and insertion: pubococcygeus, puborectalis, and iliococcygeus. The total muscle mass extends from the pubic symphysis to the coccyx and from lateral sidewall to lateral sidewall. The coccygeus is a triangular-shaped muscle that extends between both ischial spines and to the coccyx at the apex of the triangle. The levator ani muscles functioning jointly play a major role in the control of urination, in the birth process, in maintaining fecal continence, and in supporting abdominal and pelvic viscera (Figure 17.1).[1]

Urogenital Diaphragm

A second musculofascial diaphragm important in pelvic support is the more superficial diaphragm extending from the pubic symphysis to a line between the two ischial tuberosites. It supports the anterior segment of the pelvic outlet and consists of three muscle bundles, the ischiocavernosus, which extends between the pubic symphysis and the ischial tuberoscity along the pubic ramus; the bulbocavernosus, which extends between the pubic symphysis and the perineal body surrounding the vaginal outlet; and the deep transverse perineal muscle, which extends from the ischial tuberosites to the perineal body. These join with the external anal spinchter muscles that surround the rectum but blend into the perineal body. The urogenital diaphragm supports the external urethra and the introitus to the vagina. The urogenital diaphragm contains the pudendal blood vessels and

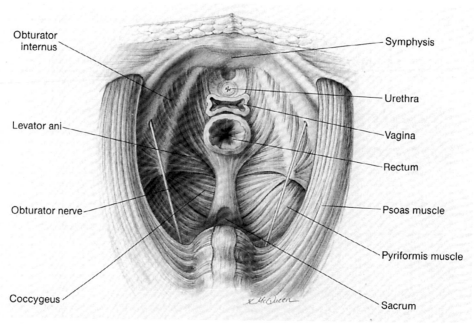

Obturator internus

Symphysis

Urethra

Levator ani

Vagina

Rectum

Obturator nerve

Psoas muscle

Pyriformis muscle

Coccygeus

Sacrum

Figure 17.1 A superior view of the pelvic diaphragm, demonstrating the levator ani and coccygeus muscles. From Herbst AL, Mishell, DR, Stenchever, MA, Droegemueller, W: Disorders of abdominal wall and pelvic support, in *Comprehensive Gynecology,* St. Louis, 2nd ed. CV Mosby, 1992, Chapt 19; with permission).

nerves, the external sphincter of the urethra, and the dorsal nerve to the clitoris. The urogenital diaphragm is extremely important in maintaining the position of the bladder neck (Figure 17.2).[1]

Supporting Ligaments

Although pelvic ligaments are called ligaments, they are really thickenings of the retroperitoneal fascia. Nonetheless, these structures tend to surround the vagina and cervix as an endopelvic fascia. The layer that separates the vagina and the cervix from the bladder is commonly called the pubocervical fascia and tends to support the bladder from herniating into the vagina. This blends laterally with the cardinal ligaments (Mackenrodt's ligaments), which extend from the lateral aspect of the upper vagina and cervix to the lateral pelvic wall bilaterally. The cardinal ligaments, as such, form the base of the broad ligament, which is a tent of peritoneum draped across the round ligament in which are found the uterine artery and vein and the ureter. The ureter transverses the cardinal ligament adjacent to the cervix. Posteriorly, the endopelvic investment fascia thickens into the uterosacral ligaments, which join the cervix to the sacrum. Within these ligaments run nerve bundles that supply the uterus and cervix. The endopelvic fascia jointly offers support to the pelvic structures that it invests and contributes, via the uterosacral ligament, to the support of the cul de sac. The round ligament extends from the fundus of the uterus into the inguinal canal and has little support function other than to help hold the uterus forward in an anteflexed position. It does, however, make up the apex of the tent of the broad ligament.[1]

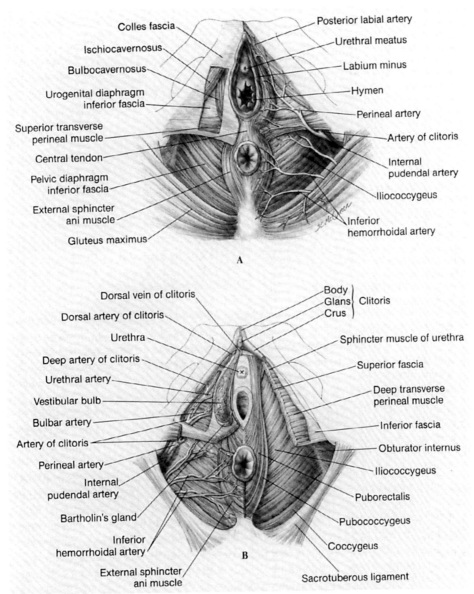

Figure 17.2 (A) Schematic view of the perineum, demonstrating superficial structures of the urogenital diaphragm.
(B) Schematic view of the perineum, demonstrating superficial structures and deeper structures showing the relationship of the levator, ani, and coccygeus muscles. (From Herbst AL, Mischell DR, Stenchever MA, Droegemueller, W: Disorders of the abdominal wall and pelvic support, in *Comprehensive Gynecology,* St. Louis, 2nd ed. CV Mosby, 1992, Chapt 19; with permission).

Changes with Estrogen Withdrawal

Estrogen withdrawal may have a profound effect on pelvic support structures. Not only does the loss of estrogen lead to atrophy of the epithelium of the vagina, bladder neck, and urethra, it also relates to the loss of elastic tissue and collagen in the endopelvic support fascia. Such changes can often be reversed, at least in part, by utilizing estrogen replacement therapy (ERT). In general ERT should be prescribed whenever patients are undergoing treatment for pelvic relaxation, unless, of course, there is a contraindication.[1]

Pelvic Support Disorders

If weakening of the pelvic support structures occurs, the resultant problem may be a urethrocele, cystocele, rectocele, enterocele, or descensus of the uterus and cervix. Often, a variety of these conditions occur in the same patient.[1]

Urethrocele and Cystocele

Weakening of the pubocervical fascia may allow for a herniation of the urethra (urethrocele), bladder neck, or bladder (cystocele) into the vagina. When the urethra and bladder neck remain supported but a cystocele develops, the patient often does not suffer from urinary incontinence. However, when the support structures beneath the urethra and bladder neck are weakened, urinary stress incontinence may be present. Women with gynecoid-type pelvises whose subpubic arches are wide may be at greatest risk for damage to the pubocervical fascia because the pressure of the fetal head at the time of vaginal delivery may be brought to full bear against this region. But women with narrower pelvic arches may be afforded a degree of protection to this structure.[2]

The symptoms associated with urethrocele and cystocele may include stress incontinence, often a feeling of urgency or a sensation of incomplete emptying after voiding, and a sensation that a structure is falling out of the vagina. The patient may be aware of a soft, bulging mass from the anterior vaginal wall and occasionally will need to replace this mass before being able to void. With strain and cough, the mass is accentuated and may remain present outside the introitus. When the physician examines such a patient, either in a standing position or in lithotomy with straining, the bulge will be apparent (Figure 17.3).[2]

Although urethroceles and cystoceles are almost always found in parous women, they have been noted in nulliparous women who have poor structural supports. This may be associated with congenital malformations or weakness of the musculature and connective tissue of the pelvic floor secondary to chronic strain, trauma, or other forces. Cystoceles are quite common, and in patients without symptoms therapy may not be required.[2]

For specific diagnosis, the patient is placed in lithotomy position, a posterior blade of a vaginal speculum is inserted to depress the posterior wall and the patient is asked to strain. The degree of cystocele and/or urethrocele may then be noted. The physician should palpate the bladder neck and estimate the degree of its support. Generally, if the bladder neck is well supported, the urethra will be, as well. In order to best assess the degree of cystocele and urethrocele, the examination is best performed with the bladder at least partially filled (100 to 250 ml).[2]

Urethroceles must be differentiated from inflammation and enlargement of the Skene's glands and from urethral diverticulum. Bladder tumors and bladder diverticula, which are both rare, may masquerade as cystoceles. Although diverticula of the urethra or the bladder may be reduced, there is generally the sensation of a mass on palpation. Inflamed Skene's glands are tender, and it may be possible to express pus from the urethra when they are palpated. Pus may be expressed

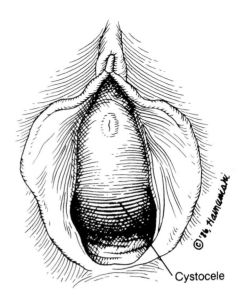

Figure 17.3 Cystocele. Herbst AL, Mishell, DR, Stenchever MA, Droegemueller, W: Disorders of abdominal wall and pelvic support, in *Comprehensive Gynecology,* St. Louis, 2nd ed. CV Mosby, 1992, Chapt 19; with permission.)

Cystocele

from urethral diverticula as well. When such is found, cultures, specifically for Chlamydia and gonococcus organisms, are appropriate. Although these organisms are less likely to be found in older than younger women, the possibility still exists.

Therapy for urethrocele and cystocele may be nonoperative or operative. The former consists of supporting the herniation of the bladder using a pessary of the Smith–Hodge or inflatable type. Occasionally, in less symptomatic women, even a large tampon may suffice. Kegel exercises (see Chapter 8) will help to strengthen pelvic floor muscles and therefore may relieve some of the symptoms of pressure but will not address the problem of endopelvic fascial damage. In postmenopausal women, estrogen should be prescribed either as a vaginal cream or systemically. This should help to strengthen pelvic support structures and improve their vascular supply. Even if a surgical procedure is contemplated, a pretherapy treatment with estrogen should improve the outcome and aid the healing process.[2]

Cystocele and urethrocele repair may be performed separately or in conjunction with repair of other pelvic relaxation problems. It is most common to at least perform a rectocele repair as well. Often, when a large cystocele with small rectocele is present, if only the cystocele is repaired, the subsequent weakening of the posterior wall will lead to a need for further repair of the posterior wall at a later date. If uterine descensus is noted, this may be addressed operatively as well. Frequently, an enterocele accompanies a cystocele and rectocele and should always be sought during the procedure. When it is present, the enterocele sac should be excised and repair affected.[2]

Anterior wall repair (colporrhaphy) is performed by incising the vaginal epithelium transversely just above the anterior lip of the cervix in the region of the bladder inflection. If a previous hysterectomy has been performed, the incision may be made 1 to 1½ cm anterior to the vaginal scar. The vagina is then incised longitudinally from the transverse incision to the level of the bladder neck. If no urethrocele is present, this is a sufficient extent for the incision. If a urethrocele is present, the incision must be continued under the urethra as well. When a longitudinal incision is complete, the cut edges of the vagina are separated by blunt and sharp dissections from the pubocervical fascia, which is attached to the bladder. This procedure is repeated on both sides, and at this point the bladder and pubocervical fascia are free of the vaginal wall. The operator then places a suture at the level of the bladder neck (Kelley stitch) bringing together the pubocervical fascia from either side (Figure 17.4). This stitch is placed in such a fashion that pubocervical fascia is sutured as far away from the cut edge as possible in parallel to the mid-line incision. No. 0 polyglycol suture is most appropriate for this closure. With the bladder neck identified and supported, the pubocervical fascia is then closed with progressive similar stitches, completely imbricating the fascia over the bladder. If a urethrocele is present, it, too, may be repaired in a similar fashion. If a major stress incontinence problem is present, the bladder neck may be further supported to the pubic symphysis using sutures that connect the perivaginal tissue on either side of the urethra to the pubic symphysis. A Pereyra or Stamey modification of the Pereyra procedure is a reasonable alternative. After completing the imbrication of the pubocervical fascia, the vaginal edges are trimmed and the vagina is closed with a row of interrupted No. 2, No. 0 polyglycol or catgut sutures.

The bladder should be drained for about 3 to 5 days postoperatively, and this may be accomplished in a number of different ways. The first would be to leave a No. 16 Foley catheter in place for 3 to 5 days, remove it, and allow the patient to try to void. If voiding occurs, to the amount of 100 to 200 ml, the patient would be catheterized for the presence of residual urine. If residual urine is found in a quantity of greater than 150 ml on two successive voidings or if the amount of voiding is less than 100 ml, the physician should consider replacing the catheter for an additional 24 to 48 hours. If residual urines are less than 150 ml on two consecutive voidings, no further steps are necessary. Occasionally, patients have difficulty voiding even after an additional 2 days and may be followed with Foley catheterization to continuous drainage into a leg bag or may have the catheter clamped and may empty it when the need to void is noted. After 5 to 7 days a further attempt to remove the catheter may be carried out. Prophylactic antibiotics are rarely necessary, but lower urinary tract infections are common in elderly women and should be treated if they occur. At the time of the removal of the catheter, the urine should be sent for culture and sensitivity.

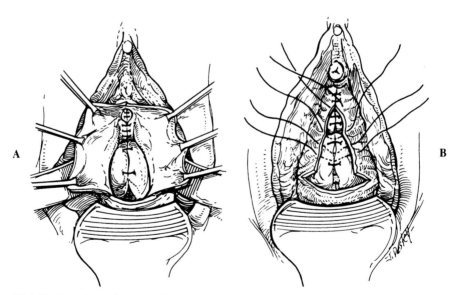

Figure 17.4 Cystourethrocele repair. (**A**) Appearance of a cystourethrocele after plication of bladder-neck and repair of cystocele; cut edges of vagina are held apart above repair.
(**B**) Repair of vagina over cystocele is noted. (From Symmonds RE: Relaxation of pelvic supports, in Benson RC (ed.): *Current Obstetrics and Gynecologic Diagnosis and Treatment,* ed. 5. Los Altos, Lange Medical Publications, 1984; with permission.)

Occasionally, patients with chronic urinary tract infections are administered prophylactic antibiotics, such as a sulfa preparation or furadantin.

Alternatives to the previously mentioned regimen of catheter control include: suprapubic catheter drainage or the placement of an infant feeding tube (No. 5) through the urethra attached to the labia with a suture. In both methods, the drainage tube can be clamped, allowing the patient to void when she can and for residual urines to be measured. The suprapubic technique is simple to use and seems to have a lower incidence of infection. However, patients may complain of extravasation of urine around the site and occasionally hematoma formation. The selection of a means of draining the bladder after repair is generally determined by the experience of the surgeon and the custom of the hospital.

Since it is imperative that healing be allowed to be completed before increasing stress and strain on the operative area, the patient must be cautioned to do no heavy lifting, straining, or prolonged standing, for at least 3 months. Estrogen therapy should be maintained and, as a rule, coitus is not resumed until the 3-month period is past, in the older woman.[2]

Rectocele

A patient with a rectocele will often complain of heaviness in the pelvis or a sensation that her rectum is falling out of her vagina. She may have constipation, and occasionally state that she needs to splint her vagina with her fingers in order to effect a bowel movement. She, too, many have a feeling of incomplete emptying of the rectum after a bowel movement.

A rectocele may be identified by retracting the anterior vaginal wall upward and having the patient strain (Figure 17.5). The rectum may bulge into the vagina and, if the rectocele is large enough, the bulge may protrude through the introitus. The physician may place one finger in the rectum and one in the vagina and palpate the hernia. The rectovaginal septum may appear to be paper thin and the entire limits of the rectocele may be palpated. If an enterocele is present, with

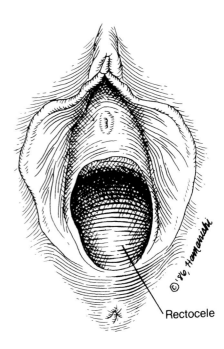

Figure 17.5 Rectocele. (From Herbst AL, Mishell DR, Stenchever MA, Droegemueller, W: Disorders of abdominal wall and pelvic support, in *Comprehensive Gynecology,* St. Louis, 2nd ed. CV Mosby, 1992, Chapt 19; with permission.)

Rectocele

straining it may be possible to differentiate this sac from the rectocele. Small enteroceles will escape detection by this method and may be only found at the time of operation.

The rectocele may be treated with pessary, Kegel exercises, and ERT in appropriate situations. As with cystocele, ERT may help tissue strength and vascularity.

Operative management (posterior colporrhaphy) is often performed at the time of an anterior colporrhaphy with or without enterocele repair or operation for descensus of the uterus. Most women with rectoceles will also have weakened perineal bodies leading to a gaping vagina and therefore will require a perineorrhaphy at the time of the procedure. Therefore, when operatively repairing a rectocele, the surgeon should estimate at the beginning of the posterior wall repair what degree of perineorrhaphy is desirable. The margins of the perineum to be narrowed are marked with Allis clamps at their extremes and the skin of the introitus between these clamps is then incised. The vaginal wall is then separated from the underlying tissue with a progressive longitudinal incision in the mid-line beginning at the introital incision and carried to the apex of the vagina above the limit of the rectocele. This is best performed with Metzenbaum scissors in a similar fashion to the cystocele repair. The vaginal wall is completely incised, the vagina is separated from the rectum by blunt and, if necessary, sharp dissections. This is continued until the operator can palpate the perirectal space on each side exposing the region of the levator ani muscles. There is little endopelvic fascia in this region. If an enterocele is present, it will generally be observable at this point. The enterocele sac, if present, must then be dissected free, as will be described later.

The operator then places a finger of the nondominant hand into the rectum using a double glove technique, while an assistant lifts up the perirectal tissue on either side. The operator then places a No. 0 suture of either nonabsorbable type (silk or dermalon) or a polyglycol slow-absorbing suture into the perirectal tissue on either side, attempting to get portions of the levator muscle. Approximately three or four of these sutures are required but, in the case of a large defect, more may be necessary. The operator should use the finger in the rectum to ensure that no suture is placed into the rectum. The sutures are then tied, interposing perirectal tissue and levator ani muscle fibers between the rectum and the vagina, thus reducing the rectocele. These sutures will also serve to tack the vagina to the levator ani area, thereby avoiding future vaginal prolapse if a hysterectomy has also been performed. The vaginal edges are then trimmed and the vagina closed with either a row of continuous or interrupted polyglycol or catgut sutures.

The perineorrhaphy is then closed by placing No. 0 polyglycol suture into the lateral margins of the transverse incision, essentially bringing bulbocavernousal muscles from either side together in the mid-line. The operator should be sure that the bulbocavernousal muscle insertions are included in the sutures by pulling on the sutures as they are placed and noting whether there is tension in the muscle bundles. The remainder of the perineal incision is then closed using a row of No. 2, No. 0 polyglycol or catgut suture in the deep tissue. The skin of the perineum may be closed with an interrupted or continuous subcutaneous suture of No. 3, No. 0 catgut.[1]

Enterocele

An enterocele is a true hernia of the peritoneal cavity from the pouch of Douglas (cul de sac) between the uterosacral ligaments and into the rectovaginal septum (Figure 17.6). The contents of an enterocele are always small bowel and may include omentum. Patients with enteroceles also note a heaviness in their pelvis and may detect a bulge coming from their introitus, frequently quite large. The enterocele is not always easy to diagnose. It may be detected as a separate bulge from a rectocele at the time of a rectovaginal examination. If large enough, it may be possible to

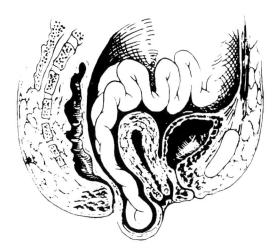

Figure 17.6 Enterocele and uterine prolapse. (From Symmonds RE: Relaxation of pelvic supports, in Benson RC (ed.): *Current Obstetrics and Gynecologic Diagnosis and Treatment*, ed. 5. Los Altos, Lange Medical Publications, 1984, with permission.)

transilluminate the sac and small bowel shadows within the sac. It may be possible to reduce the hernia, but at times the small bowel contents are fixed to the peritoneum of the sac by adhesions.

While an enterocele may be supported as part of a total prolapse using a pessary, it is most effectively treated operatively. The repair may be carried out separately or at the time of a posterior colporrhaphy. The sac is visualized as the vagina is separated from the rectum. It must be dissected free of the underlying tissue and isolated at its neck. It should be opened to ensure that all contents are replaced into the peritoneal cavity. The neck of the hernia is then sutured with a purse-string No. 0 polyglycol suture and the sac wall excised. A second purse-string suture is usually placed 1 cm below the first. In some cases where the sac neck is large, multiple, progressive purse-string sutures may be necessary.

Enteroceles often occur after abdominal or vaginal hysterectomies and generally are due to the fact that support of the pouch of Douglas is weakened. In order to prevent enteroceles at the time of hysterectomy, the uterosacral and cardinal ligaments are extremely important structures and should be incorporated into the vaginal vault repair. The ligaments from each side may be joined together.[3]

Enteroceles may also be reduced transabdominally at the time of other abdominal procedures or as a primary procedure. The sac should be reduced upward and, if uterosacral ligaments can be identified, these should be brought together in the mid-line. If uterosacral ligaments cannot be identified as with large enteroceles following previous hysterectomy, the cul de sac may be obliterated by concentric purse-string sutures in the endopelvic fascia. Care must be taken to avoid damaging the ureters, rectum, and sigmoid colon. Permanent suture or polyglycol sutures are best used for this procedure. For large or multiple recurrent enteroceles, both a vaginal and an abdominal approach may be necessary.

Pitfalls in enterocele repair that may lead to a recurrence are often related to the operator not isolating the neck of the sac adequately. This is an extremely important aspect of the procedure.[1]

Uterine Prolapse (Descensus, Procidentia)

Descensus of the uterus and cervix into or through the barrel of the vagina is often associated with injuries of the endopelvic fascia, including cardinal and uterosacral ligaments, as well as injury or relaxation of the pelvic floor muscles, particularly the levator ani muscles. Prolapse may occur because of increased intra-abdominal pressure, such as may be seen with ascites, or a large pelvic or intra-abdominal tumor superimposed on poor pelvic supports. Occasionally, sacral nerve disorders, especially injuries to S1–S4 or diabetic neuropathy may be responsible. Factors that increase tension of pelvic floor musculature, such as chronic respiratory disease, including asthma, bronchitis, and bronchiectasis, and morbid obesity may be associated. Congenital damage or relaxed pelvic floor supports may cause prolapse in young nulliparous women. Often, patients with descensus are multiparous and the problem may be related to childbirth trauma. Descensus is almost always associated with other forms of pelvic relaxation, including cystocele and rectocele. Enterocele may be present as well.[1]

Descensus is graded in the following manner: a prolapse into the upper barrel of the vagina is defined as first degree. A prolapse through the barrel of the vagina to the region of the introitus is defined as second degree. If the cervix and uterus prolapsed through the introitus, it is defined as a third-degree or total prolapse (Figure 17.7). Essentially, when a total prolapse occurs, the vagina is everted around the uterus and cervix and completely exteriorized. Often, particularly in older women not on ERT, dryness rapidly develops with thickening and chronic inflammation of the vaginal epithelium. Stasis ulcers may occur, and edema and interference with blood supply to the vaginal wall takes place. Rarely are these ulcers cancerous, but biopsies should be taken to ensure that they are not. Invariably, perineal supports are poor and the perineal body is damaged.[1]

The major symptoms noted by patients with descensus are: a feeling of heaviness or fullness, or that something is falling out of the vagina. In second-degree prolapse the cervix may be noted to be protruding from the introitus, giving the patient the impression that a tumor is bulging out of her vagina. Once total prolapse has occurred, the patient is aware that a mass is actually protruded from the introitus. Symptoms of cystocele and rectocele may also be present. With ulceration of the vaginal epithelium or of the cervix, pain and vaginal bleeding may occur. Discharge may also be present if infection has occurred.[1]

First-degree prolapse may not need therapy unless the patient is very uncomfortable. As the degree of prolapse increases and the cervix is placed at or through the introitus, discomfort is

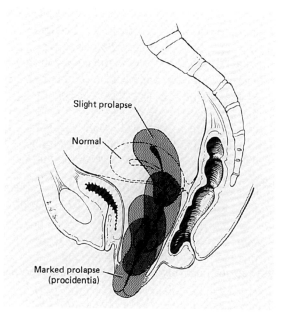

Slight prolapse

Normal

Marked prolapse
(procidentia)

Figure 17.7 Various degrees of prolapse of the uterus. (From Symmonds RE: Relaxation of pelvic supports, in Benson RC (ed.): Current obstetrics and gynecologic diagnosis and treatment, ed. 5. Los Altos, Lange Medical Publications, 1984; with permission.)

generally more severe and therapy is indicated. Medical management of such conditions involve using a pessary. This requires the replacement of the uterus and cervix to their normal position in the pelvis and the institution of support using one of these devices. Pessaries are available in various sizes and shapes. It is often necessary to consider the patient's anatomy and personal needs when selecting the appropriate pessary. This type of management is particularly of value in individuals of poor operative risk. ERT is necessary in such patients as is the case for other pelvic relaxation problems. Certainly, ERT for at least 30 days should be undertaken before considering surgical repair. Repair should not be undertaken until all ulcers of the vagina and cervix are healed. Otherwise, there is risk of infection and breakdown of the repair.

Operative repair of a prolapse of the uterus and cervix generally involves a vaginal hysterectomy with anterior and posterior colporrhaphy. At the time of hysterectomy, cardinal and uterosacral ligaments are carefully isolated so that they may be used in support of the vaginal vault. Uterosacral ligaments and cardinal ligaments should be sutured carefully to the vagina and brought together in the mid-line to support the cul de sac. This will help to prevent enterocele in the future.[1]

In some instances, a vaginal hysterectomy may not be advisable. These include previous intra-abdominal surgery for an inflammatory process, such as pelvic inflammatory disease and endometriosis. In such instances, an abdominal hysterectomy may be performed followed by a vaginal anterior and posterior colporrhaphy. Procedures that amputate the cervix and use the cardinal ligaments to support the bladder repair (Manchester procedure) may be instituted in certain situations. Most often, the best reason for performing a Manchester procedure is that the patient has an elongated cervix with a fairly well-supported uterus, and it is the cervix that is protruding from the introitus. This is seen not infrequently in elderly women.

In the very elderly, who are no longer sexually active, a simple procedure for reducing prolapse may be a partial colpocleisis. The classic procedure was described by Le Fort and involves removal of a strip of anterior and posterior walls of the vagina with closure of the margins of anterior and posterior walls to each side. This procedure may be performed with or without the presence of a uterus and cervix. When it is completed, a small vaginal canal exists on either side of the septum, which is produced by the suturing of the lateral margins of the excision. The line of dissection of the vaginal wall should be carried out to the level of the bladder neck anteriorly and to the reflection of bladder on to cervix in the depth of the vagina if the uterus is present.

Posteriorly, the dissection is carried from just inside the introitus to a position just posterior to the cervix, if the uterus is present. If the uterus is absent, the extent of the incision into the depth of the vagina should be to approximately 1 cm from the previous vaginal scar. Since the area of the bladder neck is avoided, urinary incontinence is generally not a consequence of this procedure. On the other hand, if stress urinary incontinence is a problem, bladder neck plication may be carried out as part of the procedure. After healing, a small introital area is noted that has cosmetic benefits in the older woman. Narrow canals are present on each lateral vaginal wall. If the cervix and uterus are still present and intrauterine pathology should occur, bleeding along these canals could take place, alerting the physician to the fact that a problem exists.[1]

The Goodall-Power modification of the Le Fort operation is essentially the removal of a triangular piece of vaginal wall beginning at the cervical reflection or 1 cm above the vaginal scar at the base of the triangle and the apex of the triangle just beneath the bladder neck anteriorly and just at the introitus posteriorly. The cut edges of the vaginal wall making up the base of the triangle anteriorly are sutured to the similar wall posteriorly, and the vaginal incision is then closed with a row of interrupted sutures beginning beneath the bladder neck and being carried side to side to the area of the introitus. This procedure works well for relatively small prolapses, however, the Le Fort procedure is best for larger ones.[1]

If an enterocele is found at the time of colpocleisis, it must be repaired. Failure to repair an enterocele at the time of colpocleisis will probably lead to a breakdown of the repair. In all cases, a perineorrhaphy is performed to reduce the size of the introitus.[1]

Colpocleisis to reduce a prolapse and to prevent recurrence is generally quite effective. Ridley,[4] reports no prolapse recurrence in 58 patients unless an incomplete procedure was performed. Three patients in Ridley's series developed urinary stress incontinence where none had been present preoperatively.[4]

Prolapse of the vaginal vault at some time remote to the performance of either abdominal or vaginal hysterectomy has been reported as occurring in between 0.1% and 18.2% of patients. Such a prolapse may be total and may be accompanied by cystocele, rectocele, enterocele, or some combination thereof. In examining such patients it is important to identify the upper scar of the vagina and then try to determine which contents are present within the vault (cystocele, rectocele, or enterocele). Richter,[5] reporting on 97 vaginal vault prolapses, found that 6.2% contained cystocele only, 5.1% rectocele only, 9.3% enterocele primarily, and 72% a mixture of contents.

Vaginal vault prolapse probably occurs as a continuing pelvic support weakness problem and a failure of the cardinal and uterosacral ligaments to maintain their tone or attach to the vagina. The symptoms and signs are the same as those delineated for descensus of the uterus, including pelvic heaviness, backache, and a mass protruding from the introitus. At times stress incontinence, urgency, frequency, dribbling, vaginal bleeding, or discharge (if there is an ulcer) will occur. If the mass is large, there may be difficulty in sitting or walking. Examination will help to differentiate the contents of the prolapse. Rectovaginal examination may help to delineate an enterocele from a rectocele.

In the planning of a repair of a vaginal prolapse, several principles should be kept in mind. The first is that the normal position of the vagina in a standing position is against the rectum and no more than 30 degrees from the horizontal.[6] Second, pelvic relaxation is part of a problem which dictates that an existing cystocele, rectocele, or enterocele must be repaired as part of the procedure. A third principle acknowledges that the perineal body is almost always weakened and in such individuals there should be reconstruction of this as well. The nonsurgical management of vaginal prolapse can include pessary, ERT, and the clearing up of ulcers when present. Pessaries are rarely retained in such individuals unless there is an adequate perineal body.[1]

Surgical procedures to repair a vaginal prolapse are many. They include those that use an abdominal approach, vaginal approach, or some combination thereof. If the surgeon prefers an abdominal approach, a variety of procedures are available. These include fixation of the vaginal vault to the anterior abdominal wall, to the lumbar spine, to anterior longitudinal ligaments near the sacral promontory, or to various tendinous lines in the musculature of the true pelvis or to the sacral spinus ligament. The anterior abdominal wall fixation increases the diameter of the pouch of Douglas and frequently contributes to the formation of a subsequent enterocele. Fixation to the lumbar spine or sacral promontory is often difficult to achieve directly. Most often it requires the interposition of a different material. In the past, ox fascia lata, fascial aponeurosis from the individual herself, and inert material such as mersilene have been utilized. If a stint is used, it should be covered with peritoneum, thereby rendering the stint retroperitoneal. Obliteration of the pouch of Douglas may be necessary as well to prevent a recurrent enterocele. Grafts of mersilene or Gore-Tex can be used and will be long-lasting in most cases. Sloughing of the graft from the vaginal vault in the development of a sinus tract is an occasional complication. Timmons and coworkers[3] report a 99% rate of good, long-term results in 163 patients repaired at Duke. Enterocele occurred in only 3 (2%) and recurrent urinary incontinence in 18 (11%).[7] Fixation to the sacral spinus ligament has had an encouraging degree of success.

Sacrospinus ligament fixation of the vaginal wall can be accomplished vaginally. Randall and Nichols[8] reported excellent success with both abdominal and vaginal approaches. In 18 patients treated with fixation of the vaginal wall to the sacral spinus ligament via the vaginal route, all had successful outcomes.

Although a variety of vaginal procedures have been designed, the best success has been in those situations where adequate vaginal length is maintained and the vagina is positioned against the rectum nearly parallel to the horizontal.

Morley and DeLancey[9] reported on 100 women who underwent repair of vaginal vault prolapse using the vaginal sacrospinus ligament suspension with good and lasting success. Twenty-three had only the suspension performed, whereas 67 underwent a form of colporrhaphy as well. One-year followup revealed 67 of the 71 patients available had satisfactory results, 4 had developed symptomatic cystoceles, and 3 had had a recurrent prolapse.

If a vaginal prolapse has occurred without a concordant cystocele and/or rectocele, a repair may be affected vaginally by making a transverse incision on the posterior wall of the vagina approximately 1 or 2 cm from the upper scar, separating the rectum from the vagina by blunt dissection, splitting the perirectal tissue above the sacral spinus ligament on the right, and suturing the upper end of the vaginal vault to the sacrospinus ligament using either No. 0 silk or a polyglycol suture of No. 0 strength. Generally two sutures are used. Following this the vagina is simply closed. In older women who are no longer sexually active a colpocleisis procedure may be performed.

It is important that the physician determine the desires of the patient before deciding which procedure is best suited for her needs. This can be accomplished by careful preoperative counseling. Many elderly women, although no longer sexually active, do not wish to lose the potential use of their vaginas. Therefore, the physician caring for such women should not take for granted that their current circumstance of sexual inactivity dictates a colpocleisis as the appropriate therapy.

References

1. Herbst AL, Mishell DR, Stenchever MA, Droegemueller W: Disorders of abdominal wall and pelvic support, in *Comprehensive Gynecology*. St. Louis (2d ed.) CV Mosby, 1992.
2. Herbst, AC, Mischell, DR, Stenchever, MA and Droegemueller, W.: *Comprehensive Gynecology* St. Louis, (2nd ed.) CV Mosby, 1992.
3. McCall M: Posterior culdeplasty. Surgical correction of enterocele during vaginal hysterectomy; a preliminary report. *J Am College Obstet Gynecol* 1957;6:595–602.
4. Ridley JH: Evaluation of the colpocleisis operation: A report of 58 cases. *Am J Obstet Gynecol* 1972;113:1114.
5. Richter K: Massive eversion of the vagina. Pathogenesis, diagnosis, and therapy of the true prolapse of the vaginal stump. *Clin Obstet Gynecol* 1982;25:897.
6. Peters WA III, Thornton N. Jr: Surgical anatomy of the perirectal fascia: A gynecologic perspective. *Obstet Gynecol Survey* 1987;42:605–611.
7. Timmons MC, Addison WA, Addison SB, Cavenar MG: Abdominal sacral colpopexy in 163 women with posthysterectomy vaginal vault prolapse and enterocele. Evolution of operative techniques. *J Reprod Med* 1992;37:323–327.
8. Randall CI, Nicols DH: Surgical treatment of vaginal inversion. *Obstet Gynecol* 1971;38:327.
9. Morley GW, DeLancey JOL: Sacrospinus ligament fixation for eversion of the vagina. *Am J Obstet Gynecol* 1988;158:872–881.
10. Elia G, Bergman A: Pelvic muscle exercises: When do they work? *Obstet Gynecol* 1993;81:283–286.
11. Imparato E, Aspesi G, Rovetta E, Presti M: Surgical management and prevention of vaginal vault prolapse. *Surg Gynecol Obstet* 1992;175:233–237.
12. Iosif C: Abdominal sacral colpopexy with use of synthetic mesh. *Acta Obstet Gynecol Scand* 1993;72:214–217.
13. Nichols DH: Transvaginal sacrospinus fixation. *Pelvic Surgery*. 1981;1:10.
14. Shull BL, Capen CV, Riggs MW, Kuehl TJ: Bilateral attachment of the vaginal cuff to iliococcygeus fascia: An effective method of cuff suspension. *Am J Obstet Gynecol* 1993;168:1669–1677.

Chapter 18

Vulvar and Vaginal Conditions in the Older Woman

Louis Vontver, MD

Mature women are subject to the same vulvar and vaginal conditions as younger women. There is a difference in the prevalence of certain conditions, notably atrophic changes resulting from lack of estrogen after the menopause, found predominantly in women who do not take hormone replacement therapy, and an increased incidence of malignancies and dermatoses, though the vulva and vagina are relatively rare sites for these entities. This chapter focuses on conditions that are more commonly found and emphasizes some abnormalities that occur more frequently with aging.

Normal Anatomy and Histology

The normal changes of aging include a relative loss of endogenous estrogen after the menopause. This results in vulvar atrophy with a decrease of subcutaneous fatty tissue, shrinking of the labia majora, and thinning of the vulvar dermis and epidermis, with loss of dermal elasticity. With loss of elasticity vulvar varicosities may occur. The amount of pubic hair is also decreased and small (cherry) hemangiomas may frequently be found on the labial surface (Figure 18.1).

Some authors state that there is a relative increase in the size of the clitoris due to increased testosterone as a result of increased levels of luteinizing hormones. However, more recent data do not show an increase in clitoral size with age but these authors[1] did not examine postmenopausal women. In any event, if there is true enlargement of the clitoris, that is, a clitoral index (length × width of glands in mm) greater than 35 mm[2], an exogenous or endogenous abnormal source of androgen should be sought.[2]

With loss of estrogen the vaginal epithelium also becomes thinner and loses elasticity, resulting in a diminution of vaginal diameter. The normal secretions that aid in vaginal lubrication are decreased. The thinning and a flattening of the epithelial layer together with a loss of glycogen results in a decrease in lactobacilli, lactic acid production, and a concomitant increase in the number of various bowel bacteria in the vagina. The vaginal pH also rises. All of these factors render the vagina more susceptible to irritation and lead to the common complaint of a dry vagina, susceptible to infection and injury. Atrophy often causes dyspareunia, and other vulvovaginal discomfort.[3]

The degree of atrophy of the vulva and vagina is quite variable after menopause, depending on the amount of estrogen that is produced by the peripheral conversion from adrenal androgens and, to some extent, by the persistence of coital activity. However, in many cases the loss of estrogen is great enough to induce the characteristic symptom of vaginal dryness. The loss of

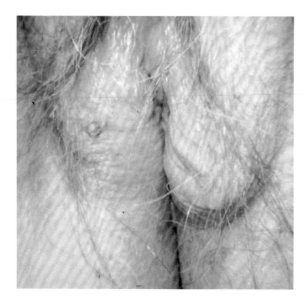

Figure 18.1 Note the loss of subcutaneous fat in the labia majora, decreased amount of hair, and the small angioma on one labia.

vaginal epithelial thickness and rugae results in a pale, erythematous vaginal epithelium that may contain small petechiae. Occasionally the atrophy is severe enough to cause bleeding. Ten to fifteen percent of postmenopausal vaginal bleeding is estimated to be due to atrophic vaginitis. Figures 18.2 and 18.3 compare the histology of the vaginal epithelium in pre- and postmenopausal patients, respectively.

In addition to the gross appearance and subjective symptom of dryness of the external genitalia and vagina resulting from the relative decrease of estrogen stimulation, cells scraped from the lateral wall of the vagina can be evaluated for estrogen effect by the maturation index (MI), or the karyopyknotic index (KI). The MI is a ratio of numbers of parabasal, intermediate, and superficial squamous cells that are seen when counting 100 vaginal epithelial cells. The KI is expressed as a percentage of superficial cells found in the total group of vaginal epithelial cells examined. As effective estrogen is lost, the MI shifts from larger numbers of superficial cells toward a larger number of intermediate and parabasal cells, and KI shows a decrease in superficial cells. Figure 18.4 is a drawing of the mature vaginal epithelium and the cells that exfoliate from it. Replacement estrogen causes reappearance of intermediate and superficial cells. Figure 18.5 demonstrates parabasal vaginal cells from the vagina of a postmenopausal woman not on estrogen replacement therapy. Figure 18.6 demonstrates cells obtained from the vagina of a woman of menstrual age.

Parabasal, intermediate, and superficial cells can easily be identified on a vaginal wet mount. Neither the MI nor KI is quantitative enough for direct correlation with the amount of circulating estrogen. They are influenced by many other factors such as other hormones and vaginal infections. However, they do correlate with patients' urinary symptoms, subjective evaluation of vaginal dryness, and vaginal mucosal atrophy as judged by visual inspection. Therefore, they provide some additional evidence of estrogen effect or lack thereof, and as they are commonly identified on a vaginal wet mount, the physiology of their appearance should be understood.[4]

In a study using a modified grading of the vaginal smear for superficial, intermediate, and parabasal cells, the clinical features that were the best predictors of vaginal atrophy on the smear were a thin body habitus and dryness on vaginal examination.[5,6]

The distal vagina, urethra, and the trigone all originate from the fetal urogenital sinus. Estrogen

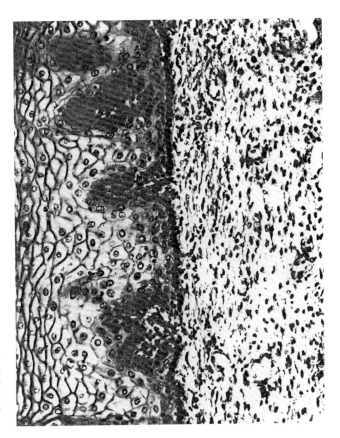

Figure 18.2 The histology of a normal, mature vagina. Note the maturation of the epithelial cells. (From de Neef: *Clinical Endocrine Cytology,* Hoeber Medical Division, 1965, Figure 1.9.)

receptors are present in high concentrations and therefore these structures respond to the loss of estrogen by becoming atrophic. Atrophy increases the frequency of symptoms of urine loss and the chance of urinary tract infection as the urethra is in proximity to an increased number of bowel flora such as *Escherichia coli,* in the vagina.[7]

The mucosa of the vagina and urethra responds to the addition of estrogen by regaining the characteristics found in menstrual age women, including increased KI and lactobacilli. The treated vagina also shows decreased bowel bacteria, and urinary symptoms are often alleviated.[8]

Atrophy of the vaginal and cervical cells may also cause atypical cells on pap smears. A short course of vaginal estrogen will cause maturation of these cells and often will result in normal PAP smears.[9]

Treatment of Atrophic Changes Secondary to Estrogen Loss

The treatment for atrophic vaginal and vulvar changes due to estrogen loss is replacing estrogen. Most studies have revealed the efficacy of either systemic or topical therapy using conjugated equine estrogens, estradiol, or estriol. Approximately equal amounts of estrogen receptors (ER) have been measured in vaginal biopsies of menstrual age and postmenopausal women. This may help explain why there is a rapid response of these cells to exogenously supplied estrogen.[10]

Very low doses of topical vaginal estrogen provide effective relief of the vaginal symptoms at low cost.[11] For example, as little as 0.5 g of conjugated estrogen cream inserted vaginally, daily

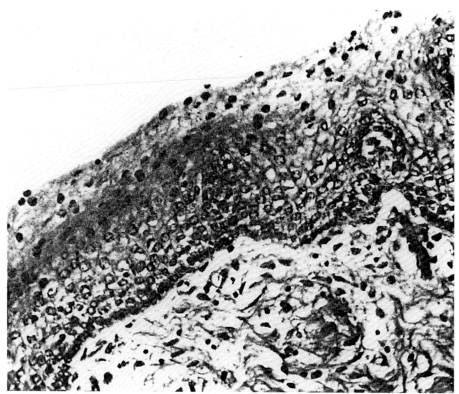

Figure 18.3 Note the layers of parabasal cells and the lack of maturation at the surface of the atrophic vaginal epithelium. (From Blaustein A (ed.): *Pathology of the Female Genital Tract,* ed 2. New York, Springer Verlag, 1982, Figure 3.5, p. 62.)

for 2 weeks and then 3 times a week in a small group of patients provided subjective relief as well as objective improvement in vaginal cytology without demonstrated endometrial proliferation. Because of the small amount of cream used, the cost was low. Similar results can be seen with vaginally administered estriol or estradiol.[12,13] The more atrophic the vagina the greater the systemic absorption of vaginally delivered estrogen and progesterone. Therefore, large amounts of vaginal estrogen can cause systemic effects.[14]

More commonly, conjugated estrogen with or without a progestin, is given orally either cyclically or continuously as hormone replacement therapy (HRT). This provides adequate estrogen support to the vaginal, vulvar, and urethral tissues and also provides protection from hot flashes, bone reabsorption, and cardiovascular diseases.[15,16] Although daily oral intake of 1.25 mg of conjugated estrogen is required to change the MI to values similar to those found in premenopausal subjects, the symptoms of vaginal dryness are usually relieved by half this amount.

Transdermal estrogen is another method of delivering systemic estrogens that is effective in relieving vulvovaginal symptoms as well as preventing bone loss.

Effects of Tamoxifen on the Vaginal Mucosa

Many older women are currently taking tamoxifen as an adjuvant therapy for breast cancer. Its pharmacology is complex. Tamoxifen acts as both an estrogen antagonist and agonist, depending

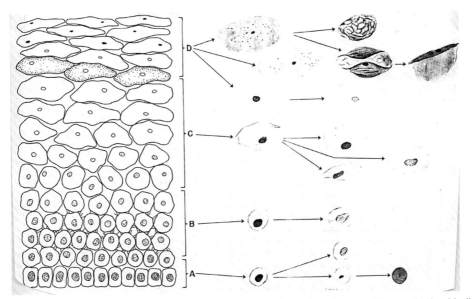

Figure 18.4 Note the different cell types that exfoliate from the various layers of the vaginal epithelium. (From de Neef: *Clinical Endocrine Cytology,* Hoeber Medical Division, 1965, Plate 3, 37.)

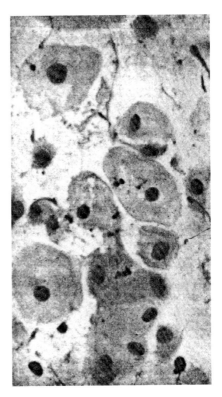

Figure 18.5 Parabasal cells. Note the amount of contour, the large amount of cytoplasm, and the large, round nucleus. (From Novak, Woodruff: *Gynecologic and Obstetric Pathology with Clinical and Endocrine Relations,* ed 8. Philadelphia, WB Saunders, 1979, Figure 34.11, p 707.)

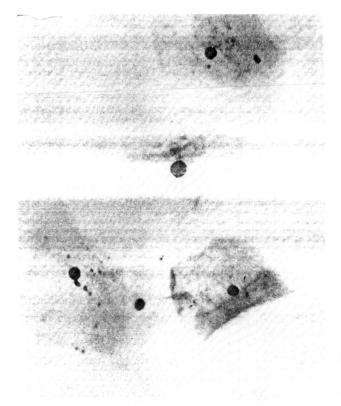

Figure 18.6 Superficial cells and an intermediate cell. (From Blaustein A. (ed.) *Pathology of the Female Genital Tract,* ed 2. New York, Springer Verlag, 1982, Figure 35.3, p. 839.)

on the species and hormonal status of the subject. Twenty milligrams a day has been shown to increase the KI in postmenopausal women. However, in premenopausal women or in women who were treated with estrogen, tamoxifen at high dosages significantly opposes the effect of estrogen on the vaginal epithelium and decreases the KI. In postmenopausal women, tamoxifen reduced the vaginal pH, changed the visual assessment of the vaginal mucosa so that it was not considered atrophic, and changed lateral vaginal smears to a estrogenized status.[17–20]

Vaginal Infections

The vagina and vulva of the older woman are subject to the same infections as a younger woman, though less frequently. The normal vaginal discharge in a woman of menstrual age is floccular, white, nonodiferous, and does not cause irritation. Atrophic vaginitis in the older woman is not a true infection but causes a dry vagina with thin mucosa, loss of rugae, decreased superficial and intermediate cells and increased pH. Such a vagina is easily infected.

Discharge due to yeast is classically white, curdy, and can be found in association with either a high or a low pH. The discharge from bacterial vaginosis tends to be gray, clear, homogenous, and watery. Trichomonas infection classically causes a gray-green, frothy discharge. However, clinical observation without microscopic aid is unsatisfactory for diagnosis because of great variation of the discharges (see Table 18.1).

The etiology of any vaginal discharge should be initially evaluated by measuring its pH, which is normally below 4.5 in women of menstrual age. Vaginal discharge due to atrophic vaginitis,

Table 18.1 Vaginitis in the Older Woman: Diagnosis and Treatment

Type of vaginitis	History	PE	pH	Wet mount (Saline and 10% KOH)	Treatment
None	No complaints	Normal	<4.5	Normal lactobacilli and normal superficial and intermediate squamous cells	None
Atrophic (may have associated infection)	Dry vagina, painful intercourse	Thin, pale vaginal wall with loss of rugae	>4.5	Few lactobacilli; few superficial cells More intermediate and parabasal cells	Topical or systemic estrogen replacement Rx concommitant infection if present
Mycotic infection	Itching with or without discharge	Curdy white discharge, red introitus	Can be < or > 4.5	Mycelia and spores on KOH prep	Imidazole
Bacterial vaginosis	Irritating discharge; amine (fishy) odor, which is worse at menses or after coitus	Homogeneous gray discharge at introitus	>4.5	Clue cells Odor with KOH	Metronidazole topical or oral, or topical clindamycin
Trichomonas	Irritating or itchy discharge with or without odor, dysuria, dyspareunia	Gray-green frothy discharge	>4.5	Motile trichomonads on saline, increased white blood cells, with or without fishy odor	Metronidazole oral
Allergic or contact	Use of douche, suppository, latex, lubricant, spermacide, etc. With or without history of allergies	White discharge	Variable	Not specific, perhaps slightly increased white blood cells May need staining for eosinophiles	Discontinue use of irritant or allergen, possible use of antihistamines and/or cromolyn sodium
Dermatosis	Lesions present elsewhere on skin or mucous membranes	Lesions elsewhere	Variable	Not specific; biopsy often needed	As indicated by diagnosis

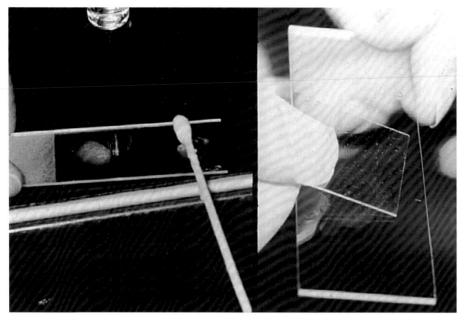

Figure 18.7 Demonstration of how to prepare a wet mount of vaginal secretion by placing two drops of saline on a clean slide, mixing it with the discharge, and covering each. One drop of the mixture has an additional drop of 10% KOH added and both are covered with a cover slip, taking care not to mix. These are then examined under low and high dry magnification.

trichomonas, and bacterial vaginosis usually has an elevated pH (above 4.5). The next step in diagnosis is microscopic examination of the discharge on a wet-mount preparation made by mixing normal saline and the vaginal discharge on a glass slide and covering it with a cover slip (Figure 18.7). The wet mount should be examined for normal lactobacilli, squamous epithelial cells, coccobacillary bacteria, trichomonas, yeast, and clue cells.

Yeast Vaginitis

Diagnosis of yeast vaginitis is aided by microscopic examination of a KOH wet-mount preparation, made by adding a drop of 10% KOH to the mixture of vaginal discharge and saline on the slide. It is a relatively insensitive test for diagnosing yeast infection, but it is adequate for most yeast infections that cause symptoms. In some cases vaginal culture for yeast may be indicated when recurrent symptoms of itching and redness make one highly suspicious of yeast even though the examination of KOH wet mounts are continuously negative. Yeast cultures require 10^3 organisms for accurate determination. If the vulva is also involved in suspected yeast infection, a scraping of vulvar epithelial cells can be prepared with KOH and warmed over a small flame. This will lyse the epithelial cells, allowing easier identification of mycelia. Most vaginal yeast infections are due to *Candida albicans,* however, other species of yeast may cause vaginal infection and some of them—such as *Candida glabrata, Candida torulopsis,* and *Candida tropicalis*—may be more resistant to the usual course of therapy. Treatment is by one of the topical imidazoles, which inhibit membrane synthesis of the yeast. Drugs include clotrimazole, miconazole, terconazole, and butaconazole in vaginal creams or suppositories once a day at bedtime for 1, 3, or 7 days, depending on the preparation (see Table 18.1). In the patient who develops frequent, recurrent symptomology, careful evaluation should be done to make sure the diagnosis is correct, because most treatment failures are due to an inaccurate initial diagnosis.[21]

If frequent, recurrent yeast infection is confirmed despite adequate initial treatment, retreatment should be instituted with a vaginal antimycotic drug daily for 14 days, or 400 mg/day of oral ketoconazole for 14 days may be used. This treatment can be followed by a maintenance dosage of topical imidazole vaginally 2 times a week, or of 100 mg/day oral of ketoconazole for several months. Studies have shown that patients receiving a monthly ketoconazole prophylaxis have approximately a 50% decrease in recurrent vulvovaginal candidiasis. However, ketoconazole is expensive and has potential liver toxicity and side effects that may limit its use.[22,23]

In addition, ketoconazole has only a slightly better clinical cure than clotrimazole with approximately the same rate of clinical recurrence after 2 months. Because the side effects (including headache, nausea, abdominal discomfort, fatigue, increased hepatic transaminases) are significantly greater with ketoconazole, local prophylaxis with topical imidazoles may be a better treatment modality, even though oral ketoconazole may be more convenient.[24]

Fluconazole, an oral antifungal preparation has been recently approved for the treatment of yeast in the vulvovaginal area. It seems to have a comparable efficacy as 7 days of daily topical cremes. It is given in a single dose of a 150 mg tablet but the 1 dose has approximately 15% @I side effects. (The Med Letter)

Because frequent vulvovaginal yeast infection is associated with diabetes, many patients with diabetes who have vaginal symptoms are often treated for yeast without being evaluated. A recent study by Rowe and coworkers[25] of recurrent vulvovaginal irritation in older women with diabetes who were treated for yeast without laboratory proof of yeast infection revealed that frequently they did not have vaginal candidiasis. Many had infection with beta hemolytic streptococcus or other bacteria. The patients who had bacterial infection had remission of their symptoms after antibiotic treatment specific for the cultured organism. The study demonstrated that *C. albicans* was not found as frequently as expected in diabetic women with vulvovaginal irritation. Therefore, the need to clearly document yeast infection before treatment is doubly important in this high-risk group in whom bacterial infection is equally probable.

Bacterial Vaginosis

Bacterial vaginosis (BV) (Figures 18.8 and 18.9) is the current term used to define an irritating vaginal discharge, diagnosed clinically by presence of at least three of the following signs (see Table 18.1):

1. Characteristic homogeneous adherent discharge

2. Vaginal pH greater than 4.5

3. Presence of clue cells (squamous epithelial cells whose margins have been obscured by adherent bacteria)

4. The production of an amine (fishy) odor when KOH is added to the vaginal fluid.

Bacterial vaginosis is due to polymicrobial overgrowth in the vagina, with loss of normal lactobacillus and an increase in the numbers of bacteriodes species, streptococcus, Gardnerella, and mobiluncus. Although Gardnerella has been implicated in BV, its presence or absence is not diagnostic, as up to 50% of women without the clinical criteria for BV may have Gardnerella in the vagina.

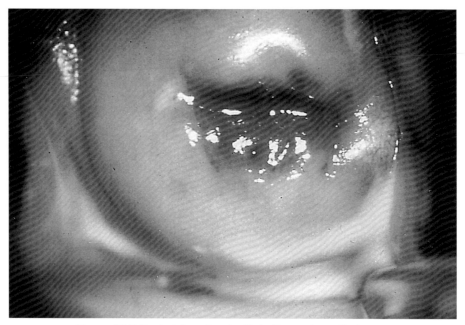

Figure 18.8 Bacterial vaginosis. Note the copious discharge.

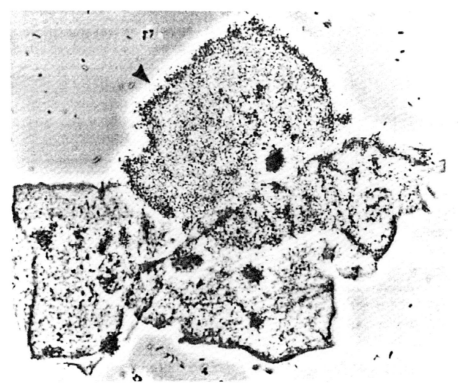

Figure 18.9 Clue cell. Note the obliteration of the cell border by adherent bacteria. (From Vontver L., Eschenbach DA: *Clin Obstet Gynecol* 1981;24:453.)

Therefore, culturing Gardnerella is of little use in the diagnosis, management, or follow-up of this disease.[26]

A similar polymicrobial overgrowth may coexist with other forms of vaginitis, especially trichomonas. BV is more commonly found in younger women and may be present in older women who maintain sexual activity, but it can also be found in women who are not sexually active. The currently recommended treatment is metronidazole, either 2 g orally in a single dose, or 2% clindamycin cream, 5 g at bedtime for 7 days, or metronidazole gel 0.75, 5 g intravaginally, 2 times a day for 5 days, or clindamycin, 300 mg orally 2 times a day for 7 days. Usual precautions regarding alcohol intake during treatment with oral metronidazole must be followed.[27]

The longer regimes have slightly better overall cure rates than the single-dose regimen but suffer from decreased compliance. However, there is a discouragingly high rate of recurrent infection, which is not well understood. Treatment of the male partner does not significantly alter the recurrence rate. In older women, the presence of BV increases the risk of posthysterectomy infections.[28]

Trichomonas Vaginitis

Although the prevalence of trichomonas infection of the vagina appears to be decreasing, and the infection is most often found in young women, it may also be present in sexually active older women. The diagnosis should be considered in any woman who gives a history of an irritating vaginal discharge and in whom a profuse discharge is found on physical examination (see Table 18.1). It is due to a flagellated protozoan, which attaches to squamous mucus membranes. The organism is sexually transmitted, usually by asymptomatic carriers. Although it classically presents with an irritating yellow, green, or gray, frothy discharge, the discharge alone is not adequate for diagnosis. A saline wet-mount preparation examined immediately is the diagnostic procedure of choice. However, the wet mount is not a very sensitive test because at least 10^4 organisms per ml of vaginal fluid are necessary to identify the protozoan. Even cultures require an innoculum of 10 to 1,000 viable organisms to achieve growth.[29]

Symptoms include an irritating discharge, with or without odor and with or without itching. Dyspareunia is common and dysuria may occur. The classic strawberry cervix and vaginal wall are rare findings that, if present, strongly suggest trichomoniasis. On wet mount the organisms, which are around the size of a polymorphonuclear leukocyte, are best recognized by their motility (Figure 18.10). Staining with various dyes adds very little to the sensitivity of the wet mount. PAP smears have a large false-positive rate. Culture is more sensitive but is costly and lacks immediacy.

Therapy is oral metronidazole, either in a 2 g single dose, which cures approximately 85% to 90% of women, or 500 mg 2 times a day for 7 days, which has about a 90% cure rate. The longer course is slightly more effective if used as directed, but patient compliance is a problem. All sex partners should be treated. Patients should avoid coitus until the patient and partner(s) are cured.[27] Metronidazole will produce a disulphiram-like effect with nausea and flushing in many patients if they consume alcohol while taking it. Occasionally, vaginal yeast infection will occur with the longer course. Clotrimazole is another possible therapy for patients who cannot take metronidazole; however, it is much less effective.[30]

Occasionally, metronidazole-resistant strains of trichomonas vaginalis have been reported. In those cases, high and prolonged doses of metronidazole (eg, 500 mg 3 times a day for 14 days) may be employed. Partners should also be treated in such cases, although this has not been unequivocally shown to be helpful.[31]

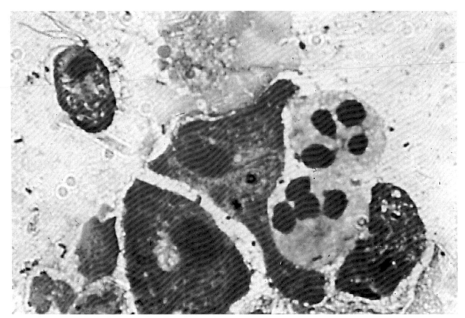

Figure 18.10 Trichomonas on a vaginal smear. Note the variation in size and shape and the presence of polymorphonuclear leukocytes.

Unusual Causes of Vaginitis

Occasionally, a patient is seen who has a persistent vaginitis that does not fit any of the previously described categories and that has not responded to numerous empirical treatments of topical and oral estrogen, steroids, antibiotics, and antimycotics. In these cases, vaginal dermatoses, such as lichen planus (which is the most common cause of erosive vaginitis) must be considered (see Table 18.1). These dermatoses often have secondary bacterial infection, which makes diagnosis more difficult. Diagnoses of lichen planus may be facilitated by finding the classic lesions on the skin. The pneumonic of purple, polygonal, planar, puritic papules will help one to remember how to identify these lesions. The surface of the papules may show a lacy, reticular pattern of whitish lines (Wickham's striae), which are due to focal epidermal thickening. This diagnostic sign is often seen on the oral buccal mucus membrane. In this condition, the vagina appears atrophic and there will be parabasal cells on the wet mount, but the condition will not respond to estrogen. Although secondary bacterial invaders may respond to topical antibiotic treatment, the underlying disease is not affected and the infection soon recurs. Other laboratory findings of the vaginal discharge in lichen planus include an alkaline pH, lack of squamous cell maturation, decreased lactobacilli, and high white blood cell count. The diagnosis is made by thinking of the disease, looking for manifestations elsewhere, and obtaining a biopsy, which reveals an infiltrate of white cells composed primarily of lymphocytes next to the dermal–epidermal junction. Treatment is by intravaginal steroids with occasional use of systemic steroids. For resistant cases, dapsone or griseofulvin have been tried with some success. Dapsone dosage is 50 to 100 mg/day, but hematologic parameters must be monitored closely while it is being used.

Pemphigoid and pemphigus may also cause red erosive areas in the vaginal mucosa. The diagnosis is made by biopsy for direct immunofluorescence, which reveals a linear band of immunoglobulin G (IgG) and/or complement 3.[32] (Figure 18.11).

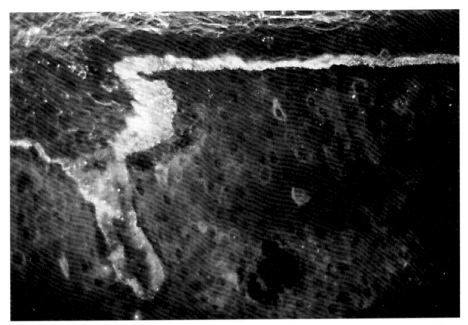

Figure 18.11 A biopsy showing a layer of complement 3 beneath the basement membrane.

Allergy has been described as a rare cause of vaginitis (see Table 18.1).[33] It is diagnosed by careful history and ruling out other causes. Diagnosis may be aided by finding eosinophilia in the vaginal exudate using Hansel staining. It is treated by removal of the offending agent. Dworetzky has reported that cromolyn instillation gave relief to one patient.[34,35]

Vulvar Abnormalities

Many of the vulvar changes and symptoms in the older woman are due to the lack of menstrual age estrogens as described previously. The symptoms of dryness and irritation can be treated by replacement estrogen taken either systemically or applied locally.

The atrophic vulvar vestibule is particularly vulnerable to coital trauma. This vulnerability can be greatly relieved by estrogens. In patients who are unable to take estrogens, personal lubricants allow sexual activity with much less irritation. Although KY jelly or vaseline is commonly used, much better vaginal lubricants such as Astroglide are available.

Other major causes of vulvar irritation are the vaginal infections discussed earlier in this chapter. Careful evaluation of any vaginal discharge and treatment of the offending organisms will often relieve the irritation on the vulva.

Although sexually transmitted diseases are less frequent in older women, they still occur and several are mentioned here, so they are not forgotten. Parasites, such as lice or scabies may be found. Viral infections, such as molluscum contagiosum, genital warts, and recurrent or even primary herpes infections can occur. Infections of Bartholin's or Skene's glands are unusual in this age group. If such an infection or mass occurs in a postmenopausal woman, biopsy is necessary to rule out the rare occurrence of carcinoma. The same holds true for any ulcerative lesion that does not heal rapidly, that is, within 2 weeks.

Yeast can cause cutaneous infection of the vulva as well as vaginitis. Elderly women who are

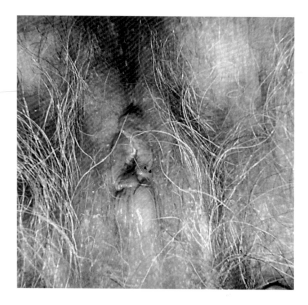

Figure 18.12 A yeast vulvovaginitis, which can easily be diagnosed by KOH prep from vaginal discharge or vulvar scrapings.

overweight, diabetic, on antibiotics, or have lost immune competency are particularly susceptible. Classically, vulvar cutaneous yeast infection presents as a symmetric erythematous lesion of the perineum, often containing satellite pustules (Figure 18.12). Evaluation should include a KOH wet mount from the vagina and/or scrapings from the vulvar skin. The scrapings should be placed on a slide with a 20% KOH and gently warmed to aid epidermal cell lysis and microscopic identification of the yeast. If these tests are negative, a culture of the scrapings from the skin should be obtained on either Sabouraud's or Nickerson's media. Treatment of cutaneous yeast requires application of a topical imidazole creme 1 or 2 times a day, usually for several weeks. Ketoconazole can be used if the infection is persistent despite the above therapy, but is costly and requires monitoring for hepatotoxicity. Fluconazole may also be used and appears to have less toxicity. Treatment often requires several weeks and should be continued for at least 1 week after all symptoms and signs are resolved.[36]

Nonneoplastic Epithelial Disorders of the Vulva

These disorders are found more commonly with increasing age. The International Society for the Study of Vulvar Disease has classified neoplastic epithelial disorders of the vulva to facilitate identification and to enhance research regarding their etiology and treatment. The classification used from 1975 to 1989 was the following:

I. Hyperplastic dystrophy

    A. Without atypia

    B. With atypia

However, because it was not appropriate to include atypia with nonneoplastic disorders, a new classification was proposed in 1989 and is the currently approved and most widely used classification. However, both classifications are in use. Being familiar with both is important during the transition. The 1989 Classification is as follows:

Nonneoplastic Epithelial Disorders of the Vulvar Skin and Mucosa

I. Squamous cell hyperplasia (formerly hyperplastic dystrophy)

II. Lichen sclerosis

III. Other dermatoses

Squamous Cell Hyperplasia

Squamous cell hyperplasia is probably the result of moisture and scratching due to itching. It is often lichenified (thickened epidermis with accentuated skinlines). Because of the variations within the vulvar environment, it may have highly variable gross appearance. Suspicious thick areas require biopsy to rule out underlying dysplasia and/or carcinoma (Figure 18.13).

The biopsy reveals squamous cell hyperplasia, hyperkeratosis, parakeratosis, and frequently an inflammatory reaction in the dermis. Treatment includes: (1) Keeping the area clean and dry, (2) stopping the itch–scratch cycle, which may require a treatment of associated vaginal discharges, and (3) applying corticosteroids. Often a mixture of a steroid with crotamiton, an antipuritic, is used (7 parts of 0.1% Valisone and 3 parts of 10% Eurax applied 2 times a day for 3 or 4 weeks has been recommended by Friedrich).[37] After the acute phase is over and the itch–scratch cycle

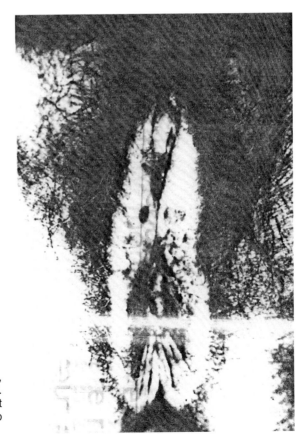

Figure 18.13 Squamous cell hyperplasia, chronic scratching has created thickening. (From Stenchever: *Office Gynecology.* St Louis, MO, Mosby, 1992, Figure 1028, p 280.)

controlled, a less potent steroid applied less frequently will often maintain near-normal state. If the vulva is weeping, the skin should be healed or initially soothed with wet soaks 4 to 6 times/day.

Lichen Sclerosis

Lichen sclerosis had many names, such as kraurosis vulvae, "primary atrophy," and atrophic leukoplakia. Lichen sclerosis may occur on many areas of the body and may be found at all ages. However, it is more common in the elderly and is often found in the anogenital region. The patient usually complains of itching, irritation, and perhaps stricture of the vulvar area and vaginal introitus. On examination, there is a classic parchment-like crinkled, white, thin-appearing epithelium that often surrounds the vagina and the anus in a figure 8 pattern (Figure 18.14). As it progresses, the labia minora may completely disappear, fissures may occur on the skin on the mid-line, and the clitoris may be completely hidden beneath the clitoral hood, which adheres to itself in the mid-line. Biopsy is diagnostic. The classic findings are epithelial thinning, hyperkeratosis, and pink-staining, acellular zone of homogeneous tissue beneath the basal layer. Frequently, areas of lichen sclerosis and squamous hyperplasia are juxtaposed.

Lichen sclerosis has been treated with the use of 2% testosterone proprionate in petrolatum applied 2 to 4 times/day for several months, after which time the dosage may be decreased for maintenance and may be continued for years. If burning or unwanted increase in libido results from the testosterone, topical application of 2% progesterone in petrolatum can be helpful. Recently, several articles have reported treatment with a high-potency steroid (clobetasol proprionate 0.05%), the effectiveness of which has been compared with testosterone and progesterone preparations. In these studies, patients treated with clobetasol responded much more quickly, had improvement in histology, and had a significant reduction in appearance of epidermal atrophy after treatment. Some of these patients have been followed nearly 2 years and have been maintained in remission with less potent topical steroids that previously were ineffective. The current first choice of therapy for vulvar lichen sclerosis appears to be this potent topical steroid. However, close follow-up is

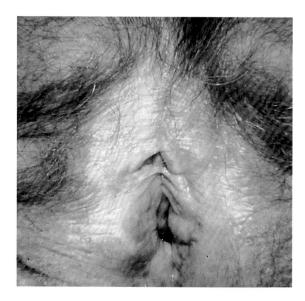

Figure 18.14 Note the thin, white epithelium surrounding the clitoral hood. On this patient the abnormality does not extend all the way around the vulva and anus.

mandatory, and caution must be exercised with use of clobetasol because of the potential for true atrophy and rebound to occur with such preparations.[38,39]

On occasion, elderly women will have fusion of the labia minora because of chronic irritation. This may cause difficulty with intercourse as well as complaints of urinary incontinence and recurrent urinary tract infections because of almost complete obliteration of the vestibule over the vaginal canal and urethra. Such extreme situations are rare and usually respond to estrogen creams or other specific local therapy but may require surgical procedures for alleviation.[40,41]

If severe itching associated with either hyperplasia or lichen sclerosis cannot be relieved by any topical medications, injection of 0.2 ml of absolute alcohol can be done under anesthesia. This is a last resort and should not be used for symptoms of burning. The alcohol is injected at intersections of a 1-cm grid, drawn as depicted in Figure 15. There is danger of sloughing of the epithelium (Figure 18.15).

Other Dermatoses

Vulvar dermatoses include manifestations of skin disorders on the vulva, such as contact or allergic dermatitis, psoriasis, lichen planus, pemphigus, and pemphigoid. They also include cutaneous manifestations of systemic disease, such as Behçet's syndrome, Crohn's disease, lupus erythemato-

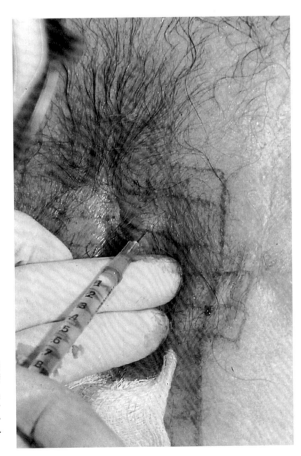

Figure 18.15 Method of injecting absolute alcohol as a last resort for symptoms of itching of the vulva. (From Kaufman R., Friedrich E., Gardner H. ed.: Benign Diseases of the Vulva and Vagina, ed. 3 Yearbook Medical Publishers, (1989) p. 319–320.

sus, and Reiters disease, which can cause vulvar ulcers. Also some malignancies may mimic dermatoses. For those reasons, diagnostic tests including skin scrapings, cultures, and biopsy, should be utilized to establish a specific diagnosis, thereby allowing a specific treatment. Many dermatoses are not curable, but can be treated with good results.

Contact or Irritant Dermatitis

McKay makes an important distinction between irritant and allergic reactions. Confusion between these leads many patients to claim they are "allergic to everything." Patient irritant reactions are common, whereas true allergies are rare. Irritant reactions are typified by immediate burning or stinging because of contact with a medication or other substance. Vesicles do not form but edema and redness may occur and last for several hours. Common irritants are soaps, some medications, particularly lidocaine and crotamiton, and some ingredients of common cremes and ointments, such as propylene glycol. These are treated by avoidance of the inciting substance, soothing with Sitz baths, Burows solution, and application of protective substances. A true allergic reaction may cause itching and blistering, may take 48 hours to develop, affects skin no matter where the allergen touches, and lasts for a longer period of time. Primary treatment is to remove the offending substance and to use topical steroids. Sometimes systemic steroids are necessary. Treatments with potent topical steroids can cause side effects, one of which is a rebound inflammatory reaction with redness and burning that gets worse when the steroid is withdrawn.[42]

Primary skin diseases of either vesicular bullous or papule squamous type are often found on the vulva as well as on other areas of the body. Occasionally, the vulva is the only site. Psoriasis has a classic clinical appearance of red plaques with a silvery white scale found on the scalp, knees, elbows, and sacrum. Because of the moisture of the vulva, the appearance may be variable and the diagnosis is facilitated by finding the classic lesions elsewhere (Figure 18.16). Psoriasis can be treated with topical hydrocortisone. Lichen planus, which has been mentioned as causing erosive vaginitis, may also be found on the vulvar skin. If it is diagnosed by biopsy, high potency topical steroids or intralesional steroids may be employed.

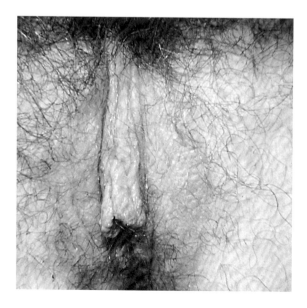

Figure 18.16 Psoriasis. This irritated vulva could be due to many causes. The diagnosis was made by the presence of classic lesions on the knees and elbows.

Vesiculo Bullous Diseases

These diseases, such as pemphigus, pemphigoid, erythema multiforme, and dermatitis herpetiformis, should have a biopsy diagnosis and treatment with steroids, immunosuppressive agents, and/or dapzone. Primary skin diseases found on the vulva or vagina are often best managed in conjunction with a dermatologist.

Systemic diseases that cause vulvar lesions include Behçet' syndrome, which is diagnosed by oral ulcers plus any two of the following: genital ulcers, uveitis, erythema nodosum, or pathergy (a sterile pustule arising in 24 to 48 hours of the site of a needle stick). If present it is treated with corticosteroids or immunosuppressive therapy. Behçet's syndrome is often overdiagnosed, particularly if a patient has aphthous ulcers of the mouth and vulva with no other criteria. If Behçet's is suspected, the patient should be evaluated by an ophthalomologist for uveitis because blindness is a long-term complication.

About one-quarter of the patients with lupus erythematosus will demonstrate mucosal lesions that may be confused with herpes simplex. Reiter's syndrome may also cause pustular or erosive mucocutaneous lesions, in conjunction with urethritis, conjunctivitis, and arthritis. Because several dermatologic conditions, such as Behçet's, Lichen planus, and Reiter's syndrome have oral and ocular manifestations, as well as genital manifestations, the mouth and eyes should be evaluated by history and physical examination whenever there is question as to the etiology of a vulvar lesion.[43]

Seborrheic Dermatitis

Seborrheic dermatitis causes chronic superficial inflammation with fine scaling and occasionally, in severe outbreaks, red or yellow-brown marginated plaques with dry or greasy scales. It is found in skin areas with many sebaceous glands, such as the scalp, nasal labial fold, sternum, groin, and gluteal cleft. Seborrhea is rarely isolated on the vulva; therefore, examine the other high-risk areas of skin. Primary treatment is with low-potency topical steroids. Ketoconazole cream has been effective in persistent cases.

Seborrheic dermatitis may be confused with moles, psoriasis, candidiasis, or Paget's disease. Evaluation for these entities should be pursued if the vulvar dermatitis does not respond.[44]

Vulvodynia

Vulvodynia is defined as chronic vulvar discomfort described by the patient as a burning rawness or irritation. It should be specifically separated from itch, which causes the patient to scratch. Vulvodynia, which is a painful irritation, prompts the patient to leave the area alone. Vulvar burning pain can be due to a vaginal secretion. Therefore, the vagina should be carefully evaluated for a vaginitis. It can also be due to one of the dermatoses that have just been described, or can be secondary to the use of medication. For example, an angiontension-connecting enzyme (ACE) inhibitor, enalapril, has been reported in one patient as causing vulvovaginal pruritis and burning at the end of urination without urinary frequency or urgency, or any vaginal discharge. The effect was postulated to be mediated by elevated levels of bradykinin, resulting in increased production of prostaglandin E_2. This report reminds us to consider medications as etiologic agents when otherwise unexplained vaginal symptoms occur in elderly patients who are often taking many different prescription drugs concurrently.

There are several other entities that may be found in the patient who has constant burning in the absence of any evidence of vaginitis or dermatoses. Recurrent genital herpes (herpes simplex virus [HSV]) should be considered, though chronic symptoms are highly unusual. HSV can be evaluated by culture of an active lesion or by specific Western blot serologies for genital herpes types I and II. If the latter is positive, it means that the patient has been exposed to herpes II, but this does not necessarily mean that her symptoms are due to HSV.

Vulvar vestibulitis is another chronic and persistent syndrome, usually found in women under 40. It is diagnosed by a burning pain created by light touch on the vulvar vestibule, often with very few objective signs, for example, redness in the vestibular area. Although several theories have been advanced as to the etiology, it is currently unknown. If a woman complains of persistent (over 6 months), severe introital pain, often preventing intercourse or the use of tampons and there is no other explanation and no pain within the vagina or outside the vestibular area, the clinical diagnosis of vestibular vulvitis should be considered.

Many treatments for vestibular vulvitis have been used with little relief. If the symptoms are mild, lubricants and/or 5% lidocaine gel on the vestibule prior to initiating intercourse may be sufficient. However, if symptoms are severe and persist, two other therapies may be tried. The first, described by Horowitz,[45] is injections of alpha-interferon, given in 12 sites around the vestibule, corresponding to the hours on a clock. One million units of recombinant interferon is diluted in 0.5 ml of saline and injected 3 times a week for 4 weeks. This treatment has a response rate of approximately 50% (Figure 18.17). The second treatment is surgical removal of the vulvar vestibule

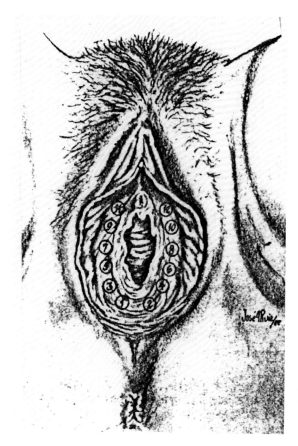

Figure 18.17 Method of interferon injection for vestibular vulvitis. (From Horowitz: Interferon therapy for condylometous vulvitis. *Obstet Gynecol* 19XX;73:446–448. Figure 1, p. 447.)

with undermining of the vaginal mucosa, which is then sutured to the perineal skin. This has a complete or significant relief in approximately 70% of the patients.

A study by Marinoff and coworkers[46] has shown that interlesional alpha-interferon used before surgery is attempted is a cost-effective method of therapy for vulvar vestibulitis.

Essential Vulvodynia

Essential or dysesthetic vulvodynia is most common in perimenopausal and postmenopausal women. It is defined as chronic vulvar burning without point tenderness on touching with a Q-tip, as occurs in patients with vulvar vestibulitis. Essential vulvodynia is not influenced by estrogen replacement therapy, but the use of a tricyclic antidepressant in small doses seems to benefit the patient over 40 years of age with constant unremitting perineal discomfort who has no obvious etiology. In older women, amitriptyline should be started at a low dose (eg, 10 mg/day) and slowly increased to 50 to 75 mg/day. Amitriptyline is likely to cause sleepiness. Other similar drugs, such as trazodone or clonazepam, may have fewer such side effects. This therapy has not been as useful in younger women (ie, under age 40), and Prozac has not been found to be helpful.[47]

Sexual Abuse of the Elderly

Sexual abuse of the elderly woman may occur more commonly than is recognized. One of the difficulties of recognition is a lack of a clear definition; however, most authorities will agree that physical sexual relationship without informed consent constitutes sexual abuse. The elderly are susceptible to abuse because they are often weak and unable to resist unwanted sexual advances. Also, they may live in an institution that has limited supervision; they may be mentally ill, so that they are unaware of or unable to inform others of abuse when it occurs. The potential for abuse should be considered when there is obvious trauma to the genital area and no clear explanation can be obtained. On the other hand, it is important to recognize dermatoses so that attendants of such patients are not unjustly suspected of mistreatment.

In cases of sexual abuse or rape, the caregiver is first responsible for the initial medical care of the victim; second, for the documentation of any injuries and evidence of rape for medical and legal purposes; and third, the long-term support of the patient's emotional needs. In the elderly woman, the possibility of pregnancy is usually low as many will be peri- or postmenopausal; however, because the possibility of sexually transmitted disease remains, appropriate cultures and baseline serologies should be obtained. The presence or absence of injuries should be recorded. Vulvar and vaginal lacerations are more likely to occur in the older woman whose introitus may be somewhat stenotic, and the vaginal walls thin.

Documentation of injuries and evidence of the attack and possible ejaculation should be obtained and the specimens cared for in a way that permits legal recourse if that avenue is pursued. Emotional support of the patient should include specific follow-up plans and return visits for evaluation of general well-being as well as for review of possible infectious disease. Some method of counseling and adequate follow-up should be routine. As is true in cases of younger women, the rape victim should be assured that she is not to blame for the occurrence.[48,49] One report emphasizing the seriousness of sexual abuse in the elderly describes a death as a result of insertion of a hand and forearm into the rectum.[50]

Female circumcision, which is practiced in several African countries by several ethnic and cultural groups, is another form of sexual abuse that is being seen more frequently in the United

States, usually in immigrants from Africa. Currently, it is more frequently noted in young women of child-bearing age and will continue to cause problems as the woman ages. The procedure varies from removal of the clitoris to removal of the vulvar vestibule, labia minora, and portions of the labia majora. The sides of the remaining vulva often grow together. The resultant deformity can cause increased urinary tract infection, sexual and psychological difficulties, and, in the younger woman, significant difficulty with child-bearing. The practice is mentioned here to increase awareness of the procedure and the potential long-term effects. Efforts to outlaw it are underway.[51]

Noninvasive Neoplastic Lesions of the Vulva and Vagina

Neoplastic diseases of the vulva and vagina are identified by having cellular atypia as opposed to those nonneoplastic lesions in which there are abnormalities without cellular atypism. However, the clinical manifestations such as itching, erosions, and lichenification, may be similar; and therefore such vulvar and vaginal lesions often require biopsy before a diagnosis is made. Vulvar intraepithelial neoplasia (VIN) may be found alone or in association with other dermatoses. In either event, the VIN should be reported as such and any other diagnoses reported separately.

VIN is classified as follows:

VIN1 — Mild dysplasia

VIN2 — Moderate dysplasia

VIN3 — Severe dysplasia or carcinoma in situ

VIN is characterized by a loss of epithelial cell maturation, associated with cellular changes of nuclear hyperchromatosis and pleomorphism, cellular crowding, and abnormal mitoses (Figure 18.18).

The lesions on the keritinized skin of the vulva may appear hyperkeratotic and white or may

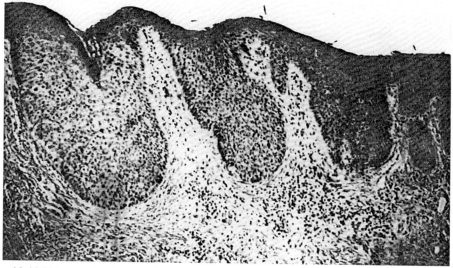

Figure 18.18 Vulvar epithelial neoplasia. Note the hyperkeratosis, cellular crowding, and atypism. (From Stenchever, *Office Gynecology* St Louis, MO, Mosby, 1992, p 286.)

be hyperpigmented in a small percentage of patients. VIN lesions on the mucous membranes may be pink or red. Pigmented lesions may be lentigo, or carcinoma in situ, melanoma, residual from inflammatory lesions, seborrheic dermatoses or other dermatoses. Biopsy should be employed if there is any question.

VIN is most commonly noted in the older woman but can develop at any age, and it appears to be increasing in frequency among younger women. It is associated with a prior history of abnormal cervical smear or cervical interepithelial neoplasia (CIN). Testing has shown that women with multicentric squamous cell neoplasia frequently have human papilloma virus (HPV) in that same area.[52]

The most common presenting symptom is pruritis, however, pain, warts, vaginal discharge are also found. Presence of a mass or bleeding is indicative of more advanced neoplasia, that is, invasive cancer. Diagnosis is facilitated by careful vulvar examination, using hand lens or colposcopy to evaluate the lesion and to guide diagnostic biopsy. VIN lesions are frequently multifocal. In such cases more than one biopsy should be obtained. Wide local excision is the most common method of therapy and close follow-up for possible recurrence is necessary.[53,54]

Vaginal Intraepithelial Neoplasia (VAIN)

Intraepithelial neoplasia of the vagina is quite rare. If present, it is usually associated with invasive carcinoma of the cervix or occurs after radiation therapy for an invasive lesion. This can appear years after the primary disease and requires recognition of this possibility and careful regular evaluations over a long period of time. Diagnosis is made by PAP smear followed by colposcopy and biopsy. Remember to perform colposcopy on the vagina carefully if PAP smears show squamous intraepithelial lesion (SIL) and the cervix is negative after careful evaluation. The management of VAIN is mainly by local excision. Excellent reviews are found in the references.

Invasive Cancer of the Vulva and Vagina

Primary invasive cancer of the vagina is extremely rare. It is most commonly found in older women and is usually of squamous cell origin. However, melanomas, sarcomas, and adenocarcinomas have been reported.

Secondary cancers of the vagina are more common. They are most often due to extensions of cancer in nearby organs. In most series, bleeding is the earliest and most common symptom. The rare occurrence of cancer in the vagina provides the reason for continuing PAP smears at approximately 2- to 3-year intervals, even in posthysterectomy patients who have had no history of prior neoplastic disease. Careful inspection and palpation of the vaginal walls at the time of examination may detect an abnormality early in its course. If an ulcer that does not heal or a nodularity is found, biopsy should be performed to determine the etiology. As mentioned above, *squamous cell carcinoma* is by far the most common of these rare tumors. Melanoma is the second most frequent type. Any grossly pigmented area in the vagina should be biopsied, especially if it is thickened.

The vulva is also a uncommon site for carcinoma. However, about 3% to 5% of all female genital malignancies are on the vulva. Most of these are found in older women. They are usually of squamous cell origin, but melanoma, Bartholin's gland adenocarcinomas, and rarely basal cell carcinomas have been reported. Any ulcer or mass palpated on the vulva of an elderly woman should be biopsied if it does not spontaneously resolve within 1 to 2 weeks.

Paget's disease is also occasionally found. Extramammary Paget's disease is a rare condition that has a predilection for the vulvar area in older women. It may be red, thickened, or white and often presents with severe pruritis. Paget's disease is usually intraepithelial but frequently extends beyond grossly visible margins. It is associated with underlying adenocarcinoma and with visceral cancers. Removal of tissue should be deep enough to detect an underlying adenocarcinoma on biopsy. The histopathology of Paget's disease is characterized by large cells, with a granular clear cytoplasm found along the base of the epidermis (Figures 18.18 and 18.19).

Grossly pigmented lesions should be removed, particularly if they present with any of the worrisome signs of melanoma, such as asymmetry, irregular borders, variegated color, a diameter greater than 0.6 cm, elevation, inflammation, or recent growth. The prognosis of a melanoma is related to its size and depth of penetration. Melanomas are staged either by Clark's or Breslow's classification (Figure 18.20).

Palpation of any mass in the area of Bartholin's gland or a Bartholin's abscess occurring in a postmenopausal woman should be completely excised and submitted for pathology to rule out invasive malignant disease.

Occasionally, a slow-growing variant of squamous cell carcinoma called verrucous carcinoma is found, and it sometimes will grow to large size before the patient is willing to present to a physician (Figure 18.22).

Urethral carcinoma is extremely rare and usually is either of squamous origin in the ductile mucosa or aednocarcinoma from the periurethral or Skene's ducts. In the elderly woman a urethral caruncle, which is a growth of vascular tissue at the urethral meatus, may be mistaken for carcinoma. If any doubt exists, a biopsy should be done.

The early diagnosis of invasive cancer of the vulva or vagina depends on remembering that it can occur. Careful visualization and palpation of the structures at the time of physical examination and early biopsy when a nonhealing ulcer or mass or other symptom is noted will verify the diagnosis. Numerous studies have shown that the elderly woman can tolerate surgical or radiation therapy for these lesions. Neither diagnosis or therapy should be withheld simply because of age.[36,55–60]

Methods of therapy for the various types and stages of tumors can be found in the references.

Conclusion

The major vulvovaginal disorders that have an increased prevalence in elderly women are atrophy from estrogen deprivation; nonneoplastic epithelial disorders, including vulvar dermatoses, which perhaps are not curable but which are uniformly treatable; and malignancies. Appropriate history, examination, and liberal use of biopsy and other tests will usually make for an accurate diagnosis. Awareness of potential for sexual abuse in the elderly woman is also important as are abnormalities associated with systemic diseases and the medications taken for them. Sexually transmitted infections may still occur but are of a much lower prevalence than in younger women. Most abnormalities of the vulva and vagina can be diagnosed and easily treated. The more complex and serious diagnoses should be referred to or managed with the appropriate specialist for long-term care.

References

1. Verkauf B, Von Thron J, O'Brien W: Clitoral size in normal women, *Obstet Gynecol* 1992;80:41–44.
2. Tagatz G, Kopher R, Nagel T, Okagaki T: The clitoral index: A bioassay of androgenic stimulation, *Obstet Gynecol* 1979;54:562–564.
3. Milsom I, Arvidsson L, Ekelund P, Molander U, Eriksson O: Factors influencing vaginal cytology, pH and bacterial flora in elderly women. *Acta Obstet Gynecol Scand,* 1993;72:286–291.

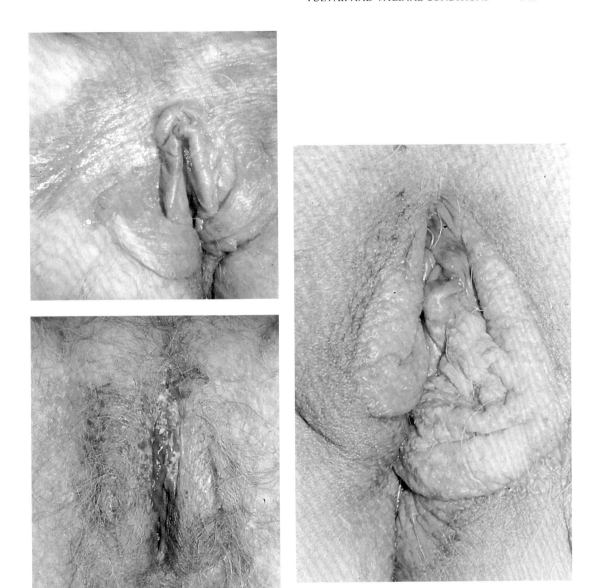

Figure 18.19 Paget's disease. These three different-appearing lesions all were proved by biopsy to be Paget's disease. This emphasizes the need for biopsy to determine the exact etiology of vulvar lesions.

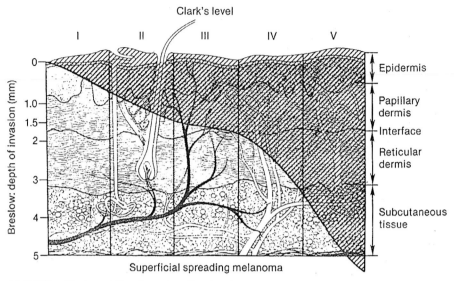

Figure 18.20 The Clark and Breslow classification for staging of melanoma. (From DiSaia & Creasman, *Clinical Gynecologic Oncology,* ed. 4 1993, Figure 818, p. 267.

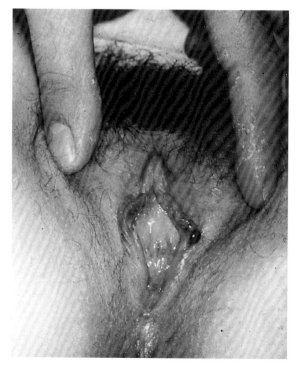

Figure 18.21 A vulvar nevus, which appears as a dark pigmented area on the vulva, which was shown by biopsy to be a nevus rather than a melanoma.

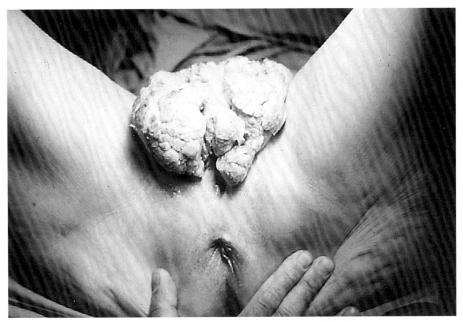

Figure 18.22 Verrucous vulvar carcinoma in an elderly woman.

4. Kramer P, Lubkin V, Potter W, Jacobs M, Labay G, Silverman P: Cyclic changes in conjunctival smears from menstruating females, *Ophthamology.* 1990;97:303–307.

5. Capewell A, McIntyre M, Elton R: Post menopausal atrophy in elderly women: Is a vaginal smear necessary for diagnosis? *Age and Ageing* 1992;21:117–120.

6. McLennan M, McLennan C: Estrogenic status of menstruating and menopausal women assessed by cervovaginal smears. *J Obstet Gynecol* 1971;37:325–331.

7. Bergman A, Karram M, Bhatian N: Changes in urethral cytology following estrogen administration. *Gynecol Obstet Invest* 1990;29:211–213.

8. Brown K, Hammond C: Urogenital atrophy. *Obstet Gynecol Clin North Am,* 1987;15:13–22.

9. Kaufman R, Friedrich E, Gardner H (ed): *Benign Diseases of the Vulva and Vagina,* ed 3. Chicago, IL, Yearbook Medical Publishers, 1989, Chapt 42, pp 319–320.

10. Perez-Lopez F, Lopez C, Alos L. Juste G, Ibanez F, Martinez-Hernandez H: Estrogen and progesterone receptors in the human vagina during the menstrual cycle, pregnancy, and post menopause. *Maturitas,* 1993;16:139–144.

11. Handa V, Bachus K, Johnston W, Robboy S, Hammond C: Vaginal administration of low-dose conjugated estrogens: Systemic absorption and effects on the endometrium. *Obstet Gynecol,* 1994;84:215–218.

212. Iosif C: Effects of protracted administration of estriol on lower genital urinary tract in post menopausal women, *Arch Gynecol Obstet* 1992;251:115–120.

13. Heimer GM, Englund D: Effects of vaginally administered estriol on post menopausal, urogenital disorders: A cytohormonal study. *Maturitas,* 1992;14:171–179.

14. Pschera H, Hjerpe A, Carlstrom K: Influence of the maturity of the vaginal epithelium upon absorption of vaginally administered estrodial 17 beta and progesterone in post menopausal women. *Gynecol Obstet Invest.* 1989;27:204–207.

15. Molader U, Milsom I, Ekelund P, Mellstrom D, Eriksson O: Effect of oral estriol on vaginal flora and cytology and urogenital symptoms in the post menopause. *Maturitas.* 1990;12:113–120.

16. Geogla F, Frumar A, Tataryn I, Lu K, Hershman J, Eggena P, Sambhi M, Judd H: Biological effects of various doses of conjugated equine estrogen in post menopausal women. *J Clin Endocrinol Metab* 1980;51:620–625.

17. Miodrag A, Eklund P, Burton R, Castleden C: Tamoxifen and partial estrogen agonism in post menopausal women. *Age Ageing,* 1991;20:52–54.

18. Eelb T, Alpern H, Grzywacz C, MacMillan R, Olson J: The effect of tamoxifen on cervical squamous maturation on papanicolaou stained cervical smears of post-menopausal women. *Cytopathology* 1990;1:263–268.

19. Boccardo F, Bruzzi P, Rubagotti A, Nicolo G, Rosso R: Estrogen-like action of tamoxifen on vaginal epithelium cancer patients. *Oncology* 1981;38:281–285.

20. Maenpaa J, Soderstrom K, Gronroos M, Taina E, Hajba A, Kangas L: Effect of poremifene on estrogen primed vaginal mucosa in post menopausal women. *J Steroid Biochem* 1990;36(3):221–223.

21. Sobel J: Epidemiology and pathogenesis of recurrent vulvovaginal candidiasis, *Obstet Gynecol,* 1985;152:924–935.

22. Sobel J, Schmitt C, Meriweather C: Clotrimazole treatment of recurrent and chronic candido-vulvovaginitis. *Obstet Gynecol* 1989;73:330–334.

23. Eschenbach D: Diagnosis and treatment of vaginitis; in *Office Gynecology,* St Louis, MO, Mosby, 1992, pp. 305–310.

24. Sobel J, Schmitt C, Stein G, Mummawn, Christiansen S, Meriweather C: Initial management of recurrent vulvo-vaginal candidaisis with oral Ketoconazole and topical chlotrimazole. *J Repro Med* 1994;39:517–520.

25. Rowe B, Logan M, Farrell I, Barnett A: Is Candidiasis the true cause of vulvovaginal irritition in women with diabetes mellitus? *J Clin Pathol* 1990;43:644–645.

26. Hillier S, Holmes K: Bacterial vaginosis, Ch 4, in STD, Holmes K et al (ed.): in STD ed 2, New York, McGraw Hill, 1990, Chapt 47, pp 547–559.

27. 1993 STD treatment guidelines: *Morbidity and Mortality* weekly reports, 1993;42:67–73.

28. Soper D, Bump R, Hurt W: Bacterial vaginosis and trichomonas vaginitis are risk factors for cuff cellulitis after abdominal hysterectomy. *Amer J Obstet Gynecol* 1990;163:1016–1023.

29. Kreiger J, Tam M, Steven C, et al: Diagnosis of Trichomonaisis: Comparison of conventional wet mount examination with cytological cultures, studies, and monoclonal antibody staining of direct specimens. *JAMA* 1988;259:1223–1227.

30. Rein M, Muller M: Trichomonas vaginalis and Trichomonaisis, in *Sexually Transmitted Diseases,* ed 2. New York, McGraw Hill, 1990, pp. 481–490. ed K. Holmes et al.

31. MacGregor J: Trichomonaisis: A common challenge in STD treatment. *STD Bull* 1989:8:3–11.

32. Habif T: A color guide to diagnosis and therapy, in *Clinical Dermatology,* ed 2. St Louis, MO, Mosby, 1990, pp. 170–175, 415–419.

33. Dworetzky M: Allergic vaginitis. *Am J OB/GYN* (letter) 1989; 161:1752–1753.

34. Haye K, Mandal D: Allergic vaginitis mimicking as bacterial vaginosis. *International J STD AIDS,* 1990;1:440–442.

35. Heckerling P: Enalapril and vulvovaginal pruritis. *Ann Intern Med* (letter) 1990;112:879–880.

36. Vontver L: Management of vulvar diseases, in Stenchever M (ed.): *Office Gynecology.* St Louis, MO, Mosby, 1992, Chapt 10, pp 258–259, 284–292.

37. Friedrich, Edward D. Vulvar disease. 2nd ed. 1983, p. 51. WB Saunders.

38. Dalziel K, Millard P, Wojnarowska F: The treatment of vulvar lichen sclerosis with a very potent topical steroid (clobetasol propionate .05 percent) creme. *Br J Dermat* 1991;124:461–464.

39. Bracco G, Carli P, Sonni L, et al: Clinical and histological effects of topical treatment of vulvar lichen sclerosis: A critical evaluation. *J Repro Med* 1994;38:37–40.

40. Chuong C, Hodgkinson C: Labial adhesions presenting as urinary incontinence in post-menopausal women. *Obstet Gynecol* 1984;64:81s–84s.

41. Johnson N, Lilford R, Sharpe D: A new surgical technique to treat refractory labial fusion in the elderly. *Am J Obstet Gynecol* 1989:161:289–290.

42. Marren P, Wojnarowska F, Powell S: Allergic contact dermatitis and vulvar dermatoses. *Br J Dermatol* 1992;126:552–556.

43. McKay M: Vulvitis and vulvovaginitis: cutaneous considerations. *Am J Obstet Gynecol* 1991;165:1176–1185.

44. McKay M: Vulvar dermatoses. *Clin Obstet Gynecol* 1991;34:614–629.

45. Horowitz B: Interferon therapy for condylomatis vulvitis. *Obstet Gynecol* 1989;73:446–448.

46. Maninoff S, Turner M, Hirsch R, Richard G: Intralesional alpha interferon: Cost-effective therapy for vulvar vestibulitis syndrome. *J Repro Med* 1993;38:19–24.

47. McKay M: Dysesthetic "essential" vulvodynia. Treatment with amitriptyline. *J Repro Med* 1993;38:9–13.

48. Stenchever M: Rape, incest and abuse, in *Comprehensive Gynecology,* St Louis, MO, Mosby, 1992, Chapt 12, pp 363–375.

49. Benbow S, Haddad P: Sexually abuse of the elderly mentally ill. *Postgrad Med* D. Mishell (ed.), 1993;69:803–807.

50. Reay D, Eisele J: Sexual abuse and death of an elderly lady by "fisting." *Am J Forensic Med Pathol* 1983;4:347–349.

51. Toubia N: Female circumcision as a public health issue. *N Engl J Med* 1994;331:712–716.

52. Beckmann A, Acker R, Christiansen A, Sherman K: Human papilloma virus infection in women with multicentric squamous cell neoplasia. *Am J Obstet Gynecol* 1991;165:1431–1437.

53. Shafi M, Luesley D, Byrne P, Samra J, Redman C, Jordan J, Rollason T: Vulgar interepithelial neoplasia: Management and outcome. *Br J Obstet Gynecol* 1989;96:1339–1344.

54. Disaia PJ, Creasman WT: Preinvasive disease of the vagina and vulva, in *Clinical Gynecologic Oncology,* ed 4. St Louis, MO, Mosby, 1993, Chapt 2.

55. Kennedy A, Flagg J, Webster K: Gynecologic cancer in the very elderly. *Gynecol Oncol,* 1989;32:49–54.

56. Kirschner C, Deserto T, Isaacs J: Surgical treatment of the elderly patient with gynecologic cancer. *Surg Gynecol Obstet* 1990;170:379–384.

57. Disaia PJ and Creasman WT: Invasive cancer of the vagina and urethra, in *Clinical Gynecologic Oncology,* ed 4. St Louis, MO, Mosby, 1993, Chapt 9.

58. Disaia PJ and Creasman WT: Invasive cancer of the vulva, in *Clinical Gynecologic Oncology,* ed 4. St Louis, MO, Mosby, 1993, Chapt 8.

59. Ragnarsson-Olding B, Johansson H, Rutquvist L, Ringborg U: Malignant melanoma of the vulva and vagina, trends in incidents, age distribution, and long-term survival amounting to 245 consecutive cases in Sweden in 1960–1984. *Cancer* 1993;71:1893–1897.

60. Brand F, Lagasse L, Fu Y, Berek EJ: Vulvovaginal melanoma, report of 7 cases in literature review. *Gynecol Oncol* 1989;33:54–60.

61. Bazin S, Bouchard C, Brisson J, Morin C, Meisels A, Fortier M: Vulvar vestibulitis syndrome: An exploratory case control study. *Obstet Gynecol* 1994;83:47–50.

62. Ricer R, Guthrie R: Allergic vaginitis: A possible new syndrome: A case report. *J Repro Med* 1988;33:781–783.

63. Mann M, Kaufman R, Brown D, Adam E: Vulvar vestibulitis: Significant clinical variables and treatment outcome. *Obstet Gynecol* 1992;79:122–125.

Chapter 19

Preoperative and Postoperative Care in the Older Woman

Joseph F. Lang, MD, and *M. Wayne Heine, MD*

The preoperative and postoperative management of the older woman is an area of growing importance to the practicing surgeon. The elderly population has previously been thought of as poor surgical candidates simply due to age alone as a co-existing variable. However, advancement in surgical care and techniques as well as improvements in anesthesia have opened up surgical solutions to problems in the elderly that previously have been treated with medical management.

The elderly population is growing at a fast rate. In the age group 65 and older women out number men by 1.5 to 1.[1] Women age 65 and older encounter a variety of problems that are amenable to surgery. In considering gynecological disorders, indications for surgery in the mature woman include genital prolapse, including urinary incontinence; cystocele, rectocele, and enterocele; malignant and premalignant conditions of the endometrium, vagina, vulva, and cervix; and ovarian tumors. Emergency surgery is much more poorly tolerated by elderly patients, therefore early diagnosis should lead to prompt surgical intervention. Delay and reluctance to operate often lead to a worsening of the underlying condition, which makes surgical intervention even more difficult.

Despite improvements in anesthesia, intra-operative monitoring, and preoperative evaluation, the elderly patient population does have an increased operative mortality.[2] The operative mortality rate for all procedures emergent and nonemergent for patients less than 60 years of age is approximately 0.9% to 1.5%, as opposed to the elderly in whom it ranges from 5% to 10%.[3,4,5] Despite evidence that age alone does not present a contraindication to surgery, increased operative and postoperative complications occur in the elderly because of the prevalence of co-morbid disease processes and the effects of age-related physiological changes.

Elderly women have an increased incidence of cardiac, renal, and pulmonary disorders as compared with their younger counterparts. These organ systems must be fully evaluated before surgery because the stress of surgery may lead to rapid deterioration in their function. Age alone causes a loss of physiological reserve in the body systems in general. However, care must be taken when attributing surgical risks to age associated changes. Goldman and coworkers as described by Frances[6] report no clear relationship between a decline in organ function and a risk of surgical complication. Chronic illness and life-style patterns, such as smoking, lead to increased surgical risks far greater than any changes in organ function caused by the aging process. Studies have demonstrated that surgical mortality is low in elderly patients who do not have underlying medical problems and in those whose underlying medical problems are under control.[7]

Actual physiological changes, however, may increase the chances or severity of a postoperative complication. These changes may also vary in the way a complication presents itself. Therefore the clinician must be astute in preoperative evaluation to discover and correct any underlying disease state. Finally, the clinician needs to be aware of normal changes associated with aging so as not to be surprised by an adverse postoperative event.

General Considerations

The preoperative assessment of the elderly woman begins when a problem that is potentially amenable to surgical interventions is first discovered. Usually there is a discussion of the various options available, including medical and surgical interventions, in light of her co-existing medical problems.

Since the elderly have been previously thought of as poor surgical candidates, many had surgery as a last resort or only in the case of emergency. Due to improvements in perioperative medicine, elective surgery is an appropriate option for the elderly woman. In fact, this population has the highest number of surgical procedures performed on them. The number of operations performed on patients in this age group has increased from fewer than 4 million in 1977 to about 6.4 million in 1987. Thus, it is the clinician's responsibility to offer a surgical solution to all amenable conditions, if the patient is a candidate. If the clinician does not perform surgery, a referral for evaluation, particularly in the presence of malignancy should be made. The operating surgeon is ultimately responsible for the appropriateness of surgery and the need for further preoperative work-up. This often involves the use of consultation with cardiologists and nephrologists.

An often-cited classification for risks of general anesthesia and for postoperative complications, is the physical status classification system of the American Society of Anesthesiologists (ASA) (Table 19.1).

This system gives the surgeon and the anesthesiologist an estimate of the patient's surgical risk and alerts them to potential problems. In an analysis of clinical anesthetic and surgical factors involved in morbidity and mortality in aged patients, no correlation was found between physical status and postoperative cardio respiratory function in general surgical patients with ASA classifications I and II. For patients with ASA status III and above, physical classification based on subjective information alone did not give enough information with which to base decisions regarding postoperative morbidity. The addition of objective quantifiable identifications of ventricular function as well as oxygen diffusing capacity measured by A-a gradient improved the predictive capabilities of the ASA classification system.

Unfortunately, this system is subject to significant interobserver disagreement.[8] Still, the ASA classification does provide a useful means of distinguishing high-risk from low-risk patients. Since most elderly fall between the II and III risk categories, the surgeon needs to appreciate the classification's limitations. The goals of preoperative evaluation are identical in patients of all ages. First identification must be made of all problems that may affect surgical risk. Second, the

Table 19.1 Physical Status Classification of the American Society of Anesthesiologists

Class	Definition
I	Healthy patient
II	Mild systemic disease, no functional limitation
III	Severe systemic disease with functional limitation
IV	Incapacitated patient
V	Moribund patient not expected to survive 24 hours with or without surgery

surgeon needs to identify those patients in whom surgical risk is excessive, precluding the procedure. Last, all medical conditions should be optimized preoperatively to minimize risk. Careful preoperative evaluation begins with the time honored detailed history and physical examination.

History and Physical Examination

Meticulous attention to detail is the only approach to obtaining a concise but complete history in the elderly patient. All existing medical problems need to be reviewed, especially those involving the cardiovascular system and the pulmonary system because these are often sites of intraoperative and postoperative complications. Of elderly patients undergoing surgery, 80% have some medical condition in addition to the surgical problem; these problems may help determine the surgical risk. Preoperative testing can be tailored to the organs or organ system most at risk from the surgery.

The surgeon must review past surgical procedures that may affect the current surgery. It is always prudent to obtain operative reports in order to review previous findings and determine the extent of previous surgical procedures, in order to avoid surprises at the time of operation. Simply relying on the patient's memory may not be adequate because patients are often unclear as to the nature of their previous surgical procedures.

In general, a careful review of family history is of less importance in the elderly patient, except in certain diseases and malignancies. In addition, the patient's habits including smoking and alcohol use should be reviewed. Intervention, if indicated, may be carried out in the interest of lowering perioperative complication and risks associated with these substances.

A detailed review of current medication use is an important part of the preoperative evaluation. All medications that the patient is currently using need to be reviewed and the indication for each medication must be sought. Patients many times are on medication with no clear reason, generally a function of habit or multiple physician involvement. Often, patients are taking medications from over-the-counter sources that may interfere with surgery or result in complications postoperatively. These medications include aspirin and ibuprofen that can cause coagulation difficulties in the perioperative period, if taken in high enough doses. Patients should understand which medications they are to continue and which they are to discontinue preoperatively. For these purposes, providing written instructions is better than reciting a verbal list. We do not generally recommend the discontinuation of hormone replacement therapy (HRT) unless there is a specific reason such as the discovery of an underlying adenocarcinoma of the endometrium. We generally continue estrogen replacement therapy (ERT) through the preoperative period and into the postoperative period, because the levels of these medications are generally physiological in terms of perimenopausal activity.

Any medication to which the patient is allergic should be clearly documented in the preoperative record. A description of the medication to which the patient is allergic as well as the type of allergic reaction experienced should be noted. Finally, there should be a review of previous surgeries in terms of anesthetic reactions. If any exist, these should be thoroughly discussed with the anesthesiologist or anesthetist involved in the patient's care.

Previous postoperative complications such as deep venous thrombosis, severe wound infections, prolonged fevers, or prolonged return of bowel function should be addressed. These problems should be understood in the context of the previous surgery as well as the current surgery. The awareness of prior surgical morbidity in a particular patient should place the surgeon on guard for the recurrence of similar untoward phenomena.

Following the detailed history, a careful physical examination is performed. A general assessment of the patient's body habitus is important since the surgical approach may be altered based on the information obtained. For example, morbidly obese patients may undergo panniculectomy to provide access to the pelvis. This is an extreme example; however, simple evaluation of the patient's weight gives information about the underlying nutritional status, which has a clear implication in postoperative recovery. After the general assessment a systematic examination should follow. Special attention should be directed to the examination of the size and presence of nodularity in the thyroid gland. Careful examination of lymph node status including the presence of enlarged supraclavicular, cervical, or axillary lymph nodes should be part of all physical examinations in the elderly woman. A breast examination is of vital importance prior to performing any surgical procedures on a elderly woman. This will allow a review of breast self-examination and will also serve to screen for disease that may take precedence over the surgery currently being planned. It is often recommended that a screening mammogram be obtained prior to any surgical procedure in an elderly female. Pulmonary and cardiac status should be evaluated; further details are given below in the individual sections regarding preoperative cardiopulmonary assessment. Careful abdominal examination including inspection, auscultation, percussion, and palpation should be made to identify any pathology not previously known. Pelvic examination to review any findings should be made at the time of the preoperative visit. Examination of the extremities for evidence of poor venous perfusion and varicosities that may place the patient at increased risk of deep venous thrombosis should be performed as well.

In general, the preoperative assessment should be made over a period of time. The preoperative assessment involves, first, a decision that surgery is a desirable alternative to medical management and second, that surgery can be performed in a safe manner in that particular patient. Serial visits in which evaluations of underlying disease states are carried out may allow time to maximize the patients presurgical condition.

An important part of the preoperative evaluation includes frank discussion of the underlying pathology, including a complete description of the planned surgical procedure. The patient should be made aware of the potential complications involved with the surgery as well as the extent of the disease process. The patient should understand what the proposed surgery involves and the modifications that may occur during the procedure. The benefits of the surgery and the expected outcome of the operation should be made clear. Alternative therapies should be discussed. These options should be documented in the patient's medical record, making it clear that the patient selected surgical intervention rather than her other alternatives.

Finally, a discussion of potential complications such as bladder, ureter, and bowel injury should be made. The patient should be viewed as a consumer, and the knowledge of risk allows the patient to be informed. This insight should allow for a better physician-patient relationship and should create an improvement in the rapport with the patient.

Cardiovascular Assessment

Noncardiac surgery in the elderly female generally does not require an extensive cardiac workup; however, there are a variety of age-related changes in the cardiovascular system that deserve mentioning. Fibrosis and degeneration of pacemaker and conducting tissue may increase the risk of conduction disturbances. In addition, there is an impaired diastolic filling due to a variety of mechanisms, including mitral valve thickening, decreased ventricular compliance, and prolonged isovolumetric relaxation. These lead to an increased risk of hypotension with surgically induced events such as dehydration, tachyarrythmias, and vasodilitory medications. Other age-related changes include decreased arterial compliance, leading to systolic hypertension and subsequent ventricular hypertrophy. The elderly also have impaired compensatory mechanism such as decreased baroreceptor sensitivity and decreased renin, angiotensin, and aldosterone secretion, which may decrease heart rate response to stress and increase the risk of hypotension. Despite the fact that cardiac output at rest is unchanged with age, maintaining cardiac output with exercise is more dependent on stroke volume as the patient ages due to lower ability to increase heart rate. Approximately 35% to 50% of postoperative deaths in the elderly population are due to myocardial disease.

How does the surgeon establish an individual risk? An excellent guide to assessing the perioperative risk of cardiac complications is the Goldman criteria. As noted in Table 19.2, information obtained by history and physical examination, the electrocardiogram (ECG), and simple laboratory studies can give an estimate of the risk for postoperative complications. The Goldman criteria are modified in the presence of known or suspected coronary artery disease. It is important to note that routine echocardiography is not generally recommended because its value in predicting postoperative complications has not been defined.

The cornerstones of preoperative cardiac evaluation are the history and physical examination. The cardiac history should focus on previous myocardial infarction, current angina, and CHF symptoms. An estimate of the patient's exercise tolerance should be determined. It is helpful to ask about the patient's ability to climb stairs or walk certain distances such as street blocks.

Table 19.2

Criteria	Points
• Age > 70	5
• MI within 6 months	10
• S3 or JVD	11
• Symptomatic Aortic Stenosis	3
• More than 5 PVC or ECG in pt. with CAD	7
• Rhythm other than sinus or sinus plus atrial premature bent in last preop EGG	7
• Emergency operation	4
• Thoracic or Abdominal	3
• Miscellaneous:	3

S3: Third heart sound
JVD: Jugular venous distension
PVC: Premature ventricular contraction

Miscellaneous:

K < 3 mEg/l	Abnormal SGOT	Cr > 3 mg/dl
BUN > 50 mg/dl	Pt. chronically bedridden	PCO_2 > 50 mm Hg
PO_2 < 60 mm Hg	HCO_3 < 20 mEg/L	Chronic liver disease

Scoring System

Risk	Life-threatening complication (%)
Low (0–5 pts)	0.7
Significant (6–12 pts)	5
Moderate (13–25 pts)	11
High (> 26 pts)	22

Kozak E: *Geriatrics* 1993;48:39–
MI, Myocardial infarction; ECG, electrocardiogram; CAD, coronary artery disease; SGOT, serum glutamate oxaloacetate transaminase; BUN, blood urea nitrogen; PCO_2, partial pressure of carbon dioxide; PO_2, partial pressure of oxygen; HCO_3, biocarbonate.

Greenberg and coauthors demonstrated in elderly patients that those who left the home two times per week had a decreased rate of cardiopulmonary complications.[10] McGerson and coauthors describe an easy method to determine exercise tolerance that was shown to be well correlated with postoperative prognosis for patients over 65 undergoing noncardiac surgery. Patients who could not bicycle supine for at least 2 minutes at a heart rate greater than 99 beats/min, had a higher rate of cardiac complications.[11]

The next step is the physical examination. Several misleading findings are noted here. Arcus senillis has been noted in the past to be a marker for arthrosclerosis; however, it is so common in patients over age of 50 that it really has no clinical utility. In addition the elderly undergo age-related stiffening of the aorta that leads to the presence of clinically insignificant systolic ejection murmurs. Last, carotid bruits in the asymptomatic patient generally indicate a risk for coronary artery disease but not an increased risk of stroke.

In general, however, the clinician needs to perform a careful cardiac examination including, blood pressure evaluation and identification of carotid bruits and murmurs. Appropriate preoperative referral should be made if indicated.

A general approach to cardiac evaluation after careful history and physical examination is an evaluation of exercise tolerance and the ECG. If the patient has good exercise tolerance and no cardiac risk factors with a normal ECG, no additional cardiac work-up is indicated. Referral to a cardiologist for evaluation is prudent if the patient has no risk factors and good exercise tolerance, but an abnormal ECG (such as Q-waves, T-wave inversions, or ventricular arrythmias); has poor exercise tolerance; or has a history of cardiac disease. The consultant can help determine if the patient needs further testing with exercise stress test, multiple gated acquisition (MUGA) scan, echocardiography, or catheterization. These more advanced recommendations are best left to an expert in the evaluation of cardiac disease. Overall, it is the job of the clinician who plans to do surgery to be diligent with the cardiac evaluation and make the appropriate referral if an indication is present.

Since nearly 40% of elderly Americans suffer from hypertension, the perioperative management of this problem deserves special attention. If surgery is considered in the elderly woman with hypertension, this disorder must be under control. A diastolic blood pressure of greater than 110 mm Hg is a contraindication to elective surgery.[13] If hypertension is discovered during the preoperative evaluation, it is best to postpone surgery until the blood pressure is brought under control with medication. Beginning new medications in the preoperative period is hazardous because of the variety of adverse drug reactions to blood pressure medications that can occur in elderly women.

The management of the hypertensive patient needs to be done with a combination of identification and perioperative medication management. If a patient is taking antihypertensive medication, it should be discontinued on the day of surgery and resumed as soon as possible after the operation. Nearly 25% of patients with hypertension have significant hypertensive episodes during the perioperative period. This is due to anesthetic agents, age-related changes in the cardiovascular system, alterations in the intravascular volume, and most importantly—pain.[14] The anesthesiologist should be aware of these problems and must manage intraoperative hypertension quickly and efficiently. Pain is the most common cause of hypertension in the postoperative hypertensive or normotensive patient. If pain has been managed, hypertensive agents such as hydralazine, hydrochlorothiazide, beta blockers (relatively contraindicated in patients with congestive heart failure, bronchospasm, and diabetes mellitus) or even nitroprusside can be used to control blood pressure. The use of a calcium channel blocker such as nifedipine is an excellent choice in elderly women. Calcium channel blockers are long-acting and are not associated with hypotension, angina, or myocardial ischemia.

Postoperative telemetry is recommended by some clinicians if the patient has any one of the following risk factors for postoperative myocardial ischemia: left ventricular hypertrophy on ECG, hypertension that requires medication for blood pressure control, diabetes mellitus, definite coronary artery disease, or the use of digoxin.[12]

Pulmonary Assessment

Complications in the pulmonary system occur in about 40% of patients postoperatively and account for approximately 20% of the preventable deaths occurring during this time period.[15] Aging produces a variety of changes in pulmonary function, as in the cardiovascular system. These changes affect perioperative management in unique ways. With aging, there are altered mechanisms of ventilation that lead to loss of elastic recoil, steepening of the chest wall, and increased ventilation-perfusion mismatch.

The FEV_1 (forced expiratory volume in one second) fails by 0.2 L per decade after the age of 20. The altered mechanics of ventilation due to aging lead to decreased vital capacity and pulmonary reserve; there is also an increased reliance on diaphragmatic breathing as well as arterial hypoxemia. Arterial oxygen pressure is a good indicator of lung function because it provides information on oxygenation, the primary function of the lungs. The arterial oxygen pressure decreases approximately 4 mm Hg each year after the age of 20.

Aging also leads to decreased ventilatory response to hypercapnia, resulting in a greater potential for ventilatory failure. Finally, aging leads to an increased risk of aspiration and infection since impaired cough reflexes, laryngeal reflexes and mucosal ciliary function reduce airway protection.[16]

The information given above seems to indicate that age-related pulmonary changes place the elderly women at significant surgical risk. However, this is not necessarily true. As mentioned, the FEV_1 declines 200 ml each decade after the age of 20, which leaves the average 80-year-old with an FEV of more than 2 L. This is well below the risk level at which pulmonary complications occur.[17] Chronic diseases and smoking exert a much greater effect than age alone. Pre-existing chronic obstructive pulmonary disease (COPD) is the most important preoperative risk factor in any age group, leading to greater than 20 times the normal complication rate postoperatively.[18] If a patient is found to have an underlying pulmonary disease on examination, she is at risk and further testing is required. By identifying the high-risk patient and taking preventive measures, the complication rate due to pulmonary problems can be significantly decreased.[19] It should be noted that the decrease in the elderly woman's pulmonary function may not be symptomatic, and objective testing may be indicated to discover an underlying change that may be hazardous in the postoperative period.

Pulmonary function testing evaluates a variety of parameters defining the quality of ventilatory functioning. The forced vital capacity (FVC) is an indication of ventilatory reserve; it represents the ability to maintain adequate pulmonary function by adequately ventilating and clearing secretions. Normal vital capacity ranges between 55 and 85 ml/kg. A minimum of 15 ml/kg or approximately 1 L is necessary for effective coughing and deep breathing to clear secretions. The FEV_1 (force expiratory volume in one second) is an indicator of airway resistance. A healthy individual expires nearly all of his or her entire vital capacity in 1 second. A patient should be able to exhale his or her vital capacity in less than 3 seconds to be able to tolerate the changes brought about by anesthesia and surgery. The normal FEV_1 is greater than 4 L and the should be greater than 2 L for elective surgery. The FEV_1 is usually expressed as the percentage of FVC, and is normally 80% of the FVC. An FEV_1 of less than 50% is an indicator of airway resistance of such magnitude that significant reduction of ventilatory reserve is present.

Pulmonary function tests have been used to assess operative risks as well as to predict postoperative pulmonary complications. Test levels that correlate with pulmonary complications and mortality include maximal breathing capacity less than 50% of predicted value, an FEV_1 less than 2 L, a partial pressure of carbon dioxide in arterial blood greater than 45 mm Hg[20] and a partial pressure of carbon dioxide of less than 60 mm Hg.

If pulmonary function tests are normal, the patient has a low risk of developing pulmonary complications. Patients with marginal values must be carefully assessed because the effects of anesthetic agents, narcotic medications, and infection may push normal functioning respiratory systems to failure.

An effective and simple evaluation of pulmonary reserve is the stair-climbing exercise. The ability to climb stairs seems to be correlated with values obtained during pulmonary function testing. For example, a patient who is unable to climb three flights of stairs probably has an FEV_1 of less than 1.7 L.[21]

Regional anesthesia is a preferred over general anesthesia for elderly patients in terms of pulmonary management. This is due to a variety of reasons, including improved PaO_2, reduced risk of atelectasis, and decreased risks of deep venous thrombosis and pulmonary embolism.[17,22–24] Thus, regional anesthesia should be an option in patients undergoing gynecologic surgical procedures if the procedure and the patient are amenable to this approach.

In a patient at low or moderate risk for pulmonary complications based on preoperative testing, incentive spirometry, humidified oxygen, position changes, early ambulation, and the avoidance of excessive use of sedative medications is indicated in the postoperative period.

If a patient is at increased risk for a pulmonary complication based on preoperative testing additional methods to reduce the risk of untoward events should be employed. These include the use of bronchodilators and antibiotics preoperatively, careful hydration, attention to operative time, prevention of aspiration, intermittent hyperventilation, and an arterial line placement for blood gas monitoring. Postoperative bronchodilator use, pulmonary therapy, monitoring, and possible short stays in the intensive care unit (ICU) are also indicated in these patients.

Endocrine Assessment

The elderly female population often presents with a variety of endocrine-related disorders. There is a 1% per year decrease in basal metabolic rate after age 30 and lean body mass gradually decreases as the amount of fatty tissue increases with age.[25]

These changes, in addition to the age-related changes in the secretion and action of insulin, lead to increased susceptibility to a variety of endocrine-related disorders. The most common and significant include diabetes mellitus, thyroid disorders, and adrenal disorders.

Glucose tolerance undergoes age-related decline. There is an increase of 1 mg/dl per decade in the fasting serum glucose and a 5 mg/dl increase in the 2 hr postprandial glucose per decade.[26] Given the age-related decrease in insulin secretion and action there are trends toward hyperglycemia with a glucose load even in elderly patients who are nondiabetic.

Approximately 70% of patients with diabetes undergoing surgery are age 50 and over, the majority of whom have type II diabetes. The problem is relative insulin resistance in these patients, and they are not as prone to ketoacidosis as type I diabetics. In many elderly women, type II diabetes mellitus of recent onset is due to obesity despite the fact they have relatively easy glucose control with either diet or oral hypoglycemic agents, these patients often have underlying atherosclerotic or cardiovascular disease. Thus, the presence of type II diabetes should alert the clinician to be aware of underlying risk for cardiovascular compromise in the perioperative period.

A variety of factors affect glucose metabolism in the perioperative period, including hormonal factors such as insulin, glucagon, cortisol, catecholamines, and growth hormone. There are also nonhormonal influences on activity such as stress and intravenous administration of dextrose-containing fluids. These factors, with the exception of insulin, tend to raise glucose levels as opposed to decreased caloric intake that occurs postoperatively, which tends to lower serum glucose levels. In general, it is difficult to predict how a given patient will respond to surgery with respect to her glycemic control. Thus, there should be careful and frequent monitoring of serum blood sugar both intraoperatively and postoperatively.

A target range of 180 to 220 mg/dl is considered adequate control in the postoperative period. This range is acceptable because it avoids hypoglycemia with a potential risk of dehydration, as well as the decreased phagocytic function that occurs in leukocytes when serum glucose levels rise above 240 mg/dl.[27]

For patients who maintain their blood sugar in the normal range with conservative methods such as diet and exercise, no extra preparation or evaluation is needed preoperatively. However, it is important to monitor these patients' blood sugar intra-operatively and postoperatively because, as indicated above, the unique situation imposed by surgery places these patients at risk for glucose abnormalities. For patients using oral hypoglycemic agents several important issues arise. It is important to know which agent is being used. For example, chlorpropamide has a long duration (approximately 60 hrs) compared with tolbutamide, the duration of which is in the range of six to twelve hours. Second is the risk of hypoglycemia when these agents are given with the reduced caloric intake in the perioperative period. A good general plan for oral hypoglycemic use in the postoperative period is as follows: (1) Oral hypoglycemic agents should be discontinued 1 day before surgery, (2) The longer-acting chlorpropamide should be discontinued at least 3 days before surgery, and (3) Serum glucose levels should be checked on the morning of surgery, which is planned ideally early in the day.[28] Insulin should be used for serum glucose levels greater than 250 mg/dl preoperatively. During surgery glucose should be checked at frequent intervals (ie, every 90 to 120 minutes). Postoperatively, sliding-scale insulin coverage should be used until the patient is tolerating an oral diet. There are a variety of opinions about the dose for sliding-scale insulin coverage. It is probably best to tailor the sliding-scale to the patient's insulin requirements, which can be quickly ascertained over several hours. An oral hypoglycemic agent should be added when the patient is tolerating a regular diet and is not at risk for hypoglycemic effects. An incremental return to the previous dose level is prudent for elderly patients who may not be eating at their usual level. Starting low and increasing slowly is a good rule of thumb.

If the patient is on insulin already, careful management is in order. The total insulin requirements will be lower on the day of surgery because the patient will, in general, have reduced or no oral intake. It is generally recommended that blood glucose be measured in the morning prior to surgery and sliding-scale coverage be given if greater than 240 mg/dl. In terms of long-acting insulin it is recommended that one third of the total usual dose be given on the morning before surgery and repeated in approximately 10 hrs. Postoperatively, in addition to the long-acting insulin, regular insulin is given in a sliding-scale fashion. Blood glucose is monitored approximately every 6 hrs. This is continued until the patient is tolerating a regular diet. From that point, the usual insulin dose is added in an incremental fashion. The clinician must be aware of the effects of postoperative stress, gastrointestinal function, and infection that can affect blood sugar, and must adjust insulin accordingly.

Despite the decline of thyroid function with aging, most patients are able to maintain the normal activity of the thyroid gland. However, elderly women often do not display the typical presenting symptoms of hypothyroidism or hyperthyroidism.[29,30]

Subclinical hypothyroidism can present with normal serum concentration of thyroid hormones but increased levels of thyroid-stimulating hormone (TSH). These patients however do well pre- and postoperatively. Patients with more severe forms of hypothyroidism have more difficulty.

Patients with significant hypothyroidism have increased rates of adverse drug reactions because they tend to metabolize drugs more slowly. In addition, they have greater sensitivity to central nervous system (CNS) depressants. These medications may result in longer periods of confusion and difficulty with arousal in elderly patients.

An important clinical implication of hypothyroidism is that such patients tend to have more intra-operative hypotension, postoperative ileus, confusion, and infections that are less often associated with fever. Patients in whom hypothyroidism is suspected or in those whom it is known preoperatively should undergo thyroid function testing. The patient should be euthyroid prior to surgery, especially in elective gynecologic procedures.

Hyperthyroidism with its common clinical presentation of tachycardia, weight loss, and heat intolerance is often not seen in the elderly woman. Patients with suspected or known hyperthyroidism should be rendered euthyroid prior to surgery. Postoperatively, patients with hyperthyroidism are at risk for hyperpyrexia, heart failure, and cardiac rhythm disturbances. Careful monitoring and continuation of thyroid medications are indicated in these patients. To convert the oral dose of levo-thyroxine to an intravenous equivalent, reduce the dose by half or give the full oral dose every other day if the patient is tolerating a regular diet.

Despite a 25% decline in its secretion due to age, cortisol is removed from the circulation at a slower rate in elderly patients. This results in normal plasma levels of cortisol.[31] Generally, elderly women undergoing gynecologic procedures or general surgical procedures should have minimal risk of adrenal insufficiency. Concern should be raised in the patient who has taken corticoid steroids for any number of indications. The steroid dosage needed to cause adrenal suppression is the equivalent of 40 mg/day or more of prednisone for 1 to 2 weeks, or more than 7.5 mg/day of prednisone given chronically. The recovery from chronic administration may take as long as 1 year. Simply stated, if a patient has taken high doses of steroids for more than 10 days within 9 months of planned surgery, supplemental steroid coverage is indicated to prevent adrenal crisis. Signs and symptoms of such crisis events are not easily noticed because they can be part of any postsurgical situation. Symptoms such as nausea, fever, and ileus may be indicative of adrenal insufficiency. Given the rather low risk of replacement, most recommend replacing corticosteriods if the patient is at risk for adrenal hypofunction. Replacement is usually 100 mg. of hydrocortisone succinate prior to surgery, then every 8 hours for approximately 24 hours. If the patient has an uneventful postoperative course, this dosage is tapered to the usual equivalent dose or completely stopped.

Nutritional Assessment

An important but often overlooked aspect of the preoperative assessment is the evaluation of nutritional status. Many elderly woman have poor eating habits, limited financial resources, or medical conditions that impair their ability to maintain adequate nutritional stores. In fact, nutritional assessment is as important as cardiac and pulmonary assessment in the elderly patient. Malnutrition is a significant source of postoperative morbidity in this patient group.[32]

Protein calorie malnutrition is seen in nearly 20% of elderly patients.[33] The major difficulties surrounding nutritional assessment include the following: (1) How does one measure nutritional status? (2) How does one manage a nutritional deficiency once it is found?

Nutritional status can be measured by both anthropometric techniques and biochemical markers. The easiest and most informative measure of nutritional status is body weight. If a patient has been seen over many visits, serial weights offer excellent insight into energy and protein reserves.

Another simple method is the tricep skinfold thickness measurement, which can be used to calculate adipose stores.[34]

Biochemical markers and anthropometric techniques are combined to obtain a creatinine and height index. This gives an approximation of the muscle mass. Creatinine is obtained with a 24-hour urine collection and an overall assessment of nutritional status is ascertained based on the value for the index. Biochemical markers alone are good at estimating protein storage and thus overall nutritional status.

Protein reserves are estimated by serum albumin and transferrin levels. Serum albumin levels less than 2.5 mg/dl are associated with increased surgical morbidity.[35] In general, signs of protein deficiency include serum albumin levels of less than 3.5 mg/dl, serum lymphocyte counts of less than 1500/mm³, serum transferrin levels decreased to less than 150 mg/dl, and lastly a loss of reaction to common skin antigens (Table 19.3).

Serumk albumin has a long half-life; therefore, a significant decrease in the albumin level may not be seen for a month after a decrease in nutritional intake. The reverse is true as well, in that attempts at nutritional improvement do not show up immediately in the serum albumin level. Transferrin is beneficial because its half-life is 8 to 10 days and nutritional replenishment will become evident in its level within 2 weeks. Unfortunately, transferrin is subject to increased turnover with illness. Changes in iron stores will also affect its level.

Malnutrition leads to involution of the T-cell producing tissue, which leads to decreased T-cell production and function. These changes result in a decrease in absolute lymphocyte count and a delayed cutaneous hypersensitivity response to skin test antigens.[36] The absolute lymphocyte count and the sensitivity testing have been used to assess nutritional status.

There is controversy over whether the serum albumin level alone is predictive of poor or adequate nutritional stores. Serum albumin levels are affected by a variety of co-factors other than poor nutrition.[37] The clinician's best approach is a combination of the above, with a careful history to obtain as good an assessment of nutritional status as possible.

An interesting attempt to guide the clinician to patients at risk for nutritional related postoperative complications is the prognostic nutritional index (PNI).[38]

Equation: PNI equals 158 minus 16.6 (ALB) minus 0.78 (TSF) minus 0.2 (TFN) minus 5.8 (DH)

where: ALB=Albumin
        TSH= Triceps skinfold thickness (cm)
        TFN= Serum transferrin
        DH= Delayed skin hypersensitivity (scale 0 to 2)

Patients with a score greater than 30% are at increased risk of postoperative complications. If it is discovered during assessment that a patient has decreased nutritional stores, attempts should

Table 19.3 Nutritional Assessment and Risk

	Mild	Moderate	Severe
Albumin	2.8–3.2 mg/dl	2.1–2.7 mg/dl	<2.1 mg/dl
TLC	1,200–2,000/mm³	800–1200/mm³	<800/mm³
Triceps skinfold		<16.5 mm	
Transferrin	175–200 mg/dl	120–175 mg/dl	<120 mg/dl
Skin tests (Candida, mumps, PPD)	10–15 mm	5–10 mm	0–5 mm

TLC, Total lymphocyte count; PPD, ????.

be made to improve the nutritional status. This is most easily accomplished through enteral feedings with supplementation. Peripheral parental nutrition can be used to augment enteral feedings or alone as hyperalimentation or total parenteral nutrition (TPN).

Nutritional recommendations need to be individualized. Preoperative nutritional support should be given as long as surgical delay does not worsen the expected outcome. Patients should receive adequate caloric and protein levels as well as micronutrients postoperatively to avoid deficiency and assist with stress induced by surgery. The surgeon needs to be vigilant for postoperative nutritional deficiencies. Feedings should begin as soon as possible by enteral routes; however, if delayed bowel function is expected, there should be no reluctance to start TPN. Consultation with dieticians or nutritionists is generally quite useful in these circumstances.

Renal Assessment

The age-related changes in the kidney are threefold. There is a generalized reduction in renal blood flow, renal mass, and renal function as a patient reaches her mid sixties.[39]

Renal mass is lost primarily in the cortex; glomerular filtration declines linearly approximately 8 ml/min per 1.73 m^2 each decade after age 30. Renal blood flow declines approximately 10% each decade.[40] Renal function also changes with age as a result of an increase in glomerular basement membrane permeability, which leads to an increase in urinary protein excretion. Hyperfiltration subsequently occurs, and eventually sclerosis. When combined with the age-induced loss of renal mass, these changes make fluid and electrolyte management more difficult in the mature female population. It should be noted that creatinine production decreases secondary to a decrease in muscle mass, which leads to a false reassurance of normal glomerular filtration rate given a "normal" serum creatinine. Age also leads to delayed response to sodium deficiency, which increases the risk of fluid overload and subsequent hyponatremia. Lastly, there is a delayed capacity to excrete salt and water, which increases the older woman's risk for fluid overload as well as hyponatremia.

Renal dysfunction is usually not obvious until uremia occurs, and the major risk for developing postoperative renal failure is pre-existing renal dysfunction. As noted above, the serum creatinine level does not necessarily provide a useful estimate of the glomerular filtration rate. Formulas are available using easily acquired values to estimate the creatinine clearance rate. The Cockcroft and Gault equation modified for older women is as follows: Creatinine clearance in mililiters per minute equals 140 minus the age (in years) times the weight (in kilograms) times 0.85; the remainder is divided by 72 times the serum creatinine. This formula may be written as follows:

$$CrCl = \frac{140 - (age) \times (weight) \times 0.85}{72 \times Creatinine}$$

This formula gives an estimate of the creatinine clearance, which allows for adjustment of dosage of renally cleared medications.

For patients undergoing gynecological procedures a urinalysis should be part of the preoperative evaluation. Most gynecological patients require transient urethral catherization during the immediate postoperative period and the presence of an infection can affect the postoperative course. In addition, the urinalysis is relatively inexpensive way to screen for underlying kidney disease not evident by history or physical examination. For example, the presence of protein may signal worsening chronic disease states such as hypertension or diabetes. Thus, we obtain a urinalysis on all the postreproductive age women on whom we operate.

Medication

It is well known that many elderly patients take a variety of medications for varying indications. Moreover, the frequency of adverse drug reactions in the elderly is at least 2 to 3 times that of their younger counterparts. The preoperative assessment period, therefore, is an excellent time to review the list of medications and to re-evaluate the need to continue. Although it is not a good time to experiment, many patients take medications prescribed by different physicians without clear indications. Given the elective nature of many gynecological procedures, a delay in surgery may be warranted if removal of a drug with potential negative side effects, especially those affecting the genitourinary system, is to be possible.

Aging has profound effects on drug absorption, distribution, and metabolism. Age-related changes in gastric acid secretion, prolonged gastric emptying, decreased intestinal blood flow and motility, can all delay drug absorption. This is one reason that the use of sublingual and transdermal estrogen replacement therapy is so effective in the elderly population. Age-related decrease in lean body mass and increase in body fat lead to a relatively prolonged effect of water-soluble drugs. Changes in renal blood flow and overall renal function, as well as the age-related decrease in hepatic blood flow and enzymatic activity, greatly affect drug metabolism. Appropriate dosage adjustments should be made in the elderly patient at risk.

Specific dosage adjustments should be made in opioids, sedatives and hypnotic medications. These medications should be given in small increments, less frequently. Careful attention to individual patient effect is required whenever any of these medications is used, especially in the perioperative period.

Screening Tests

The preoperative studies should be tailored to those needed to completely evaluate a particular organ or organ system of concern, as discovered by physical examination and history. Which tests should be ordered for a healthy, mature woman is an area of controversy from a medical and economic viewpoint. In general, a screening test should be performed when the result should denote a problem that could alter the outcome of surgery and affect perioperative management.

We prefer to obtain an ECG on all the mature women on whom we operate. ECG provides an important adjunct to the history and physical examination and helps to plan appropriate referral. A chest radiograph is also a part of preoperative assessment, especially for the older woman undergoing oncological surgery and in whom an ongoing pulmonary disease is noted.

Basic laboratory function tests include a complete blood count (CBC), electrolyte analysis, and serum glucose and creatinine levels. A CBC gives valuable information on any underlying anemia that may require evaluation. Mild anemia is a difficult problem to detect on examination alone; however, it is prevalent in the elderly population. The causes of anemia are beyond the scope of this chapter, but if discovered, a careful evaluation for underlying nutritional deficiencies, thyroid disorders, or cancer may be indicated.

Documentation of normal electrolytes and creatinine values is important preoperatively. This gives important information on the kidneys' ability to metabolize and excrete drugs and anesthetic agents. An elevated creatinine level indicates significant renal impairment in the elderly woman. It also allows for an assessment of possible renal failure or even ureteral obstruction due to uterine prolapse. The value of testing for preoperative glucose levels is undetermined; however, it may give insight into an underlying insulin resistance phenomenon. In patients with a history of diabetes mellitus, there is a need to determine preoperative glucose levels.

We perform routine urinalysis on all our mature female patients in whom we feel, based on physical examination or symptoms, are at risk for infection. If a patient is to be catheterized postoperatively it is prudent to know that no infection was present prior to the catheterization.

Routine liver function tests are not obtained because the prevalence of liver disease is generally low. However, if the planned surgery may potentially compromise hepatic function, it is not unreasonable to obtain a serum glutamate oxaloacetate transaminase (SGOT) or a serum glutamate pyruvate transaminase (SGPT) level before surgery.

Multiple studies exist to support the notion that routine screening for coagulation deficits with prothrombin time, partial thromboplastin time, and bleeding time are not valuable in predicting postoperative bleeding problems in the asymptomatic patient undergoing surgery.[45,46] It is best to direct coagulation tests to the patient who has a history of anticoagulation therapy, use of aspirin, or use of nonsteroidal anti-inflammatory drugs (NSAIDS). It should be noted that a patient who has taken daily low-dose aspirin for cardiac prophylaxis does not require coagulation testing. Coagulation tests should be sought in patients with liver disease, malabsorption, malnutrition or any other known bleeding disorder. In a patient who does not fall into one of the above risk categories, routine testing of coagulation parameters is not helpful. This is due to the fact that abnormalities in testing do not correlate with high rates of bleeding complications. That is, if the patient does not fall into one of the risk categories described above, preoperative testing does not add any further information and is not helpful in predicting whether a patient will have an intraoperative or postoperative bleeding problem.

In conclusion, in addition to the history and physical examination, we obtain a chest radiograph, an ECG, a CBC, electrolytes, creatinine, and a urinalysis on all the elderly female patients on whom we operate. We tailor further testing based on the individual patient's history and examination, thus guiding further intervention and/or referral.

Risk Assessment

Once the preoperative evaluation is complete and a detailed history, careful physical examination and follow-up diagnostic tests have been completed, a general risk assessment for the particular surgical procedure is obtained. By assessing operative risks, the clinician is attempting to determine the probability of an adverse outcome associated with a particular procedure. This is weighed against the benefit of the procedure. The clinician can only give an estimated risk based on groups with similar characteristics; the exact risk for an individual is undeterminable.

When consultation is sought, it is recommended that the consultant determine the extent of the underlying disease, the status of current medical management, and what additional intervention is necessary.

In assessing preoperative risks, Hirsch[47] describes four determinants: patient-related, procedure-related, provider-related, and anesthetic agent-related risks. First, patient-related risks include age, gender, race, socioeconomic status, surgical disease, concurrent medical disease, medication history, and nutritional status. Many of these variables are interdependent. In terms of age, there is clearly a rising perioperative death rate with age.[48] However, the female gender had lower death rates than male.[49]

Second, the procedure being performed has significant impact on the individual patient's perioperative risks. High mortality rates are seen for craniotomy, cardiac procedures, and exploratory laparotomy. Most gynecological procedures, aside from some gynecological cancer surgeries, fall into a lower risk range.

Third, interestingly, there are certain provider-related risks that can be factored into the overall risk for an individual patient. Institutional experience as a whole and the quality of nursing care may play a role for a particular procedure.[50] In general, gynecological procedures are fairly routine, being performed safely in a variety of institutions with low complication rates.

Last, concern about the choice of anesthetic affects overall risks. There is no firm data to suggest that regional anesthesia is safer than general anesthesia.[51,52] Intuitively, those patients receiving regional anesthesia should have better outcome; however, this has not necessarily been the case as shown in a variety of studies. The main point is to individualize anesthetic choice for a given patient.

Overall, the patient's risk assessment is based on underlying disease and health status because most postoperative problems occur as a result of underlying physiological dysfunction. Age-related changes to organ systems should be viewed in light of functional status. Age alone should add only a small level of risk to an otherwise healthy, mature woman. The preoperative period should be an opportunity to optimize functional status and delineate the appropriate surgical intervention to provide the patient with the best possible outcome.

Postoperative Management

Postoperative recovery begins with adequate preparation preoperatively. A well-informed patient does much better physically and mentally after surgery than one who is completely unaware or unsure of her role in the postoperative period. A frank discussion of what is expected prior to surgery in terms of intravenous (IV) line placement, use and purpose of thromboembolism deterrents and types of anesthesia to be used is always a prudent approach. The patient will be much more at ease because information gives the patient a sense of understanding and control. It is also prudent to speak with the patient about what is expected of her after surgery. The patient should be informed that her pain will be adequately controlled by whatever means with which the physician is comfortable. Avoidance of intramuscular pain medication is encouraged because it tends to cause pain itself. If available, the patient-controlled analgesia (PCA) pump is an excellent alternative that is convenient for both the patient and the hospital staff. The use of this device should be discussed preoperatively and the patient should know how to operate the machine before being dependent on it after surgery. If a bowel preparation is being used, the patient should be instructed on its method and why it is being ordered. An informed patient will more likely complete the preparation than one who does not understand why she is being made to suffer through a night long bout with diarrhea.

The patient should also be informed about when her diet will be advanced. Generalization need only be given, with the understanding that various factors may affect diet advancement. Patients should also be encouraged preoperatively to ambulate as soon as possible in the postoperative period to decrease the risk of venous thrombosis. Finally, the patient should be instructed on the use of incentive spirometry prior to surgery, so this can be used to prevent pulmonary-related complications.

Overall, the patient should be reassured that the physician will be available for her needs in the postoperative period and that everything will be done to ensure her comfort. If preoperative consultation has been obtained, the consultant should follow the patient postoperatively and offer advice about the specific organ system for which he or she is responsible.

Surgical complications can occur at any time after surgery, and not necessarily only within the first several postoperative days. Therefore, consultants should remain involved until several weeks after surgery.

Intraoperative Management

Whether age alone can be considered an independent variable affecting intraoperative morbidity has not been defined. However, aging does lead to slower re-epithelialization and fewer dermal blood vessels, which affect the rate of wound healing. In addition, older tissues may have a reduced healing capacity (due to underlying nutritional deficiencies) and impaired immune function (due to age related T-cell dysfunction).

Ideally, the operating surgeon should see the patient in the preoperative holding area prior to the administration of any premedication to provide comfort, reassurance, and answer any remaining questions. This may alleviate much anxiety. The surgeon should also see that preoperative orders have been expedited, such as the administration of antibiotics and placement of thromboembolism prevention devices, and all laboratory studies should be rechecked. The patient should be accompanied to the operating room; there, it is the surgeon's voice that the patient recognizes amidst all of the others present. Offering reassurances as the patient drifts off to sleep is a positive experience for both the physician and the patient, in addition to setting the tone for the entire operation.

The surgeon should also be involved with the positioning of the patient, taking care to avoid injury to fragile joints and to protect nerves from compressive damage, especially the peroneal nerve, which may be injured by the placement of the patient in the dorsal lithotomy position.

Intraoperative guidelines are generally applicable to all patients, not only the elderly. Speed, meticulous technique, and gentle handling of tissues are the cornerstones of surgical methodologies. Given the general slower healing elderly women may experience, we recommend the use of nonabsorbable monofilament suture on the facial closures. Care should be taken in closing the skin with either sutures or clips and adding an extra day before removal is prudent due to the slower healing in the older woman. Skin tape should be placed gently, without stretching or pulling, to avoid the damage to skin surfaces that often accompanies these final parts of the procedure.

Postoperative Care

General guidelines for postoperative care include attention to pain control, fluid and electrolyte management, and gastrointestinal and cardiopulmonary functioning.

Pain control must be viewed in light of the patient's age and ability to metabolize drugs. We avoid intramuscular injections because of the pain associated with them and the negative reinforcement they entail, as well as potential complications of bleeding and/or hematoma at the injection site. Rather, we prefer the use of patient controlled analgesia (PCA) if the patient can understand how to operate the pump. If she has been adequately counseled preoperatively, the system offers a patient a sense of control over the pain. The use of bolus dosing appears effective and avoids the complications associated with continuous dosing. These pumps can be instituted immediately upon emergence from anesthesia. Initial PCA orders may start at 1.2 mg of morphine sulfate with a lockout period of 10 to 12 minutes; appropriate adjustments can take place from there. Reduce the above dosage if oversedation occurs or decrease the interval if pain control is inadequate. Pain control is easily accomplished with modern pumps.

In general, elderly patients require lower narcotic doses, but the clinician needs to monitor the patient closely for adequacy of analgesia because this affects the overall sense of recovery. Antiemetics should be available or even given routinely with narcotic analgesics because nausea and vomiting are common postoperative complications. Compazine, 10mg IV every four hours as needed for nausea, is a good choice. Alternatively, newer antinausea medications such as ondansetron are excellent short-term alternatives.

The fluid requirements for replacement in the elderly woman need to be written in light of the age-related changes in renal function, as mentioned earlier in this chapter. Intravenous fluid should be ordered on an individualized basis rather than by generalized routine. For the usual elderly female 5% detrose in half normal saline with 20 mEq/L of potassium chloride is an appropriate replacement for standard daily needs. The rate is determined by the kilogram method. For the first 10 kilograms of bodyweight, 100 ml/kg per day, plus 50 ml/kg per day for the second 10 kilograms in bodyweight, plus 20 ml/kg per day for the remaining weight is calculated. This value is divided by 24 to give the hourly rate. This gives a more precise hourly fluid rate, avoiding the possible fluid overload in these older patients who otherwise could develop potentially life-threatening pulmonary edema. As the kidneys age, they go through a variety of changes that ultimately affect their function and make them quite susceptible to sudden failure. The clinician needs to be well aware of the factors that can accelerate renal dysfunction preoperatively (such as diabetes and hypertension) and postoperatively (such as volume depletion, obstruction, drugs, and infection). Quick action on any of the above processes may avoid an otherwise complicated prolonged postoperative recovery.

Management of drains, lines, and tubes is beyond the scope of this chapter, but suffice it to say that they should be removed as soon as possible. Unless the patient has undergone a bladder-related procedure such as an anterior colporrhaphy or a urethropexy, we generally remove the urinary catheter in the early morning of postoperative day one. Urine culture and sensitivity are usually not necessary in these patients.[53]

Suction drains are emptied every 4 hours and removed when the drain is less than approximately 25 ml/day. Nasogastric tubes are not often used for gynecological procedures. In general, if needed these tubes are left in based on the procedure performed and return of bowel sounds, not on some standardized time length. For small bowel surgery nasogastric (NG) tubes are generally removed after 2 to 3 days while large bowel processes generally require longer periods of NG suctioning. Careful attention to fluid and electrolyte status should be maintained during NG suctioning because the patients have the potential to develop metabolic alkalosis. The NG aspirate should be replaced 0.5 to 1.0 ml for every ml removed with 5% dextrose with half normal saline, and 20 mEq/L of potassium chloride. This IV fluid closely approximates gastric fluid.

Patients should be encouraged to ambulate as early as possible. This will decrease the risk of thromboembolism, urinary retention, fecal impaction, and pneumonia. If full activity is not possible, range-of-motion exercises should be prescribed.

Thromboembolism Prevention

As many as 40% of females undergoing gynecological oncology surgery experience deep venous thrombosis (DVT). The risk of a thromboembolic phenomenon increases substantially with age. The combination of gynecologic cancer surgery and older age thus puts the elderly woman at considerable risk. Benign gynecologic procedures also place patients at risk for thromboembolic complications. Nearly 40% of deaths after gynecological surgery are secondary to pulmonary emboli.[54] Risk factors associated with venous thromoembolic complications include the following: age, nonwhite race, stage of cancer, previous occurrence of DVT, lower extremity edema or venous stasis changes, lower extremity varicosities, obesity, and previous radiation therapy.[55]

There are specific factors that place a patient at high, moderate, or low risk for thromboembolic events. High-risk factors include, not surprisingly, a history of pulmonary embolism, extensive cancer surgery, and a lower extremity orthopedic procedure. The moderate-risk group include patients who are older than 40, but undergoing general surgical procedures of greater than 30 minutes duration. The low-risk group includes all patients under age 40, or those patients over age 40 who are undergoing procedures of less than 30 minutes. These risk groups have an incidence of fatal pulmonary emboli of approximately 3%, 0.3%, and less than 0.1%, respectively. When examined independently, age greater than 70 years is a risk factor for thromboembolic disease.[56] Thus, in general, the incidence of DVT for gynecological surgery varies with the presence of malignancy and type of procedure. Nononcological abdominal hysterectomy has a DVT rate of 10 to 12%. Vaginal hysterectomy has a DVT rate of 6% to 7%. If an oncologic surgery is being performed, the rate is as high as 35%.

Clearly, the elderly woman undergoing a surgical procedure, especially a gynecological surgical procedure, has a considerable risk for thromboembolic disease. DVT prevention should be a primary concern of the surgeon caring for the postmenopausal woman. There have been a variety of methods used for DVT prophylaxis including low-dose heparin, adjusted dose heparin, warfarin, and external pneumatic compression devices.

The use of low-dose heparin has been shown to be effective in prevention of DVT's only if it is started preoperatively. Heparin, 5,000 U given twice every 8 hr prior to surgery then continuing every 8 hr postoperatively, appears to be effective in deterring DVT; so does 5,000 units given 2 hr preoperatively and every 8 hr postoperatively.[57] This regimen is effective in patients with gynecological cancer, but its benefits is not necessarily noticeable in patients undergoing benign gynecological procedures. The use of low-dose heparin in this group is not necessarily warranted. Heparin even at so-called low doses is not necessarily a benign agent. It has been associated with increased surgical blood loss,[59] increased incidence of lymphocyst,[60] and considerable incidence of thrombcytopenia.[61]

Various physical techniques are available for the prevention of DVT. These include elastic stockings (TEDS: thromboembolic deterrent stockings) and external pneumatic compression hose. Elastic stockings are commonly used because of their ease and simplicity. The major drawback associated with their use is a tourniquet effect that may occur with improper fitting. Compression stockings are a more effective alternative. They compress at approximately 60 mm Hg, leading to an increase in both venous blood velocity and systemic fibrinolytic activity. Some feel the fibrinolytic activity is the real basis of their effectiveness.[61]

Overall the "right" choice of thromboembolic prophylaxis for the elderly woman undergoing gynecological surgery has not necessarily been established. In oncological cases the use of low-dose heparin or pneumatic compression hose with or without elastic stockings is indicated. In nononcological gynecological surgery the choice is less obvious because the effectiveness of any agent or device has not necessarily been demonstrated. Given that age itself is a risk factor for thrombosis, we use a combination of thigh-high elastic stockings and knee-high compression hose. These are left on until the patient is ambulating. This is a preferred alternative to the heparin because of its simplicity and ease.

Anesthesia

The management of anesthesia and the choice of anesthetic agents are generally the concerns of the anesthesiologist or anesthetist. Some practical knowledge about the anesthetic alternatives and options is presented here so that the clinician may understand some of the particulars.

Some general rules are as follows. In terms of premedication a reduction of the dose of sedative, hypnotic, and opioid drugs is indicated in the elderly due to decreased absorption distribution, metabolism, and clearance. The use of long-acting drugs with active metabolites should be avoided. Thiopental sodium tends to have an increased volume of distribution in elderly patients. The fat solubility of benzodiazepines such as diazepam and chlordiazepoxide as well as the opioid fentanyl citrate and sufentanil citrate coupled with decreased hepatic metabolism can prolong the effects of these medications. Appropriate dosage adjustment is warranted then when these agents are used. Finally, in terms of premedication there is increased potential for drug interaction in elderly patients.

The surgeon should discuss with the anesthesiologist preoperatively the various monitoring techniques that can be used during anesthesia. The best approach is that of individualization. There is no need for increased monitoring based on age alone. The use of various monitoring techniques from arterial lines to pulmonary artery catheters should be based on the severity of the age-related changes and the presence of coexisting disease.[41]

The choices of anesthesia are general, regional, and local anesthesia. Local anesthesia is easiest and best tolerated: however, often it is not adequate. The use of regional anesthesia is often the preferred alternative. Many gynecological procedures lend themselves to a regional anesthetic approach; thus, the technique is encouraged whenever it is feasible. Excellent analgesia and muscle relaxation can be achieved with most blocks, allowing surgical procedures to proceed easily and safely. In a study of high-risk elderly surgical patients, intraoperative epidural anesthesia combined with postoperative epidural opioid analgesia lead to fewer complications, shorter stays in the intensive care unit, and reduced costs compared with a similar cohort of patients undergoing general anesthesia and receiving routine postoperative parenteral narcotis.[42] It should be noted, however, in large series no apparent difference in mortality or morbidity is noted with either regional or general anesthesia.[43]

The use of hydration is an important part of the management of regional anesthesia in the elderly patient because the major complication of this technique is hypotension. However, despite the increased evidence indicating the superiority of regional anesthesia over general anesthesia, the latter technique appears to be just as well tolerated. The apparent discrepancy between regional and general techniques seems to reflect the poor monitoring and suboptimal postoperative care in older studies.[44]

A perioperative anesthetic complication that is prevalent in the elderly is hypothermia. This is defined as a drop in core temperature to less than 36°C. The elderly patient is at an increased risk due to a variety of factors, including low basal metabolic rate, peripheral vascular disease, and higher ratios of surface area to body mass. The risks of hypothermia are far-reaching. During a period of operative hypothermia, cardiac output can decrease leading to poor oxygen delivery. Postoperatively, during rewarming, oxygen consumption can increase up to 400% during shivering. This causes an increase in cardiac output and subsequently places a great demand on cardiac reserve. If cardiac reserve is already compromised, a difficult situation may arise in terms of cardiopulmonary status. All attempts should be made to prevent hypothermia, although it is a risk of surgery. Intraoperative preventive measures include decreasing patient exposure to the cool operating room environment, use of radiant warmers, efficient surgery, and accurate temperature monitoring intraoperatively and during the immediate recovery period. Thus, although hypothermia often cannot be avoided in the elderly patient, every attempt should be made to correct it as soon as it is observed.

The choice of anesthesia is best made by combined decision between the operating surgeon and the anesthesiologist, taking into account the patient's underlying medical history. Although the benefits of regional over general anesthesia are still being debated we prefer to use a regional anesthetic approach whenever applicable and feasible in an individual patient.

Infectious Disease Prophylaxis

Age itself does not place patients at increased risk for infection. Contributing factors such as concurrent illness, nutritional status, and immune status certainly exacerbate age-related effects. There is some impairment of T-cell function, which could theoretically lead to an increased infection in elderly patients. Overall, however, the same methods used for infection prophylaxis in young women should be used in the elderly female patient. To be effective, prophylactic antibiotics should be broad spectrum, that is, cover the organism most likely to be encountered. In addition they should be given within 2 hours of surgery.[62] It is generally recommended to continue the prophylaxis for two doses postoperatively. Simply continuing antibiotics indefinitely would lead to selection of resistant organisms, drug reactions, and superinfection.

The large bowel contains 1×10^{12} CFU/ml of bacteria. In fact, the bacteria in feces is estimated to contribute one-third of its dry weight. Thus, any surgery in this region has a great risk for infection. If colon surgery is contemplated or possibly involved in a planned procedure, such as an ovarian debulking surgery, adequate bowel cleansing is necessary. A standard bowel preparation includes a mechanical portion and an oral antibiotic portion. Mechanical agents include polyethylene glycol or magnesium citrate. The former is the preferred agent. Antibiotic agents include neomycin and erythromycin base. Care must be taken to provide adequate IV fluid and electrolyte support, especially in the elderly patient with underlying cardiopulmonary disease because of the dehydration and electrolyte disturbances that may occur with aggressive bowel preparations.

Postoperative Complications

Older patients face the same postoperative complications that younger patients do; however, they need to deal with these stresses with a significant decrease in reserve. Therefore, once the complication occurs, it often leads to a cascade of events that may ultimately end in the patient's death. Thus, the cornerstone of perioperative management is identification of risk. The most serious complications occur in the cardiac and pulmonary systems.

Approximately 40% of elderly patients undergoing general surgical procedures have a pulmonary complication that leads to significant postoperative morbidity. The use of incentive spirometry is an excellent aid in the prevention of atelectasis, which can lead to a collapse of large lung segments and possibly to pneumonia.[63] All patients should be instructed on the use of incentive spirometry preoperatively.

An often unexpected but dreadful complication of surgery is pulmonary embolism. Nearly 90% of all pulmonary emboli occur in patients over the age of 50,[64] and there is a steady increase with age.[65] All clinicians should keep this diagnosis in mind whenever a patient's status changes unexpectedly. Risks factors for pulmonary embolism include previous history, immobility, pelvic surgery, cancer, and—debatably—estrogen therapy. The best treatment is the prevention of DVT with either prophylactic heparin or compression devices.

Cardiac disease accounts for 35% to 50% of postoperative deaths in the elderly.[66] Myocardial infarction is the leading cause of death in patients over the age of 80 undergoing a wide variety of surgical procedures. The general principle of preoperative preparedness is applicable. Using the Goldman criteria and being aware of the individual patient's estimated risk allows for a tailored postoperative therapy. The appropriate postoperative environment, such as an ICU for a given patient, should be clearly worked out preoperatively or adjusted by intra-operative events. Any sudden change in status or slower return to baseline should be an indication for an evaluation for possible cardiac event. Myocardial infarction is often silent and may present postoperatively as a change in mental status, hypertension or arrhythmia.[67] An ECG should be performed immediately and compared with the preoperative ECG for changes. Serial enzymes including creatine phosphokinase MB fraction should be obtained immediately as well.

A common occurrence postoperatively in the elderly patient is delirium,[68] otherwise known as acute confusional state, disorientation, or sundowning. It is best treated by prevention. The incidence of postoperative confusion ranges from 7% to 15% in elderly patients.[69] Postoperative confusion is described as a fluctuation of memory, mood, attention, and self awareness, but as opposed to dementia, it is reversible. Risk factors include advanced age greater than 75 years, number of postoperative medical problems, male gender, fluid and electrolyte imbalance, cardiovascular problems, respiratory disease, overt infection, and analgesic use. This is quite a comprehensive list. Most of our patients could satisfy one or more criteria and be at risk for postoperative confusion. Also note that patients with alcohol and/or sedative hypnotic dependency should be evaluated and observed for postoperative delirium.[70]

Examination with attention to orienting the patient is an integral part of the postoperative daily visit. A sensitive, verbal nursing staff is also instrumental in avoiding patient anxiety and confusion. Reducing the amount of sedative medication such as narcotics is prudent in elderly patients prone to postoperative confusion. Delirium may present as a disorientation of time, but as opposed to dementia, a reduced level of consciousness is present. The patient usually also develops difficulty paying attention to instructions. An increase or decrease in activity may be noted. A careful evaluation of potential causes of individual patient's delirium should be made prior to the institution of therapeutic intervention. A CBC, electrolytes, blood urea nitrogen (BUN), creatinine, glucose, arterial blood gas, urinalysis, chest x-ray, and ECG should be obtained to evaluate the confusional state. Confusion may be the presenting sign for a variety of postoperative medical conditions such as infection, acute myocardial infarction, congestive heart failure, metabolic disturbances, dehydration, alcohol or sedative hypnotic withdrawal, or drug reactions such as those that occur with the use of antihistamines, opioid analgesics, phenobarbital, beta blockers, cimatadine, digoxin, diuretics, NSAIDS, and even penicillin.

Management should be directed to the underlying cause. Low doses of haloperidol (0.5 mg) is the agent of choice due to its limited anticholinergic affect and sedating abilities. Overall, the best treatment for a postoperative confusion state is prevention. This can be achieved by careful daily monitoring and frequent orienting visits by the physician and a caring hospital staff.

Laparoscopy

As the number of reports and studies on the burgeoning field of operative laparoscopy grows, special mention should be made in reference to these procedures in the mature woman. Overall, these procedures are extremely well-tolerated by elderly women, even in the advanced laparoscopic procedure such as laparoscopic-assisted vaginal hysterectomy and laparoscopic pelvic and para-aortic lymph node dissection.[71] Childers and coworkers[72] describe a cohort of patients in whom laparoscopic-assisted surgical staging procedures were performed, including laparoscopic-assisted vaginal hysterectomy, bilateral salpingo-oophorectomy, pelvic washings and pelvic and para-aortic lymphodectomy. The age range for these patients was 40 to 85 years, with a mean of 69. Of interest, however, is the finding that 41% of the patients were more than 71 years of age. The average hospital stay was 2.9 days. Clearly, these are well tolerated procedures by all age groups and further study is warranted on the postmenopausal population.

Conclusion

Overall, surgery should be considered as a viable alternative to medical management in the elderly patient. Age alone should not be considered a significant influence on operative risk. Chronic disease in association with the aging process should alert the clinician to an increased operative risk.

The preoperative period should be an opportunity to assess risk by identifying problems and addressing them by intervention or referral.

Key points to remember during the perioperative period include careful administration of medication with low starting doses and slow incremental increase, realization that the type of anesthesia generally does not alter perioperative morbidity or mortality in the elderly, and identification of malnutrition, because this is a significant cause of morbidity in elderly operative patients.

Postoperative care should focus on problems identified preoperatively, early ambulation, low but adequate doses of narcotic analgesics, patient orientation, early removal of catheters, and antibiotic prophylaxis.

A careful and meticulous approach to perioperative care should provide a rewarding postoperative experience for the older woman and reduce complication rates.

References

1. Pompei P: in Haji SN, Evan WJ (eds.) *Clinical Postreproductive Gynecology.* Norwalk, Conn, Appleton and Lange, 1993;p. 41.
2. Barber HRK, in HRK Barber (ed): *Clinical Geriatrics.* Philadelphia, JB Lippincott, 1986, p. 364.
3. Greenberg AG, Sask PP, Pridham D: *Am J Surg* 1985;150:65.
4. Furrow SC, Fowkes FGR, Lunn JN, Robertson LB: *Br J Anest* 1982;54:811.
5. Plamberg S, Hirsjavi E: *Gerontology* 1979;25:103.
6. Frances J. Jr: Goldman Dr., Brown FH, Guarnieri DN (eds.): in *Perioperative Medicine.*
7. Johnson JC: *J Am Geriatr Soc.* 1983;31:621.
8. Owen WD, Felts JA, Spiznagel EL: *Anesthesiology* 1978;49:239.
9. Goldman L, Cadera DL, Nusbaum SR: *N Engl J Med* 1977;297;845–.
10. Greenberg AG, Saik RP, Pridham D: *Am J Surg.* 1985;150:70.
11. McGerson, Hurst JM, Hertzberg VS: *Ann Intern Med.* 1985;103:832.
12. Kozak E: *Geriatrics* 1993;48:32.
13. Miller ED: *Can Anaesth Soc J.* 1985;32:542.
14. Pompei P: in Hajj SH, Evan WJ (eds.): *Clinical Postreproductive Gynecology.* Norwalk, Conn, Appleton & Lange, 1993, p. 234.
15. Seymour DG: *Gerontology* 1983;29:262.
16. Tisi G: *Am Rev Respir Dis.* 1979;119:293.
17. Johnson JC: *J Am Geriatr Soc.* 1983;31:621.
18. Stein M, Kerota GM, Simon J, Frank HA: *JAMA* 1962;181:765.
19. Houston MC, Ratcliff DG, Haj JT: *South Med J* 1987;80:1385.
20. Jackson CV: *Arch Int Med* 1988;148:2120.
21. Bolton JW, Werman DS, Haynes JL, Horning CA, Olsoen GN. Almond CH: *Chest* 1987;92:738.
22. Hole, A, Terjesen T, Breivih H: *Acta Anesthesiol Scand.* 1980;21:279.
23. Kehlet H: *Int Care Med* 1984;10:165.
24. Modig J, Borg T, Karlstrom G, Maripau E, Sahlstedt B: *Anesth Analg* 1983;62:174.
25. Evans TI: *Anest Int Care* 1973;1:319.
26. Andres R, Tobin JB: in Finch CE, Schneider EL (eds.): *Handbook of the Biology of Aging.* Van Norstrand Reinhold, 1985; p. 433.
27. McMurray JF: *Surg Clin Nor Am* 1984;64:769.
28. Skootsky SA, Glasby JA: in JS, Hacker NF (eds.): *Practical Gynecologic Oncology.* Baltimore, Williams & Wilkins, 1994; p. 575.

29. Davis, PJ, Davis FB: *Medicine* 1974;53:161.
30. Roizen MF, Hensen P, Lichtor JL, Schreider BD: *Anesthesiol Clin North Am* 1987;5:277.
31. West CD, Brown H, Simons, EL Carter PB, Kamagai LF, Englert E: *J. Clin Endocrinol Metab* 1961;21:1197.
32. Mullen JL, Buzby GP, Matthews DC: *Ann Surg* 1980;192:604.
33. Brown RB: *WJ Med* 1986;144:63.
34. Butterworth CE, Blackburn GL: *Nutrition Today,* 1974;9:1.
35. Rich MW, Keller AJ, Schechtman KB: *Am J Cardiol* 1989;63:714.
36. Heber D: in Berek JS, Hacker NF (eds.): *Practical Gynecologic Oncology.* Baltimore, Williams & Wilkins, p. 644.
37. Friedman PJ, Campbell AJ, Caradoc-Davis TH: *J Clin Exp Gerontol* 1985;7:191.
38. Mullen JL, Buzby GP, Waldman JG: *Surg Forum* 1979;30:80.
39. Cheng EY, Wang-Cheng RM: *J Clin Anesth* 1991;3:384.
40. Anderson S, Brenner BM: *J Am Geriatr Soc* 1987;35:59.
41. Cheng EY, Wang-Cheng RM: *J Clin Anesth* 1991;3:324.
42. Yeager MP, Glass DD, Neff RK: *Anesthesiol* 1987;66:729.
43. White PF: *Int Anesthesiol Clin* 1988;26:105.
44. Cote J, LaPointe P: *Can Anaesth Soc J* 1985;32:188.
45. Suchman AL, Mushlin AI: *JAMA* 1986;256:750.
46. Barber A, Green D, Gallazzo T: *Am J Med* 1985;78:761.
47. RA Hirsh: in Goldman DR, Brown FH, Guarrieri DM (eds.): *Perioperative Medicine.* New York, McGraw-Hill, 1993, pp. 9–13.
48. Marx GF, Mateo CV, Orkin LR. *Anesthesiol* 1973;39:54.
49. Cohen MM, Duncan PG, Tate RB: *JAMA* 1988;260:2859.
50. Beecher HK, Todd DP: *Ann Surg* 1954;140:2.
51. Modig J, Borg T, Karstrom G: *Anesth Analg* 1983;62:174.
52. Davis FM, Woolner DF, Frampton C: *Br J Anaesth* 1987;59:1080.
53. Michelson JD, Lotke PA: *N Eng J Med* 1988;319:321.
54. Jeffcoate TNA, Tindall VR: *Aust N.Z. J Obstet Gynecol* 1965;5:119.
55. Clarke-Pearson DL, Delong E, Synan IS: *Obstet Gynecol* 1982;69:146.
56. NIH Consensus Conference: *JAMA* 1986;256:744.
57. Clarke-Pearson DL, Delong E, Synan LS: *Obstet Gynecol* 1990;75:614.
58. Dockerty PW, Goodman JDS, Hill JG: *Br J Obstet Gynecol* 1983;70:759.
59. Piver MS, Maltetano JH, Lele SB: *Obstet Gynecol* 1983;62:127.
60. Clarke-Pearson DL: *Obstet Gynecol* 1984;64:689.
61. Allenby F, Borardman L, Pflugg JJ: *Lancet* 1976;2:1412.
62. Classen DC, Evans RS, Pestotnik RI, Burke JP: *N Engl J Med* 1992;326:281.
63. Celli BR, Rodriquez K, Snider GL: *Am Rev Resp Dis* 1984;130:12.
64. Bell WR, Smith TL: *Am Heart J* 103;239 1982;103:239.
65. Coon WW: *Arch Surg* 111;398 1976;111:398.
66. Djokovic JJ, Hedley-Whyte J, *JAMA* 1978;242:6.
67. Lubin MF, Kelly KG: in Merli, Wertz (eds.): *Medical Management of the Surgical Patient.* Philadelphia, WB Saunders, 1992, p. 364.
68. Williams-Russo P, Urquhart BL, Sharrock NE, Carlson ME: *J Am Geriatr Soc* 1992;40:759.
69. Miller HR, *Br J Psych* 1982;138:17.
70. Eryina PL, Gold SL, Meatino JL: *WJ Surg* 1993;17:192.
71. Childers JM, Hatch KD, Tran AN, Surwit EA: *Obstet Gynecol* 1993;82:741 72. Childers JM, Brzechffa PR, Hatch KD, Surwit EA: *Gynecol Oncol.* 1993;51:33.

Chapter 20

Sexuality and Aging

Julia R. Heiman, PhD

Raising sexual complaints is rarely easy for patients seeking medical care. This discomfort is magnified in older women who often believe, and have sometimes experienced, that their complaints are ignored or trivialized. There are a variety of reasons for this situation. *Cultural stereotypes* of aging include a diminution of all capacities, and older women are too often seen as desexualized and unattractive. Signs of sexuality in women beyond the child-bearing years are viewed rather suspiciously. Aging men, on the other hand, are often seen as sexually viable until they are very old or have little financial security. Overlapping with, and dependent on, cultural stereotypes is the problem that *medical training* in the area of "normal" and problematic sexuality is addressed minimally in most medical schools, and unevenly in nursing schools. As a result, capable and thoughtful health care providers are poorly trained to ask, respond to, and conceptualize the connection between a sexual disorder and broader patient health issues. An additional influence constraining the inclusion of sexual factors in patient care is the very limited *research* thus far on sex and aging. Currently there are no US population-based studies on sexual practices and problems across the life span. Nor are there broad-based longitudinal attempts to integrate biological, behavioral, and psychosocial data. This situation is currently changing, with several important studies underway looking at health issues in women and including sexuality variables. While treatment studies are more available, they leave many issues unresolved about lifetime sexuality.

The combination of factors—cultural bias, training emphasis, research limitations—interact to the disadvantage of the consultation between the health care provider and the patient. The purpose of this chapter is to provide information to help health care providers, especially those in a primary care role to be more alert to the importance of sexual complaints, to more ably conceptualize and discuss them with patients, and to efficiently formulate an integrated treatment plan.

Normal Sexual Changes with Aging

Many older adults do remain sexually active, as Brecher[1] and Comfort[2] both attest. The degree to which sex is an important source of gratification and comfort during early and middle adulthood appears to be related to how frequent and satisfying it is in later life.[3] The extent to which health decline, illness, and medications are involved with advancing age may directly decrease sexual function and satisfaction.

In Brecher's Consumer's Union nonrepresentative survey of 4,246 adults over the age of 50, most individuals were sexually active.[1] Sexually active individuals reported happier marriages than their nonsexually active counterparts. Among this sample, sex was felt to be an important component of marriage. Women did show a more marked decline than men in remaining sexually active. Masturbation frequency remained stable in women and gradually decreased in men. More marked decline in sexual interest and activity among women has been reported elsewhere. In one of the few representative samples of 956 women before and after menopause (between the ages of 38 and 54), Hallström found decreasing sexual desire and orgasmic response.[4]

Although sexual behavior decreases with aging, the changes are not universal and are characteristically variable. For example, Cutler and Garcia's study of perimenopausal and menopausal women found that since their menstrual periods had begun to change, 49% of women reported a decline in sexual activity, 38% reported no change, and 14% reported an increase.[5] Bretschneider and McCoy, studying adults between the ages of 80 and 102 years, found that intercourse was less likely with advancing age but the frequency of caressing did not change.[6] This result parallels Turner and Adam's study of 60- 85-year-old men and women, which found increasing interest in petting and masturbation but decreasing interest in coitus in older people.[7]

Attempts to integrate how sexual behavior, satisfaction, *and* relationship quality evolve together are rare. One effort along these lines comes from Hawton and coworkers in England.[8] They randomly selected a community (Oxford) sample of 436 women with partners, with 100 to 150 in each of 5 age groups between ages 35 and 59. Frequencies of sexual intercourse, orgasm, and enjoyment of sexual activity with the partner were most closely associated with younger age and better marital adjustment. However, partner's age also appeared to be an important negative influence on intercourse frequency, and relationship duration negatively impacted enjoyment of sexual activity. Women's sexual relationship satisfaction bore no relationship to age, instead being more strongly associated with marital adjustment. Psychiatric factors and gynecological symptoms were largely unrelated to sexual behavior. A modest exception to the latter was that psychiatric disorders (especially depression) were related to decreased sexual satisfaction (Table 20.1).

Barring illness, disease, and major psychosocial stressors, sexuality responses change gradually, rather than suddenly, over the years. Overall changes include slower and decreased levels of vaginal lubrication, probably due to Bartholin gland atrophy and decreased quantity of vaginal cells. Breast enlargement and sex flush responses are less noticeable during sexual arousal. Reaching orgasm takes longer and is accompanied by fewer contractions according to Masters and Johnson.[9] Some

Table 20.1 Typical Changes with Aging that Impact Sexual Functioning and Satisfaction in Women

Physical changes		Psychosocial changes
↓Estrogen and progesterone levels	→	↓Pregnancy worry
↑FSH and LH levels		↓Cultural definition of sexual attractiveness
↓Testosterone levels		↑Losses
↓Thickness and elasticity of vaginal and urinary tract tissues		↓Availability of males for relationships
↓Vaginal lubrication		↑Likelihood male partner experiencing erection problems
↓Size of uterus, vulva, cervix, ovaries		↓Family responsibilities
↑pH of vagina		
↓Number and intensity of orgasmic contractions		
↑Sexual arousal time		
↓Elasticity and smoothness of facial and body skin		
↑Likelihood of illness and medication use		

FSH, Follicle-stimulating hormone; LH, luteinizing hormone.

women may experience pain or cramping during or after orgasm. It is unclear to what extent these changes are under hormonal control. It does appear that decreased estrogens, via decreased pelvic vascular supply, are related to genital appearance changes, including the thinning and drying of vaginal mucosa, decreased fullness of the clitoris and labia majora, and reduction in pubic hair. The vagina also decreases in length and diameter and becomes more stenotic. These physical changes of the genitalia are often summarized by the term *vaginal atrophy* (see McCoy's review for further details[10]). While *vaginal atrophy* can lead to increased susceptibility to vaginal infections, vaginal tears, and inflammation, these outcomes can be avoided in most women.

Thus, the normal overall changes in sexual functioning include a decrease in the desire for and intensity of sexual response, an increase in latency to arousal and orgasm, and decreased lubrication. Fortunately, these changes are rather gradual, although some women experience menopause as a more abrupt shift. In addition, none of these changes by themselves dictate that there will be any problems or complaints with sexual functioning.

Assessing Sexual Problems

Assessing sexual problems involves two processes: (1) Getting a complete description of the problem; (2) clarifying likely biological and psychosocial contributors to the problem to formulate the best treatment intervention.

Description: Initial Information or Screening

A straightforward and descriptive system that parallels the DSM-IV[11] and related work includes the following categories:

- *Sexual Desire Disorders:* Hypoactive sexual desire disorder refers to the persistent absence of sexual feelings and desire for sexual activity. Sexual Aversion Disorder refers to persistent or recurrent aversion to and avoidance of genital contact with a sexual partner.

- *Sexual Arousal Disorders.* This disorder describes a lack of some or all physical response, as indicated by genital lubrication or vasocongestion, to sexual stimulation. If a women states she lubricates but does not feel aroused, this may be a desire problem.

- *Orgasm Problems.* Persistent delay or absence of orgasm fits into this category. Coital orgasm absence is considered a normal variation of a women's sexual response, if she is able to experience orgasm with a partner using noncoital methods.

- *Sexual Pain Disorders.* Dyspareunia refers to recurrent genital pain before, during, or after intercourse. Vaginismus refers to the involuntary spasm of the outer third of the vagina interfering with or preventing coitus.

- *Sexual Satisfaction.* If satisfaction is present despite a dysfunction, eventual referral for treatment may be in question. Partner's satisfaction is also relevant.

For each of the areas listed above, it is also useful to ask whether it has been present *lifelong or not lifelong,* is *global or situational,* and if there is more than one disorder, which is *primary.*

Each of the areas listed above needs to be probed. For example, if a woman comes in reporting lack of desire, one would conceptualize her problem differently if it was accompanied by dyspareunia, and if both disorders were current, which occurred first historically. Also, it is my impression that women seeing a physician and possibly other medical specialists may be more likely to complain of pain than the other disorders. Pain is considered a legitimate and serious symptom, worthy of a doctor's attention. If pain is the presenting complaint, it is important to probe for other areas that may have an equivalent or a greater impact on physical health and psychosocial functioning, with depression and relationship distress (including abuse) being prime examples.

The first phase of obtaining a description can occur in two ways: a written checklist or an interview, either being part of more general screening or information collection procedures. A written checklist can be brief: "Are you currently experiencing any sexual concerns or problems that you find distressing? (please circle): sexual desire; sexual arousal (including lubrication); orgasm; pain." In an interview, the same thing can be asked. Notice that two questions are being asked, which may be presented separately: Is there a sexual problem(s), and are you distressed by it (them)? The latter gets at the idea of satisfaction. As we have seen from the normative data, some women may not be concerned about a problem and feel it does not impact their lives (eg, low desire in a woman not in a relationship). Overall then the screening serves the purpose of providing a description of sexual functioning that may be a clue for other nonsexual issues (eg, depression and effects of diabetes) or may on further exploration be an area worthy of investigation in its own right.

In defining the sexual problem, it is important not to assume that a woman is heterosexual. Lesbian women often will not disclose their sexual orientation to their medical provider. One 1985 study of over 2,000 lesbian and bisexual women revealed that over 40% believed that revealing their sexual orientation to their gynecologist would impair the quality of their medical care, and one third of the sample had not revealed their sexual orientation for this reason.[12] More informally, practitioners who are sensitive to sexual orientation issues become known in a given community and tend to be sought out by lesbian women. Approximate prevalence of exclusive homosexuality in women is 1% to 2%, with occasional homosexual experience estimated at 13% to 15% of women.[13,14] Little research has been done on lesbian sexual complaints or about lesbian relationships across the life span. However, clinical reports have indicated that their sexual complaints have considerable overlap with heterosexual women, with the exception of the heterosexually biased dysfunctions such as vaginismus, which can occur among lesbians but are less cause for complaint.

Clarification: Biological and Psychosocial Factors

Sexual response and behavior are determined by complex biological and psychosocial factors. The health care provider's role is to understand the possible contributions of the various factors in order to develop treatment options. Intervention on one level will impact the others. For example, a woman in an unhappy relationship with an alcoholic partner may be more likely to report problematic side effects to a medication intervention designed to improve her sexual response. While broader social factors cannot be the main concern of the gynecologist, their presence must be recognized and appropriate referrals made to provide adequate and efficient care of a patient.

Any factors affecting vascular, neurological, or endocrine functioning can affect sexual functioning. The common physical areas to review are: menopause, chronic or acute illness, disease, medications, or surgery. Depression may be particularly implicated in desire problems and less commonly anxiety and panic disorders may contribute to sexual dysfunctions. Diabetes in women is associated with all categories of dysfunction, although type 2 has more often been associated with lubrication and orgasm problems than has type 1.[15] Still, diabetic women overall show sexual dysfunction rates of 27% to 47%, not necessarily higher than an age-matched control group.[15-17] Most important for our purposes here, postmenopausal data on diabetic women are almost nonexistent.

Hysterectomies can have physical and psychological sequelae. The type of surgery, complications, and hormonal levels after surgery are significant factors. In addition, current medications are important because they often on impact sexual response and are increasingly used by older individuals. The use of alcohol, which has acute negative effects on sexual response by decreasing physical arousal and delaying or inhibiting orgasm, may have permanent effects if used abusively and chronically.

Interpersonal psychosocial problems including historical issues—such as the effects of an affair or sexual or physical abuse—or current issues—such as job loss or stress, family problems, or changes, and marital distress—may be important. A partner's health and sexual functioning may be impairing a woman's response. In one study, 50% of 60- to 70-year-old women stated that their partners had erection difficulties.[18] Women sometimes feel rejected or even suspicious about their partner's erection problems, which in turn affects their own sexual feelings.

There is a high probability that physical and psychosocial factors interact in any given case, although with increasing age, there is increasing likelihood that medications or physical changes play a role.

Common Sexual Problems: Initial Recommendations

The most common sexual complaint of older heterosexual women is *dyspareunia*. Clarifying the onset of symptoms and their relationship to the changes in desire, arousal, and orgasm is important in deciding on further evaluation and treatment. If symptoms began before the perimenopausal period or were preceded by a period of decreasing arousal and/or decreasing attraction to the partner, other physical (eg, injury, scarring, and local or systemic medications) and psychosocial issues (eg, depression, anxiety, and relationship distress) need to be considered. If these other factors are not present and/or the symptoms appeared during the perimenopause, vaginal atrophy and lubrication diminution are likely causes to address initially. In any case, it is important to take a history covering these issues and to do a careful examination of the genital area for injury, sensitivity, scarring, or other genitourinary sources of discomfort (Table 20.2).

Several factors may prevent or correct dyspareunia. One is that there is a considerable variability in hormone levels among menopausal women, and for some women the ovaries and/or adrenal glands produce sufficient estrogen as to avoid menopausal symptoms. A second factor that appears to help maintain rapid and sufficient lubrication despite vaginal atrophy symptoms may be regular sexual activity. This finding was first suggested by Masters and Johnson (1966) who found that only 3 of 54 women over 60 showed sexual response patterns comparable to younger women.[9] These three women were the only ones who had remained consistently sexually active throughout their middle and postmenopausal years. A more carefully controlled study by Leiblum and colleagues compared sexually active and inactive postmenopausal women and found less vaginal atrophy was characteristic of the cohort who had more frequent coitus.[19] In addition, more frequent masturbation helped to slow genital atrophy. Later work by members of this research team has found that these differences may not be mediated by hormonal status.[18]

A third related factor that may influence the complaint of dyspareunia is the sexual partner who may himself be sexually dysfunctional and unable to provide coital stimulation. A number of men who experience erection disorders may also withdraw from other sexual interaction, and thus a pattern of irregular sexual activity occurs that in turn influences the possible appearance of dyspareunia in the female partner.

The usual current intervention for dyspareunia that is believed to be menopause-induced is local estrogen cream or hormone replacement therapy (HRT) that includes estrogen or an estrogen–progesterone combination, with the estrogen seen as the active agent for the vaginal atrophy condition. The alternatives are nonhormonal water soluble lubricants or short-term HRT. In some

Table 20.2 Schema for Description, Assessment, and Initial Treatment Recommendations for Sexual Problems with an Emphasis on Aging-Related Issues

Presenting Complaint
Sexual Desire Disorder: Hypoactive or aversive *Sexual Arousal Disorder:* Including lubrication *Orgasmic Disorder* *Sexual Pain:* Dyspareunia, Vaginismus *Other Sexual Disorders* *Sexual Dissatisfaction*

Assessment Evaluation
Problem description: Lifelong or not, generalized or situational, onset, relationship to other sexual disorders. *Biological factors:* History and current illness, disease, surgery, medications, alcohol and substance use, endocrine status, neuroendocrine problems. Laboratory tests are indicated for illness, endocrine status. Examination of genitals and related areas if sexual pain is present. *Psychosocial Factors:* Acute or chronic stress, knowledge and attitudes on aging, menopause, values (including religion), negative body image, illness, surgery, aging, body weight, history of physical or sexual abuse, relationship distress, role strain at work or in family, partner's pressure, partner's illness, change in partner's sexual appeal/interest.

Treatment options	
When Sx appear primarily related to biological factors	When Sx appear primarily psychosocial
For endocrine disorders, consider hormone replacement therapy. For depression and anxiety, discuss medication and/or therapy, with sexual side effects of medications in mind. For other illnesses, diseases (diabetes, multiple sclerosis), treat medically with discussion of sexual consequences of illness and treatment. For medication-caused sexual problems, consult as needed to change type, dosage, or administration time. For pain disorders, attempt to alleviate with genital lubricant, hormone replacement therapy, low dose of antidepressants, as indicated. If problem appears complex, biologically and psychosocially maintained, **or** there is minimal or no change with biological treatment, refer to appropriate specialist.	Provide information on sexual desire, book references on menopause, other self-help references. Suggest patient discuss problem with partner, unless relationship is unsafe. Refer for consultation or therapy to individual, couples, or group therapist for sexual, relationship, pain, adjustment issues around stress, illness, depression, and anxiety.

cases, resumption of regular sexual activity while using a lubricant may help diminish the need for its continued use. The appropriateness of estrogen for a given woman, and the growing research on the multiple health implications of estrogen use, is beyond the scope of this chapter. At the present time a careful consideration of each individual woman's risks and benefits, discussed with her, is the safest recommended basis for treatment intervention. Different women may find more or less risk acceptable, depending on the importance of sex to their lives combined with the importance of the other systems affected by HPT.

Other physical interventions for dyspareunia may be topical or systemic corrections of local infections or irritations. Low doses of certain antidepressants may also be helpful if the pain is not helped by other means or is chronic. This level of antidepressant medication does not necessarily imply that the woman is depressed (because the dosage is not considered therapeutic for depression), and thus the sexual side effects such as delayed orgasm and decreased desire are usually minimal. Consultation with a professional who is knowledgeable about and up to date on medications and who is aware of sexual side effects is valuable.

If the dyspareunia appears to be related primarily to psychosocial factors or the physically-based interventions fail to alleviate symptoms, referral to a sexual disorders specialist may be effective. Psychological interventions can be useful to help manage pain symptoms by helping the woman relax and refocus her attention during nongenital and genital touching. It is not uncommon to include the partner in this type of treatment, given the importance of a partner's understanding of the problem and involvement in the outcome. It is also typical to initially avoid direct genital touching, which involves a partner's awareness and understanding of the rationale and cooperation. Effectiveness of treatment for the disorder for individuals and couples varies from approximately 40% to 70%, with longer duration of symptoms and degree of relationship distress accounting for the less successful outcome statistics.

Another common sexual complaint in older women is the loss of sexual desire, *hypoactive sexual desire*. This is a very heterogeneous disorder that may have as its etiology in an individual problem (physical and psychogenic illnesses, such as diabetes, depression, and anxiety, medications, or surgery) or in interpersonal problems (eg, relationship distress, or partner's health). Some decrease in desire is expected with aging so that it is important to ask about current versus past levels (excluding the first year of any love relationship, which may be unusually high) to understand how sudden and severe the change is in order to recommend appropriate treatment or to reassure the patient. A number of women find that their lack of desire is related to feeling less desirable due to the aging process or finding that their partner is less sexually appealing. A percentage of women feel more desire possibly due to a combination of hormonal (greater ratios of androgens to estrogens) and social (eg, more time, more sleep, and no children) changes.

The endocrine causes of low desire are only partially substantiated. The estrogens that are prescribed in a HRT regimen may somewhat improve sexual desire, initially due to improvement of vaginal lubrication and decreases in hot flashes, itching, and depression. However, research by Mathur and coworkers has shown that after several months of taking estrogen replacement therapy, women showed a 30% reduction in testosterone.[20] While there is no systematic body of research on which to base firm conclusions about the role of androgens in women, Greenblatt has suggested that low doses of testosterone may help with problems of low desire.[21] Other studies have shown that women who are postmenopausal but still have their ovaries show variable levels of androgens. In some women, androgen levels increase postmenopausally; in others, androgens decrease dramatically. Research by Sherwin Gelfand has shown that women who have their ovaries removed during hysterectomy report lower levels of desire, arousal, and fantasies when taking placebo or estrogen compared with women with the same surgery who were taking testosterone or a testosterone-estrogen combination. The latter group's sexual behavior was in fact similar to a group of women who had hysterectomies without ovarian removal.[22–25]

Although it is not unusual for women to take testosterone, there is limited data on effective but safe dosages especially with reference to cardiovascular disease, and there is no long-term follow-up data. For women with clear androgen deficiencies such as those produced by bilateral oophorectomy or chemotherapy, Kaplan and Owett have recommended low doses of testosterone to replace or restore androgen levels.[26] While not stating recommended doses except to note that, for one patient, 15 mgm of testosterone enanthate in aqueous solution (bimonthly injections) restored libido and orgasmic response with no signs of virilization. As of this writing, the clinical use of androgens is best embarked on with clear cautions to and attentive monitoring of the patient.

Other treatments for low sexual desire could include antidepressants if the patient has depressive symptoms. However, women who wish to minimize medication use, whose general health may mitigate against further medications, or who want to avoid the sexual side effects of most medications may want to consider brief (15 to 20 sessions) therapy for depression. Research has shown essentially equivalent effects of medications and psychotherapy for depression.[27]

Other chemical treatments, as reviewed by Segraves, such as yohimbine and dopamine agonists appear to carry more of a placebo than a direct effect on low desire.[28] Minimal research exists on the effect of these compounds on women's sexuality.

Patients may also benefit from information, because everyone carries expectations about how much desire is enough. A woman might be informed that there are no current norms for sexual desire at different ages. Normally, with the exception of notable emotional or physical stress, desire should be expected to gradually rather than suddenly decline. There are no data on the percentage of couples who stop having sexual activity while maintaining a good relationship, but it does occur, and as Blumstein and Schwartz have shown, may be more common in lesbian couples.[29]

Barring a medical disorder or solution, individual or couple's therapy can be recommended. Although no controlled treatment studies of low desire have been published, we have an estimate of effectiveness from the clinical literature. However, this literature does not focus on older couples. Kilmann and coworkers found a success rate of 50%,[30] and Rosen and Leiblum have noted that better outcomes have been associated with the absence of global and lifelong sexual desire disorder and strong commitment to the relationship.[31] Treatment duration usually varies from 15 to 45 sessions. This disorder is one of the more difficult sexual complaints to treat with psychotherapy, perhaps because it is more often linked to more general relationship problems.

Other sexual problems, *arousal, orgasm, sexual aversion,* and *vaginismus* problems are less frequent complaints, except as consequences of pain or desire disorders, in older than in younger women. Decreased lubrication may be more correlated with a decreased sense of subjective than genital sexual arousal in older women. A minority of women who report pain during or after orgasm, a complaint that is not considered to be dyspareunia, appears to be helped by HRT. For the other dysfunctions, after eliminating possible physiological contributions, referral to a specialist may be indicated because these conditions are relatively successfully treated with psychotherapy (see Heiman[32]).

Other Important Concerns Related to Sexuality and Aging

Two other areas that are important in the aging process with respect to sexuality are hysterectomies and dementia.

Hysterectomy and Sexuality

As of the early 1980s, the lifetime prevalence of hysterectomy in the United States (outnumbering western Europe by at least fourfold) appeared to level off at between 50% and 60%, and it was the second most common operation performed on women.[33] For hysterectomies that include bilateral ovariectomy, vaginal dryness, dyspareunia, and loss of libido are common. However, loss of libido can occur even when the ovaries are retained. Libido loss may occur in 50% of women and has been documented to last 5 years or more beyond the operation. As mentioned earlier, estrogen alone does not necessarily help low sexual desire, although it often helps dyspareunia problems.

Kilkku's research in Scandinavia has found that when comparing married women with complete versus supracervical hysterectomies, the latter group experienced a lower incidence of painful coitus and sexual activity was more frequent. Libido did not differ, but women with complete hysterectomies suffered a substantial loss in the capacity for orgasm.[34,35] Other work has suggested that hysterectomy, particularly if it includes ovariectomy, may decrease orgasm capacity. This decision must balance the likelihood of, for example, ovarian and cervical cancer risk against any advantages of organ retention. This is an area that is underresearched with less than adequately controlled studies overall, thus contributing toward a more medically conservative solution—that is, more organ removal to avoid possible disease.

In summary, hysterectomy does appear to impact sexual functioning, in some cases only for 6 months, in other cases for many years. Some of its effects can be tempered with ovarian retention or HRT; however, no treatment decision is without disadvantage and some risk, of which each woman must be aware.

Dementia

Dementia is a common disease. According to Jorm, it affects 2% of adults between 65 and 69 years of age and 40% of those over 90.[36] Although it is not a woman-specific illness, women in industrialized countries live longer and thus make up a larger proportion of the very old. Dementia is associated with a range of sexual problems, but the research is so limited that it is often difficult to be sure that the sexual problems are caused by dementia. Sexual acting out, referring to sexual acts such as masturbation or genital fondling in public, is in fact uncommon. Burns and coworkers found sexual acting out in only 7% of an Alzheimer's sample of 178 patients.[37] False sexual allegations about others may occur, secondary to broader delusions or hallucinations; however, the possibility that the allegations may be true must be considered. There is no clear indication as to whether loss of sexual interest or, alternatively, increased demands for sex are more common in demented patients compared with persons without dementia of the same age. However, sexual disinhibition does appear to be associated with the severity of dementia in patients with Alzheimer's disease. Sexual disinhibition is also a recognized feature of frontal lobe lesions, and thus it may be relevant to subtypes of dementia affecting the frontal lobes including Pick's disease and alcoholic dementia. Temporal lobe damage has also been associated with hypersexuality, as has the use of certain medications such as levodopa. Excessive sexuality is less often reported in women, but this may be a reporting bias.

The treatment for sexual problems in patients suffering from dementia is rarely discussed, but Haddad and Benbow have summarized various attempts.[38,39] One is the reduction or removal of substances causing sexual problems. Another is to use drugs such as benzodiazepines and neuroleptics (when patients present with nonsexual symptoms as well those for which these drugs may be useful), progestogens, estrogens, antiandrogens, and luteinizing hormone—releasing hormone (LHRH) antagonists. In general, due to ethical dilemmas, these drugs are recommended only when sexual disinhibition is a major problem or other treatments have failed, and in combination with a psychosocial approach. Psychosocial approaches include gentle and repeated discussion with a patient as to why problem sexual behavior is unacceptable, attention to the staff's behavior if a person is in an institutional setting, or working with the spouse of the patient. Certainly, the partner of demented patients suffer in a variety of ways, including the loss of a sexual partner both physically and cognitively. Discussing sexuality with the partner can illuminate possible solutions in dealing with the spouse's sexual behavior and the caregiver's own touching and sexual needs.

Referring to a Specialist

The primary care practitioner cannot be expected to keep pace with all of the options needed to competently treat an area as biopsychosocially complex as sexual disorder. Knowing when and how to refer to a specialist will avoid ineffective consultations and unnecessary treatment.

When to Refer

Conditions particularly suitable for making a referral include the following:

1. Diagnostic uncertainty or descriptive complexity. Long-term, multiply influenced sexual disorders may benefit from a referral to provide additional expertise or a second opinion. This is particularly useful early in evaluation and treatment in order to save patients the time and money of inappropriate or unnecessary treatments.

2. Factors surrounding a sexual problem appear to be in an area where the primary care provider has less expertise. Typical examples are psychological and interpersonal factors, including those consequent to a disease, surgery, illness or even a normal aging process that appears to be adequately medically treated. For example, women who are relieved to have hysterectomy may still experience related psychological reactions, as may their partners. Similarly, menopause raises a number of psychosocial issues that may not necessarily automatically resolve with time.

3. Symptom intensity or severity. Ongoing depression that interferes with functioning and relationship-threatening interpersonal problems deserve the attention of a specialist who may effect more rapid improvement.

Methods of Referral

A referral for a second opinion, consultation, or treatment is more likely to be followed up under two conditions: (1) the manner and message of presenting the referral and (2) the availability of names of experts who are thorough and efficient.

With respect to presenting the referral to the patient, briefly explain why you believe this would be valuable to their care (eg, complexity, beyond your expertise, and ultimate efficiency of treatment). If referring to a nonmedical specialist, remind the patient that mind and body are linked in both normal and problematic sexual functioning. In patients with genital pain, let them know that psychological interventions have been found to be important in controlling pain along with medical monitoring, which will continue. For referral to a marital or relationship therapist, it may be reassuring to mention that distressed relationships take a toll on individual family members, health (including increased clinic visits), working efficiency, and general functioning (see the review by Burman and Margolin[40]). The message patients need to hear is that a given referral will increase the likelihood that the problem will be dealt with more quickly and thoroughly, minimizing loss of health and life quality.

Having an updated short list of specialists with expertise in sexuality, endocrinology, psychotherapy, psychology, and relationship distress is useful. The nature of feedback is also important. Written reports take longer and may bear a cost to patients. In some cases, patients may refuse information exchange between professionals if they accept a referral and reveal information about themselves or their partners that they do not wish to be shared with other professionals or made part of their medical record. Even in these cases, which are not that common, referral can often give feedback on nonsensitive material.

The above referral issues have been discussed from a patient-centered perspective, meaning what is in the patient's best interests. As managed care companies have greater input into referral approval and specialist pools, methods and options may be reduced for access to specialists. Having a selection of consultants that the primary care provider considers high quality may nevertheless ultimately save time and resources in dealing with sexual problems.

Treatment Examples

Case One: Long-term Dyspareunia and Nonsexual Genital Pain

Ms. L., a 48-year-old woman, complained of 3 years of dyspareunia as well as pain during genital stroking by her husband during foreplay or tissue contact by herself after urination. Her gynecologist identified soreness at 10:00 on the introitus with Q-tip stimulation. Her endocrine levels were nonmenopausal; periods rather short but regular. Ms. L. viewed herself as sensitive to pain, often overwhelmed, perfectionistic, and controlling. Her husband agreed with this description, and also viewed himself as being somewhat clumsy and insensitive about her needs earlier in the relationship. Ms. L. had trouble sleeping but no other vegetative depressive symptoms. Both were committed to the marriage and to their 10- and 12-year-old children. There had been no intercourse in 18 months, although she manually stimulated Mr. L. to orgasm about once every 6 weeks. Infrequent affectionate touching occurred at nonsexual times as well due to her fear of pain and his fear of rejection. She was orgasmic but had decreased desire. Treatment gynecologically included topical cortisone for two weeks, plus a trial of low-dose antidepressants for the pain and sleep. Pain during daily activities and self-touch decreased to almost zero—although she occasionally felt sensitive—and sleep improved. Her gynecologist referred her for individual therapy for the sexual issues. There she revealed family issues, no sexual abuse, conditioned pain response, and unresolved angry feelings toward her husband around their early sexual relationship. She was cooperative with genital self-exploration to explore for positively and negatively sensitive areas. After four sessions alone, her husband joined the therapy to work on first nonsexual and then sexual touching. She also independently decided to increase her exercise and lose the 40 pounds she had gained after her last pregnancy, even though her husband had not been bothered by her weight. Progress was very difficult and rather slow (23 sessions over 49 weeks), the couple was able to increase affectionate touching and to gradually resume occasional intercourse, with Ms. L. being in control of the tempo. Important ingredients of this work were: (a) Medical attempts, initially frustrating but eventually successful, to reduce the ongoing daily genital area pain, (b) a gradual approach toward addressing the sexual pain that included involving her husband, beginning with no sexual touch and analyzing the problems it revealed (miscommunication, control issues, the need for her own time, her mistrust of him being sensitive to her), having lidocaine cream as a backup, but in fact not used, and encouraging her control of the sexual interaction in order to avoid pain or stop contact when pain appeared. The couple was pleased overall with their progress.

Case Two: Loss of Sexual Desire

Ms. M. sought treatment at 59 for loss of sexual desire with her partner of 16 years. Ms. M. was orgasmic and masturbated once a week but found it a "depressing and unsatisfying discharge of energy." She was 7 years postmenopause and had experienced loss of lubrication. She was healthy and on no medications. She had decided not to use estrogens but had used nonhormonal lubricants. She reported that 9 years earlier her partner had gone through a major crisis for 4 years at work in which a colleague had brought a lawsuit. Despondent and depressed, the partner withdrew emotionally and physically and did not want to be touched. Sex ceased completely, after having been frequent and enjoyable for both. When they came to therapy, sexual contact to orgasm had occurred 3 to 4 times a year until 2 years prior when it stopped altogether.

While she empathized with her partner's crisis, she was angry and hurt at "going through menopause alone." She also felt "dropped" out of his interest and his attention to her. She coped by increasing her work intensity, but she felt "dead" without sex.

She was not depressed. Her partner had been in therapy and was no longer depressed. Both were interested in improving sex but if necessary would continue their marriage without sex, as they were very committed to each other. She was opposed to any medical interventions, probably because of her own mother's hysterectomy resulting in complications, infection, and multiple corrective surgeries. However, she did agree to a gynecological examination, which was negative except for small fibroids and menopausal vaginal atrophy.

Therapy consisted of 15 sessions over 25 weeks with assignments of nonsexual, brief touching only when both were willing. This built up some trust between the couple. The fact that they had articulated that they could be satisfied if sex did not change helped to reduce the anxiety and pressure in moving into genital touching and response. By the tenth session, they were touching outside of sexual contact several times a week and touching to orgasm about once a week. Intercourse had occurred twice in the month and, though tentative, was quite satisfying. However, they preferred the nonintercourse activity and felt that this was a sufficiently positive outcome for them. Her desire had increased modestly and her avoidance decreased more substantially as her partner's attention and sensitivity became more clearly expressed.

Concluding Remarks

A woman's sexuality does change with increasing age, the change being gradual unless there is a sudden alteration in her life such as surgery, illness, or loss of her partner. When problems do present in sexuality, they are often amenable to biological, psychosocial, or combined interventions. This chapter has underscored the value of the primary care provider being educated with respect to resisting sociocultural pressures to see older women as nonsexual and to overcome any omissions in his or her own training that might have minimized or discounted the potential importance of sexual and relationship distress to a woman's overall health. It is rather likely that, if the emphasis on women's health issues continues, over the next 20 years our knowledge and research base on aging, sexuality, and health in women will expand. Hopefully, we will be prepared to receive that knowledge, appreciate its complexity, and, when called upon, to take thoughtful therapeutic action.

References

1. Brecher EM: *Love, Sex and Aging: A Consumer's Union Report.* Boston, Little, Brown, 1984.
2. Comfort A: *A Good Age.* New York, Crown Publishers, 1976.
3. George LK, Weiler SJ: *Sexuality in middle and late life. The effects of age, cohort, and gender. Arch Gen Psychiat* 1981;38:919–923.
4. Hallström T: *Mental Disorders and Sexuality in the Climaterie.* Göteborg, Scandinavian University Books, 1973.
5. Cutler WB, Garcia CR, McCoy N: *Perimenopausal sexuality. Arch Sex Behav* 1987;16:225–234.
6. Bretschneider JD, McCoy NL: *Sexual interest and behavior in health 80–102 year old. Arch Sex Behav* 1988;17:109–129.
7. Turner BF, Adams CG: *Reported change in preferred sexual activity over the adult years. J Sex Res* 1988;25:289–303.
8. Hawton K, Gath D, Day A: *Sexual function in a community sample of middle-aged women with partners. Effects of age, marital, socioeconomic, psychiatric, gynecological, and menopausal factors. Arch Sex Behav* 1994;23:375–395.
9. Masters WH, and Johnson VE: *Human Sexual Response,* Boston, Little, Brown, 1966.
10. McCoy NL, in Sitruk-Ware R, Utian WH (eds.): *The Menopause and Hormonal Replacement Therapy: Facts and Controversies.* New York, Marcel Dekker, 1991, pp. 73–100.
11. American Psychiatric Association: *Diagnostic and Statistic Manual of Mental Disorders,* ed 4. Washington, DC, American Psychiatric Association, 1994.
12. Smith EM, Johnson SR, Guenther SM: *Health care attitudes and experiences during gynecologic care among lesbians and bisexuals. Amer J Public Health* 1985;75:1085–1987.
13. Kinsey AC, Pomeroy WB, Martin CE, Gebhard PH: *Sexual Behavior in the Human Female.* Philadelpha, WB Saunders, 1953.

14. Gagnon J, Simon W: *Sexual Conduct: The Social Sources of Human Sexuality.* Chicago, Aldine, 1973.
15. Schriener-Engel P, Schiavi RL, Vietorisz D, Smith H: *J Psychosom Res,* 1987;1:141–.
16. Jensen SB: *Diabetic sexual dysfunction: A comparative study of 160 insulin treated diabetic men and women and an age matched control group. Arch Sex Behav* 1981;10:493–504.
17. Newman AS, Bartelson AD: *J Behav Med* 1986;9:261–.
18. Bachman GA, Leiblum SR: *Maturitas* 1991;13:43–.
19. Leiblum G, Bachmann G, Kemmann E, Colburn D, Swartzman L: *The sexual functioning of elderly hypertensive women. JAMA* 1983;2198–.
20. Mathur RS, Landgrebe SC, Moody LO, Semmens JP, Williamson HO: *The effect of estrogen treatment on plasma concentrations of steroid hormones, gonadotropins, prolactin and sex hormone-binding globulin in post-menopausal women. Maturitas* 1985;7:129–133.
21. Greenblatt RD: *The use of androgens in the menopause and toher gynecologic disorders. Obstet Gynecol Clin North Am* 1987;14:257–268.
22. Sherwin BB, Gelfand MM: *Sex steroids and affect in the surgical menopause: a double-blind cross-over study. Psychoneuroendocrinology* 1985;10:325–335.
23. Sherwin BB, Gelfand MM, Bender W: *Androgen enhances sexual motivation in females: a prospective, crossover study of sex steroid administration in the surgical menopause. Psychosom Med* 1985;47:339–351.
24. Sherwin BB, Gelfand MM: *The role of androgen in the maintenance of sexual functioning in oophorectomized women. Psychosom Med* 1987;49:397–409.
25. Sherwin BB: *Ann Rev Sex Rres* 1991;2:181–.
26. Kaplan HS, Owett T: *The female andorgen deficiency syndrome. J Sex Mar Ther* 1993;19:3–14.
27. Hollon SD, Shelton RC, Loosen PT: *Cognitive therapy and pharmacotherapy for depression. J Consult Clin Psych* 1991;59:88–99.
28. Segraves RT: Leiblum SR, Rosen RC (eds.): in *Sexual Desire Disorders.* Guilford Press, New York, 1988, pp. 313–347.
29. Blumstein P, Schwartz P: American Couples, New York, Morrow, 1983.
30. Kilmann PR, Boland JP, Norton SP, Davidson E, Cald C: *J Sex Mar Ther* 1986;12:116–.
31. Rosen RC, Leiblum SR: in Rosen RC, Leiblum SR (eds.): *Principles and Practice of Sex Therapy,* ed 2. New York, Guilford, 1989, pp. 19–47.
32. Heiman J: Lemcke D, Marshall L, Cowley Pattison D, (eds.): in *Women's Health Care.* New York, Appleton & Lange, in press.
33. Cutler WB: *Hysterectomy: Before and After.* New York, Harper & Row, 1988.
34. Kilkku P: *Supravaginal uterine amputation vs hysterectomy: effects on libido and orgasm. Acta Obstet Gynecol Scand* 1983;62:141–152.
35. Kilkku P, Gronroos M, Hiroven T, Rauramo L: *Supravaginal uterine amputation vs hysterectomy. Effects on coital frequency and dyspareunia. Acta Obstet Gynecol Scand* 1983;62:147–145.
36. Jorm AF: *The Epidemiology of Alzheimer's Disease,* London, Chapman & Hall, 1990, pp. 54–76.
37. Burns A, Jacoby R, Levy R: *Psychiatric phenomena in Alzheimer's disease IV: Disorders of behavior. Brit J Psychiat* 1990;157:86–94.
38. Haddad, PM, Benbow SM: *Int J Ger Psychiatry* 1993;8:547–.
39. Haddad PM, Benbow SM: *Intl J Ger Psychiatry* 1993;8:631–.
40. Burman B, Margolin G: *Analysis of the association between marital relationships and health problems. An international perspective. Psych Bul* 1992;112:39–63.

Index